Life stage group	Potassium (g/d)	Chloride (g/d)	Calcium (mg/d)	Phosphorus (mg/d)	Magnesium (mg/d)	Iron (mg/d)	Zinc (mg/d)	Selenium (µg/d)	Iodine (µg/d)	Copper (µg/d)	Manganese (mg/d)	Fluoride (mg/d)	Chromium (µg/d)	Molybdenum (µg/d)	Water (L/d)[8]
Infants															
0-6 mo	0.4*	0.18*	200	100*	30*	0.27*	2*	15*	110*	200*	0.003*	0.01*	0.2*	2*	0.7*
7-12 mo	0.7*	0.57*	260	275*	75*	11	3*	20*	130*	220*	0.6*	0.5*	5.5*	3*	0.8*
Children															
1-3 y	3.0*	1.5*	700	460	80	7	3	20	90	340	1.2*	0.7*	11*	17	1.3*
4-8 y	3.8*	1.9*	1,000	500	130	10	5	30	90	440	1.5*	1*	15*	22	1.7*
Males															
9-13 y	4.5*	2.3*	1,300	1,250	240	8	8	40	120	700	1.9*	2*	25*	34	2.4*
14-18 y	4.7*	2.3*	1,300	1,250	410	11	11	55	150	890	2.2*	3*	35*	43	3.3*
19-30 y	4.7*	2.3*	1,000	700	400	8	11	55	150	900	2.3*	4*	35*	45	3.7*
31-50 y	4.7*	2.3*	1,000	700	420	8	11	55	150	900	2.3*	4*	35*	45	3.7*
51-70 y	4.7*	2.0*	1,200	700	420	8	11	55	150	900	2.3*	4*	30*	45	3.7*
>70 y	4.7*	1.8*	1,200	700	420	8	11	55	150	900	2.3*	4*	30*	45	3.7*
Females															
9-13 y	4.5*	2.3*	1,300	1,250	240	8	8	40	120	700	1.6*	2*	21*	34	2.1*
14-18 y	4.7*	2.3*	1,300	1,250	360	15	9	55	150	890	1.6*	3*	24*	43	2.3*
19-30 y	4.7*	2.3*	1,000	700	310	18	8	55	150	900	1.8*	3*	25*	45	2.7*
31-50 y	4.7*	2.3*	1,000	700	320	18	8	55	150	900	1.8*	3*	25*	45	2.7*
51-70 y	4.7*	2.0*	1,200	700	320	8	8	55	150	900	1.8*	3*	20*	45	2.7*
>70 y	4.7*	1.8*	1,200	700	320	8	8	55	150	900	1.8*	3*	20*	45	2.7*
Pregnancy															
≤18 y	4.7*	2.3*	1,300	1,250	400	27	12	60	220	1,000	2.0*	3*	29*	50	3.0*
19-30 y	4.7*	2.3*	1,000	700	350	27	11	60	220	1,000	2.0*	3*	30*	50	3.0*
31-50 y	4.7*	2.3*	1,000	700	360	27	11	60	220	1,000	2.0*	3*	30*	50	3.0*
Lactation															
≤18 y	5.1*	2.3	1,300	1,250	360	10	13	70	290	1,300	2.6*	3*	44*	50	3.8*
19-30 y	5.1*	2.3	1,000	700	310	9	12	70	290	1,300	2.6*	3*	45*	50	3.8*
31-50 y	5.1*	2.3	1,000	700	320	9	12	70	290	1,300	2.6*	3*	45*	50	3.8*

Sources: Data compiled from *Dietary Reference Intakes for Calcium, Phosphorus, Magnesium, Vitamin D, and Fluoride.* Washington, DC: National Academies Press; 1997. *Dietary Reference Intakes for Thiamin, Riboflavin, Niacin, Vitamin B_6, Folate, Vitamin B_{12}, Pantothenic Acid, Biotin, and Choline.* Washington, DC: National Academies Press; 1998. *Dietary Reference Intakes for Vitamin C, Vitamin E, Selenium, and Carotenoids.* Washington, DC: National Academies Press; 2000. *Dietary Reference Intakes for Vitamin A, Vitamin K, Arsenic, Boron, Chromium, Copper, Iron, Manganese, Molybdenum, Nickel, Silicon, Vanadium, and Zinc.* Washington, DC: National Academies Press; 2000. *Dietary Reference Intakes for Water, Potassium, Sodium, Chloride, and Sulfate.* Food and Nutrition Board. Washington, DC: National Academies Press; 2005. *Dietary Reference Intakes for Calcium and Vitamin D.* Washington, DC: National Academies Press; 2011. These reports may be accessed via http://nap.edu.

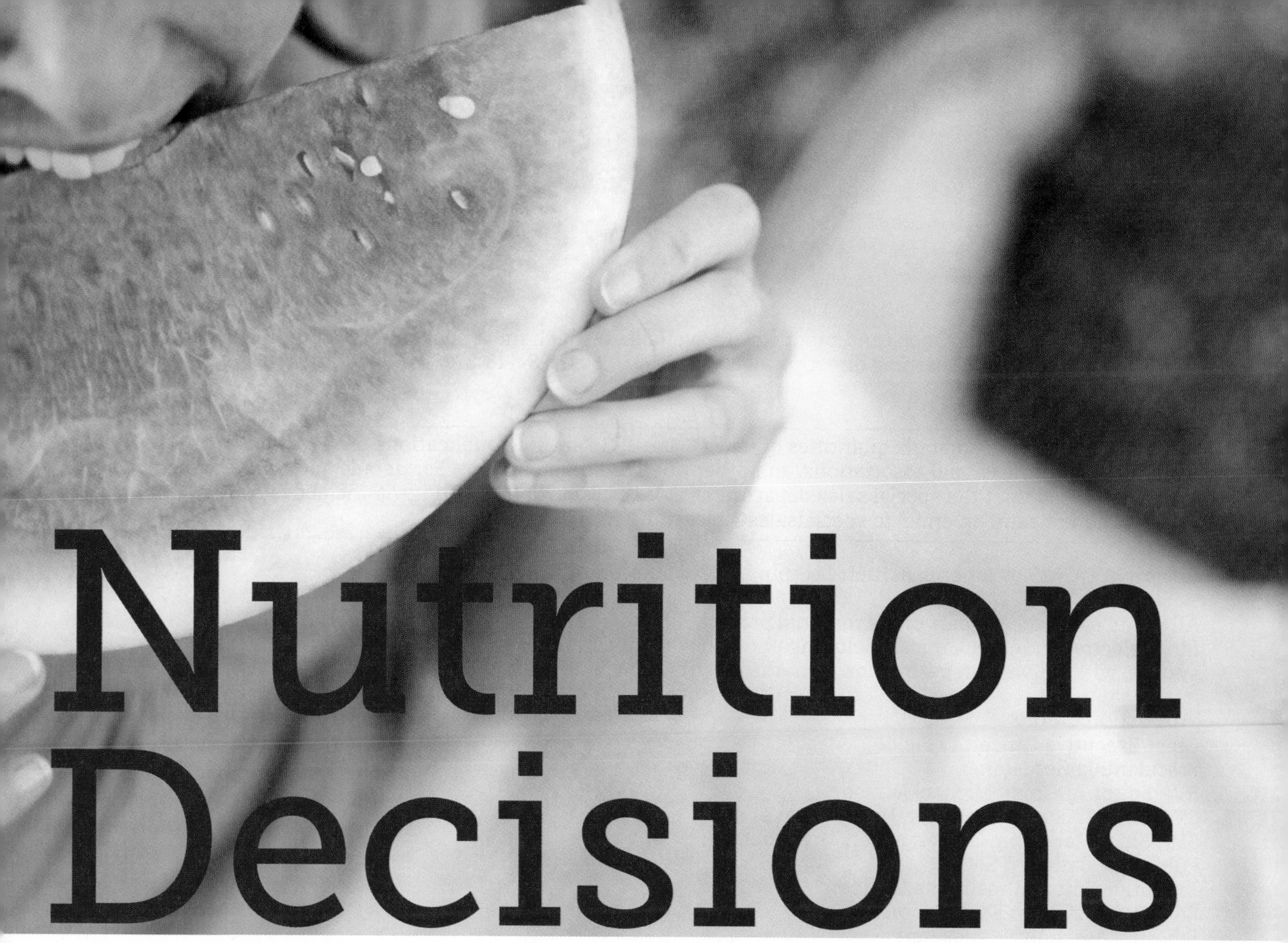

Nutrition Decisions

EAT SMART, MOVE MORE

CAROLYN DUNN, PhD
Professor and Nutrition Specialist
Associate State Program Leader, Family and Consumer Sciences
North Carolina Cooperative Extension Service
North Carolina State University
Raleigh, North Carolina

JONES & BARTLETT
LEARNING

World Headquarters
Jones & Bartlett Learning
5 Wall Street
Burlington, MA 01803
978-443-5000
info@jblearning.com
www.jblearning.com

Jones & Bartlett Learning books and products are available through most bookstores and online booksellers. To contact Jones & Bartlett Learning directly, call 800-832-0034, fax 978-443-8000, or visit our website, www.jblearning.com.

Substantial discounts on bulk quantities of Jones & Bartlett Learning publications are available to corporations, professional associations, and other qualified organizations. For details and specific discount information, contact the special sales department at Jones & Bartlett Learning via the above contact information or send an email to specialsales@jblearning.com.

Production Credits
Chief Executive Officer: Ty Field
President: James Homer
SVP, Editor-in-Chief: Michael Johnson
SVP, Chief Technology Officer: Dean Fossella
SVP, Chief Marketing Officer: Alison M. Pendergast
Publisher: Cathleen Sether
Executive Editor: Shoshanna Goldberg
Editorial Assistant: Sean Coombs
Editorial Assistant: Agnes Burt
Production Manager: Julie Champagne Bolduc
Production Assistant: Emma Krosschell
Marketing Manager: Jody Yeskey
V.P., Manufacturing and Inventory Control: Therese Connell
Composition: Publishers' Design and Production Services, Inc.
Cover Design: Kristin E. Parker
Rights and Photo Research Manager: Katherine Crighton
Photo Researcher: Sarah Cebulski
Cover Image: © Ty Milford/Aurora O. Collection: Aurora Photos, Inc./age fotostock
Printing and Binding: Courier Companies
Cover Printing: Courier Companies

To order this product, use ISBN: 978-1-4496-5295-1

Library of Congress Cataloging-in-Publication Data
Dunn, Carolyn, PhD.
Nutrition decisions : eat smart, move more / by Carolyn Dunn.
p. cm.
Includes bibliographical references and index.
ISBN 978-0-7637-8376-1 — ISBN 0-7637-8376-5
1. Nutrition—Textbooks. 2. Health. 3. Diet. 4. Physical fitness—Nutritional aspects. I. Title.
RA784.D863 2013
613.7—dc23

2011044885

6048
Printed in the United States of America
16 15 14 13 12 10 9 8 7 6 5 4 3 2 1

This book is dedicated to
Betty Cook, Kay Ann Friedrich, and Dr. Marilyn Stuber.
Meredith College was fortunate to have you as faculty;
I am honored to call you my mentors.

Brief Contents

Contents

Features

Try Something New

Which Side Are You On?

How Policy and Environment Affect My Choices

Personal Health Check

Special Report

Green and Healthy

Preface

You are keenly aware that eating smart and moving more are two of the most important things for overall good health. Putting that knowledge into action and helping students make eating smart and moving more part of their everyday life is another story. Life's challenges—work, school, family, friends—all vie for their time and attention. Too often, their own health takes a back seat. I believe that if students could feel the power, energy, and vitality that eating smart and moving more bring, they would make them part of their life forever. That is where this book comes in. Learning about the concepts of healthy eating and physical activity is, of course, the first step. This book goes beyond the facts and offers practical ways to put knowledge to work immediately. As the title indicates, it starts with decisions that are often motivated by what students think is possible or doable. This book provides them with the skills they need to make eating healthy and being active doable, no matter how busy they are.

This book is for anyone who wants to eat better, move more, and achieve and maintain a healthy weight. It is written for the English major who has gained 20 pounds since high school; for the nursing major who knows that he needs to find a way to become more physically active; and for the business major who lost her father to heart disease and knows that what she eats and how she moves impact her health. Regardless of the major, prior knowledge of nutrition, or where students are in their own journey to good health, this book is a guide to eating smart and moving more. I have worked my entire career to create meaningful messages and ways to reach people with information about healthy eating and physical activity habits. This book is the culmination of much of that work. The concepts in this book will help students make decisions that move them on a path to health by eating smart and moving more.

Nutrition Decisions is unique in that it challenges students to align their eating and physical activity behaviors with what they are learning. Each chapter starts with a story that illustrates the struggles we all face in trying to eat smart and move more in our everyday lives. *Nutrition Decisions* is designed not only to inform but also to empower and provide motivation to put knowledge into practice. Special features throughout the book will help to navigate some of the controversial issues in nutrition and physical activity, check one's own health status, try something new, learn how eating healthy and being physically active can also help the environment, explore how policies and the environment in which we live affects health, and help students take a small or large step toward eating smart and moving more.

The Pedagogy

Nutrition Decisions focuses on teaching behavioral change, personal decision-making, and up-to-date scientific concepts in a number of dynamic ways. The interactive approach addresses different learning styles and makes it the ideal text to ensure a high likelihood of student success. Throughout the text, the material engages students in considering their own behavior in light of the knowledge they are gaining. The following pedagogical aids appear in most of the chapters.

Personal Health Check

Tracking eating habits, examining physical activity, and knowing weight, blood pressure, or risk for diabetes can provide insight into the student's personal health status. The Personal Health Check feature will guide students to "check" their own behavior or health status based on the chapter content. This knowledge will help them set goals to move toward better health.

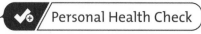

Personal Health Check

Your BMI and Daily Calorie Needs

What Is Your BMI?

To assess your personal BMI you need two pieces of information: your height without shoes and your weight in pounds. Use the equation presented in the sidebar earlier in this chapter to calculate your BMI. Then use the color-coded BMI chart in Figure 12.1 to see into what category your BMI falls. You can also find several BMI calculators online. If you are in the overweight or obese category, how many pounds would you need to lose to be in the healthy weight category?

How Many Calories Do You Need Each Day?

Your **basal metabolic rate (BMR)** and physical activity level dictate the number of calories you need each day. Your BMR is the number of calories that you need at rest to keep your body alive. These are the calories needed to keep you breathing, your heart beating, your temperature normal, and all body systems functioning. Your BMR is affected by several factors.[71] Genetics dictates some of what your BMR will be. Some people simply have a faster metabolism than others. Gender also affects BMR, with males having a higher BMR than females. Body fatness greatly effects BMR; the more muscle you have, the higher your BMR. Age effects BMR as well. As you get older, your BMR will decrease; however, some of this depends on how much lean body mass you lose as you age. Finally, diet can affect BMR. If you are on a low-calorie diet, your BMR will decrease. The body is able to sense when calories are at a deficit and slows everything down to conserve energy. This safety mechanism helped keep us alive thousands of years ago when we had to hunt for food. In times of low food intake, our bodies held on to every calorie it could in order to survive until food would be available again. Today, even though food is readily available, perhaps even too available, our bodies still have this mechanism. This is one reason why ultra-low-calorie diets are not recommended.

The other factor that dictates the number of calories you need each day is your physical activity level. Your daily physical activity level includes all the times you move your body in a given day. On one end of the spectrum would be someone who sits at a desk all day and moves very little to someone who is training for an athletic event or does manual labor most of the day. The *Dietary Guidelines for Americans* has ranges of calories based on gender, age, and activity level.[72]

Estimate of Daily Calorie Needs

This table estimates the number of calories that you need each day. It is only an estimate; individual calorie needs vary based on body size, gender, and activity level.

		Activity Level		
Gender	Age	Sedentary	Moderately Active	Active
Female	19–30	1,800–2,000	2,000–2,200	2,400
	31–50	1,800	2,000	2,200
	51+	1,600	1,800	2,000–2,200
Male	19–30	2,400–2,600	2,000–2,200	3,000
	31–50	2,200–2,400	2,400–2,600	2,800–3,000
	51+	2,000–2,200	2,200–2,400	2,400–2,800

Source: P Britten, K Marcoe, S Yamini, C Davis. Development of food intake patterns for the MyPyramid Food Guidance System. *J Nutr Educ Behav.* 2006;38(6 Suppl):S78–S92.

Try Something New

Choose Low-Fat Dressings

Salads are a great way to add lots of vegetables to your diet. They also can be a low-fat addition; that is, unless you drown them in high-fat dressing. Many low-fat and fat-free dressings are available in restaurants and grocery stores. When you eat out, ask for low-fat or fat-free dressing. At home, try making your own fat-free dressing. Experiment with your own favorites. It will keep for several days in the refrigerator.

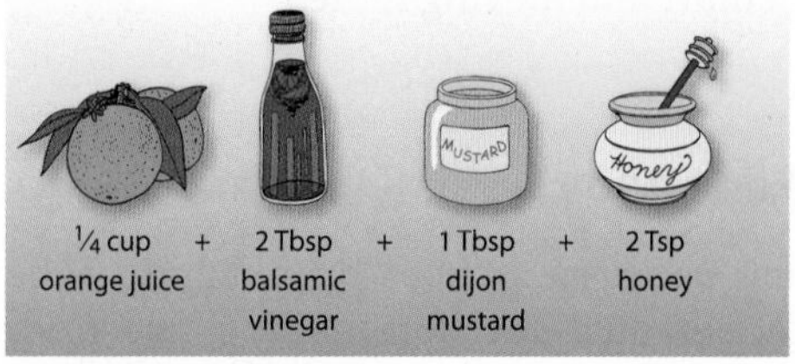
Mustard
Honey
¼ cup orange juice
+
2 Tbsp balsamic vinegar
+
1 Tbsp dijon mustard
+
2 Tsp honey

Make Your Own Oil-Free Dressing
Blend the ingredients together in a small container. It will keep for several days in the refrigerator.

Try Something New

There are countless opportunities to eat healthy and be active. Have your students ever eaten kohlrabi? How about quinoa? Sometimes, however, we get stuck in a rut eating the same foods or doing the same activity. Try Something New will provide ideas for new foods or new activities to keep students motivated.

Which Side Are You On?

Nutrition and physical activity can sometimes be complicated and confusing. Which is better, wild salmon or farm raised? Is organic always better? Is sugar better than high fructose corn syrup? What about detox diets—are they healthy? The Which Side Are You On? section presents unbiased facts about controversial topics. When there are two distinct sides to a situation, both sides will be presented with the most compelling research from each point of view to help students make up their own minds based on the facts.

Which Side Are You On?

Organic or Conventional Milk?

Organic milk is now widely available in most grocery stores across the country. Should you spend the extra money for milk that is certified organic? Is it more nutritious or safer than conventional milk? Controversy surrounds the answers to these questions, and depending on who you talk to organic milk is either a must buy for consumers or a waste of money. Let's take a closer look.

According to the U.S. Department of Agriculture, milk can only be labeled "organic" if the cows have been fed exclusively organic feed, have not been given synthetic hormones, have not been given antibiotics, are kept in pens with adequate space, and are allowed access to the outdoors.

Proponents of organic milk argue that these standards make the milk safer than conventional milk by controlling the antibiotic and hormone levels in the milk. Some people feel that giving cows fewer hormones and antibiotics results in milk that is safer. You can find much information on the Web about the improved safety of organic milk, but note that most of it is not supported by scientific evidence. Milk—conventional and organic—is one of the most tested foods on the grocery store shelf. Studies have found no meaningful difference in hormone or antibiotic content of organic versus conventional milk.[51]

What about nutritional composition? This is an easier one for you, the consumer, to check. A quick look at the nutrition labels on conventional and organic milk will reveal that they are identical with respect to their vitamin, mineral, and protein content. Fat content is also similar based on the type of milk in question.

One difference between organic and conventional milk is price. The higher cost for farms to follow the guidelines required to be certified organic means that organic milk carries a higher price tag.

Safety is similar, and nutrition is similar—why then does the demand for organic milk continue to increase, with an estimated 25% more certified organic cows each year since 2000?[52] Many consumers believe, in spite of evidence to the contrary, that organic milk is a safer and more wholesome product. Consumers also may make the organic choice based on how animals that are certified organic are treated, having access to pasture and less crowded conditions. Another reason to choose organic would be to support organic farming practices that are more environmentally friendly. Ultimately, the decision is up to you as to your choice of milk, organic or conventional. If cost is a factor, conventionally produced milk may be a better choice, because it delivers the same nutritional punch.

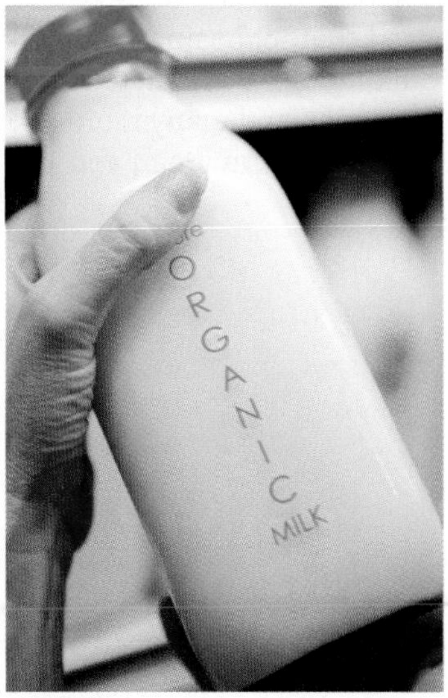

Organic Milk
"Organic" can only be used on the label if the cows have been fed exclusively organic feed, have not been given synthetic hormones, have not been given antibiotics, are kept in pens with adequate space, and are allowed access to the outdoors.

How Policy and Environment Affect My Choices

Finding the Trans Fats

Hydrogenation is a process by which hydrogen is bubbled through a liquid fat such as soybean or corn oil. This process breaks some of the double bonds between the carbons and attaches hydrogen to the bonds. The once polyunsaturated oil is now partially hydrogenated. The process of hydrogenation turns the liquid oil into a solid or semisolid spread. The high cost of butter in the 1950s and 1960s led to the commercialization of making liquid vegetable oil solid so that it could be used as a spread. Later, the realization that polyunsaturated fats were heart-healthy made hydrogenated spreads even more popular. An added benefit to these hydrogenated fats was that they added shelf life to processed foods such as crackers, snack foods, and cookies.

Butter and lard were out and margarine was in—that is until we learned more about the types of fats that were being produced by the hydrogenation process. The hydrogenation of oils produces fatty acids with a trans configuration. Trans fats increase LDL cholesterol and decrease HDL cholesterol in the blood, thus increasing the risk of heart disease.[39–48] Trans fats increase the risk of heart disease more than any other single nutrient, with a substantial risk at even low levels of consumption.[39]

To assist consumers in locating trans fats in their foods, the FDA now requires the Nutrition Facts panel to include trans fats in a separate line under saturated fat. As a result of this requirement, many manufacturers have removed some or all of the trans fats from their products.

A word of caution about what's on the label. With consumer interest in consuming "trans fat free" at a peak, manufacturers begun putting the words "contains 0 grams of trans fat per serving" on the label. Does this statement ensure that you are consuming a trans fat–free product? No, it does not, and here is why: If a product has 0.5 grams or less of trans fats per serving, the amount can be rounded down to 0 grams of trans fat per serving, hence the wording of the claim to read "0 grams of trans fat PER SERVING." So, for example, if you had a product that has 0.5 grams of trans fat per tablespoon and you had 3 tablespoons, you would be getting 1.5 grams of trans fat. Hardly trans fat free! The only way to see if a product really is trans fat free is to read the ingredient label. If the product contains an ingredient that is hydrogenated or partially hydrogenated, such as partially hydrogenated soybean oil or hydrogenated cottonseed oil, it is not trans fat free. If the word *hydrogenated* is in the ingredient list, it has at least some trans fat in the product.

Another source of trans fats in the American diet is restaurant food. Restaurants, for the most part, do not have to reveal the type of fat they use in cooking and often use hydrogenated oils. To further protect the public from unhealthy trans fats, New York City and California have banned the use of trans fats in restaurants. Other cities and states are sure to follow as the public becomes savvier about the dangers of trans fats.

The requirement of labeling foods with the amount of trans fat in the product and the ban of use of trans fat in restaurants are examples of how policy change can affect the health of the population. Consumers now have an easy way to know how much trans fats are in the foods they buy. The even bolder step of banning trans fats in restaurants further protects consumers from unknowingly consuming harmful trans fats.

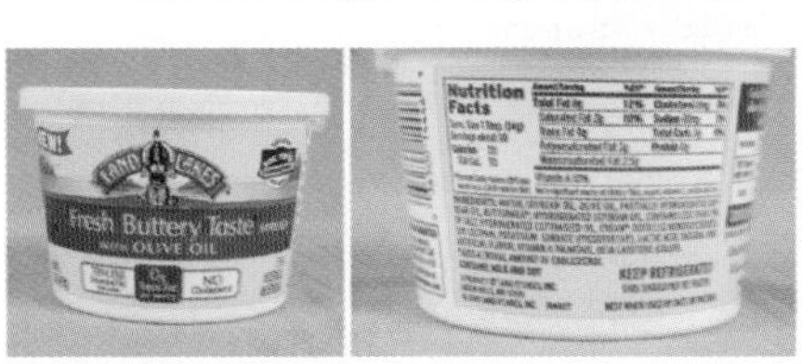

Zero Trans Fat
Zero grams of trans fat per serving does not always mean trans fat free. Look for the word *hydrogenated* in the ingredient list. This indicates that the product has trans fat.

How Policy and Environment Affect My Choices

Many factors affect our ability to eat smart and move more. Knowledge is a good first step, but it is only the beginning. We must live in an environment that supports healthy eating and physical activity. Imagine if there are no sidewalks or safe places to be active, or all that is available in a 1-mile radius of campus is fast food. How Policy and Environment Affect My Choices explores current policy and environmental issues that play a role in healthy eating and physical activity. It discusses how important our surroundings are to being healthy and how policy change is a powerful tool to create environments that support positive health behaviors.

Green and Healthy

Is there a relationship between eating healthy and helping the environment? There are many choices related to eating and physical activity that can have a very positive effect on the environment. Green and Healthy discusses how eating a more plant-based diet, choosing local foods, walking or biking instead of using your car, and many more behaviors can be both green and healthy.

Green and Healthy

Tap Water or Bottled Water?

Water should be your number one beverage of choice. But where that water should come from, the tap or a bottle, is not so clear-cut. The debate over bottled water or tap water includes issues related to water quality, safety, taste, convenience, and, of course, the environment.

Many different types of bottled water are available. The FDA oversees what bottled water can be called and the safety and quality of bottled water. The **Environmental Protection Agency (EPA)** has regulatory oversight for tap water under the Safe Drinking Water Act. Each time the EPA changes or establishes a new standard for drinking water, the FDA either adopts it for bottled water or suggests that the standard is not necessary for bottled water in order to protect the public health. As a result, the standards for bottled water and tap water are very similar.[8] Tap water may have one thing that bottled water doesn't—fluoride. Many municipalities treat their water with fluoride to prevent tooth decay. Oftentimes, fluoride is not added to bottled water or the fluoride has been removed if the water has been purified or distilled. Some bottled water does have fluoride added; if so, this will be indicated on the label. If you drink primarily bottled water without fluoride you should consult your dentist to see if a supplement is in order.

Taste is another factor when answering the question of "bottle or tap?" Water varies from town to town, city to city, and even within a municipality. Water from one location may taste better than that from a different location. If you don't like the taste of your tap water, you probably are not going to drink it. Filtering the water or choosing bottled water may be a better option to encourage you to make water your beverage of choice.

The most prevalent reason that people choose bottled water over tap is convenience. It is easy to grab a bottle of water and go. You can keep it in the car, at your desk at work or school, in your backpack, or in your gym locker.

Finally, what about all the plastic water bottles? Plastic bottles are not environmentally friendly. Several issues are at play here: making the bottles, transporting the bottles, and disposing of the bottles. It takes over 17 million barrels of oil to make the number of water bottles needed in the United States for one year. Then the bottles have to be transported, which means more oil. Finally, only about 15% of bottles get recycled, leaving 85% to sit in the landfill. The Pacific Institute, an independent think tank, estimates that the total amount of energy embedded in the use of one bottle of water can be as high as the equivalent of filling a plastic bottle one quarter full with oil.[8] The Pacific Institute also estimates that it takes about 3 liters of water to make 1 liter of bottled water. This is due to the water used in producing the bottles, transportation, and refrigeration.

So, why demonize bottled water? Why not pick on soda bottles or other plastic containers? The huge increase in the use of bottled water over the last five years is one reason. The other and more compelling reason is that there is an easy alternative: buy a reusable bottle and fill it from the tap. This will save oil, water, and the landfill and keep more money in your wallet.

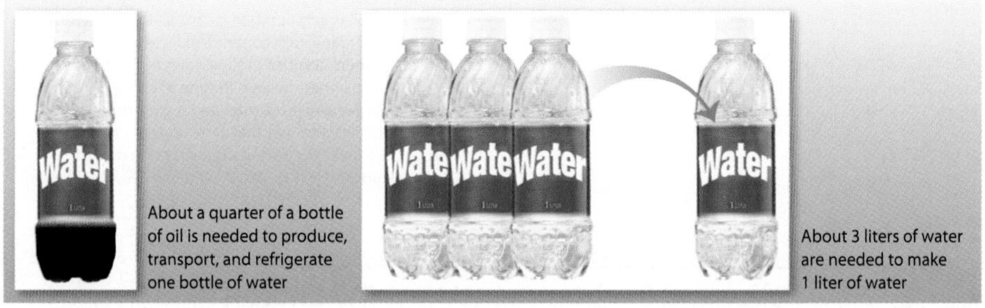
Water
About a quarter of a bottle of oil is needed to produce, transport, and refrigerate one bottle of water
About 3 liters of water are needed to make 1 liter of water

Oil and Water Used in Production of Bottled Water

Special Report

Food Allergies

A **food allergy** is an abnormal immune system response in which the body produces an antibody to a food. These antibodies are proteins that work against a particular food and enter your bloodstream after the food is digested. From there, the antibodies go to target organs, such as the skin or nose, and cause an allergic reaction. If you consume a food to which you are allergic, your body's immune system reacts to that food, resulting in side effects such as sneezing, a rash, or, in severe cases, anaphylactic shock. Allergic reactions to foods can take place within a few minutes to as long as an hour after ingesting the offending food. Persons with food allergies must be very careful not to consume the offending food. Severe food allergies can be very dangerous and can even cause death if not treated immediately.

The most common foods that cause allergic reactions are milk, eggs, peanuts, tree nuts, soy, fish, shellfish, and wheat. These eight foods account for almost all food allergies. Mild food allergies can be treated with an antihistamine or a bronchodilator. Severe reactions, including difficulty breathing or anaphylactic shock, require treatment with epinephrine. There is no cure for food allergies; the best method for managing food allergies is by way of strict avoidance of any food that triggers a reaction.[22]

True food allergies are somewhat rare, affecting only a small percentage of the population. Only about 2% of the adult population and 4–8% of children have food allergies.[23,24] Adults usually keep their allergies for life; however, some children may outgrow their food allergy. Allergies to milk, egg, or soy are more likely to be outgrown than an allergy to peanuts.

Diagnosis of a food allergy is a multistep process. The healthcare provider will first rule out any other health problems, starting with a detailed history about the person's reaction to certain foods. Some healthcare providers will get a diet history to get more details about the pattern of food consumption that may be causing a problem. Sometimes an elimination diet is prescribed, whereby certain foods are removed from the diet to see if symptoms subside. If the history or elimination diet suggests a specific food allergy, a scratch test may be performed. With a scratch test, an extract of the food is placed on the skin and then the skin is scratched with a needle. Swelling or redness may be a sign of an allergic reaction. A blood test can be done in the case of extreme allergies and the possibility of anaphylactic reactions. A blood test may be able to measure the presence of a food-specific antibody in the blood.

More common than food allergies, and often mislabeled as food allergies, are food intolerances and/or food aversions. A **food intolerance** is a reaction to a specific food that does not involve the immune system. An example of this would be lactose intolerance in those who lack the enzyme lactase, which breaks down milk proteins. Even more common are **food aversions**, which are foods that you would prefer not to consume. These may be foods that you know do not agree with you or that you simply do not like; if so, you have an aversion to that food, not a food allergy.

Special Report

Special Reports go beyond the basics to help students understand the *how* and *why* of some of the most interesting topics related to nutrition and physical activity. How nutrition or physical activity relate to chronic disease, how to eat for optimal athletic performance, how to navigate the sea of nutrition information on the Internet, and the truth about low-carbohydrate diets are just a few of the topics covered in depth as a Special Report.

Spotlight on Vitamins and Minerals: Fluoride

Fluoride protects against dental caries (cavities). Fluoride is commonly added to community water supplies and is found in most toothpaste. Community water fluoridation is an effective, safe, and inexpensive way to prevent tooth decay. Fluoridation of community water supplies has been credited with reducing tooth decay by 50–60% in the United States since the 1940s. Children and adults who are at low risk of dental decay can stay cavity-free through frequent exposure to small amounts of fluoride. This can be achieved by drinking fluoridated water and using a fluoride toothpaste twice daily. Children and adults at high risk of dental decay

Spotlight on Vitamins and Minerals

Vitamins and minerals are critical for optimal health. Where vitamins and minerals are found in food, what their functions are, what happens if there is not enough or too much are all questions that are featured in the Spotlight on Vitamins and Minerals.

Ready to Make a Change

Are you ready to make a change, small or large, in your overall health and well-being? Using some of the information provided in this chapter is a great place to start.

I commit to a small first step. Eat when you are hungry, not because of external cues. Pay attention to your level of hunger prior to eating.

I am ready to take the next step and make a medium change. What effect do food ads have on your consumption of food? Next time you are in front of the TV and a food ad comes on, analyze the effects that ad has on your hunger.

Ready to Make a Change

Making changes in eating and physical activity is not always easy. Sometimes it may seem like an all-or-none proposition. However, making even small changes to eat smart and move more can add up to big benefits. Ready to Make a Change highlights the first step students can take to eat smart or move more, and if they are ready to go further, the next steps toward making a medium or even a large change based on current eating or physical activity patterns. Whatever students choose, it will be a step toward better health.

Myth Versus Fact

Myth: Hunger and appetite are the same.

Fact: Hunger is the physiological drive to eat; appetite is the desire to eat. You may have an appetite for apple pie if you smell it baking but not have a physiological need for food.

Myth: Food ads don't have an impact on what you eat if you just ignore them.

Fact: Food advertisers use powerful food consumption cues in their ads. Research shows that many of the food ads you see on television can cause you to eat more than you would have otherwise.

Myth: Healthy foods cost too much.

Fact: It is true that some healthy foods are more expensive than cheap high-calorie foods. However, a well-

Myth Versus Fact

There are many common myths or misperceptions about healthy eating and physical activity. The Myth Versus Fact section reviews chapter content, pointing out the facts based on available evidence and dispelling some of the myths about eating smart and moving more.

TERMS

Generally Regarded as Safe (GRAS) Designation that a substance that is added to food is considered safe by experts. Any substance added to food must meet this standard.

acceptable daily intake (ADI) The amount of a substance in food (food additives) or drinking water that can be ingested on a daily basis over a lifetime without an appreciable health risk.

Key Terms

Key terms appear bold in the text and definitions are conveniently provided in separate boxes. These terms can also be found in the glossary.

The Integrated Learning and Teaching Package

Integrating the text and ancillaries is crucial to achieving the full educational benefit. Based on feedback from instructors and students, Jones & Bartlett Learning offers the following supplements:

Dietary analysis software is an important component of the behavioral change and personal decision-making focus. ***EatRight Analysis***, developed by ESHA Research, enables students to analyze their diets by calculating their nutrition intake and comparing it to recommended intake levels. It is available online (http://eatright.jblearning.com) and in a CD-ROM format.

Contact your Nutrition Representative for discount package opportunities.

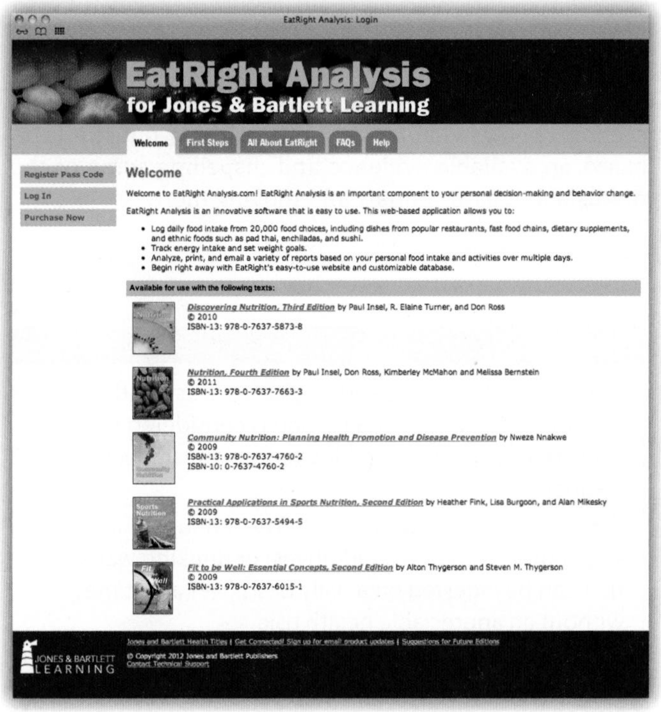

The **Instructor's Media CD** is a comprehensive teaching resource available to adopters of the book. It includes:

- PowerPoint Lecture Presentation Slides
- An Image and Table Bank providing art and tables that can be imported into PowerPoint presentations, tests, or used to create transparencies

A Test Bank is available as a free instructor download. All materials are formatted for online course management systems. Contact your Nutrition Account Specialist at http://jblearning.com.

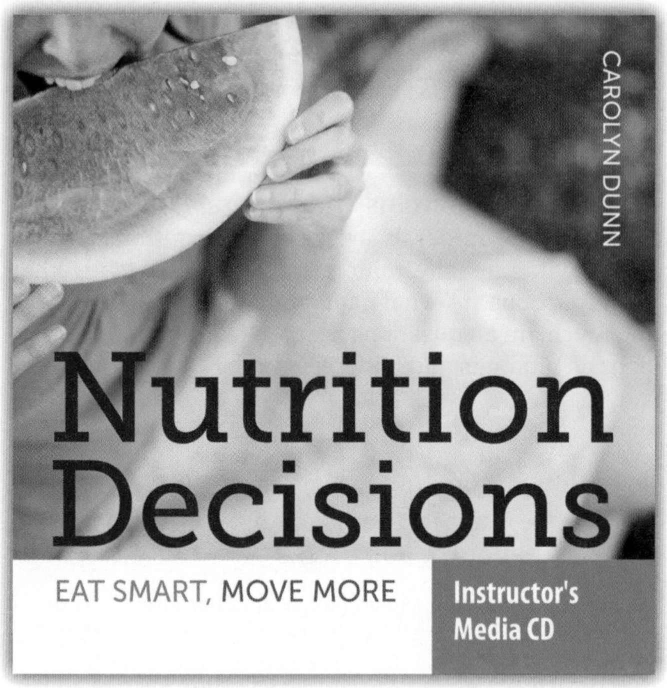

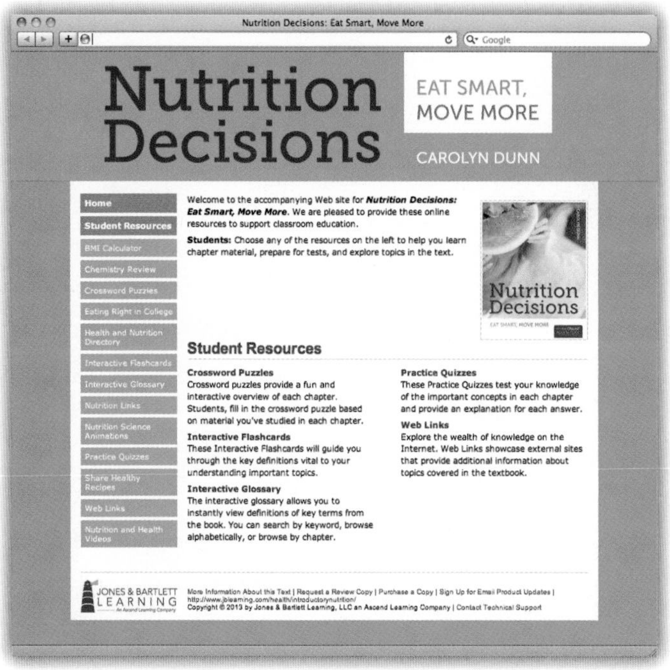

The **companion website** for *Nutrition Decisions*, **go.jblearning.com/Dunn**, offers students and instructors an unprecedented degree of integration between the text and the online world through many useful study tools, activities, and supplementary health information. This interactive and informative website is accessible to students through the redeemable access code provided in every new text.

A ***Decision-Making Workbook*** is included at the back of each book, and contains exercises and activities to help motivate students to improve and enhance their health and well-being. The workbook activities include:

- Personal Health Check: Students can check their health status based on the content of the chapter.
- Try Something New: Students are encouraged to try a new food, activity, or technique to help them eat smart or move more.
- Critical Analysis: Questions designed to get students to think about the concepts presented in the chapter are provided. The answers to these thought-provoking questions require research and reading on subjects related to eating smart and moving more.
- Test Your Skills: Students can follow suggestions of activities that they can do to test the skills learned in the chapter (e.g., comparing breakfast cereals in the grocery store).

Acknowledgments

Thank you to my wonderful family and friends for their support and love throughout the writing of this book. Your encouragement as I embarked on this new endeavor means more than I can say. Thank you to Cathy Thomas for her expert review of this text and for her support and guidance throughout the project; you are amazing. Thank you to Linda Dunn for her careful review. She is more than my sister; she is, most affectionately, the grammar police. Thanks for all the commas. Finally, thank you to Shoshanna Goldberg, Julie Bolduc, and the Jones & Bartlett Learning Health team for believing in this project and for all of your help every step of the way.

I would also like to thank the following reviewers whose insight helped make this book possible:

Carmen Blakely-Adams, MEd, RD, LD, Kent State University
Starr L. Eaddy, PhD, CHES, St. Francis College
Dr. Nancy Graves, RD, LD, University of Houston
Elizabeth Nicklay, LAT, CSCS, Luther College
Veronica J. Oates, PhD, RD, LDN, Tennessee State University
Dr. Angie Parker, Anthem College Online
Janet L. Roberts, MAT, CMA (AAMA), CHES, Western Oregon University
Long Wang, PhD, Syracuse University

About the Author

Carolyn Dunn's passion for food, nutrition, and fitness started more than 25 years ago. While working on her bachelor's degree, she began to study the connection between food and health. After receiving a BS in nutrition from Meredith College, she attended graduate school at the University of North Carolina at Greensboro where she earned an MS and PhD. For the past 20 years she has been on faculty at North Carolina State University where she develops nutrition education materials and messages that help people eat smart and move more. All of her work is done with one goal in mind: to help people live better, healthier lives. She works with partners across the nation to change policy and create environments where healthy eating and physical activity are possible. She loves to cook, especially with local foods, and enjoys running, cycling, and strength training.

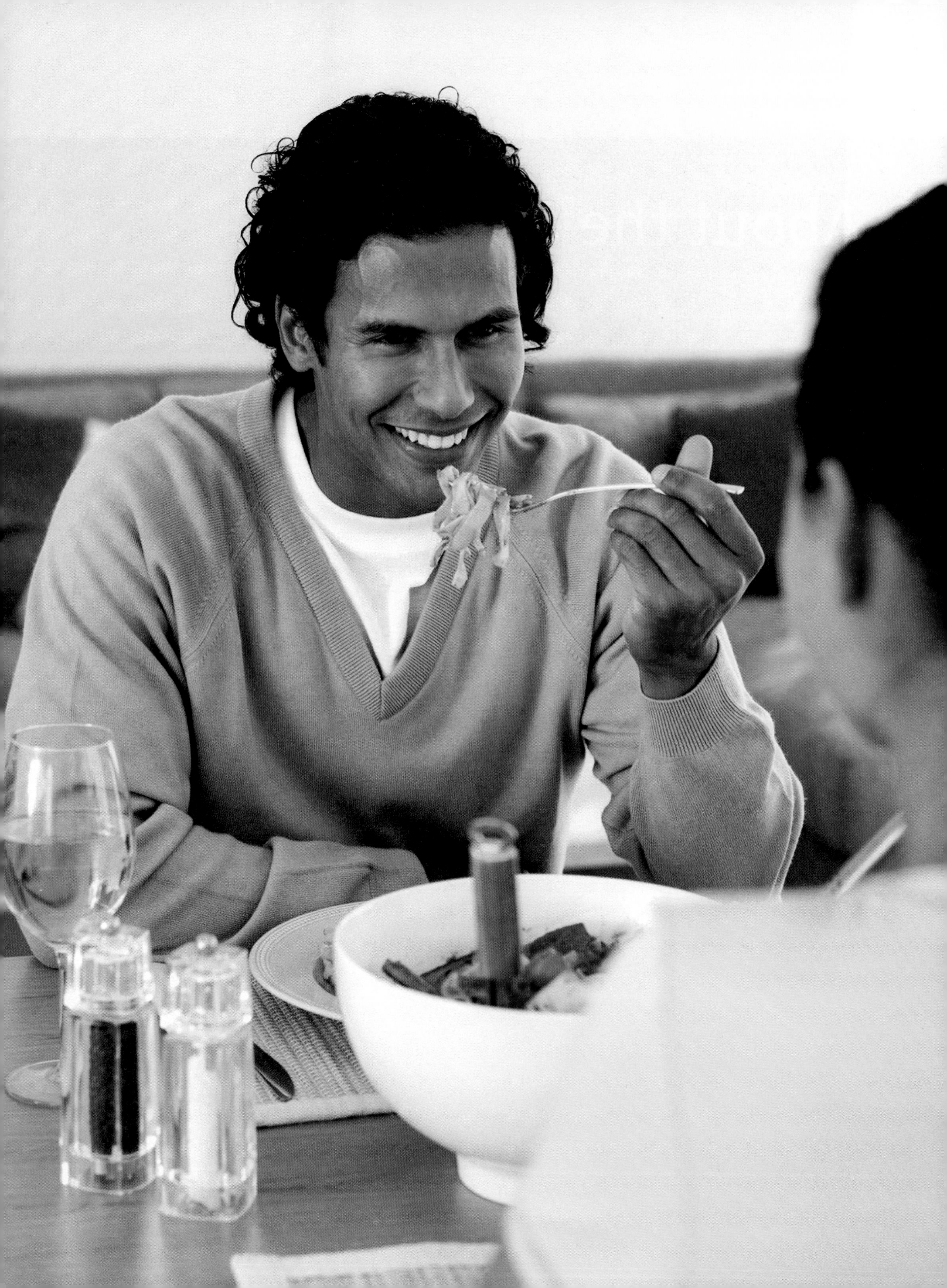

Chapter 1

Food: Why You Eat What You Eat

Key Messages

- Many factors influence your choice of foods.
- The taste of different foods influences what you choose to eat.
- Your environment and lifestyle influence your food choices.
- Food advertising has an impact on what foods you choose to eat.
- The six classes of nutrients are carbohydrates, proteins, fats, vitamins, minerals, and water.

Food and eating are fundamental aspects of life. Everyone eats to live. Food provides the nutrients needed to sustain life. The foods you choose have a profound impact on your overall health. Food, however, is much more than just a collection of nutrients. Most people not only eat to live, but live to eat. Eating is a unique joy, from a simple peanut butter sandwich with the rich taste of peanuts to a gourmet meal at a special restaurant to celebrate a life event. Eating is one of the greatest and most fulfilling pleasures in life.

What shapes your food choices? How do taste, your thoughts and feelings about food, and your environment affect your food choices? And what about nutrition, does it have an impact on what foods you choose?

Nutrition is the science behind the foods you eat. **Nutrition** is the relationship between health and the food you eat. Learning more about nutrition can help you choose foods for their potential to help you achieve better health. This chapter will examine the many influences on how you choose the foods you eat.

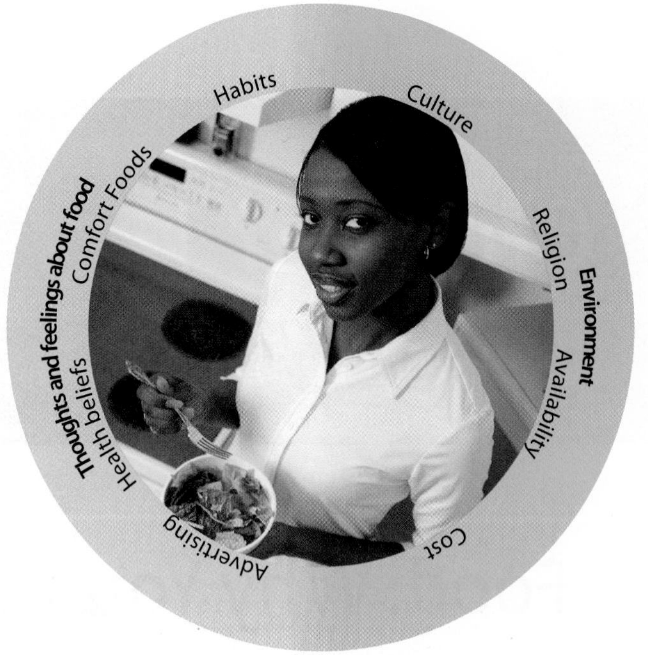

■ **Figure 1.1**
Why You Eat the Foods You Eat

Story

Sam is in his final year of college and is looking forward to graduation. He has received a job offer and will be moving to the Midwest. This will be a big change for Sam, because he has always lived in the South. While he was in the Midwest for his interview, he noticed that they had some different foods that he was not used to. He saw some unfamiliar foods when he visited a local grocery store.

Sam started thinking about what he usually ate. He could only come up with a short list of foods. The demands of college had really limited him with respect to eating a wide variety of foods. Sam's food choices were usually based on time and taste. He always shopped for groceries at the convenience store near campus. It didn't carry many fruits and vegetables and had limited choices. It was the only store within walking distance, which was important because Sam didn't have a car. How can Sam begin to expand his repertoire of foods when he makes the move from college to his new job?

Why You Eat the Foods You Eat

Why you eat is simple; it is a biological need. You have to eat to survive. **Hunger** may drive when and how much you eat, but **appetite** comes into play as well. However, what you eat and why you choose the foods you do is a bit more complex. Multiple factors influence what foods you select. Your choice of foods is driven by a complex mixture of what tastes good to you; what you are used to; your culture, religion, and health beliefs; and your thoughts and feelings about food (**Figure 1.1**).

Taste

The number one reason most people give for why they eat the foods they eat is taste. Palatability, how a food agrees with your palate, has a strong influence over what you choose to eat. What tastes good to you may not taste good to someone else. Ask 10 people their favorite food, and you are likely to get 10 different answers. What is palatable to you now as an adult may be different than it was when you were a child. Tastes change over time and can be learned. Strong flavors such as blue cheese and coffee are not usually popular with children but are among many adults' favorites.

Exposure to different flavors can influence what you consider to be palatable. You may learn to like certain foods only after you eat them several times. If you moved to another part of the country or another part of the world, you would have to adapt to new foods. Foods that you initially found to be unusual or unpleasant may become your new favorites after you continue to be exposed to them.

TERMS

nutrition The science of food and its components, including food's relationship to health and disease.

hunger The physiological drive to eat.

appetite The physiological desire to eat; not always accompanied by hunger.

Try Something New

External Cues to Eat

You have just had lunch, and you feel full. On your walk back to class, you pass a bakery and are struck by the smell of warm chocolate chip cookies. The familiar smell causes your mouth to water. Before you know it, you are diving into a bag of just-baked goodness. Were you driven by hunger to eat, or did the smell of something you knew would taste good stimulate your appetite? How susceptible are you to external cues to eat?

Often, external stimuli to eat, such as smelling, seeing, or even talking about food, override your need for calories. In other words, you may eat because the food tastes good, not because you are hungry. Even though you may salivate at the sight of a favorite food, it does not mean you should eat it. External cues may be signaling you to eat, but are you really hungry?

Keep track of how hungry you are each time you eat for the next few days. Use the hunger scale below as a guide. This will help you be more mindful of eating when you are hungry, not just when you are prompted to by external cues.

1. **Weak and light-headed** — your stomach is churning
2. **Ravenous** — you are irritable and cannot concentrate
3. **Hungry** — your stomach is rumbling
4. **Slightly hungry** — beginning to feel the signs of hunger
5. **Neutral** — you could eat more but are not hungry
6. **Satisfied** — perfectly comfortable
7. **Full** — a little uncomfortable
8. **Stuffed** — uncomfortably full
9. **Bloated** — need to loosen clothing
10. **Nauseous** — so full you may be sick

Hunger Scale

You should only eat when you are at a 1, 2, 3, or 4 on the scale. Put down your fork when you get to a 5 or 6.

Taste is one of your five senses. The taste and smell of a food together make up the flavor of that food. You are able to detect the flavor of a substance thanks to the taste buds that are concentrated on your tongue. The five basic flavor profiles are sweet, bitter, sour, salty, and umami (**Figure 1.2**). Sweetness in a food generally suggests that sugar is present. You are born with a propensity toward sweetness. You are most sensitive to bitter tastes, which is why strong bitter flavors can be off-putting. Balanced bitterness, such as that found in beer, coffee, and olives, is acceptable to most people. Sour taste signals the presence of acidity. Adding acid to foods, such as lemon on fish or vinegar in salad dressing, can introduce a bright flavor that most people enjoy. A salty flavor means that sodium is present. Salt brings out the flavor in food. The level of saltiness that is pleasing will vary from person to person.

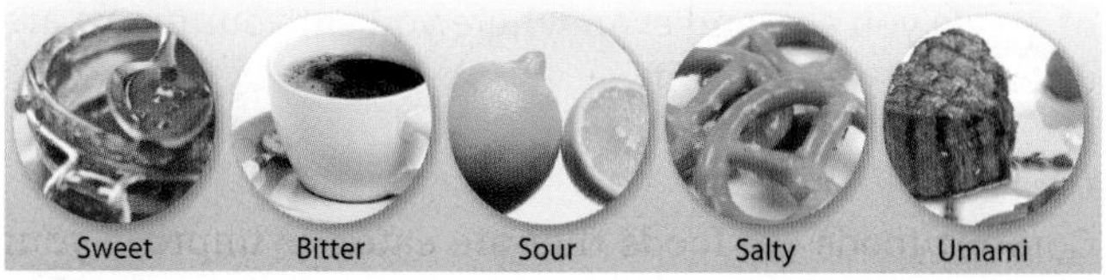

■ **Figure 1.2**

The Five Flavor Profiles

However, most people like some level of salt in food. Unlike sugar, you are not born liking the taste of salt; it is learned through exposure to salted foods. The final flavor profile is umami. *Umami* means "good flavor" or "good taste" in Japanese. It is an early, rich, savory flavor, such as is found in meat, cheese, and mushrooms.

Other sensations of taste also influence what you eat. The tongue and mouth can sense the texture of foods. You may prefer soft or crunchy foods or prefer not to eat foods with a certain mouthfeel. In fact, how a food feels in your mouth can influence whether you like that food. Fattiness is a profile found in foods that have a certain mouthfeel. The taste of full-fat ice cream is difficult to replicate without the fat. A well-marbled steak has a very different taste than a lean cut. The mouthfeel is changed greatly when the fat is decreased. Dryness, such as the astringency of dry wine or unripe fruit, is a taste profile. Coolness is present in foods that have mint or menthol. When you eat foods that have chili peppers, you get the sensation of heat or spiciness.

Taste is also affected by how food looks on the plate. You have probably heard the saying that you eat first with your eyes. Foods that are well presented and look appetizing are more likely to be pleasing to your palate.

Thoughts and Feelings About Food

How we feel about certain foods can influence whether we consume them. Your thoughts and feelings about foods are influenced by what you are used to eating, what foods make you feel good, health beliefs about food, and advertising designed to influence the foods you choose.

Habits

What you eat now is likely similar to what you ate when you were younger. It is what you are used to, and it is familiar. You may eat the same foods each day for breakfast, such as cereal, milk, and coffee. You choose this each day because it is familiar; you don't even have to think about what you are going to eat. Most people eat a very limited number of foods. Trips to the grocery store are often routine, with the same basic foods purchased each trip. You probably have your favorite items at the restaurants you frequent. When you eat your meals, the number of meals you eat, and even where you eat your meals are often done out of habit.

Comfort Foods

Comfort foods are foods that are eaten to improve your mood or to make you feel better. They give you comfort or a sense of well-being. Comfort foods are almost always foods that are familiar to you and that bring back fond memories of celebrations or happy occasions. They often carry some emotional significance and remind you of someone or some place. Comfort foods are usually filling and homey, such as chocolate cake, apple pie, meat loaf, macaroni and cheese, or pasta (**Figure 1.3**). What you consider comfort food will be shaped by your experiences and your culture. Males generally consider warm, hearty foods such as steak, casseroles, and soups as comfort foods. Females are more likely to choose chocolate or ice cream as comfort foods. People younger than age 55 are more likely to choose potato chips or cookies as comfort foods.[1] Whatever your age or gender, there is surely a food that you consider your comfort food.

Health Beliefs

Your food choices can also be influenced by what you believe will impact your health. If you believe that your health can be positively or negatively affected by the foods you eat, which it certainly can, then you are more likely to consider how healthy a food is when making food choices.[2] For example, say that you are faced with a choice of fried or baked chicken. You would prefer the fried chicken, but you know that it contains more fat and calories than the baked chicken. You choose the baked chicken because you believe that it is healthier. Whether people act on their health beliefs is based on how strong those beliefs are and how vulnerable they believe they are to the potential consequences. For example, a 20-year-old may know that the fried chicken has more fat and calories than the baked chicken, but thinks that the potential consequences, if any, are far into the future. Another 20-year-old whose father just had a heart attack and knows that he needs to lose a few pounds may be more motivated to make a food choice based on the health belief that fried foods are less healthy than baked ones.

Current health status may also influence food choices. If you have been diagnosed with a health problem whose treatment includes changes in your diet, you may be motivated to choose foods according to the recommendations you have been provided. For example, if you are being treated for acid reflux, you may avoid spicy, high-acid foods. Your belief that these foods will worsen your condition influences the foods you choose.

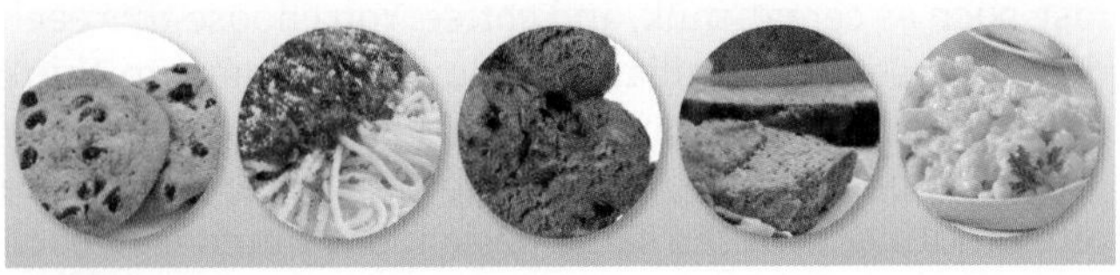

■ **Figure 1.3**
What Is Your Comfort Food?

Advertising

Billions of dollars are spent on advertising foods and beverages each year. Whether it is in print, on television, or on the Internet, the vast majority of advertising is for high-fat, high-sugar foods and beverages and fast food.[3,4] Advertisers use aggressive and sometimes deceptive tactics to encourage you to purchase their products. They use strategies to pull at your heartstrings and remind you of happy times. Attractive models are shown having fun and eating the foods they are selling. Advertisers often promote their foods or beverages as being perfect for your lifestyle, fun, and exciting and that you will be "one of the crowd" if you consume it. They try to send the message that "If you buy and eat or drink our product, you too will be attractive, happy, accepted, and cool." All of these tactics are designed to evoke positive emotions to encourage you to purchase their products.

Companies are increasingly using product placement as an advertising strategy. Product placement is a form of advertising where brand-name foods and beverages are placed in a movie or television show. Product placement subtly advertises products as they become props for the characters. The character in a movie is not just eating at a restaurant, but is eating at a McDonald's. A character in a television show is not just eating a candy bar, but is eating a brand-name candy bar with the logo front and center. Product placement is designed to encourage you to buy a particular product or eat at a certain restaurant. Product placement has been around for decades; however, it has become more popular in recent years. If you have a DVR you can skip most commercials on TV, but if a product is in a show the advertisers still have your attention.

Does all this advertising sway you to consume certain products? Does it encourage you to eat more? Many researchers believe that it does. Advertisers often say that their advertising is to promote their brand and to get you to choose their brand over the competitor's. This may be true, but the ads also encourage food consumption in general. Advertising for food and beverages communicates potentially powerful food consumption cues.[4–6] The subtle effects of food advertising on what you eat and how much you eat are usually outside of your own awareness or intention.[7] Research confirms that external cues such as food advertisements have a significant influence on food consumption behaviors. The evidence suggests that advertising for food has a direct causal link between greater consumption of food in general, not just of the food being advertised.[6]

Advertising tactics are certainly powerful and can be used to encourage consumption of healthy foods as well. Campaigns to encourage consumption of milk, cheese, fruits and vegetables, or other healthy foods are also seen

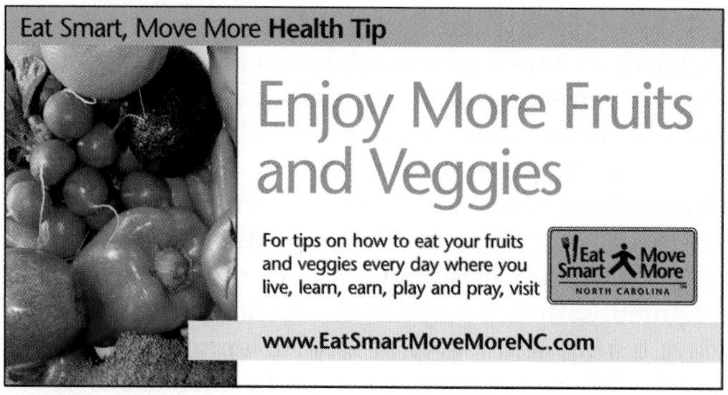

Figure 1.4

Advertisement for Fruits and Vegetables

The number of ads for healthy foods pales in comparison to the number for high-fat, high-calorie foods and beverages.

Source: © Eat Smart, Move More, North Carolina.

on billboards, in magazines, and on television (**Figure 1.4**). Although these campaigns can have a positive effect on consumption, the funding is only in the millions, not the billions that are spent yearly on advertising high-fat, high-calorie foods and beverages.[3]

Lifestyle

Your lifestyle has a major impact on your food choices. How you spend your time and how that time is allotted to what is most important to you will impact what you eat. Your lifestyle is most likely very fast paced, with multiple demands from friends, school, work, and family. Food may be eaten on the run or from a drive-thru window. Your choice of foods may be based on how quick they are to acquire and to eat. Your need to grab or prepare something quick may cause you to make choices that you may not have made otherwise. This may mean a frozen dinner prepared in minutes in the microwave or a trip to a fast-food restaurant. Eating at school or on your way to work may mean choosing between the best of several not-so-healthy choices just because that is what is available in the time you have allotted.

Your ability to plan meals as well as your food preparation skill level will also affect what you choose to eat. You may buy already prepared or partially prepared foods because you don't feel that you have the cooking skills to make food from scratch. For example, you may rely heavily on frozen meals that only require microwaving, as opposed to preparing grilled chicken, salad, and vegetables.

Which Side Are You On?

Advertising to Children

Is it fair to market foods to children, many of whom are too young to understand that companies are trying to sell a product that may not be healthy for them? Or, is it the right of companies to persuade children to purchase their products?

An estimated $2 billion is spent on marketing foods and beverages to children.[8] By far, the largest medium for advertising to children is television. Other methods include radio, magazines, product packaging, and in-store displays. Advertisers are increasingly using nontraditional marketing methods, including school-based marketing, product placement in movies and video games, toy giveaways, and logo placement almost everywhere and anywhere. Marketing techniques may also include promotion of a product by a celebrity spokesperson or a familiar cartoon character.

Young children may not understand that food companies are trying to sell them a product or that they may use persuasive techniques to get them to want their product. Very young children may not know the difference between the cartoon they are watching and the commercials.[9,10]

Most of what is marketed directly to children is unhealthy foods of poor nutritional quality.[8,11] Children view an average of 21 food ads on television each day, plus many other messages delivered through the Internet, at schools, on food packages, and in video game and movie product placement.[12]

Although parents are, of course, ultimately responsible for what their children eat, their messages to eat healthy pale in comparison to the billions spent by the food industry to promote their products. The amount of money spent and the number of messages to buy a certain product place an undue burden on parents to feed their children a healthy diet.

Because of the effect of food marketing on children's diets and their health, as well as the vast amount of marketing aimed at children, the Federal Trade Commission (FTC) has recommended that companies that market food or beverages to children should adopt meaningful nutrition-based standards for marketing their products.[8] The FTC currently allows companies to self-regulate with regard to food advertisements. Although some companies are beginning to set policies about advertising to children, most nutrition professionals feel that too few have policies and those that do don't go far enough to protect children from advertisers' persuasive tactics.[13] With so few companies adopting positive practices to market to children, government regulation may be required. What do you think? Do advertisers have the right to market to everyone, or should there be tighter regulations that protect children from the marketing of unhealthy foods?

Environment

Your environment plays a role in the foods you choose. Your culture or religion may have special foods that are important or that are forbidden. You may have limited foods available to you in your area. Your lifestyle, the importance you put on food, your food preparation skills, and the time that you have to devote to food and food preparation will influence your choices. Finally, cost will greatly impact what you choose to eat on a regular basis.

Culture

Your culture is a set of shared values and practices that characterize the group or community to which you belong. It may be your nation of origin or where you grew up. Whatever your culture is, it no doubt influences your food choices. It helps you define your attitudes about food. What foods you consider "good to eat" can be influenced by your culture and are often introduced in childhood and are associated with family. Food symbolizes many aspects of your culture and is a vehicle for social relations. You can expand your views by education and exposure to other cultures. You may become familiar with or even prefer foods from a culture other than your own.

Your culture will dictate to some extent what is appropriate to eat. Most Americans would never dream of eating horse meat or insects. However, these foods are acceptable in other cultures. Rotting shark is not usually found on the menu in North America, but is considered a delicacy in Iceland. You may have never heard of pouteen; however, this dish of french fries, gravy, and cheese curds is popular in Canada.

Food may have symbolic meaning in a culture. Some foods may symbolize wealth or celebration. Generally, Americans are thought of as meat and potato eaters. Although the size and diversity of America challenges you to name a "typical American meal," a steak and a baked potato or a hamburger and french fries are decidedly American. Similarly, a typical Japanese meal would be fish and rice; a typical Mexican meal would be beans and rice; and a typical German meal would be sausages and cabbage.

When people move from other countries to the United States, they will begin to adopt new foods. However, food is usually the last thing to change.[14] This is why in most cities you will find grocery stores that offer traditional Asian, Mexican, or European foods. People want to continue to consume what they are used to. They may slowly incorporate more American foods into their diet but continue to consume foods from their culture of origin.

Religion

Food is an important part of many religious customs and traditions. Beliefs about food, foods that are forbidden, and foods that are encouraged shape many of the world's religions. Christianity, Buddhism, Hinduism, Islam, and Judaism all have different food laws and customs. However, within each religion there is wide variation as to the interpretation of the laws and level of adherence.

Most Christian denominations do not have strict dietary laws. Most Christians consume a mixed diet of meat, dairy, produce, and grains. Although it is acceptable within the Christian faith to be vegetarian, it is not required. Catholics may fast or abstain from meat on Fridays during Lent. Seventh Day Adventists are encouraged to follow a vegetarian diet for health reasons. Those Seventh Day Adventists who do eat meat usually do not consume pork.

Islam has many dietary laws. Muslims believe that the way they eat is fundamentally about obeying God. Allowed foods are referred to as being *halal*. Forbidden foods, called *haram*, include pork, meat not slaughtered in the prescribed Islamic way, and alcohol. Although meat is allowed if slaughtered properly, many Muslims are vegetarian. Muslims, according to Islamic law, should avoid restaurants that serve forbidden food and alcohol. They also should not sit at a table where alcohol is being served. Islamic law also encourages Muslims to eat only when hungry, not to eat in excess, and to remember those who are hungry when they are eating.

Hinduism forbids meat, fish, poultry, and eggs in an effort to practice nonviolence. Some Hindus do consume meat, but almost all avoid beef. Strict Hindus also do not consume alcohol, caffeine, garlic, or onions. Many Hindus observe fasts, or *vrat*, on special occasions or holidays as a way to focus their mind and connect with God by practicing self-control. Generally, fruits, nuts, and milk are allowed during most fasts, based on local customs and beliefs.

Buddhism has no set dietary law; however, a number of food practices are common among Buddhists. Buddhists practice *ahimsa*, or nonviolence. As a result, many Buddhists are vegetarian. Some Buddhists practice Zen cooking and prepare food as part of their spiritual experience. Buddhist cooks sometimes use seitan as a meat substitute. Seitan is a product made from wheat gluten that is similar in texture to meat.

Judaism has many dietary laws. However, the degree of adherence to these dietary laws varies greatly. The Jewish practice of keeping kosher is to only eat foods that are "fit" or "proper" according to Jewish dietary law. Pork is forbidden, as are birds of prey, shellfish, or fish without fins and scales (no shark or squid). Dairy and meat are never mixed in the same meal. You may have seen kosher symbols on foods in the grocery store. This symbol means that the food has been inspected by a kosher-certifying agency and has been prepared in a way that complies with Jewish law. Although the number of Jews who "keep kosher" all the time is relatively small, the food laws continue to be an important part of Judaism, especially during religious holidays.

How Policy and Environment Affect My Choices

Food Deserts

The term **food desert** has been coined to mean a large area where mainstream grocery stores are absent or a long distance from the population center. Food deserts exist across the United States, but are primarily found in low-income neighborhoods in both urban and rural areas.[15,16] Living in a food desert has a profound impact on people's food choices.

More than 2 million families in the United States live more than 1 mile from a grocery store and do not have access to a vehicle. An additional 3 million households live 0.5 to 1 mile from a grocery store and do not have access to a vehicle.[17] Lack of transportation may force people who live in food deserts to purchase their food from drug stores, convenience stores, or smaller food outlets. These stores have limited selections, and many do not offer fresh fruits and vegetables. Food from these stores is often more expensive than that found in mainstream grocery stores. In addition, mainstream grocery stores in inner city and rural areas may charge more for food than those in suburban neighborhoods, in part, because operating costs are higher.[18]

Policy change is one solution to encouraging full-service supermarkets to locate in food deserts. Offering low-interest loans or assistance with rezoning are possible strategies to increase the number of supermarkets in such areas, giving more people access to healthy, affordable food.

Availability

Having access to a full-service supermarket greatly affects your food choices.[19] More than likely, you have easy access to a full-service supermarket that carries a large variety of foods. These stores stock multiple choices within each food category. If you are shopping for ground beef, a full-service supermarket will offer regular, lean, and extra lean options. What you chose is up to you, but all varieties are available. The store offers you a variety of food options.

Low-income neighborhoods are often served by smaller independent grocery stores or convenience stores. These stores may not stock fresh fruits and vegetables or offer them in very limited varieties and quantities. Smaller stores are less likely to offer healthy alternatives such as whole-grain breads, low-sugar canned fruits, or lean ground meats.[20] If you lived in a neighborhood served by these smaller stores and lacked transportation to shop at a larger store, your food choices would be limited.

Access to farmers' markets or farm stands also has an impact on what you choose to eat. If you have a farmers' market near your school, work, or home, you may be more likely to stop and purchase fresh foods from local farmers. Placing farm stands in neighborhoods where fresh fruits and vegetables had not typically been readily available has been shown to increase fruit and vegetable consumption.[21]

Cost

Food costs represent a significant proportion of most people's budget. The money you have to purchase foods will certainly impact what you choose to buy. The cost of food is second only to taste as the most important factor affecting your food choices.[28]

Healthier foods such as whole-grain products, low-fat dairy, low-fat meats, and fresh fruits and vegetables are higher in cost compared to other foods.[29] The low cost of high-fat, high-sugar processed foods are believed to be a direct consequence of U.S. agricultural policy over the past 30 years.[30] Corn and soybean crops are subsidized, so they cost less than nonsubsidized crops such as fruits and vegetables. Over the past 15 years, fruits and vegetables have led all other food categories in retail price increases, making processed products less costly than produce.[31] The high cost of fruits and vegetables may impact your consumption of these foods, especially if your food budget is tight.[32]

TERMS

food desert Area that lacks access to affordable fruits, vegetables, whole grains, low-fat milk, and other foods that make up the full range of a healthy diet.

Personal Health Check

What Influences Your Food Choices?

You now understand the many influences on your food choices. Examine what most influences your selection of food. Have you become a creature of habit, eating the same things day in and day out just because that is what you have always eaten? Have you allowed a tight food budget to send you to the fast-food restaurant more than you should instead of taking the time to prepare simple foods at home? Once you examine what affects your food choices, break out of your mold and expand your choices to include foods you may have never tried or take a trip to a nearby farm stand where you have never shopped. If you often use prepared foods, try making them yourself some of the time. Expanding your food choices will help you have a more varied, exciting diet.

Special Report

World and Domestic Hunger

World Hunger

The Food and Agriculture Organization of the United Nations estimates that globally 925 million people are **undernourished.**[22] This figure marks a slight improvement from previous years; however, the number remains unacceptably high.

Hunger and **malnutrition** are the underlying causes of more than half of all child deaths, killing nearly 6 million children each year.[23] Most of the world's hungry live in developing countries. The region with the most undernourished people continues to be Asia and the Pacific.

The world currently produces enough food to meet the calorie needs of every person on the planet. Why then are so many people around the globe hungry? Inequitable allocation of resources due to social, political, racial, and ethnocentrism underlie much of the world's hunger. Poverty is well recognized as the root cause of hunger. Many factors contribute to poverty, including greed, overpopulation, unemployment, political and civil unrest, and the lack of resources to produce food or goods for sale.[24,25]

At most risk for hunger are the poor and victims of catastrophes. The rural poor in developing countries likely have no electricity, no safe drinking water, and poor sanitation. Urban poor live in overcrowded conditions without access to affordable food. Floods, drought, earthquakes, and other natural disasters increase the chances of hunger, especially in disadvantaged countries. Hunger can lead to even greater poverty, further compromising a person's ability to work and learn. Conflict is also a cause of hunger. People in war-torn areas such as Sudan or Somalia face hunger or starvation due to lack of adequate food.

Solutions to World Hunger

Many organizations and governments around the world are working to address hunger.

Agencies provide access to clean water and direct food-based relief to countries with high levels of hunger. Strategies to address global hunger also include providing people the opportunity to produce food for local consumption. In addition, efforts include strategies to address poverty. These efforts include access to training to promote self-reliance and access to loans to start small businesses.

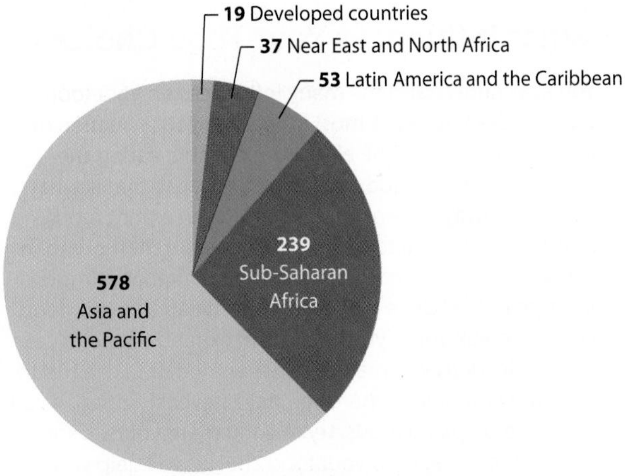

Rates of Global Hunger Are Unacceptably High

Source: © FAO, Food and Agriculture Organization of the United Nations.

Hunger in America

Hunger is not limited to developing countries. It is also an issue in the United States and other developed countries. Hunger in developed countries is often categorized as **food insecurity.** Food-insecure households have reduced food intake at times due to lack of money or other resources for food. Families that are food insecure don't have money at the end of the week or month to buy enough food, so one or more members of the family eats less or not at all until the next paycheck. An estimated 50 million people in the United States live in food-insecure households, including 17 million children.[26] The budget constraints that low-income households face due to low wages, underemployment, unemployment, or illness often lead to food insecurity and hunger.

The Hunger–Obesity Connection

All segments of the U.S. population are affected by obesity. Obesity rates are high in all socioeconomic and racial groups. However, low-income and food-insecure people are especially vulnerable to obesity due to the additional risk factors associated with poverty. When you think of obesity you generally think of excess food, not too little food. However, hunger and obesity can coexist in the same individual, family, or community.

People with limited resources often do not have access to affordable healthy foods. They may buy their foods from convenience stores or corner stores where food is more expensive and fresh fruits and vegetables are not available or limited (for more on food deserts, see "How Policy and Environment Affect My Choices"). In an attempt to stretch their food dollar, they may purchase cheap, energy-dense foods instead of fruits, vegetables, and whole grains. People who experience food insecurity may overconsume when food is available. This can result in chronic ups and downs in food intake, which can contribute to weight gain. Women are particularly vulnerable to this if they must limit their food intake to provide for their children. Food insecurity and poverty also increase stress in children and adults. Stress has been shown to increase the risk of obesity through hormonal and metabolic changes as well as unhealthy eating.[27]

Solutions to Domestic Food Insecurity

Many organizations and agencies are working to decrease food insecurity. **Food banks** collect food from manufactures, growers, restaurants, and individuals and distribute it to those in need. **Gleaning** projects make fresh fruits and vegetables available to food-insecure households. **Meals on Wheels** and **congregate nutrition sites** provide food for the elderly and homebound. Federal programs working to decrease the incidence of food insecurity include the **National School Lunch Program (NSLP)**, the **National School Breakfast Program (NSPB)**, the **Women Infant and Children Program (WIC)**, the **Supplemental Nutrition Assistance Program (SNAP)**, and the **Expanded Food and Nutrition Education Program (EFNEP).**

TERMS

undernourished Underconsumption of calories or nutrients that leads to disease or susceptibility to disease.

hunger A term used to describe the problem of lack of food and nutrients.

malnutrition Under- or overconsumption of energy or nutrients, resulting in compromised health.

food insecurity Uncertainty of having or inability to acquire enough food to meet the needs of all members of the household due to insufficient money or other resources for food.

food bank An agency or center that collects food and distributes it to the needy.

gleaning The act of collecting useful leftover crops from the fields or orchards that have been commercially harvested.

Meals on Wheels A nonprofit organization that delivers hot meals to the elderly and homebound.

congregate nutrition sites Provide hot lunches to seniors aged 60 and older.

National School Lunch Program (NSLP) A federally funded program that provides free or reduced-price school lunches to eligible students based on family income levels.

National School Breakfast Program (NSBP) A federally funded program that provides cash assistance to states to operate nonprofit breakfast programs in schools and residential childcare institutions.

Women Infant and Children Program (WIC) A federally funded program that provides nutritious foods, nutrition education, and referrals and access to health care to low-income pregnant women, new mothers, and infants and children at nutritional risk. WIC participants now receive a new healthier WIC food package that includes, fruits, vegetables, low-fat milk, and whole-grain bread.

Supplemental Nutrition Assistance Program (SNAP) Formerly called Food Stamps, this federal assistance program provides low-income people funds to purchase food.

Expanded Food and Nutrition Education Program (EFNEP) A federally funded educational program conducted through the Cooperative Extension Service in every state and U.S. territory. Families receive education about nutrition, food safety, and how to make the most of their food dollar.

Researchers compared two different week's worth of groceries. The healthier basket of groceries cost more because of the higher cost for whole grains, lean ground beef, and skinless poultry.[20] People who spend more for food are more likely to have a healthy diet.[33]

Does this mean that an unhealthy diet is a given if your budget for food is limited? Absolutely not, but it may mean that you have to prepare more foods yourself and choose carefully. Large improvements can be achieved without increasing spending on food.[33] A well-planned menu that uses simple whole foods instead of already prepared convenience foods can be lower in cost and healthier.[34] Plant-based protein sources such as dried beans and peas are among the healthiest and most economical in the supermarket. Even with the increase in cost of fresh fruits and vegetables over the past 15 years, you can still fit them into your food budget. It is estimated that you can get the recommended servings of fruits and vegetables each day for under a dollar.[35]

Introduction of the Nutrients

You have a need to consume food for biological reasons. The **nutrients** that you need to live are contained in the foods you eat (see **Figure 1.5**).

One of the reasons you need food is for the energy, or **calories**, it contains. You get calories from the energy-providing nutrients, which are **carbohydrates**, **proteins**, and **fats** (alcohol also contains calories) (**Figure 1.6**).

In their pure form, carbohydrates and proteins contain 4 calories per gram; fats 9 calories per gram, and alcohol 7 calories per gram. All of the motions of your body, both voluntary and involuntary, require energy. Your body breaks down food to provide the energy it needs for your heart to beat, for your legs to walk across campus, or for your hands to send a text message.

TERMS

nutrients Substances in food that the body uses for energy, growth, tissue repair, or regulation of body processes.

calories A unit used to measure energy in foods and beverages.

carbohydrates Organic compounds that contain carbon, hydrogen, and oxygen. Carbohydrates include sugars, starches, and fiber. They are a major source of energy for your body.

proteins Organic compounds that contain carbon, hydrogen, nitrogen, and oxygen. Proteins differ from other energy-providing nutrients in that they contain nitrogen. Proteins are made of smaller building blocks called amino acids. Proteins can provide energy but are unique in their function of maintaining body structure and regulating many processes in the body.

fats Organic compounds that contain carbon, hydrogen, and oxygen. Fats provide structure for your cells, carry fat-soluble vitamins into your body, and are a component of many hormones.

Energy-providing nutrients
- Carbohydrates
- Proteins
- Fats

Vitamins
The two classes of vitamins are fat soluble and water soluble.
Fat-soluble vitamins: Vitamins A, D, E, and K
Water-soluble vitamins: Vitamin C, B vitamins
Thiamin (B_1), riboflavin (B_2), niacin (B_3), vitamin B_6, vitamin B_{12}, folate, pantothenic acid, biotin

Minerals
The two classes of minerals are macrominerals that are needed in the body in relatively high amounts and microminerals (trace minerals) that are needed in only very small amounts.
Macrominerals: Sodium, chloride, potassium, calcium, phosphorus, magnesium
Microminerals: Iron, zinc, copper, manganese, molybdenum, selenium, iodine, fluoride, chromium, phosphorus

Water

■ **Figure 1.5**
Classes of Nutrients

In addition to the energy-providing nutrients, you also need **vitamins** and **minerals** to help regulate body functions. Water, the most important nutrient, is also needed. In fact, you can survive for several weeks without food, but only a few days without water.

TERMS

vitamins Organic substances that help regulate hundreds of processes in the body. Although they provide no energy, they help your body use the energy in the foods you eat.

minerals Inorganic substances that help regulate body processes and provide structure to the body.

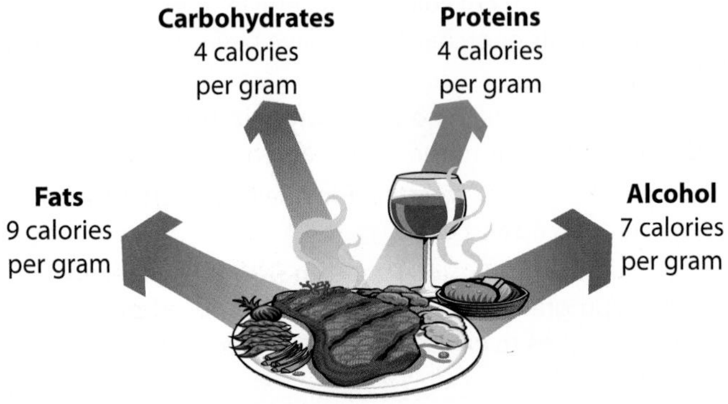

■ **Figure 1.6**
Calories in Energy-Providing Nutrients

Ready to Make a Change

Are you ready to make a change, small or large, in your overall health and well-being? Using some of the information provided in this chapter is a great place to start.

I commit to a small first step. Eat when you are hungry, not because of external cues. Pay attention to your level of hunger prior to eating.

I am ready to take the next step and make a medium change. What effect do food ads have on your consumption of food? Next time you are in front of the TV and a food ad comes on, analyze the effects that ad has on your hunger.

I have been making changes for some time and am ready to make a large change in my overall health. Expand your food-shopping environment. Shop at a full-service grocery store, if possible. Smaller independent stores have fewer options and can be higher in cost. Try farm stands or farmers' markets to further expand your options.

Myth Versus Fact

Myth: Hunger and appetite are the same.

Fact: Hunger is the physiological drive to eat; appetite is the desire to eat. You may have an appetite for apple pie if you smell it baking but not have a physiological need for food.

Myth: Food ads don't have an impact on what you eat if you just ignore them.

Fact: Food advertisers use powerful food consumption cues in their ads. Research shows that many of the food ads you see on television can cause you to eat more than you would have otherwise.

Myth: Healthy foods cost too much.

Fact: It is true that some healthy foods are more expensive than cheap high-calorie foods. However, a well-planned menu that uses simple whole foods instead of already prepared convenience foods can be lower in cost and healthier.

Myth: Hunger is only a problem in developing countries.

Fact: Hunger and food insecurity are problems across the globe, including in developed countries.

Myth: People are hungry across the globe because there is not enough food.

Fact: Enough food is available to supply everyone with the calories they need. The problem of hunger is related to poverty and inequitable distribution of resources.

Back to the Story

Sam is no different from most people. When he started college, he most likely continued to eat what he was used to eating as a child. The fast pace of studying and working to pay for college didn't leave much time for experimenting with different foods. Sam's lack of access to a full-service grocery store further limited his choices. Sam will soon have an opportunity to expand his food repertoire in a new place. Even though he will still be living in the same country, the food cultures of the Midwest and South are very different. Sam can take advantage of this and ask native Midwesterners to introduce him to foods that are common in that region. Because Sam will have a car, he will be able to shop at a full-service grocery store that has many more choices than the small store near campus where he shopped when he was a student. He can visit a local farmers' market or farm stand to see what local fruits and vegetables are available.

References

1. Wansink B, Cheney MM, Chan N. Exploring comfort food preferences across age and gender. *Physiol Behav.* 2003;79:739–747.
2. Wardle J, Haase AM, Steptoe A, Nillapun M, Jonwutiwes K, Bellisle F. Gender differences in food choice: the contribution of health beliefs and dieting. *Ann Behav Med.* 2004;27(2):107–116.
3. California Pan-Ethnic Health Network and Consumers Union. Out of balance, marketing of soda, candy, snacks and fast foods drown out healthful messages.

September 2005. http://www.consumersunion.org/pdf/OutofBalance.pdf. Accessed April 16, 2011.
4. Harrison K, Marske AL. Nutritional content of foods advertised during the television programs children watch most. *Am J Pub Health*. 2005;95(9):1568–1574.
5. Folta SC, Goldberg JP, Economos C, Bell R, Meltzer R. Food advertising targeted at school-age children: a content analysis. *J Nutr Ed Behav*. 2006;38:244–248.
6. Harris JL, Bargh JA, Brownell KD. Priming effects of television food advertising on eating behavior. *Health Psychol*. 2009;28(4):404–413.
7. Bargh JA, Morsella E. The unconscious mind. *Persp Psychol Sci*. 2008;3:73–79.
8. Federal Trade Commission. *Marketing Food to Children and Adolescents: A Review of Industry Expenditures, Activities, and Self-Regulation, A Report to Congress*. Washington, DC: Federal Trade Commission, 2008.
9. Institute of Medicine. *Food Marketing to Children: Threat or Opportunity?* Washington, DC: National Academies Press, 2006.
10. Kunkel D, Wilcox B, Cantor J, Palmer E, Linn S, Dowrick P. *Psychological Issues in the Increasing Commercialization of Childhood. Report of the APA Task Force on Advertising and Children*. Washington, DC: American Psychological Association, 2004.
11. Batada A, Wootan MG. *Better-For-Who? Revisiting Company Promises of Food Marketing to Children*. Washington, DC: Center for Science in the Public Interest, 2009.
12. Gantz W, Schwartz N, Angelini JR, Rideout V. *Food for Thought: Television Food Advertising to Children in the United States*. Menlo Park, CA: Kaiser Family Foundation, 2007.
13. Center for Science in the Public Interest. Report card on food-marketing policies: an analysis of food and entertainment company policies regarding food and beverage marketing to children. 2010. http://www.cspinet.org/new/pdf/marketingreportcard.pdf. Accessed April 19, 2011.
14. Kittler PG, Sucher KP. *Food and Culture*. 5th ed. Belmont, CA: Thompson Higher Education, 2008.
15. Beaulac J, Kristjansson E, Cummins S. A systematic review of food deserts, 1966–2007. *Prev Chron Dis*. 2009;6(3). http://cdc/gov/pcd. Accessed April 18, 2010.
16. Larson NI, Story MT, Nelson MC. Neighborhood environments: disparities in access to healthy food in the US. *Am J Prev Med*. 2008;36(1):74–81.
17. VerPloeg M, Breneman V, Farrigan T, et al. *Access to Affordable and Nutritious Food—Measuring and Understanding Food Deserts and Their Consequences: Report to Congress*. USDA Administrative Publication AP-036. 2009. http://www.ers.usda.gov/Publications/AP/AP036. Accessed April 28, 2011.
18. Kaufman PR, MacDonald JM, Lutz SM, Smallwood DM. *Do the Poor Pay More for Food? Item Selection and Price Differences Affect Low-Income Household Food Costs*. 1997. Agricultural Economic Report No. 759. http://ddr.nal.usda.gov/bitstream/10113/34238/1/CAT10841003.pdf. Accessed April 2011
19. Story M, Kaphingst KM, Robinson-O'Brien R, Glanz K. Creating healthy food and eating environments: Policy and environmental approaches. *Annu Rev Pub Hlth*. 2008;29:253–272.
20. Jetter KM, Cassady DL. The availability and cost of healthier food alternatives. *Am J Prev Med*. 2006;30(1):38–44.
21. Larsen K, Gilliland J. A farmers' market in a food desert: Evaluation impacts on the price and availably of healthy food. *Health & Place*. 2009;15(4):1158–1162.
22. Food and Agriculture Organization of the United Nations. Hunger. http://fao.org/hunger. Accessed April 18, 2011.
23. Food and Agriculture Organization of the United Nations. *The State of Food Insecurity in the World. Eradicating World Hunger—Key to Achieving The Millennium Development Goals*. Rome: Food and Agriculture Organization, 2005.
24. American Dietetic Association. Position of the American Dietetic Association: Addressing world hunger, malnutrition and food insecurity. *J Am Diet Assoc*. 2003;103(8):1046–1057.
25. Boyle, M. Community nutrition with an international perspective. In: Boyle M., ed. *Community Nutrition in Action: An Entrepreneurial Approach*. 3rd ed. Belmont, CA: Wadsworth/Thompson Learning, 2003:373–410.
26. United States Department of Agriculture, Economic Research Service. Food security in the United States: Key statistics and graphics. http://www.ers.usda.gov/Briefing/FoodSecurity/stats_graphs.htm. Updated January 14, 2011. Accessed April 18, 2011.
27. Food Research and Action Center. Hunger and obesity? Making the connection. http://frac.org/newsity/wp-content/uploads/2009/05/prardox.pdf. Updated February 2010. Accessed April 19, 2011.
28. Glanz K, Basil M, Maibach E, Goldberg J, Snyder D. Why Americans eat what they do: taste, nutrition, cost, convenience, and weight control concerns as influences on food consumption. *J Am Diet Assoc*. 1998;98:1118–1126.
29. Cassady D, Jetter KM, Culp J. Is price a barrier in eating more fruits and vegetables for low-income families? *J Am Diet Assoc*. 2007;107(11):1909–1915.
30. Muller M. A healthier, smarter food system. Institute for Agriculture and Trade Policy. 2006. http://www.iatp.org/iatp/library/admin/uploadedfiles/Healthier_Smarter_Food_System_A.pdf. Accessed April 18, 2011.
31. Putnam J. Major trends in the US food supply. *Food Rev*. 2000;23:13.
32. Ard JD, Fitzpatrick S, Desmond RA, Bryce SS, Pisu M, Allison DB, Franklin F, Baskin ML. The impact of cost on the availability of fruits and vegetables in the homes of schoolchildren in Birmingham, Alabama. *Am J Public Health*. 2007;97:367–372.

33. Bernstein AM, Bloom DE, Rosner BA, Franz M, Willett W. Relation of food cost to healthfulness of diet among US women. *Am J Clin Nutr*. 210;92(5):1197–1203.
34. McDermott AJ, Stephens MB. Cost of eating: Whole foods versus convenience foods in a low-income model. *Fam Med*. 2010;42(4):280–284.
35. United States Department of Agriculture, Economic Research Service. How much do Americans pay for fruits and vegetables? http://www.ers.usda.gov/Publications/AIB790. Updated July 20, 2004. Accessed April 18, 2011.

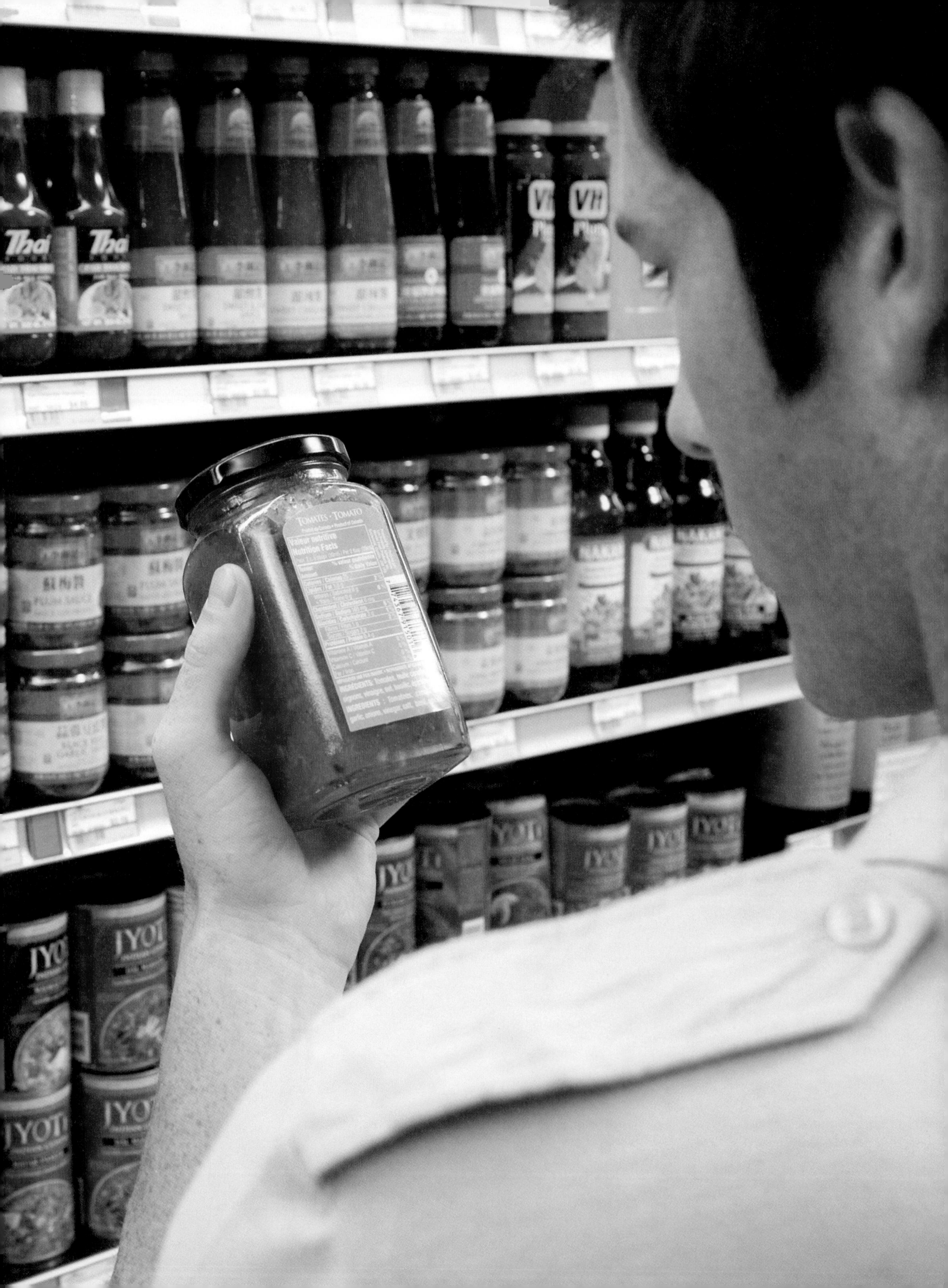
Thai
VH
Tomates · Tomato
Valeur nutritive
Nutrition Facts
INGREDIENTS
JYOTI

Chapter 2

Eat Healthy: Tools to Help You Choose

Key Messages

- The *Dietary Guidelines for Americans* provide science-based recommendations on healthy eating and physical activity to help you achieve and maintain a healthy weight and reduce the risk of chronic disease.
- Food labels provide information to help you choose foods wisely.
- MyPlate provides information about what your plate should look like as well as what specific foods you should eat each day.
- Dietary Reference Intakes (DRIs) provide recommended daily nutrient requirements for most nutrients.

Every day you are bombarded with information about food and nutrition from sources such as websites; computer applications; flyers in grocery stores; and, of course, family and friends. "Don't eat this; eat that instead." "Don't eat too much of this; make sure to get plenty of that." Often what you hear from one source will contradict what you just heard from another. Who is right? Where do you turn for reliable information about healthy eating and physical activity so that you can make an informed decision? Where can you go for unbiased information that is based on scientific research, not just the latest fad aimed at selling a product? Fortunately, several reliable tools are available to help you make wise choices with regard to your food intake and physical activity. In this chapter, you'll discover the *Dietary Guidelines for Americans*, MyPlate, dietary standards, and food labels and learn how you can put these tools to work to help you achieve better health through healthy eating and physical activity.

Story

Kenji is a freshman in college. She is excited to be away from home and starting school. She has always been healthy, but has never given much thought to what she eats. She wants to stay healthy and has an interest in eating a healthy diet. She has checked the Internet to get some help in choosing healthy foods now that she is in charge of all of her meals. She has found an overwhelming amount of information on what to eat, too much information, in fact, and lots of contradictory messages. All she wants is a simple guide to help her shop for healthy foods that she can prepare and to make healthier choices when eating out. Where can Kenji turn for some simple guidance?

Dietary Guidelines for Americans

In 1980, the **United States Department of Agriculture (USDA)** and **Department of Health and Human Services (DHHS)** jointly released the first ***Dietary Guidelines for Americans***. These guidelines are updated every five years (**Figure 2.1**).

The *Dietary Guidelines for Americans* focus on health promotion and disease prevention for adults and children older than 2 years of age. Past releases of the *Dietary Guidelines for Americans* provided guidance for healthy people only. However, the 2010 release recognizes the large percentage of the population who are overweight or obese and/or at risk for various chronic diseases. Thus, the 2010 edition of the *Dietary Guidelines for Americans* is intended for all people ages 2 years and older, including those who are at increased risk of chronic diseases. The recommendations presented by the *Dietary Guidelines for Americans* will be discussed in detail throughout this text.

How the *Dietary Guidelines for Americans* Are Developed

The development of the *Dietary Guidelines for Americans* begins with the appointment of the Dietary Guidelines Advisory Committee (DGAC). This external panel is composed of scientists and scholars from around the country who specialize in nutrition, physiology, medicine, and physical activity. The DGAC conducts a thorough review of all scientific information on diet, physical activity, and health. It uses a systematic method to review the scientific literature, giving more weight to studies that are conducted using rigorous scientific methods. The DGAC categorizes the strength of the evidence in the literature as **strong evidence**, **moderate evidence**, or **limited evidence**. The DGAC's report presents a thorough review of the most up-to-date findings on nutrition, physical activity, and health issues.

The process used by the DGAC for the 2010 *Dietary Guidelines for Americans* was open to the public. It posted meeting minutes and drafts of the report online. Public comment was encouraged throughout the DGAC's deliberations. The USDA and the DHHS use the DGAC report, along with comments from the public and various federal agencies, to create the *Dietary Guidelines for Americans*.

TERMS

United States Department of Agriculture (USDA) The federal agency that is responsible for the development and execution of policy on farming, agriculture, and food. The agency ensures that the United States has a safe food supply and that natural resources are protected.

Department of Health and Human Services (DHHS) The primary federal agency for protecting the health of all Americans and for providing essential human services.

Dietary Guidelines for Americans Provide evidence-based nutrition information and advice for people age 2 and older. It serves as the basis for federal food and nutrition education programs.

strong evidence Reflects consistent, convincing findings derived from studies that use a robust methodology and that are relevant to the population of interest.

moderate evidence Reflects somewhat less evidence or less consistent evidence. The body of evidence may include studies of weaker design and/or some inconsistency in results. The studies may be susceptible to some bias, but not enough to invalidate the results, or the body of evidence may not be as generalizable to the population of interest.

limited evidence Reflects either a small number of studies, studies of weak design, and/or inconsistent results.

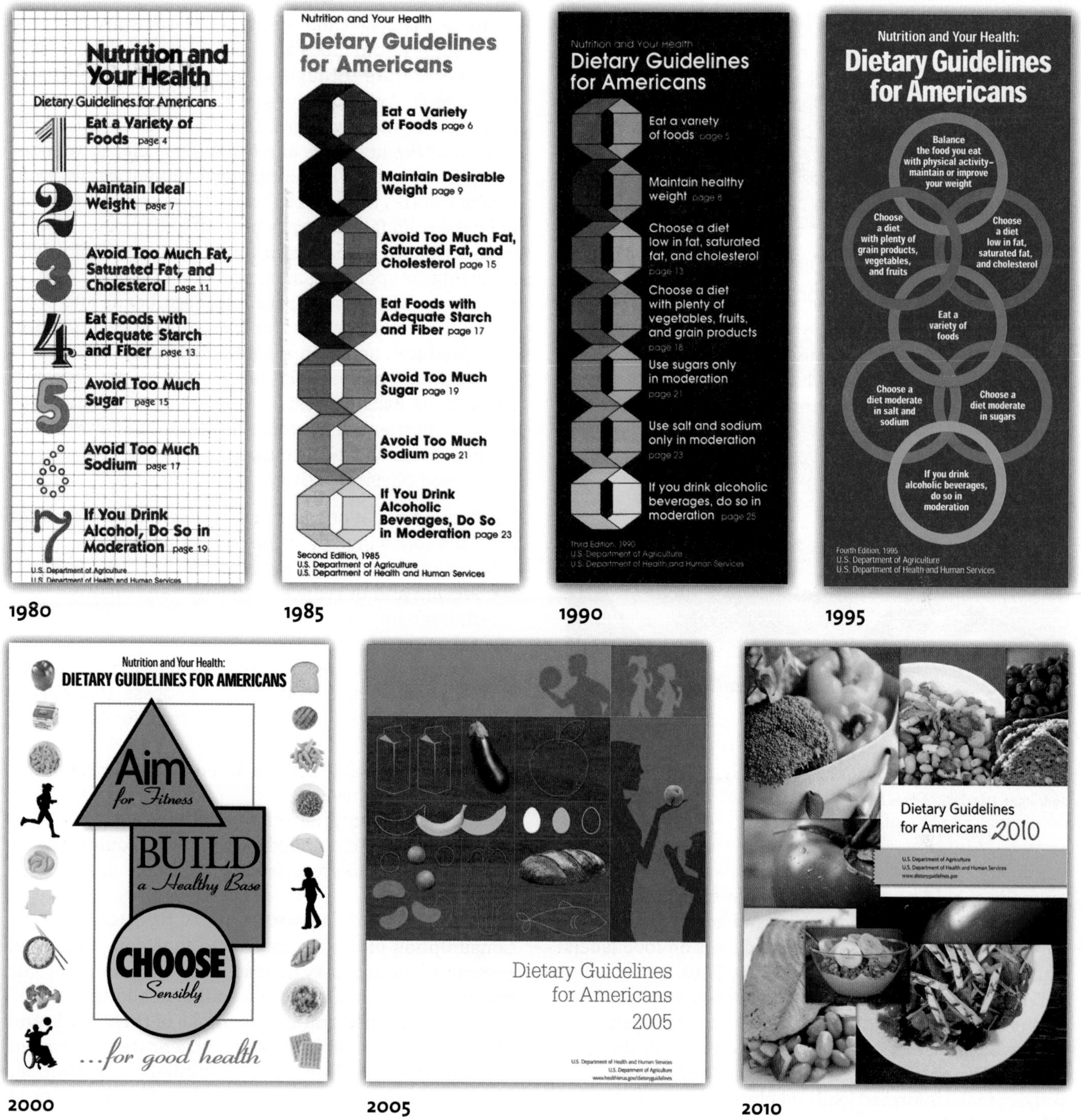

■ **Figure 2.1**

Dietary Guidelines for Americans from 1980 to Present

Source: © U.S. Department of Health and Human Services and U.S. Department of Agriculture. Dietary Guidelines for Americans, 1980–2010. 1st–7th Edition, Washington, DC: U.S. Government Printing Office. Available at: http://www.health.gov/dietaryguidelines/history.htm. Accessed September 6, 2011.

How the Recommendations in the *Dietary Guidelines for Americans* Are Used

The recommendations in the *Dietary Guidelines for Americans* are used to develop nutrition education and communication messages and materials. All publications or media campaigns supported by the federal government are required by law to be consistent with the *Dietary Guidelines for Americans*. The *Dietary Guidelines for Americans* aid policy makers in the design and implementation of nutrition-related programs. For example, the National Child Nutrition Program that governs what is served in schools is guided by the *Dietary Guidelines for Americans*. The *Dietary Guidelines for Americans* also have the potential to guide health and nutrition claims on foods. Statements

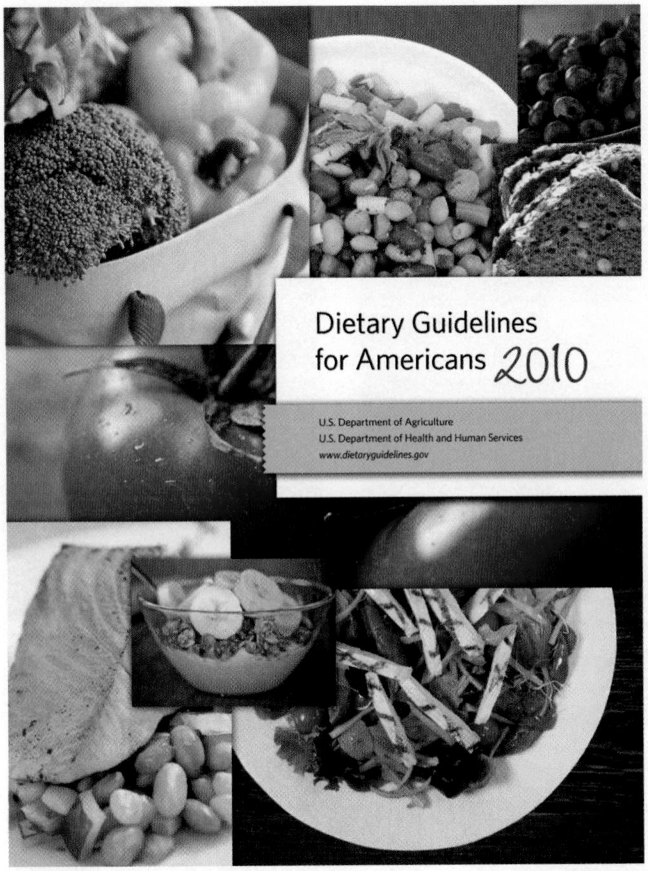

Figure 2.2

Dietary Guidelines for Americans 2010

Source: © U.S. Department of Health and Human Services and U.S. Department of Agriculture. Dietary Guidelines for Americans, 2010.

on foods should be phrased in a manner that allows for consumers to understand a claim and how it fits into the context of the total diet. By law, all claims on food labels must be based on scientific evidence. Thus, recommendations in the *Dietary Guidelines for Americans* based on strong evidence may influence claims on food labels. The *Dietary Guidelines for Americans* provide you with the best information on what constitutes a healthy diet so that you can make informed food and physical activity choices (**Figure 2.2**).

Recommendations

The *Dietary Guidelines for Americans* provide recommendations so that you can attain and maintain a healthy weight, reduce your risk of chronic disease, and achieve overall health. The recommendations are based not only on the latest research, but also take into account food preferences, cultural traditions, and customs of the diverse population of the United States.

Balancing Calories to Manage Weight High rates of overweight and obesity in all subgroups of the U.S. population indicate a need for **calorie balance** to manage weight. To decrease overweight and obesity, Americans must decrease total calories from foods and beverages and increase calorie expenditure through physical activity. The *Dietary Guidelines for Americans* suggest that you select **nutrient-dense** foods and beverages. The term *nutrient dense* indicates that the nutrients and other beneficial substances in a particular food have not been "diluted" by the addition of calories from added solid fats, sugars, or starches or by the solid fats naturally present in the foods. Ideally, nutrient-dense foods are in forms that retain naturally occurring components, such as dietary fiber. All vegetables, fruits, whole grains, seafood, eggs, beans and peas, unsalted nuts and seeds, fat-free and low-fat milk and milk products, and lean meats and poultry—when prepared without adding solid fats or sugars—are nutrient-dense foods. Balancing calories to manage weight requires selecting nutrient-dense foods and beverages from a variety of sources as well as choosing a variety of strategies to increase physical activity.

Key Recommendations The *Dietary Guidelines for Americans* offer the following key recommendations for balancing calories and managing weight:

- Prevent and/or reduce overweight and obesity through improved eating and physical activity behaviors.
- Control total calorie intake to manage body weight. For people who are overweight or obese, this will mean consuming fewer calories from foods and beverages.
- Increase physical activity and reduce time spent in sedentary behaviors.
- Maintain appropriate calorie balance during each stage of life—childhood, adolescence, adulthood, pregnancy and breastfeeding, and older age.

Foods and Food Components to Reduce

Consumption of certain foods and food components in excessive amounts may increase the risk of some chronic diseases. These foods include sodium, solid fats, added sugars, and refined grains. The intake of these foods and food components often replace nutrient-dense forms of foods in the diet. This makes it difficult to get proper nutrients without getting more calories than you need each day.

TERMS

calorie balance The balance between calories consumed in foods and beverages and calories expended through physical activity and metabolic processes.

nutrient dense Foods and beverages that provide vitamins, minerals, and other substances and that may have positive health effects with relatively few calories.

Key Recommendations The *Dietary Guidelines for Americans* offer the following key recommendations for reducing intake of certain foods and food components:

- Reduce daily sodium intake to less than 2,300 milligrams (mg) and further reduce intake to 1,500 mg among persons who are 51 and older and those of any age who are African American (due to a genetic predisposition for hypertension) or who have hypertension, diabetes, or chronic kidney disease. The 1,500-mg recommendation applies to about half of the U.S. population, including children and the majority of adults.
- Consume less than 10% of calories from saturated fatty acids by replacing them with monounsaturated and polyunsaturated fatty acids.
- Consume less than 300 mg per day of dietary cholesterol.
- Keep trans fatty acid consumption as low as possible, especially by limiting foods that contain synthetic sources of trans fats, such as partially hydrogenated oils, and by limiting other solid fats.
- Reduce the intake of calories form solid fats and added sugars.
- Limit the consumption of foods that contain refined grains and those that contain solid fats, added sugars, and added sodium.
- If alcohol is consumed, it should be consumed in moderation—up to one drink per day for women and two drinks per day for men—and only by adults of legal drinking age.

Dietary Guidelines for Special Populations

The *Dietary Guidelines for Americans* apply to all Americans age 2 and older. In addition, they offer some recommendations for specific populations.

Women capable of becoming pregnant

- Choose foods that supply heme iron (iron from meat sources), which is more readily absorbed by the body, additional iron sources, and enhancers of iron absorption, such as vitamin C–rich foods.
- Consume 400 micrograms (mcg) per day of synthetic folic acid (from fortified foods and/or supplements) in addition to food forms of folate from a varied diet.

Women who are pregnant or breastfeeding

- Consume 8–12 ounces of seafood per week from a variety of seafood types.
- Due to their high methyl mercury content, limit white (albacore) tuna to 6 ounces per week and do not eat the following four types of fish: tilefish, shark, swordfish, and king mackerel.
- If pregnant, take an iron supplement, as recommended by an obstetrician or other healthcare provider.

Individuals ages 50 years and older

- Consume foods fortified with vitamin B_{12}, such as fortified cereals, or dietary supplements.

Foods and Nutrients to Increase

A number of foods known to have a positive impact on overall health are not consumed in adequate amounts in most American's diets. You should increase your consumption of certain foods as part of an overall healthy diet while staying within the calories you need each day.

Key Recommendations The *Dietary Guidelines for Americans* offer the following key recommendations for increasing your intake of certain foods and food components:

- Increase vegetable and fruit intake.
- Eat a variety of vegetables, especially dark-green, red, and orange vegetables, as well as beans and peas.
- Consume at least half of all grains as whole grains. Increase whole-grain intake by replacing refined grains with whole grains.
- Increase intake of fat-free or low-fat milk and milk products, such as milk, yogurt, cheese, or fortified soy beverages.
- Choose a variety of protein foods, which include seafood, lean meat and poultry, eggs, beans and peas, soy products, and unsalted nuts and seeds.
- Increase the amount and variety of seafood consumed by choosing seafood in place of some meat and poultry.
- Replace protein foods that are higher in solid fats with choices that are lower in solid fats and calories and/or sources of oils.
- Use oils to replace solid fats where possible.
- Choose foods that provide more potassium, dietary fiber, calcium, and vitamin D, which are nutrients of concern in American diets. These foods include vegetables, fruits, whole grains, and milk and milk products.

Building Healthy Eating Patterns

Building a healthy diet means putting together all of the recommendations of what to eat more of and what to eat less of to create an eating pattern that supports optimal health.

Key Recommendations The *Dietary Guidelines for Americans* offer the following key recommendations for building healthy eating patterns:

- Select an eating pattern that meets nutrient needs over time at an appropriate calorie level.
- Account for all foods and beverages consumed and assess how they fit within a total healthy eating pattern.
- Follow food safety recommendations when preparing and eating foods to reduce the risk of foodborne illness.

What Do the *Dietary Guidelines for Americans* Say About Supplements?

A fundamental premise of the *Dietary Guidelines for Americans* is that nutrients should come primarily from foods. Foods in their natural form contain vitamins, minerals, fiber, and other naturally occurring substances that may have positive health effects.

There is not sufficient evidence to support a recommendation for or against the use of a multivitamin/multimineral supplement in the primary prevention of chronic disease. The evidence does support supplementation of combinations of certain nutrients in special populations. For example, supplementation of calcium and vitamin D in postmenopausal women reduces the risk of osteoporosis. You should aim to meet your nutritional needs through foods as opposed to supplements. If you choose to use supplements, discuss this with a healthcare provider to establish your need supplements and the correct dosage.

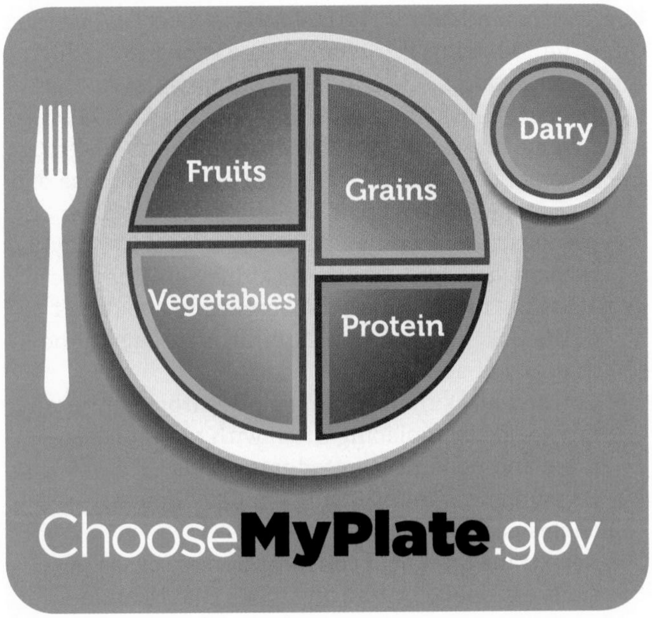

Figure 2.3

MyPlate

The MyPlate graphic indicates that half of your plate should be fruits and vegetables.

Source: Courtesy of USDA.

MyPlate

MyPlate was developed by the USDA and replaces MyPyramid as a tool to help you choose a healthy diet (**Figure 2.3**). The MyPlate graphic shows that half of your plate should be fruits and vegetables; less than one-quarter should be protein foods, such as meat, beans, or eggs; and more than one-quarter of your plate should be grain products. The MyPlate graphic is part of a larger communications initiative that is based on the 2010 *Dietary Guidelines for Americans* to help people make better food choices. The MyPlate graphic illustrates the five food groups using a familiar mealtime visual, a place setting.

Additional information beyond the graphic is available at www.ChooseMyPlate.gov. The website is an interactive web-based educational tool based on the latest science-based information on nutrition and physical activity.[2] Basic messages about healthy eating and physical activity are the core of the information provided at www.ChooseMyPlate.gov (**Figure 2.4**).

The website includes the following interactive tools:

- **Daily Food Plan.** You can use this tool to find the kinds and amounts of foods that you should eat each day. You enter your age, gender, and activity level and then the site provides a plan based on an appropriate calorie level. The food plan includes specific daily amounts from each food groups and a limit for fats, added sugars, and alcohol (discretionary calories).
- **Food Planner.** The Food Planner plans meals and menus based on your personal information and the foods you like to eat.
- **Food Tracker.** This online dietary and physical activity assessment tool provides you with information on the quality of your current diet.
- **MyFood-a-pedia.** This tool provides quick access to the calories contained in common foods (**Figure 2.5**).

Personal Health Check

Food Tracker

Tracking what you eat and how you move even for a few days will give you an estimate of how you are doing with respect to eating healthy and being active. It will give you a starting point from which you can begin to make any needed changes to improve the healthfulness of the foods you select and your physical activity level. Use the Food Tracker at www.ChooseMyPlate.gov for a few days and see how you do. Because the tracker is based on your age, gender, weight, height, and activity level, you will have a personalized account of how close your diet and activity levels are to what is recommended for good health.

TERMS

MyPlate A graphic that illustrates the five food groups using a familiar mealtime visual—a place setting. The graphic is part of a larger communications initiative to help consumers make better food choices. MyPlate is designed to remind you to eat healthfully.

10 tips
Nutrition Education Series

liven up your meals with vegetables and fruits

ChooseMyPlate.gov

10 tips to improve your meals with vegetables and fruits

Discover the many benefits of adding vegetables and fruits to your meals. They are low in fat and calories, while providing fiber and other key nutrients. Most Americans should eat more than 3 cups—and for some, up to 6 cups—of vegetables and fruits each day. Vegetables and fruits don't just add nutrition to meals. They can also add color, flavor, and texture. Explore these creative ways to bring healthy foods to your table.

1 fire up the grill
Use the grill to cook vegetables and fruits. Try grilling mushrooms, carrots, peppers, or potatoes on a kabob skewer. Brush with oil to keep them from drying out. Grilled fruits like peaches, pineapple, or mangos add great flavor to a cookout.

2 expand the flavor of your casseroles
Mix vegetables such as sauteed onions, peas, pinto beans, or tomatoes into your favorite dish for that extra flavor.

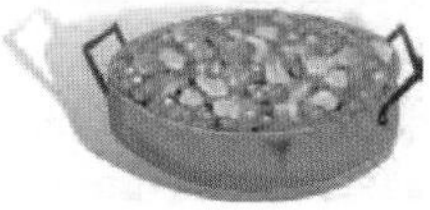

3 planning something Italian?
Add extra vegetables to your pasta dish. Slip some peppers, spinach, red beans, onions, or cherry tomatoes into your traditional tomato sauce. Vegetables provide texture and low-calorie bulk that satisfies.

4 get creative with your salad
Toss in shredded carrots, strawberries, spinach, watercress, orange segments, or sweet peas for a flavorful, fun salad.

5 salad bars aren't just for salads
Try eating sliced fruit from the salad bar as your dessert when dining out. This will help you avoid any baked desserts that are high in calories.

6 get in on the stir-frying fun
Try something new! Stir-fry your veggies—like broccoli, carrots, sugar snap peas, mushrooms, or green beans—for a quick-and-easy addition to any meal.

7 add them to your sandwiches
Whether it is a sandwich or wrap, vegetables make great additions to both. Try sliced tomatoes, romaine lettuce, or avocado on your everday sandwich or wrap for extra flavor.

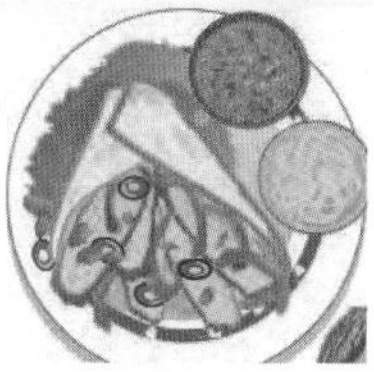

8 be creative with your baked goods
Add apples, bananas, blueberries, or pears to your favorite muffin recipe for a treat.

9 make a tasty fruit smoothie
For dessert, blend strawberries, blueberries, or raspberries with frozen bananas and 100% fruit juice for a delicious frozen fruit smoothie.

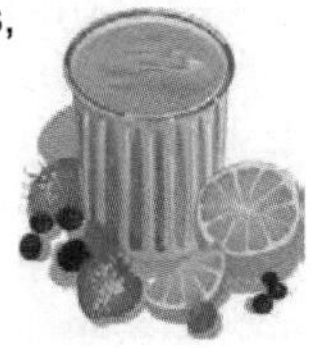

10 liven up an omelet
Boost the color and flavor of your morning omelet with vegetables. Simply chop, saute, and add them to the egg as it cooks. Try combining different vegetables, such as mushrooms, spinach, onions, or bell peppers.

USDA Center for Nutrition Policy and Promotion

Go to www.ChooseMyPlate.gov for more information.

DG TipSheet No. 10
June 2011
USDA is an equal opportunity provider and employer.

■ **Figure 2.4**
MyPlate Basic Messages

Source: © ChooseMyPlate.gov, USDA, Center for Nutrition Policy and Promotion.

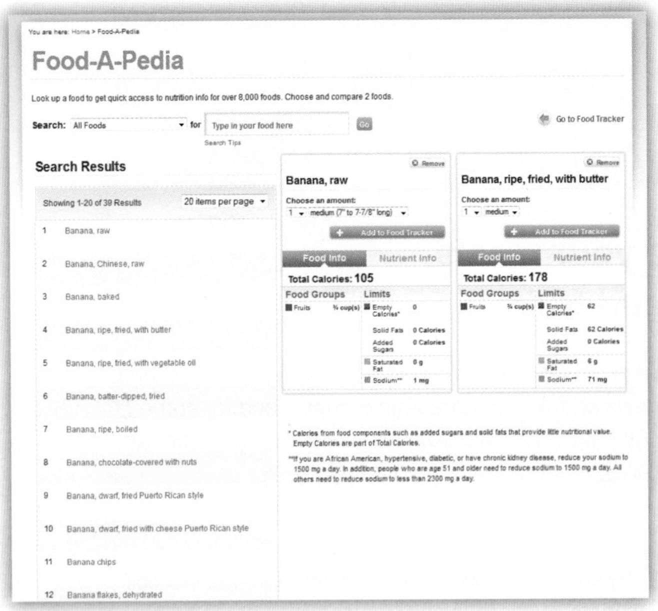

■ **Figure 2.5**

MyFood-a-pedia

The MyFood-a-pedia interactive tool found at www.ChooseMyPlate.gov can be used to find the calories in common foods. It also specifies how different foods count toward meeting the foods you need each day.

Source: Courtesy of the USDA.

Recommended Nutrient Intake

The *Dietary Guidelines for Americans* and MyPlate suggest specific foods to include in your diet and foods you should limit. Guidance is also available as to how much of specific nutrients you should consume each day. The **Food and Nutrition Board** of the National Academy of Sciences partners with **Health Canada** to set standards for nutrient intake. This body of nutrition scientists reviews all available scientific data to determine the **Dietary Reference Intakes (DRIs)** (**Figure 2.6**). The DRIs provide recommended nutrient intakes and are a set of four reference values: **Estimated Average Requirement (EAR)**, **Recommended Dietary Allowance (RDA)**, **Adequate Intake (AI)**, and **Tolerable Upper Intake Level (UL)**.[3] The DRIs also provide information on **Estimated Energy Expenditure (EEE)** and **Acceptable Macronutrient Distribution Ranges (AMDRs)**.

Estimated Average Requirement

The EAR is the average daily nutrient intake level estimated to meet the requirements of 50% of healthy people of a particular life stage (age) and gender group. For each nutrient, this level is based on an indicator of what would be considered adequate in the diet. It may be based on level of a particular nutrient in the blood or other indicator of adequacy.

Recommended Dietary Allowance

The RDA is set using the EAR and is the average daily dietary intake needed to meet the nutrient requirements of nearly all (97–98%) healthy people of a particular life stage and gender group. It is a mathematical calculation based on the EAR. If there is not enough scientific data to set an EAR for a nutrient, that nutrient will not have an RDA. Because the RDA is set high enough to include almost all individuals, your actual need for a nutrient may be lower than the RDA. Consuming nutrients at or near the RDA will more than likely meet your needs for that nutrient.

Adequate Intake

If there is not enough scientific data to set an EAR for a nutrient, an AI is established. An AI level is based on

TERMS

Food and Nutrition Board Group that studies issues of national and global importance on the safety and adequacy of the U.S. food supply; establishes principles and guidelines for good nutrition; and provides authoritative judgment on the relationships among food intake, nutrition, and health maintenance and disease prevention.

Health Canada A federal department responsible for helping Canadians maintain and improve their health, while respecting individual choices and circumstances.

Dietary Reference Intakes (DRIs) Nutrition recommendations used in the United States and Canada.

Estimated Average Requirement (EAR) Average daily nutrient intake level estimated to meet the needs of 50% of the people in a particular age/gender group.

Recommended Dietary Allowance (RDA) Daily dietary intake level of a nutrient sufficient to meet requirements for 97–98% of healthy individuals in a particular age/gender group.

Adequate Intake (AI) Used when there is no RDA established, but some data support an amount of a nutrient that is believed to be adequate for most people.

Tolerable Upper Intake Level (UL) Set to caution against excessive intake of nutrients that can be harmful in large amounts.

Estimated Energy Expenditure (EEE) The amount of energy you use to carry out bodily functions and activity.

Acceptable Macronutrient Distribution Ranges (AMDRs) A set of values for carbohydrates, fat, and protein expressed as a percentage of total daily calorie intake. Ranges of intake are set to be consistent with the reduction of risk of chronic disease.

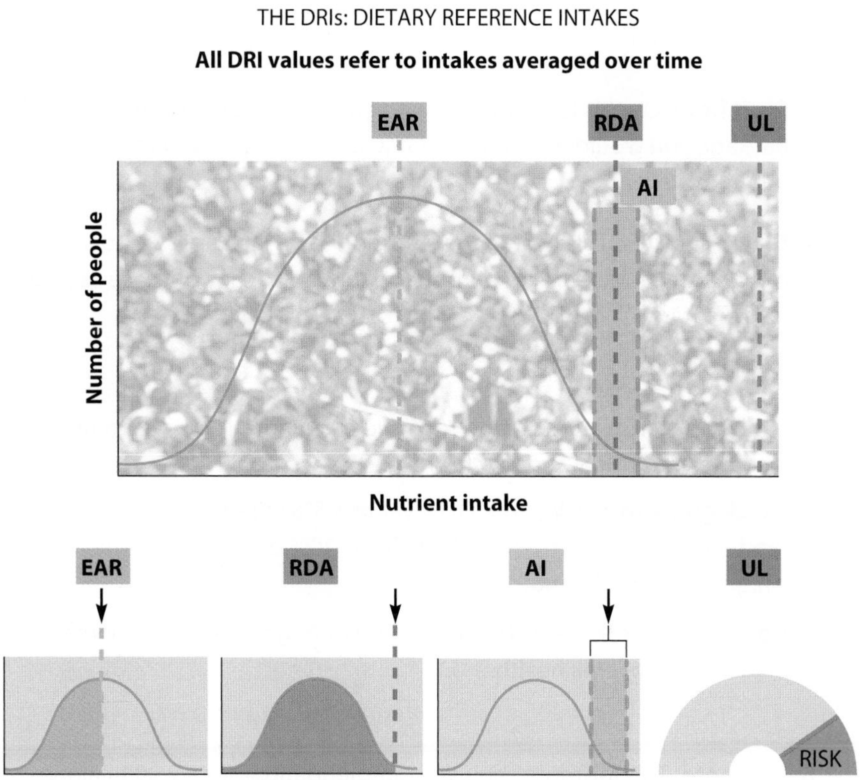

The **Estimated Average Requirement** is the nutrient intake level estimated to meet the needs of 50% of the individuals in a life-stage and gender group.

The **Recommended Dietary Allowance** is the nutrient intake level that is sufficient to meet the needs of 97–98% of the individuals in a life-stage and gender group. The RDA is calculated from the EAR.

Adequate Intake is based upon expert estimates of nutrient intake by a defined group of healthy people. These estimates are used when there is insufficient scientific evidence to establish an EAR. AI is not equivalent to RDA.

Tolerable Upper Intake Level is the maximum level of daily nutrient intake that poses little risk of adverse health effects to almost all of the individuals in a defined group. In most cases, supplements must be consumed to reach a UL.

Figure 2.6

Dietary Reference Intakes

The Dietary Reference Intakes (DRIs) are a set of dietary standards that include Estimated Average Requirements (EARs), Recommended Daily Allowances (RDAs), Adequate Intakes (AIs), and Tolerable Upper Intake Levels (ULs).

observed or experimentally determined estimates of nutrient intake by a group of healthy people. AI levels should be considered a target for a specific nutrient as opposed to a recommendation. All DRI values for infants are based on breast milk, because not enough scientific studies have been conducted in that age group to establish an EAR.

Tolerable Upper Intake Level

UIs are the highest average daily nutrient intake level that will most likely pose no risk to your health. If intake of a nutrient is consistently above the UL, there is the potential for negative effects on health. The UIs are most helpful in assessing the healthfulness of consumption of supplements that may contain large amounts of individual nutrients.

Estimated Energy Requirement

EER is the amount of energy (calories) you need to maintain energy balance. The number of calories you need is based on your gender, weight, height, age, and physical activity level.

Acceptable Macronutrient Distribution Ranges

Where your calories come from has an impact on your overall health. The AMDRs are set to allow for consumption of adequate essential nutrients as well as protect you from chronic disease.[4] The AMDRs are expressed as a percentage of total calorie intake (**Table 2.1**).

Food Labeling

One of the best ways to be mindful of exactly what you are eating is to become a label reader. People who use food labels know more about the foods they eat and have healthier diets.[5–9] Most food packages have several different labels that can help you learn more about what's inside. By law, all foods must indicate the name of the food and the name of the manufacturer, packer, or distributor, including its address. The quantity of the contents must also be displayed. The Nutrition Facts label, sometimes called the Nutrition Facts panel, and the ingredients list provide you with the information you need to know to decide if it goes from the grocery store shelf into your cart. Manufacturers also may include health or nutrition claims on the food package. Understanding what these claims mean can help you make better decisions about the foods you choose.

Table 2.1

Acceptable Macronutrient Distribution Ranges for Adults

Macronutrient	Percent of Daily Calorie Intake
Fat	20–35%
Carbohydrate	45–65%
Protein	10–35%

Source: Data from Institute of Medicine, Food and Nutrition Board. *Dietary Reference Intakes for Energy, Carbohydrate, Fiber, Fat, Fatty Acids, Cholesterol, Protein, and Amino Acids.* Washington, DC: National Academies Press, 2005.

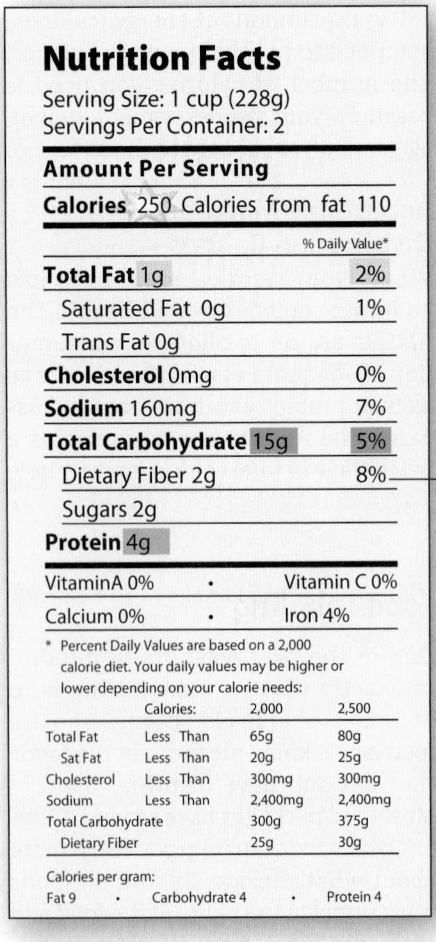

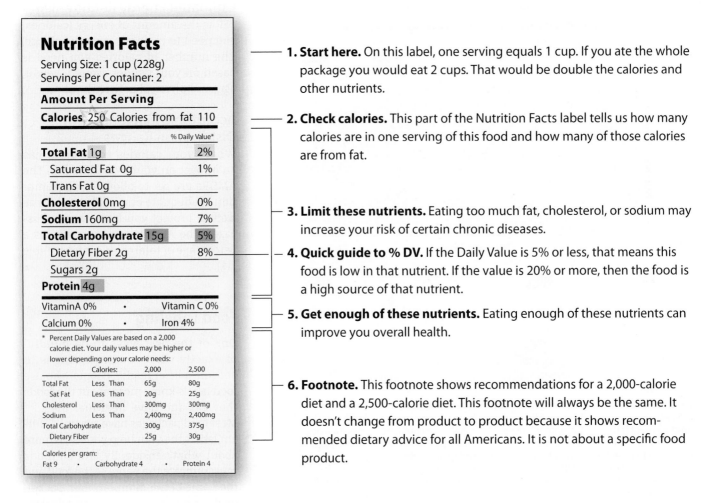

1. **Start here.** On this label, one serving equals 1 cup. If you ate the whole package you would eat 2 cups. That would be double the calories and other nutrients.
2. **Check calories.** This part of the Nutrition Facts label tells us how many calories are in one serving of this food and how many of those calories are from fat.
3. **Limit these nutrients.** Eating too much fat, cholesterol, or sodium may increase your risk of certain chronic diseases.
4. **Quick guide to % DV.** If the Daily Value is 5% or less, that means this food is low in that nutrient. If the value is 20% or more, then the food is a high source of that nutrient.
5. **Get enough of these nutrients.** Eating enough of these nutrients can improve you overall health.
6. **Footnote.** This footnote shows recommendations for a 2,000-calorie diet and a 2,500-calorie diet. This footnote will always be the same. It doesn't change from product to product because it shows recommended dietary advice for all Americans. It is not about a specific food product.

Figure 2.7
Nutrition Facts Label

Nutrition Facts Label

In 1990, the Nutrition Labeling and Education Act was signed into law. This federal law required most packaged foods to have nutrition information on the package by 1995. Thanks to this law, today the **Food and Drug Administration (FDA)** requires that almost all packaged foods have a Nutrition Facts label (small packages and manufactures with a small production may be exempt from having a Nutrition Facts label) (**Figure 2.7**). That's the good news. The bad news is that the label can be confusing if you don't know what the items on the label mean.

Serving Size and Servings per Container One of the most important pieces of information on the Nutrition Facts label is serving size. This tells you how much of that food the information presented on the Nutrition Facts panel is based upon. The FDA has recommended serving sizes for hundreds of foods. The manufacturer must use the prescribed serving size so that you can compare similar products without having to calculate for different serving sizes. The serving size will not always be what you consume; you must keep that in mind when reviewing the rest of the information on the label. For example, if a serving size on a box of crackers is 1 ounce or 6 crackers and you know that you usually consume 12 crackers, all

TERMS

Food and Drug Administration (FDA) The federal agency that has oversight for the approval of new drugs, medical devices, cosmetics, and food additives. Provides regulation and oversight for food labeling. The FDA is also responsible for advancing the public health by helping to speed innovations that make medicines and foods more effective, safer, and more affordable and aiding the public in getting the accurate, science-based information they need to use medicines and foods to improve their health.

of the nutrition information presented would need to be doubled to estimate what you consumed. This portion of the Nutrition Facts label also shows the servings per container. This is also helpful in estimating what you actually consume versus the serving size that is listed on the label. If you eat the entire container and there are three servings in the package, then you ate three servings, and everything on the label will need to be tripled to estimate what you consumed. Sometimes packages that appear to be appropriate to consume in one sitting contain more than one serving.

Calories and Calories from Fat Calories are listed for one serving of the food in the package, not the entire package. To estimate the number of calories that this food provides, you will need to use both the calorie information and the serving size. For example, if you had a bowl of cereal that was 2 cups and the cereal had 110 calories per 1 cup serving, then you ate 220 calories, not the 110 listed on the Nutrition Facts label. Calories from fat are presented to help you see how many of the calories in that product are from fat.

Nutrients In addition to calories and calories from fat, the Nutrition Facts label must include total fat, saturated fat, trans fat, cholesterol, sodium, total carbohydrate, dietary fiber, sugars, protein, vitamin A, vitamin C, calcium, and iron. Other nutrients must be listed if the manufacturer makes a claim about that nutrient. For example, if a claim is made about a cereal being high in vitamin D, then the vitamin D content must be listed in the Nutrition Facts label.

Footnote Perhaps one of the most misunderstood parts of the Nutrition Facts label is the footnote on the bottom of the label. This footnote is a guide to what is recommended with respect to nutrient intake for a 2,000- and 2,500-calorie diet. It is a guide for what you should be consuming. The footnote will always be the same; it does not change from product to product, and it does not provide any information about that specific food.

% Daily Values The % Daily Value is calculated based on what constitutes a healthy diet. These values are based on a 2,000-calorie diet, which would be an appropriate calorie level for moderately active women or sedentary men. If your recommended caloric intake differs, you will need to take that into consideration when using the % Daily Values. However, regardless of your own calorie intake the % Daily Value provides an estimate of that food's contribution to your diet. The % Daily Value helps you determine if a serving of food is high or low in a particular nutrient. If the Daily Value is 5% or less, then the food is considered to be low in that nutrient. If the Daily Value is 20% or more, then the food is considered to be a good source of that nutrient.

You can use the % Daily Value to see how a food fits into your overall diet. For example, if you consumed a food with a total fat % Daily Value of 30, then you know that you have eaten 30% of the fat that you need all day. If you eat two servings of that food, you have eaten over half of the fat you need for the day. You can use the % Daily Value to make sure that you get enough of certain nutrients as well. For example, if a food has a % Daily Value for fiber of 0%, then you know that it is not contributing at all to the fiber that you need each day. You can also use the % Daily Value to easily compare two similar foods. If you wanted to purchase a cereal that was a good source of fiber, you could compare cereals using the % Daily Value for fiber. You can use the % Daily Value to make trade-offs in your diet as well. Say that you check the label of your favorite snack cracker and see that the % Daily Value for total fat is 20%. After a quick scan of the cracker isle, you find a similar product that has a % Daily Value of 0% for fat, so it is clearly a lower-fat choice. Keep in mind that just because a single food has a % Daily Value that is relatively high in nutrients that you want to get less of, such as total fat, you don't have to give up that food altogether. You will just need to balance it with foods that are lower in fat at other times in the day.

Nutrients Without % Daily Values You will notice that trans fats, sugars, and protein do not have a % Daily Value. There is not enough information to provide a % Daily Value for trans fats. The amount consumed should be as low as possible based on scientific evidence of the relationship between trans fat consumption and increased risk of heart disease. Protein has no % Daily Value unless a claim of "high protein" is made or the food is specifically for infants and children younger than age 4. Protein consumption for adults and children older than 4 years is not considered to be a public health concern, so no % Daily Value is given. Sugars also do not have a % Daily Value. There is no recommendation for the total amount of sugar that should be consumed in a day. It is important to keep in mind that sugars listed on the Nutrition Facts panel include naturally occurring sugars (such as those in milk or fruit) as well as those that are added. You can use the grams of sugar figure in the Nutrition Facts panel to compare similar products such as cereal, breakfast bars, or yogurt to select a lower-sugar option.

Ingredient List

The nutrients contained in a food are clearly spelled out in the Nutrition Facts label but what is really in the food? The answer to that is available on the ingredient list. The ingredients must be listed on all foods with the exception of raw agricultural commodities such as fresh fruits and vegetables. Ingredients in the foods are listed in order by weight, with the ingredient present in the largest amount listed first. All ingredients used in processing must be listed.

Any substance that is added to food is subject to review by the FDA. All substances that are added to food

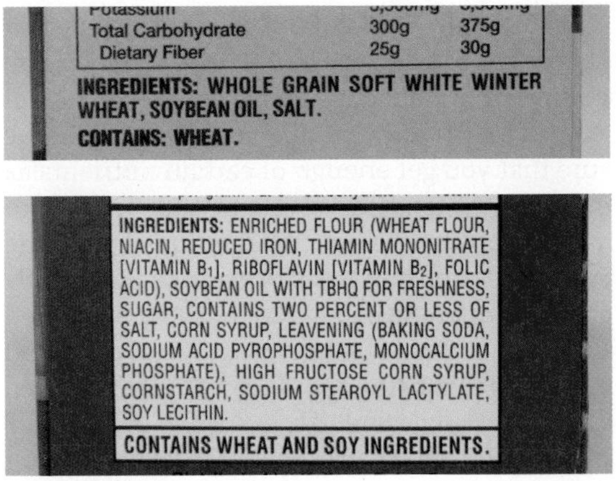

■ **Figure 2.8**

Ingredient List

One way to use the ingredient list is to choose products with fewer and simpler ingredients.

must be generally recognized among qualified experts as **Generally Recognized as Safe (GRAS)**. Food additives must meet the **acceptable daily intake (ADI)**, which is the amount that can be ingested daily without appreciable health risks.

Choose foods with as few ingredients as possible. If you are choosing a cracker and one brand has 25 ingredients, some of which you cannot pronounce, and another brand has whole wheat, corn oil, and salt, you may want to choose the simpler product (**Figure 2.8**). Choose foods that are what they are supposed to be; a cereal should be cereal, not sugar. If you are choosing a breakfast cereal and the first ingredient is sugar, you may want to choose another option. At times, the ingredient list can be deceiving. Manufacturers can list individual ingredients that really are the same thing. For example, corn oil, cottonseed oil, and peanut oil are all pure sources of fat. If a food contains all three, they may be dispersed in the ingredient list, but if you put them all together you would see that they contribute greatly to the nutrient make up of that food. The same is true for sugar. Sugar, molasses, corn syrup, and rice syrup are all pure sources of sugar. Listed separately on the label they may appear further down on the ingredient list, but if grouped together sugar could very well be the number one or two ingredient in that food (**Figure 2.9**).

TERMS

Generally Regarded as Safe (GRAS) Designation that a substance that is added to food is considered safe by experts. Any substance added to food must meet this standard.

acceptable daily intake (ADI) The amount of a substance in food (food additives) or drinking water that can be ingested on a daily basis over a lifetime without an appreciable health risk.

Try Something New

Compare Your Choices

Next time you are at the grocery store choose one food that you buy on a regular basis and examine the Nutrition Facts panel. A good place to start would be breakfast cereal or yogurt. Check out the serving size, calories per serving, and % Daily Value for fat and sodium. Compare that product to similar products. Does the product you usually consume have more or less of any nutrient than you thought? Were there products that were similar that may be a better choice for your overall diet? If so, give the new product a try; you may be willing to make a trade-off to make your usual choice the healthier choice.

Nutrient Content Claims

Laws govern what food manufacturers can say about the nutrient content of their products. The FDA has developed specific definitions that apply to terms such as *low fat*, *reduced calorie*, or *unsalted* (**Figure 2.10**). This protects you from misleading claims and makes it easier for you to compare similar products with the same nutrition claim.

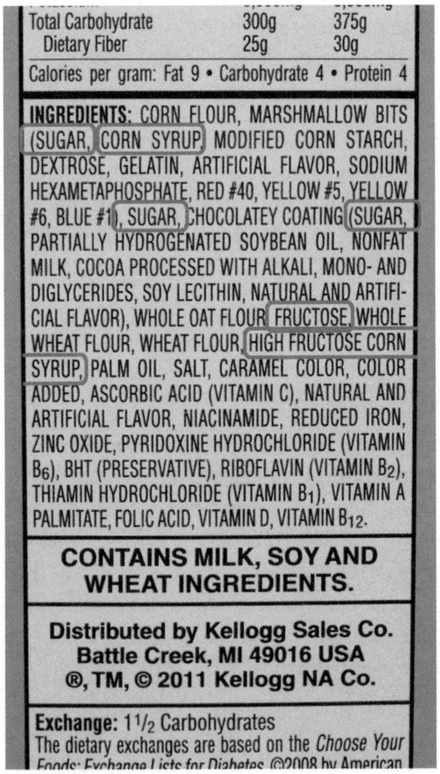

Total Carbohydrate 300g 375g
Dietary Fiber 25g 30g
Calories per gram: Fat 9 • Carbohydrate 4 • Protein 4
INGREDIENTS: CORN FLOUR, MARSHMALLOW BITS (SUGAR, CORN SYRUP, MODIFIED CORN STARCH, DEXTROSE, GELATIN, ARTIFICIAL FLAVOR, SODIUM HEXAMETAPHOSPHATE, RED #40, YELLOW #5, YELLOW #6, BLUE #1), SUGAR, CHOCOLATEY COATING (SUGAR, PARTIALLY HYDROGENATED SOYBEAN OIL, NONFAT MILK, COCOA PROCESSED WITH ALKALI, MONO- AND DIGLYCERIDES, SOY LECITHIN, NATURAL AND ARTIFICIAL FLAVOR), WHOLE OAT FLOUR, FRUCTOSE, WHOLE WHEAT FLOUR, WHEAT FLOUR, HIGH FRUCTOSE CORN SYRUP, PALM OIL, SALT, CARAMEL COLOR, COLOR ADDED, ASCORBIC ACID (VITAMIN C), NATURAL AND ARTIFICIAL FLAVOR, NIACINAMIDE, REDUCED IRON, ZINC OXIDE, PYRIDOXINE HYDROCHLORIDE (VITAMIN B_6), BHT (PRESERVATIVE), RIBOFLAVIN (VITAMIN B_2), THIAMIN HYDROCHLORIDE (VITAMIN B_1), VITAMIN A PALMITATE, FOLIC ACID, VITAMIN D, VITAMIN B_{12}.
CONTAINS MILK, SOY AND WHEAT INGREDIENTS.
Distributed by Kellogg Sales Co. Battle Creek, MI 49016 USA ®, TM, © 2011 Kellogg NA Co.
Exchange: 1 1/2 Carbohydrates
The dietary exchanges are based on the Choose Your

■ **Figure 2.9**

Ingredient List for a High-Sugar Cereal

The first ingredient is corn flour; however, on closer inspection you see sugar listed several different ways. If all of the sugars were grouped together, sugar may have been the number one ingredient in this breakfast cereal.

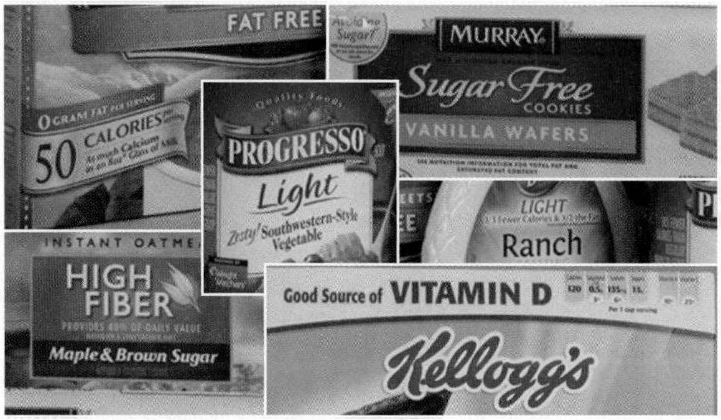

■ **Figure 2.10**
Nutrient Claims on Food Packages

The FDA defines commonly used terms (**Table 2.2**); manufacturers must meet the definition to use the claim on the label.

Health Claims

Statements linking consumption of a food or nutrient to certain health outcomes are referred to as *health claims*. The FDA has strict guidelines as to what health claims can and cannot be made and what qualifies a food to make such a claim. Whether a health claim can be made is based on a body of scientific evidence that supports the claim. The health claim must be made in simple language that most consumers can understand and must only imply that the food or nutrient might reduce risk of a certain disease (**Figure 2.11**). If a manufacturer makes a claim about a certain nutrient in that food, the food must have at least a 20% Daily Value of that nutrient. For example, if the manufacturer makes an allowable health claim about calcium and osteoporosis, that food must have a % Daily Value for calcium of at least 20%.

Two categories of health claims are allowed by the FDA. The first category is for health claims with significant scientific agreement (SSA).[10] SSA health claims are

Table 2.2

Nutrient Content Claims

Claim	Definition
Calorie free	Less than 5 calories per serving.
Low calorie	Less than 40 calories per serving.
Light or lite	At least one-third fewer calories per serving than a comparison food or contains no more than half the fat per serving of a comparison food. If a food has 50% or more of its calorie from fat, the reduction must be at least 50% of the fat. Can be used if the food is low calorie and low fat and sodium is reduced by 50%.
Reduced calorie	Contains 25% less calories than the regular product.
Fat free or nonfat	Less than 0.5 g of fat per serving.
Low fat	3 g or less of fat per serving.
Percent fat free	A claim made on a low-fat or fat-free product that accurately reflects the amount of fat present in 100 g of food (e.g., a food with 4 g of fat per 100 g would be 96% fat free).
Reduced fat	Contains 25% less fat than the regular product.
Saturated fat free	Less than 0.5 g of saturated fat and less than 0.5 g trans fat per serving.
Low saturated fat	1 g or less saturated fat per serving and less than 0.5 g trans fat per serving
Cholesterol free	Less than 2 mg cholesterol and 2 g or less saturated fat per serving.
Low cholesterol	20 mg or less cholesterol and 2 g or less saturated fat per serving.
Extra lean	Less than 5 g fat, 2 g saturated fat, and 95 mg of cholesterol per serving and per 100 g.
Lean	Less than 10 g fat, 4 g saturated fat, and 95 mg cholesterol per serving and per 100 g.
Sugar free	Less than 0.5 g of sugars per serving.
Salt or sodium free	Less than 5 mg per serving.
Very low sodium	35 mg or less of sodium per serving.
Low sodium	140 mg or less of sodium per serving.
Unsalted	No salt added during processing. To be able to use this term, the product must normally be prepared with salt and the label must note that the product is not a sodium-free food if it does not meet the requirements for sodium free.
Enriched or fortified	Has been nutritionally altered so that one serving provides at least 10% more of the % Daily Value of a nutrient than the comparison food.
High, rich in, excellent source of	Contains at least 20% of the % Daily Value for that nutrient.
Good source, contains, provides	Contains 10–19% of the % Daily Value for that nutrient.
More or extra	Contains at least 10% more per serving of the % Daily Value of a nutrient than comparison food.
Fresh	Foods in their raw state, cannot be used on food that has been frozen, cooked, or that contains preservatives.
Fresh frozen	Foods that have been quickly frozen in their raw state.

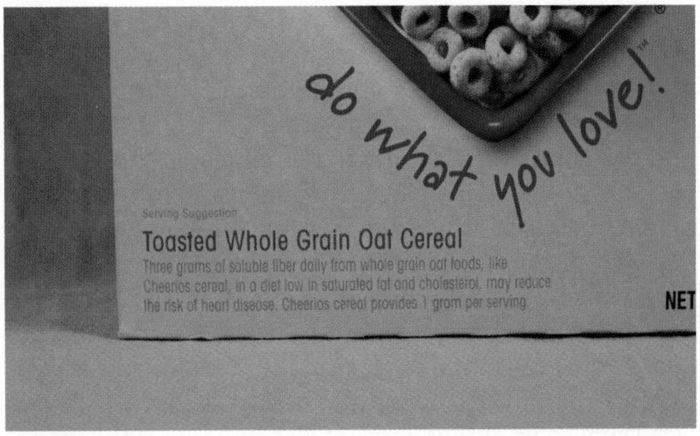

■ **Figure 2.11**

Health Claims Approved by the FDA Are Allowed on the Food Package

supported by a large body of scientific evidence that points to the consumption of a particular food or nutrient and its relationship with reduction of disease (**Table 2.3**). The second category of health claims is qualified health claims.[16] With these claims, some evidence suggests a relationship between consumption and reduction of disease, but the evidence is not yet conclusive. If a manufacturer uses a qualified health claim, the label must also state that "Although there is scientific evidence supporting the claim, the evidence is not conclusive."

Table 2.3

Health Claims That Are Allowed on Food Packages

Health Claims with Significant Scientific Agreement	Selected Qualified Health Claims[1]
Calcium and vitamin D and reduced risk of osteoporosis	Green tea and reduced risk of cancer
Low-fat diet and reduced risk of heart disease	Calcium and reduced risk of colon/rectal cancer
Low saturated fat and cholesterol intake and reduced risk of heart disease	Selenium and reduced risk of cancer
Sugar alcohols and reduced risk of dental decay	Antioxidant vitamins and reduced risk of cancer
Fiber-containing fruits, vegetables, and whole grains and reduced risk of cancer	Tomatoes/tomato sauce and reduced risk of prostate, ovarian, gastric, and pancreatic cancer
Soluble fiber in fruits, vegetables, and whole grains and reduced risk of heart disease	Nuts and reduced risk of heart disease
Folic acid and reduced risk of fetal neural tube defects	Walnuts and reduced risk of heart disease
Fruit- and vegetable-rich diet and reduced risk of cancer	Calcium and reduced risk of hypertension
Low-sodium foods and reduced risk of hypertension	Omega-3 fatty acids and reduced risk of heart disease
Soy protein and reduced risk of heart disease	
Plant stanols and sterols and decreased risk of heart disease	

[1]Must also use the following disclaimer: "Although there is scientific evidence supporting the claim, the evidence is not conclusive."

How Policy and Environment Affect My Choices

Nutrition Labeling for Meat and Poultry

Most of the foods in the grocery store have the Nutrition Facts label that helps you better understand the nutrition content of the foods you buy. Meat and poultry, however, have been exempt from this requirement, until now. As of January 2012, a rule passed by the USDA's Food Safety and Inspection Service requires that single-ingredient muscle cuts (beef, pork, lamb, and veal) and ground meat and poultry products have a Nutrition Facts label.[11] The new label will be similar to the label on other foods and will include calories, calories from fat, total fat, saturated fat, cholesterol, and sodium. The rule applies to the 40 most common cuts of meat and poultry; for example, chicken breast would have a label but chicken tenders might not. Thanks to this new rule, you will be able to know at the point of purchase the calories and fat in the meat or poultry you choose. This change in policy from a voluntary system where only a few meats were labeled with their nutrition content to a meat counter filled with products with nutrition information is a big step forward in helping you be informed about what you are eating. The new policy will allow you to compare products right in the grocery store so that you can make more informed choices.

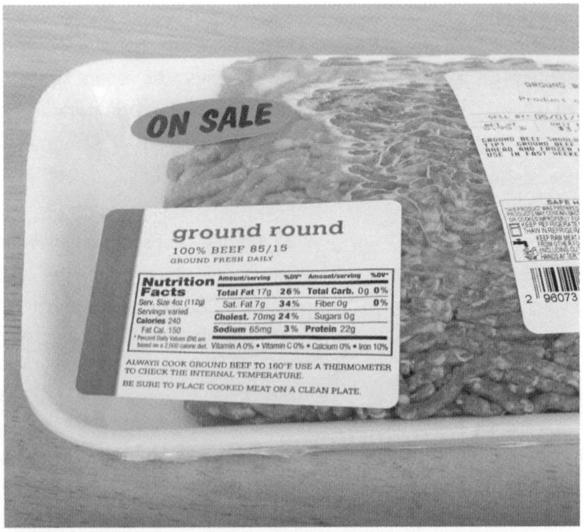

Nutrition Facts Label on Meat

The most common cuts of meat and poultry will soon be required to have the Nutrition Facts label.

Which Side Are You On?

Front-of-Package Labeling

The use of symbols that summarize key nutritional aspects and characteristics of food products has seen substantial growth over the past few years. These symbols and nutrition rating systems are referred to as *front-of-package labeling*. One example of such a system is the Traffic Light system in use in the United Kingdom.[15] These symbols may be on the actual package of food or on shelf tags where the product's price is displayed. These systems have been developed by food manufacturers, retailers, and health organizations and are intended to help consumers make healthier choices.[13]

These systems are not regulated by the FDA and are not without controversy. More than a dozen systems have been developed over the years. Similar products may have different front-of-package labeling systems with different messages. This may, in fact, be more confusing than no front-of-package labeling at all. Because front-of-package systems are not regulated, manufacturers may promote a single nutrient that their food is high or low in while the overall product is unhealthy. For example, a product may be labeled as being free of trans fats but be high in saturated and total fat; another product may be labeled as being high in fiber but have high levels of added sugar. One product that has been singled out as an example of why front-of-package labels need to be regulated is Froot Loops. Froot Loops received the Smart Choices program's green check mark. A closer examination of the cereal revealed that the first ingredient is sugar; in fact 40% of the product is sugar. This prompted consumer groups and the news media to ask why this food, and others like it, would receive a seal of approval such as the Smart Choice mark. The Smart Choices program is not currently conducting active operations,[14] but similar systems remain in place.

The Grocery Manufacturers Association has developed a voluntary system called Nutrition Keys.[15] This system places calories and key nutrients, such as sodium, clearly on the front of the package. The system is certainly accurate; however, it does not provide the consumer with any additional information or guidance than could be found on the Nutrition Facts label. Is this an improvement over what is already available to consumers and is mandated by law? Many nutrition and health experts feel that a nutrition guidance system that helps consumers choose foods more wisely is needed; a system that would be regulated by the FDA so that manufacturers and retailers who want to sell their product could not manipulate the truth.

The confusion in the marketplace, the potential to mislead consumers, and the sheer number of systems has prompted the FDA to take a closer look at front-of-package labeling. A report by the Institute of Medicine is the first step in the FDA's process to regulate front-of-package labels.[12] This report indicates that front-of-package labeling schemes should move away from systems that mostly provide nutrition information to a system that provides guidance about the healthfulness (or lack of) in a food. Rather than telling the consumer how much sodium, saturated fat, trans fat, etc., are in a food, the new front-of-package system should help consumer interpret nutrition information. The goal of the proposed system would be not only to inform consumers about detailed nutrition content, but to also encourage healthier choices. The authors of the report concluded that this could be better achieved by a simple front-of-package symbol that could cue consumers as to which foods are healthier. The Institute of Medicine's report suggests a scheme that would include calories per serving and a rating system of zero to three "nutritional points" for saturated and trans fats, sodium, and

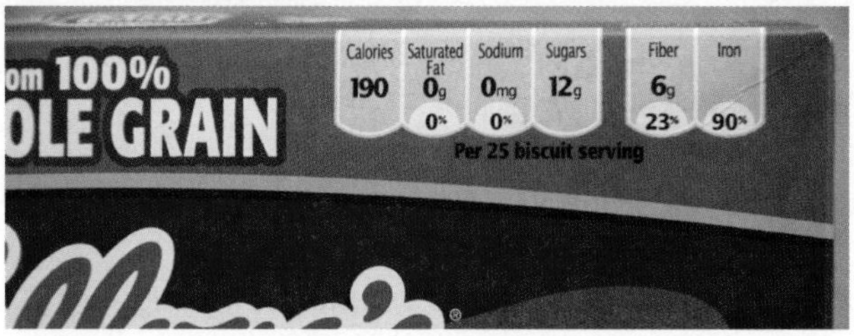
Calories Saturated Fat Sodium Sugars Fiber Iron
190
0g 0%
0mg 0%
12g
6g 23%
90%
Per 25 biscuit serving
100%
OLE GRAIN

Nutrition Keys Front-of-Package Label
The Nutrition Keys is a voluntary front-of-package labeling system designed by the Grocery Manufacturers Association. It provides similar information as can be found on the Nutrition Facts label.

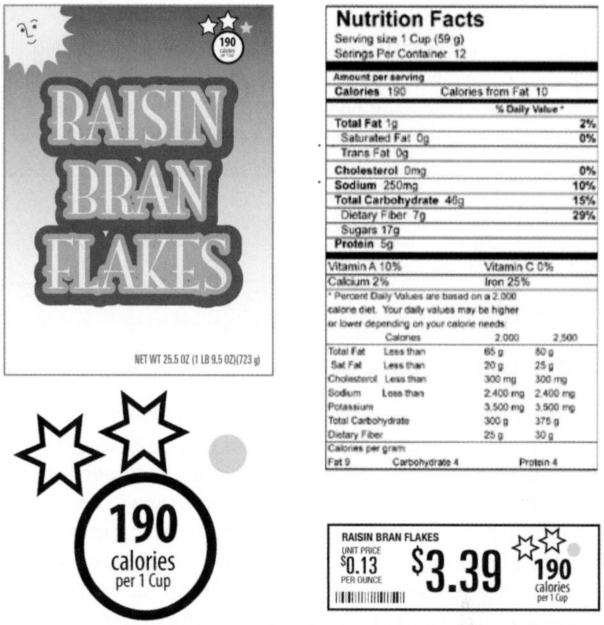
RAISIN BRAN FLAKES
190
NET WT 25.5 OZ (1 LB 9.5 OZ)(723 g)
Nutrition Facts
Serving size 1 Cup (59 g)
Serings Per Container 12
Amount per serving
Calories 190 Calories from Fat 10
% Daily Value *
Total Fat 1g 2%
Saturated Fat 0g 0%
Trans Fat 0g
Cholesterol 0mg 0%
Sodium 250mg 10%
Total Carbohydrate 46g 15%
Dietary Fiber 7g 29%
Sugars 17g
Protein 5g
Vitamin A 10% Vitamin C 0%
Calcium 2% Iron 25%
* Percent Daily Values are based on a 2,000 calorie diet. Your daily values may be higher or lower depending on your calorie needs:
Calories 2,000 2,500
Total Fat Less than 65 g 80 g
Sat Fat Less than 20 g 25 g
Cholesterol Less than 300 mg 300 mg
Sodium Less than 2,400 mg 2,400 mg
Potassium 3,500 mg 3,500 mg
Total Carbohydrate 300 g 375 g
Dietary Fiber 25 g 30 g
Calories per gram
Fat 9 Carbohydrate 4 Protein 4
190 calories per 1 Cup
RAISIN BRAN FLAKES
UNIT PRICE $0.13 PER OUNCE
$3.39
190 calories per 1 Cup

Institute of Medicine's Suggestion for Front-of-Package Label
This example includes calories per serving and a nutrient component rating symbol. It illustrates how this could be seen on the front of the package, the shelf tag, and the Nutrition Facts Panel. This was provided by the Institute of Medicine as an example only. They are encouraging input from regulators and the food industry to design the final front-of-package labeling system.

Source: Institute of Medicine. *Examination of front-of-package nutrition rating systems and symbols: promoting healthier choices.* Washington, DC: The National Academies Press, 2011.

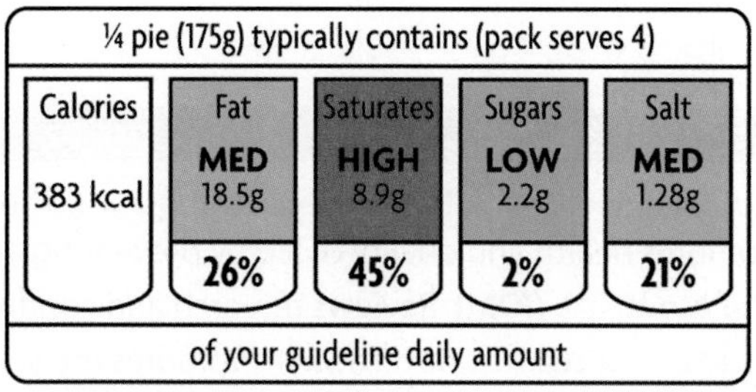

UK Traffic Light Food Label
The front-of-package labeling system in the UK is the Traffic Light. It indicates if a food is low, medium, or high in fat, saturated fat, sugar, and salt. Red means high; choose these foods less often and/or eat them in smaller quantities. Yellow means it is OK to have these foods sometimes, but if you have a choice try to go for green. Green means it is a healthier choice.

Source: © Department of Health, UK.

(continues)

added sugars. The more points a food receives, the healthier it is. The report also recommended that there should be only one front-of-package labeling system regulated by the FDA.

The Institute of Medicine's recommendations to FDA were criticized by food manufacturers as too interpretive and untested. However, consumer groups such as Center for Science in the Public Interest support the suggestions with some reservations about it not including other nutrients of importance such as fiber and protein. The FDA will now review the report and decide whether to implement the recommendations.

No front-of-package labeling system that is available or that could be designed would be perfect. However, it is possible to design a system that would at least help you, the consumer, choose healthier options that may improve your health. What do you think? Do you think there is a need for a better front-of-package labeling system?

Special Report

How to Interpret Nutrition Claims

Secret formulas, potions, exercises designed to melt fat away with no effort, the list goes on of claims for products and routines that can keep you younger, thinner, healthier, and prevent disease. How do you tell fact from fiction in the world of nutrition and health? Thanks to the Internet, information is available on virtually every topic. How do you sift out the not so good, not so credible claims from accurate information? There are no regulations about posting misinformation on the Internet. Just because information is posted does not make it correct or based in science. Here are a few steps to take that can help you get to the truth.

Make Your Search Engine Your Friend

If you hear about the latest nutrition claim to help you lose weight or stay healthy, search on it, but don't just put the claim in the search box. See what reputable scientific organizations have to say about the claim in question. Rely on the **Centers for Disease Control and Prevention (CDC)**, the **Institute of Medicine (IOM)**, the DHHS, the USDA, the **American Medical Association (AMA)**, the **National Center for Complementary and Alternative Medicine (NCCAM)**, the National Institutes of Health (NIH), or other reputable scientific groups to help you get to the truth. For example, if your friend said that eating off of a smaller plate could help you eat less and you want to find out if that is a legitimate recommendation, search on "eat on small plates" and add "CDC" or "USDA" in your search. This will bring up information on their sites related to the claim. You will find that it is indeed a strategy that is recommended for eating less.

Go Beyond the Headlines

What makes a good headline is not always the whole truth. Read the whole story and find out if the recommendation is based on a large body of evidence or just one research study or a testimonial from one person. It takes more than one study to prove the validity of a nutrition or physical activity claim.

If It Sounds Too Good to Be True, It Probably Is

Scientists all over the world have devoted their lives to finding the foods, nutrients, and eating and activity patterns that promote health. If there were a short cut or magic pill to good health, it would be on the cover of magazines and newspapers. If a recommendation sounds too good to be true, it more than likely is.

Watch the Sales Pitch

The fact that a product is being sold does not automatically make it bad. You can, however, learn a lot from the sales techniques used. If the product is promoted as a "secret formula" or is a product that the medical and scientific communities do not want you to know about, steer clear. Also, beware of products whose sales pitch indicates that the scientific or medical communities are bad or incompetent.

Ask an Expert

If you are still having trouble understanding a nutrition claim or recommendation, ask an expert. Ask a healthcare provider what he or she knows about the claim. You could check with faculty in your college or university's nutrition department or with a healthcare provider at an on-campus clinic.

TERMS

Centers for Disease Control and Prevention (CDC) The federal agency that tracks and investigates public health trends. Promotes health and quality of life by preventing and controlling disease, injury, and disability.

Institute of Medicine (IOM) Reviews research and conducts policy studies on health issues.

American Medical Association (AMA) Promotes the science and art of medicine. Disseminates information to its members and to the public on critical health issues.

National Center for Complementary and Alternative Medicine (NCCAM) The federal government's lead agency for scientific research on the diverse medical and healthcare systems, practices, and products that are not generally considered part of conventional medicine.

Ready to Make a Change

Are you ready to make a change, small or large, in your overall health and well-being? Using some of the tools outlined in this chapter is a great place to start.

I commit to a small first step. Use the Nutrition Facts label. When you shop for food or buy food from a convenience store, pay attention to the Nutrition Facts label. Use the label to choose foods that are lower in fat, saturated fat, and sodium.

I am ready to take the next step and make a medium change. In addition to using the Nutrition Facts label, check the ingredient list of the foods you buy. Are you buying too many products with long lists of hard-to-pronounce ingredients? Check similar foods to see if there is a trade-off you can make to a product that has fewer, simpler ingredients.

I have been making changes for some time and am ready to make a large change in my overall health. Use the Food Tracker at www.ChooseMyPlate.gov for one week. Based on your results, make changes to align your diet with what is suggested in your Food Tracker plan.

Myth Versus Fact

Myth: The *Dietary Guidelines for Americans* are based on expert opinion as to what is healthy.

Fact: The *Dietary Guidelines for Americans* are based on scientific literature that is interpreted for its strength of evidence. A strong body of scientific evidence is needed for a recommendation to be part of the *Dietary Guidelines for Americans.*

Myth: Sodium recommendations are the same throughout life.

Fact: The 2010 *Dietary Guidelines for Americans* set forth a new sodium guideline of 2,300 mg per day. However, the guideline is 1,500 mg per day for adults 51 and older and those of any age who are African American or who have hypertension, diabetes, or chronic kidney disease.

Myth: MyPlate is a graphic that is used in educational programs and on food packages.

Fact: MyPlate includes a graphic, but it is much more than just an image. It is an interactive web-based educational tool that helps you choose a healthy diet.

Myth: To avoid being deficient in a nutrient, you need to consume the RDA on most days.

Fact: The RDA is set to include almost all (97–98%) people. Your actual requirement may be lower. Consume at or near the RDA on most days and you will more than likely be getting plenty of that nutrient.

Myth: Manufacturers can place a nutrition claim on the label as long as they can back it up with research.

Fact: The FDA decides what health claims can be placed on the label. A manufacturer cannot use a health claim not approved by the FDA.

Myth: Look at the Nutrition Facts label to see how many calories you are eating.

Fact: The Nutrition Facts label can help you estimate the number of calories you are getting from that food. You will need to look at calories and serving size. If you eat a portion than is twice what is listed for one serving, you will need to also double the calories listed.

Back to the Story

A host of tools are available that you could recommend to Kenji to help her make smart choices about eating and physical activity. She could start with www.ChooseMyPlate.gov and get a personalized estimate of what she should be eating. She may also want to use the MyPlate Meal Planner to help with a weekly meal plan. She should learn to read the Nutrition Facts label and ingredient label so that when she shops she will have nutrition information at her fingertips. What else would you recommend for Kenji?

References

1. US Department of Agriculture and US Department of Health and Human Services. *Dietary Guidelines for Americans, 2010*. 7th ed. Washington, DC: US Government Printing Office, 2010.
2. US Department of Agriculture. www.ChooseMyPlate.gov. Updated June 14, 2011. Accessed June 23, 2011.
3. Institute of Medicine, Food and Nutrition Board. *Dietary Reference Intakes: The Essential Guild to Nutrient Requirements*. Washington, DC: The National Academies Press, 2006.
4. Institute of Medicine, Food and Nutrition Board. *Dietary Reference Intakes for Energy, Carbohydrate, Fiber, Fat, Fatty Acids, Cholesterol, Protein, and Amino Acids*. Washington, DC: National Academies Press, 2005.
5. Neuhouser M, Kristal AR, Patterson RE. Use of food nutrition labels is associated with lower fat intake. *J Am Diet Assoc*. 1999;99:45–50,53.
6. Post RE, Mainous AG, Diaz VA, Matheson EM, Everett CJ. Use of the nutrition facts label in chronic disease management: results from the National Health and Nutrition Examination Survey. *J Am Diet Assoc*. 2010;110(4):628–632.
7. Variyam JN. Do nutrition labels improve dietary outcomes? *Health Econ*. 2008;17(6):695–708.
8. Mandal B. Use of food labels as a weight loss behavior. *J Consum Aff*. 2010;44(3):516–527.
9. Satia JA, Galanko JA, Neuhouser ML. Food nutrition label use is associated with demographic, behavioral, and psychosocial factors and dietary intake among African Americans in North Carolina. *J Am Diet Assoc*. 2005;105(3):392–402.
10. Food and Drug Administration. Health claims meeting significant scientific agreement. http://www.fda.gov/food/labelingnutrition/labelclaims/healthclaimsmeetingsignificantscientificagreementssa/default.htm. Updated January 5, 2011. Accessed April 7, 2011.
11. US Department of Agriculture, Food Safety and Inspection Service. Regulations and policies. http://www.fsis.usda.gov/regulations_&_Policies/Nutrition_Labeling/

index.asp. Updated February 9, 2011. Accessed April 7, 2011.

12. Food Standards Agency. Front-of-pack Traffic Light signpost labeling technical guidance. November 2007, Issue 2. http://www.food.gov.uk/multimedia/pdfs/frontofpackguidance2.pdf. Accessed April 8, 2011.
13. Institute of Medicine. 2011. *Examination of Front-of-Package Nutrition Rating Systems and Symbols: Promoting Healthier Choices*. Washington, DC: The National Academies Press, 2011.
14. Smart Choices Program. http://www.smartchoicesprogram.com. Accessed April 8, 2011.
15. Grocery Manufacturers Association. Food and beverage industry launches nutrition keys front-of-pack nutrition labeling initiative to inform consumers and combat obesity. http://www.gmaonline.org/news-events/newsroom/food-and-beverage-industry-launches-nutrition-keys-front-of-pack-nutrition-/. Accessed April 8, 2011.
16. Food and Drug Administration. Qualified health claims. http://www.fda.gov/Food/LabelingNutrition/LabelClaims/QualifiedHealthClaims/default.htm. Updated July 27, 2010. Accessed April 7, 2011.

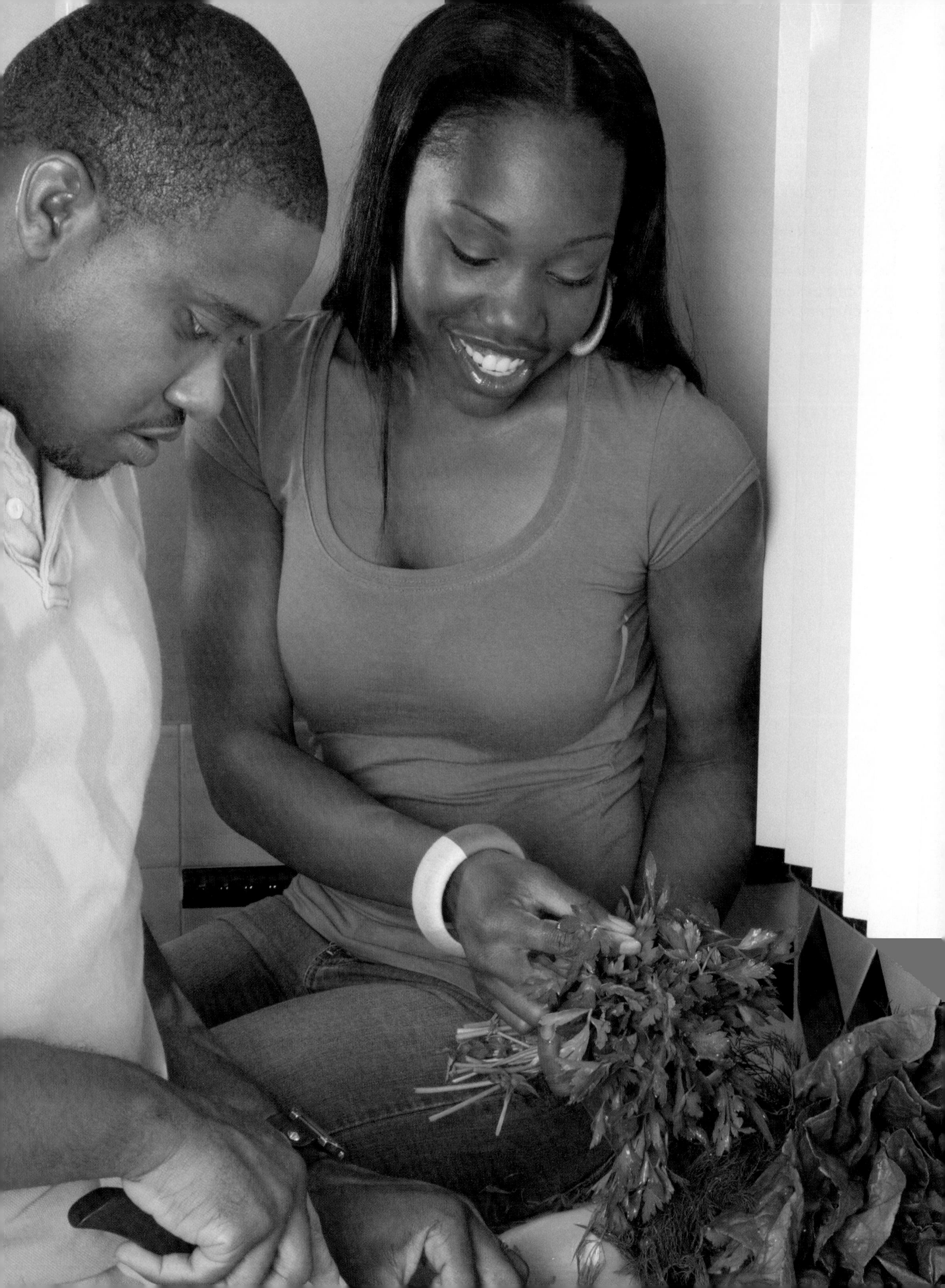

Chapter 3

Eating Out or Eating In: Where You Eat Affects What You Eat

Key Messages

- Americans are eating more meals away from home than ever before.
- Eating out generally means eating more calories, more fat, less fiber, and fewer fruits and vegetables.
- Fast-food consumption is associated with higher body weight.
- Preparing and eating more meals at home is a good strategy to improve your overall diet.

It's your birthday and you go to your favorite restaurant to celebrate, you get a promotion at work and your partner takes you to the best restaurant in town, to relax you go to the neighborhood burger hangout. Eating out used to be for special occasions. Birthdays, anniversaries, and graduations were celebrated with a special meal at a special restaurant. We still hold many of life's celebrations at restaurants, but something has changed. Over the past 20 years, restaurants have gone from an occasional treat to a daily part of life for many people. Fast food, take out, delivery, delis, and family-style restaurants are everywhere. The demand for quick food prepared by someone else has increased dramatically; according to many Americans, there is simply no time for anything else. Quick and right now has replaced home-cooked and healthy for many meals. The car has replaced the dinner table as the venue for many of our meals. How has this change from meals prepared at home to meals prepared in a restaurant impacted your health? Are we in such a hurry as a nation that simple meals prepared at home are to forever be replaced by the number one combo meal? This chapter will explore these questions as well as provide tips to help you prepare and eat more meals at home.

Story

Linda is a busy, 20-year-old full-time college student. She works part time at a local boutique. Linda has 8 AM classes on Monday, Wednesday, and Friday. On those days, for breakfast she gets a sausage biscuit and coffee from a fast-food restaurant on her way to class. The other mornings she has a toaster pastry or bowl of cereal. Lunch is almost always on campus at the student union, where there is a food court. She usually sticks with a burger or burrito—whatever is quickest. On days she has to work, she usually skips lunch altogether. Dinner depends on her schedule. If she is studying, she will grab two slices of pizza on her way to the library. On nights that she has time, she will cook. Linda has limited food preparation skills, so her at-home meals rely heavily on frozen foods or convenience foods—macaroni and cheese from a box is a typical meal. Once or twice a week, Linda and her friends will go to a sit-down restaurant. They usually go to one of the chain restaurants near campus. Linda graduates in a couple of years. She is concerned that her eating habits are not what they should be now, let alone for the rest of her life. What suggestions could you give Linda to help her create lifelong eating habits that include preparing and eating more meals at home?

Where America Eats

Americans are eating more meals than ever from some form of a restaurant. The number of restaurants has doubled over the past 20 years; today, there are an estimated 945,000 restaurants in the United States.[1] On any given

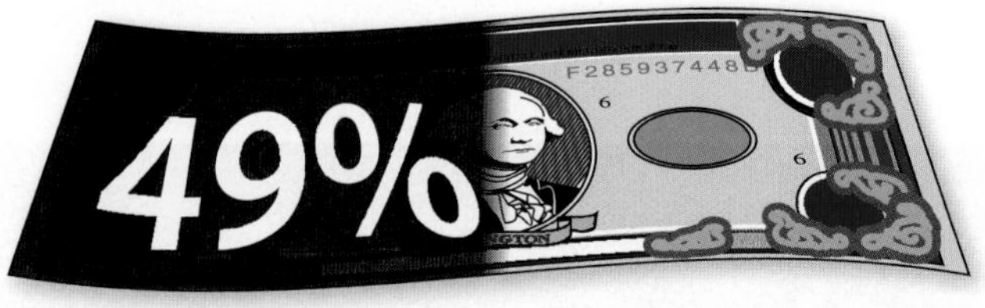

■ **Figure 3.1**

Almost Half of Money Spent on Food Is for Foods Prepared Away from Home

Source: USDA, Economic Research Service, Food Expenditure Series. http://www.ers.usda.gov/Briefing/CPIFoodandexpenditures/data/. Accessed March 3, 2010.

day, almost half of all U.S. adults will eat a restaurant meal.[2] Restaurants are a $580 billion per year industry, and the restaurant industry continues to get more of your food dollar. In the 1970s, only about 30% of your food dollar went to foods away from home; today almost half your food dollar is spent on away-from-home food from some type of restaurant (**Figure 3.1**).[3,4]

Much of the away-from-home food dollar is spent on fast food. Fast-food restaurants represent one of the largest segments of the food industry, with over 200,000 restaurants and $120 billion in sales in the United States.[5,6] Fast-food restaurants are noted for their short food preparation time; oftentimes the food is already prepared prior to you even ordering it. Although rising energy costs have slowed the growth of the number of fast-food outlets since 2006, more fast-food restaurants continue to be built in order to satisfy the public's desire for quick meals. You can find fast food on almost every corner in the country. Fast food is available in most cities and towns as well as in airports, shopping malls, discount stores, school cafeterias, and worksites. With so many fast-food outlets, it is no surprise that every day one in four Americans eats a fast-food meal.

Almost 75% of Americans usually eat out at least once a week, and an estimated 23% of our meals are from restaurants.[4,7] However, when we add foods purchased as take out from restaurants, fast-food outlets, or grocery store delis, that number goes up to 40%. So, regardless of where they are eaten, almost half of all meals are prepared away from the home. When you add the use of convenience foods that are highly processed, the number gets even higher, 65%. That only leaves 32% of our meals being simple meals made without highly processed convenience foods. The graphic in **Figure 3.2** shows the category "from scratch," which is just a simple meal of vegetables, fruit, lean meat, and grains prepared and eaten at home.[7]

What You Eat When You Eat Out

The increased frequency of eating foods prepared outside the home undeniably has a significant influence on eating behavior.[2] Hundreds of millions of people buy food from a restaurant or fast-food restaurant every day without giv-

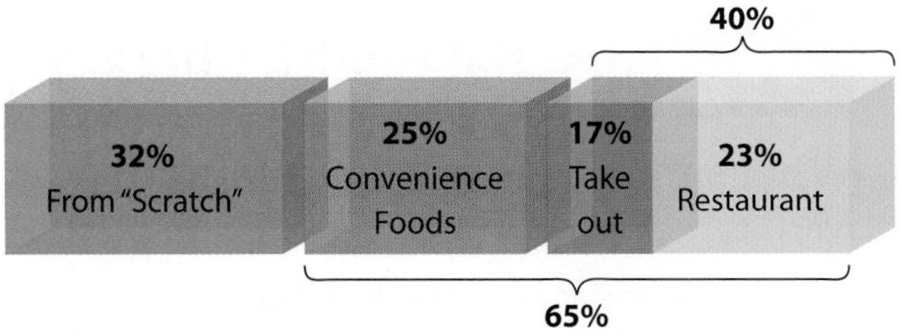

Figure 3.2

What Is America Eating?

Source: Data from Sloan EA. What, when, and where America eats. *Food Technology* 2006;January:18–27.

ing it much thought. They just pull up to the table or drive thru and order their meal without giving any thought to what the food may be doing to their bodies or how it may be affecting their health. With so many meals prepared away from home, how does it affect what you eat?

What do you eat when you go out? The most popular foods ordered in restaurants, which include those eaten at the restaurant and as take out, do not vary greatly by gender or age. For men, the number one ordered food is a burger, followed by french fries and pizza. For women and young adults, the number one food is french fries, followed by a burger and pizza. Younger children go for the french fries, pizza, and chicken nuggets.[8] Although there is nothing wrong with any of these foods in moderation, the rate at which Americans go out to eat coupled with the items being ordered most frequently presents a high-fat, high-calorie problem.

Away-from-home food accounts for about a quarter of our eating occasions, but contributes 34% of our daily calories. This suggests that away-from-home foods are higher in calories than at-home meals. In fact, a growing body of evidence suggests that when we eat out we are likely to eat more calories than we need.[9]

People who eat out more often are more likely to be at an unhealthy weight.[9] Although some restaurants are now offering healthier options, eating simple foods prepared at home provides more control over how food is prepared and how much is served. Even if you are careful when you eat out, eating out often means larger portions, more calories, more fat, fewer fruits and vegetables, fewer whole grains, fewer low-fat dairy products, and less fiber.[2,9–11] Eating foods prepared at home is associated with healthier dietary intake patterns, including more fruits and vegetables, fewer fried foods, and fewer soft drinks.[11–15] **Figure 3.3** shows some common restaurant meals and the calories they contain. Are you surprised at how many calories some of these meals have?

Fast food is one of the most popular types of away-from-home food.[16–18] Fast food is quick and relatively inexpensive. The low cost of fast food allows even families on a very limited food budget to consume it.[19] Because fast food is usually high in fat and calories and low in essential nutrients, it has a negative effect on overall diet quality.[20] (See **Figure 3.4**.) It should be no surprise that consumption

Chipotle Mexican Grill

Burrito with Rice, Black Beans, Chicken, Cheese, and Guacamole

980 calories
41 grams of fat

This burrito is made with healthy rice, black beans, and grilled chicken. At first glance it should be an ok choice, but because it is huge it has almost 1,000 calories! Even healthy foods in large quantities can add up to too many calories. Split this with a friend or save half for another meal and you have a healthier restaurant choice.

Pizzeria Uno

Individual Deep-dish Pizza with Cheese and Tomato

1,740 calories
120 grams of fat

This individual deep-dish pizza actually has three servings. Eat the whole pie and you will get more fat than you need in two days. For a healthier choice, choose thin crust pizza instead of deep dish. Choose vegetable toppings or plain cheese (not double cheese) and have just a couple of slices.

Applebee's

Oriental Grilled Chicken Salad, Regular Size

1,250 calories
76 grams of fat

How can a salad with grilled chicken have so many calories? The dressing alone contributes over 600 calories, and this salad has fried noodles as a topping. Order this salad with the dressing on the side so you can control the amount, and ask for a lower-fat dressing. Or, you can order a lower-calorie item.

Olive Garden

Spaghetti with Meatballs

1,110 calories
50 grams of fat

You followed the rules and steered clear of cream sauce and still ended up with over 1,000 calories. Add a couple of breadsticks and salad, and your meal will easily top 1,500 calories. The problem, again, is the size of the portion. Keep the salad, cut the breadstick down to one, and share the meal with a friend for a more reasonable 700-calorie meal.

Ruby Tuesday

Turkey Burger

699 calories
39 grams of fat

Turkey burgers are not always low in fat and calories. Why is this turkey burger with no mayonnaise, fries, or side dishes almost 700 calories? Big patties and huge buns add up to lots of calories. There are no doubt many other lower-calorie choices on a menu. If you must have the turkey burger, leave the bun off or share the sandwich with a friend.

Figure 3.3

Common Restaurant Meals and Suggestions for Better Choices

Source: Data from Chipotle Mexican Grill. http://www.chipotle.com/en-us/menu/nutritional_information/nutritional_information.aspx. Accessed April 11, 2011.

Pizzeria Uno Corporation. http://www.unos.com/nutrition.php. Accessed April 11, 2011.

Applebees IP LLC. http://www.applebees.com/downloads/nutritional_info.html. Accessed April 11, 2011.

Darden Concepts Incorporated. www.olivegarden.com/menus/printable/NutritionInformation.pdf. Accessed April 10, 2011.

Ruby Tuesday Incorporated. www.rubytuesday.com/assets/menu/pdf/informational/nutrition.pdf. Accessed April 10, 2011.

Sandwiches
- Cheeseburger (McDonald's): 300
- Filet-O-Fish (McDonald's): 380
- Premium Grilled Chicken Classic Sandwich (McDonald's): 420
- Whopper (Burger King): 670
- Double Quarter Pounder with Cheese (McDonald's): 740
- Quad Stack (Burger King): 930

Fries
- Small fries (McDonald's): 230
- Medium fries (McDonald's): 350
- Large fries (McDonald's) 500

Salads
- Southwest Salad with Grilled Chicken (McDonald's): 320, add 60 for croutons and 100 for Southwest dressing
- Tendercrisp Garden Salad (Burger King): 670

Combo Meals
- Double Cheeseburger Value Meal with medium drink and medium fries (McDonald's): 1,030
- Tendergrill Chicken Value Meal with small drink and small fries (Burger King): 1,040
- Whopper Value Meal with large drink and large fries (Burger King): 1,600

Figure 3.4

Calories in Common Fast-Food Menu Items

Source: Data from McDonald's Corporation. http://www.mcdonalds.com/us/en/food/food_quality/nutrition_choices.html. Accessed April 10, 2011.

Burger King Corporation. http://www.bk.com/en/us/menu-nutrition/index.html. Accessed April 10, 2011.

of fast food has been linked to an increased risk of overweight and obesity. The more often you eat fast food, the more likely you are to be overweight or obese.[11,21–24] Eating even one fast-food meal per week reduces the likelihood of having an overall healthy diet.[23] How many fast-food restaurants there are in your neighborhood also influences how often you eat fast food. Those who live in neighborhoods with a high concentration of restaurants tend to eat more fast food, and thus are more likely to have unhealthy diets overall.[23] Fast foods are heavily marketed on television, billboards, and in print ads.

Large Portions

One of the reasons foods offered in restaurants are too high in fat and calories is the size of the portions that are served. The amount we eat is as important as what we eat. Americans are eating larger portions than ever before. Many of these large portions are foods eaten away from home; restaurant portions, fast-food items, snack foods, and soft drinks have all gotten larger.[25] Portion sizes have increased significantly over the past 20 years for people in all age groups, and they continue to get larger.[26,27] This continuing trend of super-sizing, huge portions, all-you-can-eat buffets, and extra-large single servings has contributed to expanding waistlines.

Personal Health Check

What's in Your Favorite Restaurant Meals?

You don't have to stop eating out altogether to eat healthy. Prepare and eat more meals at home, and when you do go out choose healthy options. A good way to start is to find out how your favorite meals eaten away from home stack up nutritionally. Write down the three restaurants you go to most and list what you usually order. Use the Internet to find out the calories and fat in your favorite meals. If you choose a local restaurant without nutritional information, you may have to choose a similar meal from a chain restaurant that offers nutritional information. If the meals that you normally order are higher in calories than they should be, look for other menu items that you could order instead. Check the restaurant's website to see if it offers any healthy alternatives; many do. Now you are ready to dine out without breaking the calorie bank.

Portions, of course, impact the total number of calories consumed. This would not be a problem if you were able to recognize, both physically and psychologically, that you have eaten more calories than you need and compensate for it later in the day by eating less. However, studies have found that you simply do not compensate for large portions.[28,29] In fact, when served large portions you eat more calories than you need over time.[29]

It is also difficult to properly gauge portion sizes. Most people do not correctly assess how much they are eating. They tend to underestimate the amount of food that they have consumed and end up consuming more than they need.[30–32] When you are served large portions, you tend to eat more food and, therefore, more calories. Even if you don't eat the entire portion you eat more than you would have if you had been served a smaller portion, regardless of how hungry you are.[33–37] If you are served a large portion in a restaurant, you will eat, on average, 30–50% more than if you were served a smaller portion.[38] The same holds true for large-sized packages. If you are serving yourself from a large-size package, you may eat 20–40% more.[39] Even if the food being served is not very tasty, such as stale popcorn, larger servings add up to increased consumption.[40] The bottom line is that, regardless of hunger or quality of food, you eat more when you are served more or serve yourself out of a large-size package.

Large portions and packages cause you to eat more; they also cause **portion distortion**. Your perception of what

TERMS

portion distortion The perception that large portions are appropriate amounts to eat at one sitting; caused by the increase in portions served primarily in restaurants and fast-food outlets.

a normal portion should be is influenced by what you are usually served. Portion distortion begins at a very early age. Even preschool children are influenced by being fed large servings early in life.[41–43] Larger portions at restaurants have affected the amount of food you put on your plate at home.[25] Single-serving bags that really contain two or more servings make you think that is what you should eat in one sitting (**Figure 3.5**). You get used to seeing huge pieces of chicken, giant steaks, mountains of mashed potatoes, or pounds of pasta; so when you go to serve your plate, a smaller portion doesn't look like enough. Portion distortion continues to affect what is served in restaurants; patrons expect huge portions because that is what they are used to being served. Our distorted view on what constitutes a normal serving is certainly affecting our waistlines.

Tips for Right-sizing Your Portions

The following tips can help you right-size your portions:

- ***Measure your portions.*** The best way to get a handle on portion sizes is to measure and/or weigh your food. You can use measuring cups or a small kitchen scale. You don't have to do this forever; just do it for a few days or a week. This will help reset your internal cues as to what a serving should look like on your plate or in your bowl. If you are away from home, use your hand to estimate portion sizes (**Figure 3.6**).
- ***Don't serve family style.*** Serve your plate in the kitchen. Don't put serving bowls on the table. You often eat more than you need when you serve your plate at the table and have serving dishes sitting on the table for seconds and thirds. Serve yourself a reasonable portion, eat slowly, and enjoy your meal.
- ***Don't eat directly from containers or bags.*** Put a reasonable amount of food into a bowl or container and leave the rest of the package in the pantry. Package snacks in small bags for portion-controlled snacking or buy small 100-calorie packs.
- ***Use smaller plates, bowls, and glasses.*** Like our portions, dinner plates have gotten larger over time. Some dinner plates are 2–3 inches larger than in the past. Using smaller plates will help you control portion sizes.
- ***Be mindful of how much you are eating.*** The best way to break the cycle of portion distortion is to be mindful of how much you are eating. Think about what you are eating and how much. Don't eat while doing other things, such as watching TV or driving.

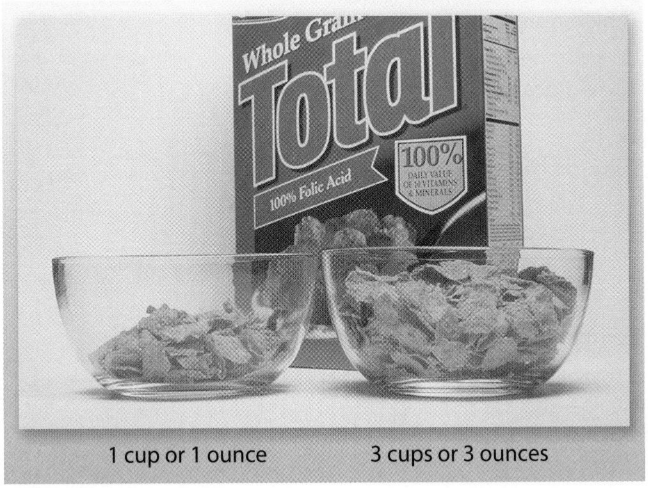

■ **Figure 3.5**

The Amount You Eat Is Often More Than One Serving

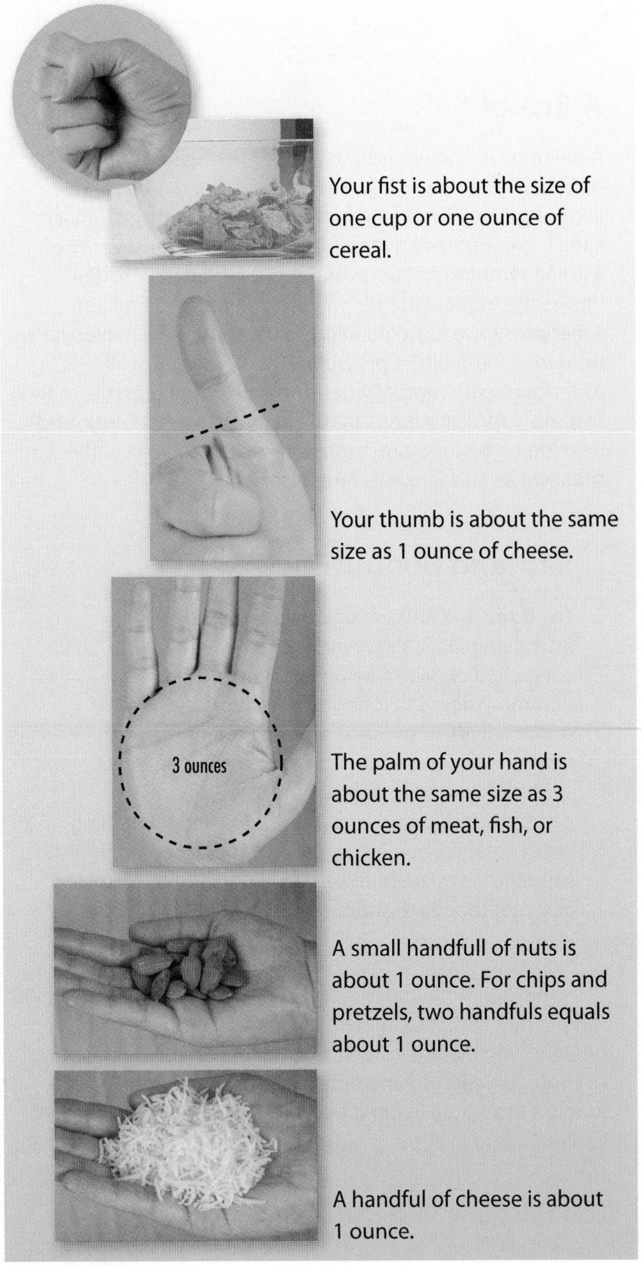
Your fist is about the size of one cup or one ounce of cereal.
Your thumb is about the same size as 1 ounce of cheese.
3 ounces
The palm of your hand is about the same size as 3 ounces of meat, fish, or chicken.
A small handfull of nuts is about 1 ounce. For chips and pretzels, two handfuls equals about 1 ounce.
A handful of cheese is about 1 ounce.

■ **Figure 3.6**

The Secret to Serving Size Is in Your Hand

Special Report

A Sea of Salt

A diet high in sodium (salt) is a major risk factor for heart disease and stroke.[44–48] A high-sodium diet has been associated with increased blood pressure, obesity, stomach cancer, osteoporosis, kidney stones, and greater severity of asthma symptoms.[49] On average, the higher your sodium intake, the higher your blood pressure. About 65 million Americans have high blood pressure; another 45 million have borderline high blood pressure.[50,51] About 90% of all Americans will eventually develop high blood pressure in their lifetime.[52] African Americans are at an even greater risk, and develop high blood pressure more often and at an earlier age than whites and Mexican Americans.[53]

Salt and Sodium

The terms *salt* and *sodium* are often used interchangeably. However, they are not the same. Salt is composed of two minerals: sodium and chloride. Common table salt is about 60% chloride and 40% sodium. It is the sodium content of food that is of concern with respect to high blood pressure. Most of the sodium in your diet comes from salt. Sodium is necessary in the body and plays a role in maintaining water balance. However, getting enough sodium is not something you need to be concerned about. Almost all of us get too much sodium.

The recommendations for sodium consumption are 2,300 mg per day, or 1,500 mg per day for African Americans; persons with diabetes, heart disease, or high blood pressure; or those 51 years old and older. To put the recommended amount of sodium in perspective, 2,300 mg is the amount of sodium found in about 1 teaspoon of salt. Nearly all Americans consume too much sodium, on average about 4,000 mg per day.[44,54]

You might think that the best way to decrease the sodium in your diet is to simply put down the saltshaker. Although not salting your food is a good step, the vast majority of sodium in the diet—about 77%—comes from processed foods and foods eaten outside the home (see the figure).[55–57]

The salt in these foods is already added, so even if you never touch the saltshaker, you are already swimming in a sea of salt. Many restaurant meals provide more than the amount of sodium you need in the whole day. Although sodium content varies depending on the restaurant and on exactly what you order, a hamburger and fries from a fast-food restaurant can have 1,500 mg or more of sodium. A couple of slices of cheese pizza can have as much as 1,500 mg of sodium.

Decreasing the number of meals eaten outside the home and decreasing your use of processed foods is the best way to decrease sodium in your diet. Read the label on packaged foods to see just how much sodium is in the product.

Steps to Reduce Sodium

The following tips can help you reduce your sodium intake:

- Reduce the number of meals eaten away from home.
- Reduce the number of processed foods eaten, such as frozen dinners, canned soups, and lunchmeats.
- Read the food label to find brands that have cut at least some of the salt.
- Choose condiments carefully and use sparingly. Items such as ketchup, salad dressing, marinades, or soy sauce may contain a lot of sodium.
- Choose more fresh foods such as fruits, vegetables, and meats that are not processed.
- Drain and rinse canned vegetables and beans.
- Season foods with herbs and spices instead of salt.

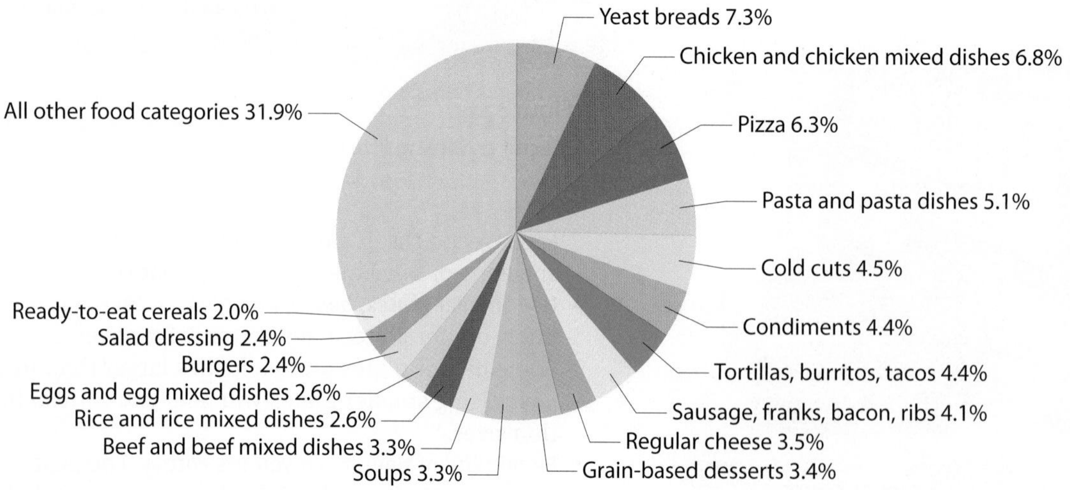

Sources of Sodium in Your Diet

Source: National Cancer Institute. Sources of Sodium in the Diets of the U.S. Population Ages 2 Years and Older, NHANES 2005–2006. Risk Factor Monitoring and Methods, Cancer Control and Population Sciences. http://riskfactor.cancer.gov/diet/foodsources/sodium/table1a.html. Accessed April 10, 2011.

Use Spices and Herbs Instead of Salt to Add Flavor Without Adding Sodium

	Appetizers	Soups	Salads and Dressings	Vegetables	Eggs and Cheese	Meats and Sauces	Poultry and Fish	Desserts and Baked Goods
Allspice	Pickles, relishes, cocktail meatballs, pickled beets, fruit compote	Green pea, vegetable beef, minestrone, asparagus, tomato	Cottage cheese, fruit salad, cheese dressing	Eggplant, spinach, beets, squash, turnips, red cabbage, carrots	Egg casserole, cream cheese	Beef stew, meat loaf, hamburgers, baked ham, roast lamb, pot roast, cranberry sauce, meat gravies, tomato sauce	Boiled fish, oyster stew	Mincemeat, tapioca and chocolate puddings, spice cake, fruit cake, baked bananas, cookies, pie
Bay Leaves	Hot tomato juice, pickles, pickled beets	Bouillon, bouillabaisse, fish chowders, lobster bisque, vegetable, minestrone, oxtail, potato, tomato, turtle	Seafood salad, tomato aspic, chicken aspic, beet salad, French dressing	Potatoes, artichokes, carrots, beets, eggplant, lentils, onions, rice, squash, zucchini	Eggs creole	Beef stew, meat pie, curried beef, pot roast, roast beef, veal, meat sauces, lamb, spare ribs, gravies	Capon, chicken salad, a la king, fricassee, turkey (roast), boiled shrimp and lobster, fish stews, baked salmon	
Caraway	Soft cheese spreads, pickles	Cream soups, clam chowder, borscht, vegetable	Potato salad, sour cream dressing, spiced vinegar, cole slaw	Cabbage, cauliflower, potatoes, carrots, onions, turnips, broccoli, Brussels sprouts, sauerkraut	Cottage cheese, cream cheese	Sauerbraten, roast pork, beef a la mode, liver, kidney stew	Tuna fish casserole, roast goose	Rye bread, muffins, rolls, coffee cakes, cookies, loaf cake
Cayenne	Deviled eggs, seafood sauces, cottage and cream cheese dips and spreads, avocado dip	Clam and oyster stews, fish chowder, cream soups, shrimp gumbo, vegetable	Tuna, shrimp, chicken, macaroni, seafood, mayonnaise, thousand island dressing, sour cream dressing	Green beans, lima beans, cauliflower, cut corn, kale, broccoli	Welsh rarebit, egg dishes, cheese soufflé, cottage and cream cheese	Pork chops, veal stew, ham croquettes, barbecued beef, sandwich fillings, meat sauces	Creamed chicken and croquettes, oysters, shrimp, poached salmon, tuna salad	
Celery Seed (salt, flakes, seeds)	Deviled eggs, ham spread, tomato juice, kraut juice, cream cheese spread, pickles	Cream of celery or tomato, fish chowders and bisques, vegetable, bean, potato, bouillon	Cole slaw, potato, egg, tuna, vegetable, kidney beans, salad dressings, sour cream dressing	Cabbage, stewed tomatoes, potatoes, cauliflower, turnips, braised lettuce	Welsh rarebit, boiled and fried eggs, cheese casserole, omelets, cheese sauce, deviled eggs	Meat loaf, pot roast, meat stews, short ribs of beef, braised lamb	Chicken croquettes, fish stew, chicken pie, oyster stew, stuffings	Rolls, biscuits, salty breads
Chili Powder	Avocado and cheese dips, seafood cocktail sauce	Corn soup, pepperpot, fish and clam chowders, tomato, bean, shrimp gumbo, vegetable, chili soup	French dressing, kidney bean salad, thousand island dressing, chili sauce	Vegetable relishes, green peas, eggplant, rice, tomatoes, corn Mexicali, green beans, lima beans	Omelets, soufflés, casseroles, boiled and scrambled eggs, cheese sauces, rarebits	Chili con carne, arroz con pollo, tamales, meat loaf, hamburgers, stews, sauces	Creamed seafood, shrimp, chicken and rice, chicken pie	
Cinnamon (ground and stick)	Cinnamon toast, sweet gherkins, hot spiced beverages, pickled fruits		Fruit salad, dressings for fruit salads	Sweet potatoes, squash, pumpkins, spinach, turnips, green beans, beets, parsnips		Pork chops, ham, sauce for pork and lamb	Boiled chicken (stick cinnamon), boiled fish, special chicken and fish recipes	Chocolate and rice pudding, stewed fruits, apple desserts, buns, coffee cake, muffins, spice cake, molasses cookies
Cloves (whole and ground)	Sweet gherkins, pickled fruits, hot spiced wines, fruit punch	Beef, bean, cream of tomato, cream of pea, mulligatawny	Toppings for fruit salads	Beets, baked beans, candied sweet potatoes, squash		(Whole) Ham and pork roast, sauces, gravies, sausage, boiled tongue	Baked fish, chicken a la king, roast or smothered chicken, chicken croquettes	Preserved and stewed fruits, apple, mince and pumpkin pies, chocolate rice and tapioca pudding, stewed pears
Curry Powder	Tomato juice, sauce for dips, sweet pickles, deviled eggs, salted nuts	Clam and fish chowders, tomato soup, cream of mushroom, oyster stew	Fruit and meat salads, mayonnaise, French dressing	Rice, creamed onions, creamed potatoes, carrots, corn, celery, lima beans	Sauce for eggs, deviled eggs, cottage cheese, cream cheese, cheese sauce	Curried lamb, veal croquettes, stews	Chicken croquettes, chicken hash, curried chicken and turkey, fish croquettes, shrimp	
Dill	Cottage cheese, anchovy spread, cheddar cheese spread, pickles, sour cream dips, stuffed eggs	Split pea soup, cream of tomato, navy bean, borscht, chicken, lobster bisque, turkey, fish chowder	Cole slaw, cucumber, green bean, lettuce, mixed green, potato, seafood, mayonnaise, sour cream, French dressing	Carrots, beets, cabbage, lima beans, green beans, turnips, eggplant, cauliflower, zucchini squash	Deviled eggs, omelets, scrambled eggs, cottage cheese, cream cheese, macaroni	Beef: Pot roast, corned, stew, barbecued, hamburger; lamb chops or stew, roast pork	Chicken pie, creamed chicken, baked halibut, mackerel, salmon, creamed lobster, boiled and creamed shrimp	

(continues)

Use Spices and Herbs Instead of Salt to Add Flavor Without Adding Sodium *(Continued)*

	Appetizers	Soups	Salads and Dressings	Vegetables	Eggs and Cheese	Meats and Sauces	Poultry and Fish	Desserts and Baked Goods
Ginger (ground)	Pickles, broiled grapefruit, chutney	Bean soup, onion, potato	Ginger pears, French dressing	Beets, carrots, squash, baked beans	Cheese dishes	Broiled beef, lamb, veal, pot roast, stews, chopped beef	Roast chicken, squab, Cornish hen, sautéed chicken	Ginger bread, cakes, cookies, pumpkin pie, custards, baked, stewed, preserved fruits, Indian pudding
Marjoram	Fruit punch, cream and cottage cheese dips, cheddar cheese spreads, pickles	Onion soup, clam, oyster, Boston clam chowder, minestrone, oxtail, spinach	Mixed green salad, asparagus, chicken, fruit, seafood	Carrots, eggplant, peas, spinach, string beans, onions, summer squash, tomatoes, celery, broccoli, Brussels sprouts	Omelets, soufflés, creamed eggs, scrambled, cheese sauce, cheese soufflé, rarebits, cheese straws	Roast beef, pork, veal, stews, meat pies, loaf, pot roast, short ribs, spare ribs	Chicken croquettes, duck, goose, pheasant, guinea hen, codfish balls, halibut, salmon loaf, shad roe	
Mustard (ground)	Pickles, pickled onions, ham spreads, Chinese hot sauce, hot English mustard, deviled eggs	Lobster bisque, bean, onion	Egg salad, shrimp, lobster, potato, fruit, salad dressings	Asparagus, beets, broccoli, Brussels sprouts, cabbage, onions, green beans, potatoes, baked beans	Deviled eggs, casseroles, cheese sauces, cream cheese	Baked ham, kidneys, pickled meat, sauces	Shrimp, creamed and stewed oysters, boiled fish, fish sauces	Molasses cookies, gingerbread
Oregano	Cheese spreads, pizza, vegetable juice, avocado dip, creamed and cottage cheese spreads	Bean, vegetable, tomato, lentil, minestrone, navy bean, onion, spinach	Salad dressings, seafood, avocado, green bean, mixed green, potato, tomato, tomato aspic	Peas, onions, potatoes, spinach, green beans, stewed tomatoes, mushrooms	Creamed eggs, omelets, scrambled eggs, cheese sauce, soufflé, cottage, cream, string, rarebits	Swiss steak, beef stew, broiled and roast lamb, meat loaf, sauces, gravies, spare ribs, veal scallopini	Chicken cacciatore, sauté, roast, guinea hen, pheasant, stuffed fish, boiled shrimp, clams	
Paprika	Canapés, deviled eggs, cream cheese spreads, stuffed celery, seafood creamed, seafood cocktails	Cream soups, chicken soup, chowders	Cole slaw, potato salad, mayonnaise, French dressing	Cauliflower, potatoes, celery, creamed vegetables	Deviled eggs, scrambled eggs, Welsh rarebit, cottage cheese, cheese and egg dishes	Hungarian goulash, ham, gravies	Poultry and seafood dishes, shellfish, fried chicken	
Poppy Seed	Cheese spreads, cottage cheese, cheese dips	Onion soup	Green salads, salad dressing	Peas, potatoes, rutabaga, sweet potatoes, carrots, zucchini	Fried and scrambled eggs, omelets, cottage cheese	Noodle dishes		Coffee cake, cookies, pie crusts, bread, rolls, pastries
Rosemary	Deviled eggs, pickles, sour cream dips	Mock turtle, chicken, lentil, minestrone, split pea, spinach, chowders	Meat salad, fruit salad	Peas, potatoes, mushrooms, onions, celery, lima beans, green beans, broccoli, cucumbers	Deviled eggs, omelets, soufflés	Roast and broiled lamb, beef, pork, veal, beef stew, pie, pot roast, Swiss steak, spare ribs	Capon, chicken fricassee, sauté, roast pheasant, partridge, quail, salmon, baked halibut, baked sole	
Saffron		Chicken, bouillabaisse, lobster bisque, turkey	Seafood salads	Rice	Scrambled eggs	Gravy for roast chicken, roast turkey, roast veal, Spanish sauce, rabbit	Arroz con pollo, bouillabaisse, chicken stew, chicken fricassee, creamed lobster, baked halibut, sole	Rolls, breads, buns, cake, frostings and icings
Sage	Cheese spreads	Consommé, fish and corn chowders, cream soups, asparagus, chicken, cream of tomato, minestrone, turkey	Salad greens, salad dressings	Brussels sprouts, onions, lima beans, peas, tomatoes, carrots, eggplant, winter squash, turnips	Creamed eggs, soufflés, cheese sauce, rarebits, egg and cheese casseroles, cottage and cream cheese	Beef: barbeque, stew, pie, roast, pot roast; barbecued lamb, roast veal, pork, veal stew	Capon, chicken stuffing, goose, duck	
Sesame Seed	Soft cheeses	Most soups	Cole slaw, salad dressings	Asparagus, green beans, tomatoes, spinach, noodle and vegetable casseroles, potatoes, rice	Cream cheese	Meat pies, Hawaiian ham steak	Fried chicken, chicken casseroles, fish	Top dressings on pies, cookies, coffee cake, rolls, breads, buns, crumpets
Tarragon	Vegetable juice cocktail, liver paté, herb butters, cheese spreads, seafood cocktails, stuffed eggs, pickles	Bean, chicken consommé, seafood chowders and bisques, mushroom, pea, tomato, turtle	Asparagus, celery, chicken, cole slaw, cucumber, egg, green bean, kidney bean, mixed green, tomato	Asparagus, beans, broccoli, cabbage, cauliflower, celery root, mushrooms, potatoes, spinach, tomatoes	Deviled eggs, omelets, scrambled eggs, cottage cheese	Most marinades, broiled steak, pot roast, braised lamb, lamb stew, veal stew, bearnaise sauce, brown garlic	Chicken, chicken sauté, broiled chicken, turkey, duck, broiled halibut, baked salmon, trout, tuna, broiled lobster	

How Policy and Environment Affect My Choices

Healthy Eating at Meetings and Gatherings

Pastry trays, donuts, fried chicken, huge desserts—foods that are offered at meetings or gatherings are not always healthy. When you are part of a captive audience, the foods selected for you may not always be healthy. Sometimes you don't have a choice but to eat what is chosen for you. Organizations can adopt a policy that encourages serving healthy foods at meetings or gatherings. It does not mean that special foods are off the menu; it just means that healthy options are available and that meeting planners are mindful of making healthy choices available. Healthy food policies are not limited to businesses; they can also be adopted by faith organizations, clubs, and even groups of friends. The following figure is a sample policy that can be used to encourage serving healthy foods. You can customize it for your group and area. It will allow you to highlight vendors or restaurants that have made the commitment to offer healthier items. Changes such as this can help make healthy eating the easy choice.

Sample Healthy Foods Policy

- For use within any organization/agency or community group where foods or beverages are served.

Whereas:

- ________________________ (*fill in your worksite, church, school, etc., name here*) is concerned about the health of our ________________ (*employees, members*);

Whereas:

- People have become more and more interested in eating smart and moving more;

Whereas:

- Heart disease, cancer and stroke—the top three causes of death in North Carolina—are largely affected by what we eat and how physically active we are;

Whereas:

- Foods such as fruits, vegetables, whole grain breads and pastas, and low-fat dairy products are better choices for preventing many diseases;

Therefore:

- Effective __________ (*today's date*), it is the policy of ________________________ (*fill in your organization's name*) that all activities and events (examples of events may include: meetings, potluck events, catered events, community sponsored events, like health fairs, etc.) sponsored or supported by this organization will always include opportunities for healthy foods and beverages by:
- Purchasing and serving one or more of these healthier items:
  Fruits and/or vegetables—Examples include fresh, frozen, canned or dried fruits (such as grapefruit, oranges, apples, raisins or 100% fruit juices), and fresh, frozen, or canned vegetables
  Low-fat milk and dairy products—Examples include skim/nonfat or 1% milk (also lactose-free); low-fat and fat-free yogurt; cheese and ice cream; and calcium-fortified soy beverages
  Foods made from grains (like wheat, rice , and oats), especially whole grains—Examples include low-fat whole-wheat crackers, bread and pasta; whole-grain ready-to-eat cereal; low-fat baked tortilla chips; pita bread
  Water
- Identifying healthy eating opportunities
  Examples include identification of restaurants, caterers and farmer's markets, where healthy food choices are readily available.
- Providing encouragement from group leadership to enjoy healthy foods
  Examples include community promotion of healthy lifestyles, group leadership being role models for healthy food choices.

Signature ________________________________ Title ____________________

Name of Organization, Church, Community Group, Worksite, School, Health Care Facility

____

Date __________

Source: Eat Smart, Move More, North Carolina. http://www.eatsmartmovemorenc.com. Accessed April 11, 2011.

- ***Be wary of single-serving packages.*** Many single-serving packages may actually be two or more servings. A bag of chips from a convenience store may be advertised as a single-serving but in reality be multiple servings. Read the label to see just how much food you are getting.

Strategies to Help You Eat Healthy When You Eat Out

Preparing and eating more meals at home is important to help you eat healthier. However, when you do eat out, you can use the following strategies to make better choices.

Prepare Before You Go

Check the menu before you go so that you can plan what you will order. Many restaurants post their menus online. Check the restaurant's website for nutrition information. Think about what would be a smart choice to order. Choose a restaurant that offers healthy options.

Think Before You Order

Think about how hungry you are. Read the menu carefully. Try not to order more food than you need.

Control Portions

Take advantage of large restaurant sizes and split an entrée with a friend or family member. Order an appetizer instead of an entrée. Take part of your meal home. You may want to ask for the to-go container at the beginning of your meal so you are not tempted to eat more than you need. Don't order the large size of an entrée, sandwich, or side; if you do, share with a friend or family member.

Choose Healthier Options

Avoid menu items with words like crispy, creamy, sautéed, pan-fried, buttery, breaded, sauced, or stuffed. These items will generally be higher in calories and fat. Choose simple foods. Generally, the more preparation a menu item requires, the more calories and fat are added. Order food the way you want it. Don't be afraid to ask for it prepared differently than is stated on the menu or ask for different side items. For example, if you don't see a simple grilled chicken breast on the menu but you do see chicken dishes with cheese or sauce, ask if you can have a chicken breast without sauce or sauce on the side. If the side dish offered with your meal is fries, ask if there is anything you can substitute, such as a small salad, steamed vegetables, or a baked potato. **Table 3.1** offers suggestions for healthy dining at ethnic restaurants.

Choosing low-fat condiments is a great way to cut fat and calories. Ask for low-fat or fat-free salad dressing. If that is not available, ask for the dressing on the side so you can control the amount. Try salsa with a baked potato instead of sour cream or butter. Choose mustard instead of mayonnaise on sandwiches.

Use the Fork Method

Salads are a great way to get more vegetables in your diet, until you kill them with high-fat dressing. You can easily add hundreds of calories to a salad with just a few tablespoons of dressing. Use the fork method for dressing. Ask for dressing on the side. Dip your fork into the dressing, and then load your fork with salad. You may be surprised how little dressing you need.

Choose pasta dishes with tomato sauces instead of cream sauces. An order of Fettuccini Alfredo has over 1,000 calories, whereas an order of spaghetti with marinara sauce has about half that many. Choose foods that are baked, grilled, broiled, poached, or steamed. A general rule of thumb is that when you fry fish or chicken you double the calories.

If you are eating at a buffet restaurant, fill up on low-calorie salad and vegetables. Choose smaller portions of

Table 3.1

Healthier Options at Popular Ethnic Restaurants

Chinese Restaurants

- Choose entrees with lots of vegetables, such as chicken with vegetables (make sure the chicken is not breaded and fried). Moo goo gai pan (chicken and vegetables in a clear sauce) has just 270 calories per cup versus 400 calories per cup of sweet and sour chicken (fried chicken with just a few vegetables).
- Choose steamed foods. Fried foods like egg rolls and wontons are high in fat and calories. One egg roll can have as many as 200 calories.
- Choose steamed rice. Fried rice can have double the calories and fat of steamed rice.

Mexican Restaurants

- Be an especially careful diner. A typical meal at a Mexican restaurant can tip the scales at over 1,000 calories.
- Order your entrée without cheese or ask them to go light on the cheese.
- Go easy on the chip basket. Fried tortilla chips are loaded with fat.
- Choose chicken dishes that are grilled instead of fried.
- Choose plain rice and black beans instead of refried beans.
- Choose salsa or picante sauce over guacamole or sour cream.
- Choose soft corn or flour tortillas instead of fried tortillas, such as you find in chimichangas or hard tacos.

Italian Restaurants

- Choose red instead of cream sauces.
- Control pasta portions by sharing or asking for half an order.
- Order grilled meat or fish instead of breaded and fried items, such as chicken or eggplant Parmesan.
- Order thin-crust pizza with lots of vegetables and no extra cheese.

Which Side Are You On?

Menu Labeling: Good Idea for Consumers or Unnecessary Burden on Restaurants?

You are now aware of the number of meals eaten outside the home. With so many meals eaten at restaurants and fast-food outlets, what you eat when you eat out significantly contributes to your overall health.

How do you know how many calories or grams of fat you are eating when you eat out? Health advocates suggest that menu labeling can help consumers choose healthier options when dining out. Menu labeling puts nutrition information on the menu or menu boards so that the information is available at the point of decision and purchase.

Many restaurants already provide this type of information to consumers, but it is often on websites or posters that are not readily accessible at the time of order. Several policies have been proposed at the local, state, and national levels to require chain restaurants that have multiple outlets to provide this information. California, New York City, and Philadelphia all have laws that require menu labeling. Several national chains have voluntarily started using menu labeling. Subway was the first large chain to add calories to its menus; Panera Bread and Yum! Brands (KFC, Taco Bell, Pizza Hut, Long John Silver's, and A&W) now provide menu labeling. Many other restaurant chains are considering implementing menu labeling nationwide.

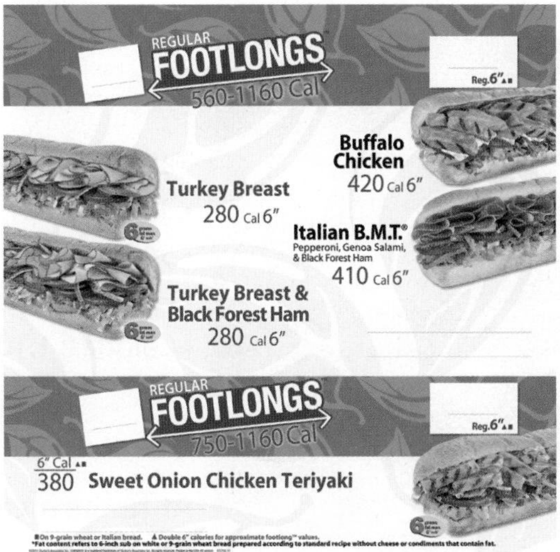
REGULAR
FOOTLONGS
560-1160 Cal
Reg.6"
Buffalo Chicken
420 Cal 6"
Turkey Breast
280 Cal 6"
Italian B.M.T.®
Pepperoni, Genoa Salami, & Black Forest Ham
410 Cal 6"
Turkey Breast & Black Forest Ham
280 Cal 6"
REGULAR
FOOTLONGS
750-1160 Cal
Reg.6"
6" Cal
380 Sweet Onion Chicken Teriyaki

Subway Labels the Menu Board with the Calories for Each Sandwich

Source: © Subway/Franchise World Headquarters.

Most consumers want menu labeling; as many as 83% of Americans support menu labeling.[58] However, the food industry's support of legislation to mandate menu labeling is mixed. Some in the food industry argue that they already provide nutritional information in brochures or on the Web; that most people know how many calories are in foods commonly served in restaurants; that it is not the government's role to regulate restaurants in this manner; that it will be costly and could put restaurants out of business; and that it is not the solution to obesity. Let's look at each of these arguments.

Nutrition information for many restaurants is available on their website. Some restaurants even have brochures or posters with nutrition information at the restaurant. However, people need the information when they order to help them make their selection. One study examined how often consumers consulted on-premises nutritional information. Almost no one (0.1%) used the brochure or poster provided by the restaurant to check the calories of the food they were about to order.[59] In contrast, when the calories were posted on the menu board or menu, consumers ate fewer calories and were less likely to order high-calorie menu items.[60,61]

Estimating calories in restaurant meals is very difficult. You do not know how the food is prepared or exactly how much of any given ingredient is added. Who would think that a single restaurant meal could have one-half to an entire day's worth of calories, that a tuna salad sandwich could have more calories than a roast beef sandwich, or that a specialty coffee drink could have over 1,000 calories? Too often, diners underestimate the number of calories and overestimate the healthfulness of menu items.[62–64] On average, 90% of people underestimate the number of calories in restaurant meals by hundreds of calories.[61] Even nutrition professionals have problems accurately estimating the number of calories in restaurant meals.[65]

Some people feel that it is not the government's role to regulate restaurants in this manner and that it will put a financial burden on restaurants. However, the government requires many businesses to disclose what is in their products. Consumers expect to see ingredients and nutrition information on packaged foods. Even cosmetic products are required to disclose specific contents.

The restaurant industry argues that menu labeling is not feasible because of constantly changing menus and special orders. They argue further that it is costly and will put smaller restaurants out of business. However, menu labeling applies only to standard menu items. If you order your Big Mac or Whopper with extra cheese, you will have to use the basic calories for the regular sandwich and know you are getting more calories thanks to your special request. As to the cost to restaurants, most already have the nutritional information; changing the menu boards or menus is a one-time cost. Current proposals only require chain restaurants to label menus with nutritional information, not small restaurants that may not be able to afford it.

Finally, there is the argument that eating out is not the sole cause of obesity and that simply labeling foods in restaurants will not solve the problem. Obesity is a complex issue with many contributing factors, and it will take actions from many groups and a variety of strategies to effectively reduce its incidence. However, menu labeling can be part of the solution. It will educate consumers as to the calories in common menu items, making it easier to make informed

(continues)

decisions when eating out. It has been estimated that even if only a small percentage of consumers chose differently based on menu labeling, it could have a sizable positive impact on obesity.[66]

The Patient Protection and Affordable Care Act of 2010 requires restaurants and similar retail food establishments with 20 or more locations, including drive thrus, to list calorie content information for standard menu items on restaurant menus and menu boards. The FDA is in charge of the implementation of this law and is working to collect information from consumers and the food industry. When menu labeling will be required has not yet been determined.

Now that you know the potential benefits of menu labeling, do you think it is a good idea to require chain restaurants to provide menu labeling? When it is available, how would it impact your choices at restaurants?

lean, grilled meats, and skip the potato bar that offers high-fat cheese sauce, chili, bacon, and butter.

Desserts are another way to pick up lots of calories. Most restaurant desserts are loaded with calories. Sorbet or fresh fruit are good low-fat choices that are offered by some restaurants. If you must have the death by chocolate, crème brule, or strawberry cheesecake, order one for the table and have just a bite or two.

Prepare and Eat More Meals at Home

So, why are we going to talk about cooking in a class on nutrition and wellness? Eating and preparing more meals at home is a critical step in improving your diet. It is very difficult to eat healthy if many of your meals are eaten away from home (**Figure 3.7**). Further, relying on highly processed convenience foods is not healthy either. That leaves simple foods that you prepare yourself. If you don't know how to cook, then you should learn. Cooking doesn't have to take a lot of time, it is healthier, and it can even save you money.

10 Keys to Cooking Smart

You don't have to be a TV-ready chef or make gourmet meals. Just learn the basics. Here are some suggestions to get you started:

1. *Keep it simple.* It's important to remember that simple is best. Use simple cooking techniques, simple ingredients, simple recipes, and simple menu planning. Learn to make just a few simple meals and build your repertoire from there.
2. *Make room to cook.* If you don't have space on your countertop to cook, then cooking will not be a pleasant experience. You don't need a large kitchen, just an uncluttered one with at least a little counter space. Clear your counter of unnecessary clutter such as decorator items, mail, or small appliances that are not used daily. Keep as much of the kitchen counter as possible clear for food preparation so that when it is time to cook you don't have to stop and make room each time.
3. *Clean as you go.* Waiting until the end of the meal to do any cleaning will quickly cause your cooking area to become cluttered. Clean pots, pans, bowls, and cooking utensils as you use them. If you have a small space, you may even choose to dry and put away items as you use them.
4. Mise en place *(pronounced "meez ahn plahs")*. The literal translation of this French phrase is "everything in place." In commercial kitchens, chefs put everything they will need in place when preparing for the night. For the home cook, it means to get organized before you begin. Assemble all the ingredients and equipment you need. Think of *mise en place* as an organized, enjoyable way to prepare food, instead of preparing food in chaos with unneeded stress.

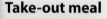

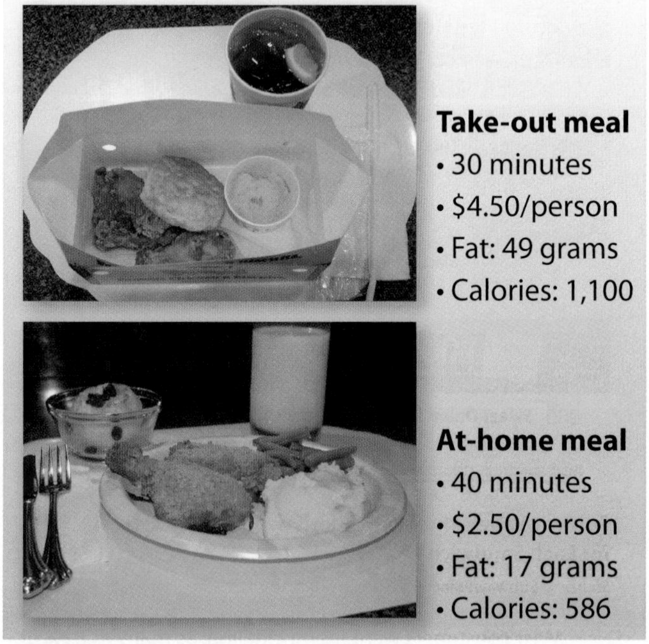
Take-out meal
• 30 minutes
• $4.50/person
• Fat: 49 grams
• Calories: 1,100
At-home meal
• 40 minutes
• $2.50/person
• Fat: 17 grams
• Calories: 586

■ **Figure 3.7**

At-Home Meal Versus Take-out Meal

Preparing simple meals at home does not have to be complicated. The at-home meal consists of oven-fried chicken, canned green beans, mashed potatoes cooked in the microwave, and a microwaved baked apple. It took only 40 minutes to prepare, with only about half of that hands-on time. The take-out meal took 30 minutes to go and get the meal from the drive thru. The two biggest differences are the cost and the nutritional value.

5. *Develop your own style.* Wherever you live, you'll have access to a variety of wonderful foods. Develop your own style of cooking. Cooking can be a way to express your individuality.
6. *Go slow.* Give yourself time to develop the cooking skills you need. A number of resources are available on the Internet and in your community that can help you develop basic cooking skills. You can also ask a friend or family member who cooks to offer you some pointers. Don't be overly ambitious when you first start cooking. If you have never made a recipe before or are trying a technique for the first time, give yourself a little extra time. Mistakes happen; even experienced cooks make mistakes. Learn from your mistakes and try again.
7. *Trust your instincts.* Use your instincts of smell, taste, and touch. Use a recipe as a guide. If it calls for 1 teaspoon of salt and the dish tastes good with half that, then great; if it calls for rosemary and that is not a favorite of yours, substitute something else or leave it out. Use your instincts to make food the way you want it. One of the best things about making meals at home is that you are in charge.
8. *Organize your recipes.* Recipes thrown into a drawer in no particular order will not be used. Find a system that works for you to organize your recipes. You may like a card file or a three-ring binder. It does not matter as long as you create a system that enables you to find your recipes when you need them.
9. *Find the joy.* Look for the joy in cooking. Make food for yourself, friends, and family. Nothing says love any louder. Even if it is just a meal for you, try to enjoy the process. Think of cooking as something you get to do for yourself and others, not as a chore. Keep it interesting by continually trying new techniques and foods.
10. *Plan.* The most important key for cooking smart is to plan. If you don't plan, you will probably not have the foods you need to cook dinner and will most likely be frustrated and end up going out or ordering in. Set aside just 30 minutes a week, which is all you need to plan your meals for the week. Make a list of the main dish and side dishes you will make for each day of the week. Find what works for you. You may just want to plan a few days at a time. Select recipes with few ingredients. It does not have to be complicated to be healthy and delicious.

Importance of Family Meals

When you think of a family meal, you might envision a scene of a family gathered around a big table awaiting the serving of a large turkey at Thanksgiving. Family meals are not something that should be reserved for special occasions. Eating simple meals together as a family has been shown to have many positive effects. Families who eat together at home eat more fruits and vegetables, fewer fried foods, and less soda and saturated fat.[67,68] Regular family meals also contribute to the formation of healthy eating habits in children.[69,70] The evidence suggests that the more children eat meals together as a family, the less likely they are to be overweight.[71] Family meals also benefit older children and adolescents. As the number of family meals eaten together increases, so do grade point averages and self-esteem. Having family meals together has also been found to decrease depression; suicide attempts; and tobacco, alcohol, and marijuana use.[72]

Try Something New

Make a Weekly Plan

How do you decide what you are going to eat for dinner? Often a plan can make the difference between having a healthy meal or reaching for fast food. Making a weekly plan for at least your evening meal will help you steer clear of unhealthy options like the number one value meal from a fast-food restaurant. Once you get the hang of it, it does not take too much time or effort. The time you do invest pays big dividends in meals that promote health and help you maintain a healthy weight.

Start by making a list of the simple, healthy entrees and side dishes that you know how to make and that you and your family and friends enjoy. Sometime during the week, set aside 30 minutes to plan for the next week. Make a list of the main dish and the side dishes that you will make each day of the week. You may make roast chicken on Sunday and then plan to eat the leftovers ("planned-overs") on Wednesday. If you know your week will be especially hectic, you may want to cook more than one meal ahead of time so that it is ready to reheat and eat.

For inspiration, look at cookbooks, websites, or grocery store flyers. Keep it simple; choose recipes with five or fewer ingredients. Choose one-pot entrees, such as stir-fry or stew. Use time savers such as bagged salad or precut or frozen vegetables. Be sure to include quick dinner ideas as part of your plan. Each week, you could have one night that is soup and sandwich and/or one night that is a cheese omelet and toast. Now that you have your plan for the week, make your shopping list so you will have the foods you need on hand to follow your plan.

Plan for Leftovers: "Planned-Overs"

Leftovers sometimes get a bad reputation. Leftovers can become "planned-overs" and make your week a lot less hectic in the kitchen. Making extra of an entrée or side dish and incorporating it into another meal is a great way to save time and money. You may have more time on one day of the week that you could cook several items that you will eat on another day. Some foods taste even better the next day, after the flavors have had a chance to mix and develop. Foods like soups or stews often taste better the next day.

Think of the remaining food as an ingredient, not the same food a second time around. Tonight's roast chicken can be reinvented into chicken quesadillas tomorrow night. That same leftover roast chicken can be added to a green salad for lunch or chopped and mixed with celery, walnuts, and grapes for chicken salad.

Freezing foods allows you to have precooked meals that you can pull out on a busy weeknight and serve. If a recipe makes eight servings and you only need two or four, prepare the full recipe and freeze the extra for later in the month. Place the frozen food in the refrigerator to thaw the night before and then reheat it for a quick dinner when you get home from work or school. You may want to freeze individual portions to control portion size.

Shop Smart

Make time in your schedule to shop for the foods you need each week. It may be better for you to shop more or less often; decide what works for you. Visit local farmers' markets or farm stands for lower prices and better quality. Make a list of the things you need for the week. Be a label-reader. This is the best way to learn about what you are eating.

Buy simple foods. Heavily processed foods or frozen foods that mimic restaurant take-out are not much better than eating out, because they can contain lots of calories and fat. One rule of thumb is to shop on the perimeter of the store. This is where you will find the fresh fruits and vegetables, meats, and dairy. The less processed the better. The best part about preparing more meals at home is that you are in control. You don't have to rely on boxed or frozen dinners that are highly processed.

Time Savers Plenty of time-savers are available that you can add to your shopping list. The produce department offers bagged salads, precut fruits and vegetables, and other items that are ready to use with no preparation. Canned or frozen fruits and vegetables can be prepared in a flash. Choose varieties without added sauce, butter, or sugar. The meat department now has many cuts of boneless, skinless chicken; pork; or beef that can be prepared in minutes.

Money Savers You can eat healthy and still save money. If you shop with a list, you will be less likely to buy things you don't need and will buy the things you do need to prepare more meals at home. Before you complete your list, check what you have on hand. Check the pantry, refrigerator, and freezer. Don't forget to keep the basics on hand. They can allow for quick changes to your menu and provide snacks or easy breakfasts and lunches.

Try Something New

Create Your Perfect Pantry

A well-stocked pantry is key for quick, healthy meals. Even if you only have a small space, a pantry stocked with staples that can easily be turned into a simple meal may make the difference between a home-cooked dinner and a call for pizza delivery. Your refrigerator and freezer can supply additional ingredients for quick meals. You should keep items on hand that you use on a regular basis. Here are some suggestions to get you started.

Dry or Canned Foods

- Canned beans
- Canned chicken
- Canned fruit
- Canned tuna or salmon
- Canned vegetables
- Nuts
- Pasta
- Rice
- Soup
- Spaghetti sauce

Freezer Foods

- Chicken
- Fruit
- Ground beef
- Vegetables
- Whole-grain bread

Refrigerator Foods

- Bag salad
- Cheese
- Eggs
- Fruit
- Milk
- Vegetables
- Yogurt

Condiments and Spices

- Olive oil
- Pepper
- Salt
- Spices (three or four of your favorites)
- Vegetable oil
- Vinegar

Use foods that are in-season. In-season foods are often cheaper. However, if they are not, remember that canned fruits and vegetables are just as healthy and can provide needed nutrition for your family.

Check the newspaper or in-store flyers for sale items. If you had planned on having broccoli but you see that cabbage is on sale, make a quick change to save money. If an item is on sale that you normally buy every week, you may want to stock up. If you find a sale on a main dish food item such as meat or poultry that is just too good to pass up, consider changing your menu.

Use unit pricing to select the best value.
The largest size is not always the best value. Using unit pricing, we can see that the large can of tuna is 19 cents per ounce, whereas the small can of tuna is only 11 cents per ounce.

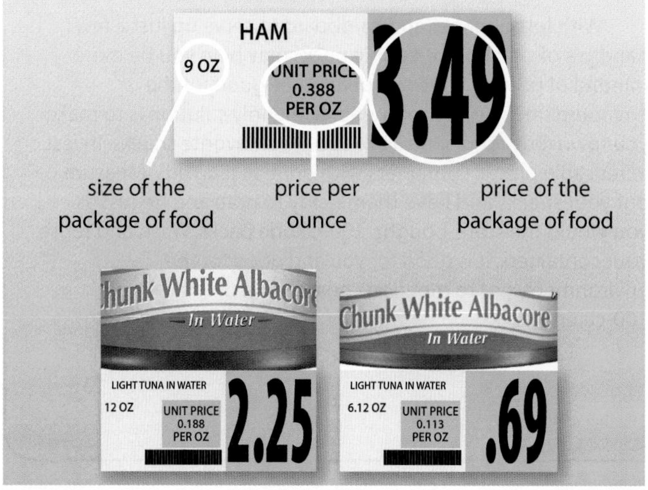

■ **Figure 3.8**
Use Unit Pricing to Select the Best Value

Using coupons can also save you money if you use them wisely. When you shop, look for coupons along the store aisles. Many grocery stores have coupons either on the back of a receipt or as a separate receipt when you check out. Local newspapers generally have a couple of food coupon flyers in the paper each week. You can also find coupons in magazines and on the Internet.

Have a special place, such as an envelope or a drawer, to store the coupons you save. Check your coupons each week to see if you have any for items on your shopping list. Be sure to keep track of the expiration dates for coupons. If you have some coupons that will expire, you may want to adjust your menu to help you use the coupon. Many stores have double or even triple coupon days. This is a good day to shop if you are a coupon clipper.

Be savvy when using coupons. Buying the largest size of an item is not always the best buy. Use unit pricing to find the best value (**Figure 3.8**). Only use coupons for foods you would buy as part of your week's worth of food. Don't buy an item just because you have a coupon.

Pack It to Go

Many of you are more than likely on the go most of the day. That may mean that fast food, vending machines, and skipping meals is your norm. None of these are consistent with good health. You already know the pitfalls of too much fast food. Vending machine items are often high-calorie, unhealthy options. Skipping meals is not a good idea either. Skipping meals can lead to binge eating and weight gain. People who eat fewer times during the day are heavier than those who eat regular meals.[73] Eating regularly will help you maintain a high metabolic rate and burn more calories. Eating regularly also helps you con-

For Fast Food, Go Slow

One of the fastest ways to have an entire meal prepared when you get home from work or school is to use a slow cooker, which is also called a crock pot. You can buy a slow cooker at a discount store for under $20. In the morning, place chicken, vegetables, stock, and spices in the slow cooker; when you come home, your meal is ready. It will only take one try to make you a slow cooker fan. If you are on a tight food budget, try dried beans. For about $2, you have a whole pot of low-fat, high-fiber, high-protein beans that cook while you are away. Slow-cooker recipes are readily available on the Internet. Here is one to get you started.

CROCK POT CHICKEN AND VEGETABLES

Ingredients

- 1 cup fresh mushrooms, sliced
- 2 carrots, sliced
- 2 onions, sliced
- 2 celery ribs, cut in 1 inch pieces
- 6 boneless, skinless chicken breast halves (about 1.5 pounds)
- 1 cup water
- 1/2 cup white wine (or 1/2 cup additional water)
- 1/2 teaspoon dried basil
- 2 teaspoons dried parsley
- Dash of red pepper flacks
- Black pepper, to taste
- Salt, to taste

Instructions

1. Combine the vegetables in the crock pot.
2. Place chicken on top of vegetables.
3. Mix together the remaining ingredients and pour over chicken.
4. Cook on high 4–5 hours.

Notes

- This dish can be served as a stew or you may choose to strain the broth and serve it on the side as you would gravy.
- This is a low-fat alternative to heavy chicken gravy made with fat and flour.
- The vegetables in this dish can be doubled; increase cooking time by about one hour.
- Rice is a nice complement to this dish.

Nutrition Information per Serving

(Makes 6 servings) Made with 1/2 teaspoon salt.

Calories **190** | Total Fat **3.5 g** | Saturated Fat **1 g** | Protein **28 g** | Carbohydrates **7 g** | Fiber **2 g** | Sodium **280 mg**

An Easy Slow-Cooker Recipe

Green and Healthy

Make Your Own 100-Calorie Packs

You have no doubt seen the 100-calorie packages of snacks. These 100-calorie packs portion out exactly 100 calories of crackers, cookies, candy, or chips. They make portion control easy. No more guessing about how many crackers is a serving or worrying about eating too many cookies out of the large box. Do these 100-calorie packs help you consume fewer snacks? The evidence suggests that they do. Research on 100-calorie packs compared to eating out of the regular-size box found that the preportioned packs helped people consume less. Even if they ate more than one package, it was less than when they ate out of the regular-size box. Also, after they were exposed to the 100-calorie packs and saw what 100 calories of a given food looked like, they ate less when making their own portion choices.[74]

With lots of paper and cardboard to serve up just a few handfuls of snacks, 100-calorie packs may help you be more mindful of portion control, but are they good for the environment? The environmentally friendly solution is to make your own. Buy regular-size boxes of your favorite snacks. Invest in reusable plastic containers with tight-sealing lids. Measure out your snacks and have them ready to grab and go just as you would the store-bought, 100-calorie packs. Wash and reuse your containers. It is good for you and good for the environment, not to mention cheaper than buying the 100-calorie packs.

trol your appetite. When you do not eat for a prolonged period of time, like when you skip a meal, your body goes into starvation mode, and your metabolism slows down to preserve energy. An alternative to unhealthy options or to not eating at all is to take it with you. Carrying a small cooler with snacks and/or a meal is a great way to take control over what you eat throughout the day. If you have healthy choices throughout the day, you will not be tempted by the vending machine, convenience store, or fast-food outlet.

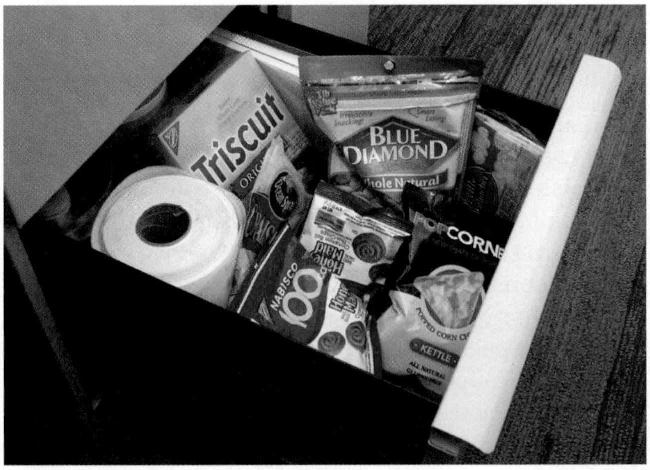

■ **Figure 3.10**

Keep a Healthy Snack in Your Desk, Locker, or Backpack

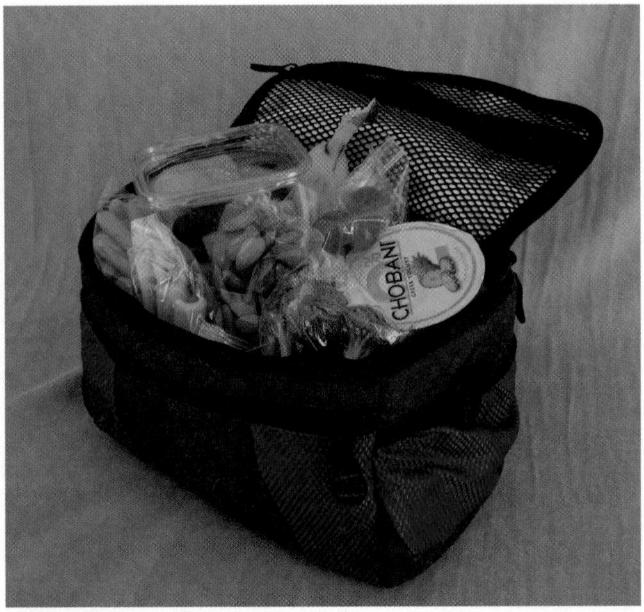

■ **Figure 3.9**

Take Healthy Foods with You

A small cooler with a freezer pack and healthy foods will keep you away from fast food and the vending machine.

Packing healthy foods to go does not have to be difficult. Get a small cooler with a couple of freezer packs to keep it cold (**Figure 3.9**). Throw in fruit, vegetables, a sandwich, cheese and crackers, a pudding cup, yogurt, or leftovers from the night before. Be sure to pack water in an eco-friendly bottle so that you don't hit the vending machine for high-calorie beverages.

In addition, keep a healthy snack bag in your car, desk, locker, or backpack. Fill a large zipper-top bag with granola bars, low-fat crackers, raisins, nuts, or small bags of unsweetened cereal (**Figure 3.10**). This is great for emergencies when you have to work or study late or need a snack before your evening workout. Just a few minutes to plan your own "to go" foods will help you steer clear of unhealthy options.

Green and Healthy

Paper or Plastic?

Today, the question of paper or plastic is rarely asked. Four out of five grocery bags are now plastic, so the choice is usually made for you—plastic. Which is better for the environment, paper or plastic? Let's examine both. Then you can make your own green decision.

About 1 billion plastic grocery bags are used in the United States each year. The number used worldwide is a staggering 500 billion, or 1 million bags a minute.[75] Plastic grocery bags are cheap, about a penny a bag. Because they are so inexpensive, more are often used than needed. Bananas, one bag; dish soap, another bag; a loaf of bread gets its own bag; what may have fit into one or two bags may get loaded into four or five.

The production of plastic bags requires energy and water. It takes about 12 million barrels of oil to produce the bags used in the United States alone. What happens to the bags after they are brought home from the grocery or convenience store? Only about 5% are recycled.[75] Recycled bags are melted and made into other plastics, such as plastic lumber. About half of the rest of the bags are burned to generate energy. This has its downside as well. Inks and additives in the plastic cause the emission of toxins (dioxins and heavy metals) into the environment. Manufacturers continue to increase their use of nontoxic inks, but the ash from the bags once they are burned is a toxic substance that must be disposed in a toxic waste dump. Bags that are not recycled or burned for energy end up in the landfill where they stay, and stay. Although there is no consensus on how long it takes a plastic bag to break down, most experts agree that, conservatively, it is hundreds of years. This means that the first plastic bags introduced in 1977 that were put into landfills are still there. Even if plastic bags are repurposed around the house for trashcan liners, book bags, or animal waste, many ultimately end up in the landfill.

Paper grocery bags must be the right choice. Not so fast, let's examine paper grocery bags and their impact on the environment. Paper bags are made from trees, and lots of them. Harvesting and transporting tress as well as the actual paper production requires oil and water. One paper bag requires 1 gallon of water, nearly 50 times the amount required for a plastic bag. Paper bags require more resources to produce than plastic ones, but they are more recyclable.[75] About 40% of paper bags are recycled, and those that do end up in the landfill will degrade. Paper bags are more expensive than plastic, about 4 cents compared to a penny, so retailers may not use as many.

Both types of bags take a lot of resources to produce, more resources to recycle, and many end up in the landfill. Not an easy choice. What can we do about all the bags that we need to bring home food, beverages, and other household goods? Some countries have begun taxing bags to encourage consumers to use fewer or to bring bags from home. Although there is not a tax on bags in the United States or Canada, it does point to an easy solution to the question of paper or plastic. The answer is neither. Bring your own reusable bag. You can find them everywhere for about $1 each. Buy a couple and keep them in your car. You now have the green solution to paper or plastic.

Ready to Make a Change

Are you ready to make a change, small or large, in where you eat most of your meals? Make the commitment to take the first step. Whether it is a small, medium, or large change, it is a step in the right direction toward healthier behaviors.

I commit to a small first step. Decrease the number of times you eat at a restaurant or fast-food outlet. Assess how many times you eat out each week. Make the commitment to reduce that number by half. Instead, plan simple healthy meals at home.

I am ready to take the next step and make a medium change. Eat out only once or twice a week and pack food from home for lunch and snacks during the day. Having food with you during the day is really a eat-smart survival kit. Because you'll have healthy foods that you have made, you won't have to rely on fast food or processed food from vending machines or convenience stores.

I have been making changes for some time and am ready to make a large change in eating and preparing more meals at home. Plan meals for the week and follow your plan. Use whatever system works for you; a white board on the refrigerator, notes in your planner or smartphone, or something you devise for yourself. Planning meals helps you be mindful of the foods you are eating and makes shopping for the week much easier. You will have the foods you need on hand to follow through on your weekly plan.

Myth Versus Fact

Myth: If I want to decease the sodium in my diet, all I need to do is put down the saltshaker.

Fact: Steering clear of the saltshaker is a step in the right direction to decrease sodium. However, most of the sodium in your diet comes from processed foods and foods eaten in restaurants. Even if you don't salt your food, the salt is already in there. Decrease the frequency that you eat out and use fewer processed foods to really decrease sodium in your diet.

Myth: It is easy to estimate the number of calories in foods served in restaurants. You don't need a label to know how many calories they have.

Fact: Even nutrition professionals have a hard time accurately estimating the calories in restaurant meals. If they were labeled with the number of calories they contain, you would be able to choose a healthier meal.

Myth: Eating out most meals is OK as long as you choose healthy options.

Fact: When you eat out, choosing healthy options will certainly help. However, even if you are a careful diner you will have trouble eating healthy if most of your meals are eaten in restaurants or fast-food outlets.

Myth: If you are served and eat a large portion, you will just make up for that by eating less at the next meal or over the next day or so.

Fact: You do not compensate for larger portions by eating less the rest of the day. In fact, when served large portions, you eat more calories than you need over time.

Myth: I don't have time to cook.

Fact: Cooking simple meals at home does not have to take much longer than going through the drive thru. Planning makes it happen. Make the time to prepare healthy foods for yourself and your family and friends. You are worth the effort.

Myth: Eating snacks out of the box is ok if you are careful not to consume too much.

Fact: Eating snacks out of a large box is not a good idea. You will most likely end up consuming more than you need and probably more than you think. Portion out snacks into a smaller container so you know how much you are eating.

Myth: Paper bags are a better choice for the environment over plastic.

Fact: Neither is really a great choice for the environment. Bring reusable bags from home to carry your purchases to be truly environmentally friendly.

Back to the Story

Linda is not unlike many college students—busy and with no time to eat healthy, or so she thinks. Linda can make some small changes that will add up to big health rewards. She will be able to function better as a student, she will have more energy, and she may even have more money in her pocket.

Linda is eating breakfast, which is good. However, fast-food restaurants offer very few healthy choices for breakfast. She is better off with a bowl of cereal. If she needs something to grab and go, she can take a peanut butter sandwich or a low-fat granola bar and fruit. For lunch, she needs to get into the habit of packing her snacks and lunch. It will keep her from skipping meals and will also save money, because she will not be stopping by the food court at school. She should grab a small cooler and pack it with yogurt, fruit, a sandwich, and water. She could even pack it the night before. If she knows that she is going to be out during the dinner hour as well, she can pack even more food so that the pizza she usually grabs becomes a once-a-week occurrence instead of what she eats on most nights.

On the nights she cooks at home, she can expand her repertoire to include healthier items like stir-fry vegetables or grilled chicken. Relying on heavily processed convenience foods is not much better than eating out. If she lacks the skills to cook, she can find a beginning cooking class in her community or find a friend or family member who cooks to help her with some basics. The once or twice a week that Linda eats out with friends is a great time for her to practice her skills of eating healthy at a restaurant. She may want to ask one of her friends to split a meal with her to save money as well as get a more reasonable portion.

References

1. National Restaurant Association. Facts at a glance. http://www.restaurant.org/research/facts/. Accessed March 3, 2010.
2. French SA, Story M, Jeffery RW. Environmental influences on eating and physical activity. *Ann Rev Public Health*. 2001;22:309–335.
3. USDA, Economic Research Service. Food expenditure series. http://www.ers.usda.gov/Briefing/CPIFoodandexpenditures/data/. Updated September 3, 2008. Accessed March 3, 2010.
4. Hayden S, Blisard N, Jolliffe D. *Let's Eat Out: Americans Weigh Taste, Convenience, and Nutrition*. USDA, Economic Research Service, 2006. Economic Information Bulletin no. 19.
5. Schlosser E. *Fast Food Nation*. New York: Houghton Mifflin, 2001.
6. Hoovers. Industry overview: fast food and quick service restaurants. http://www.hoovers.com/fast-food-and-quickservice-restaurants/--ID__269--/free-ind-fr-profile-basic.xhtml. Accessed March 3, 2010.
7. Sloan EA. What, when, and where America eats. *Food Technology*. 2006;January:18–27.
8. NPD Group. The NPD Group releases findings from its 20th annual report on eating patterns in America. http://www.npd.com/press/releases/press_051006.html. Updated October 6, 2005. Accessed April 11, 2011.
9. The Keystone Center. The Keystone Forum on away from home foods final report: opportunities for preventing weight gain and obesity. May 2006. http://www.keystone.org. Accessed April 10, 2007.
10. Frazao E, Ed. America's eating habits: changes and consequences. USDA. Economic Research Service. http://www.ers.usda.gov/publications/aib750/. Updated May 1, 1999. Accessed March 4, 2010.
11. Gutherie JF, Lin BH, Frazao E. Role of food prepared away from home in the American diet, 1977–78 versus 1994–96: changes and consequences. *J Nutr Edu Behav*. 2002;34:140–150.
12. Gillman MW, Rifas-Shiman SL, Frazier AL, et al. Family dinner and diet quality among older children and adolescents. *Arch Fam Med*. 2000;9:235–240.
13. McLaughlin C, Tarasuk V, Kreiger N. An examination of at-home food preparation skills among low-income, food-insecure women. *J Am Diet Assoc*. 2003;103:1506–1512.
14. Neumark-Sztainer D, Hannan PJ, Story M, Croll J, Perry C. Family meal patterns: Associations with sociodemographic characteristics and improved dietary intake among adolescents. *J Am Diet Assoc*. 2003;103:317–322.
15. Kant AK, Graubard BI. Eating out in America, 1987–2000: trends and nutritional correlates. *Prev Med*. 2003:38(2):243–249.
16. US Department of Labor, Bureau of Labor Statistics. Average annual expenditures and characteristics of all consumer units, consumer expenditure survey, 1993–2001. http://www.bls.gov/cex. Accessed March 4, 2010.
17. French SA, Harnack L, Jeffery RE. Fast food restaurant use among women in Pound of Prevention study: dietary, behavioral and demographic correlates. *Int J Obes Relat Metab Disord*. 2000;24:1353–1359.
18. French SA. Pricing affects food choices. *J Nutr*. 2003;133:841S–843S.
19. You W, Zhang G, Davy BM, Carlson A, Lin BH. Food consumed away from home can be a part of a healthy and affordable diet. *J Nutr*. 2009;139:1994–1999.
20. Paeratakul S, Ferdinand DP, Champagne CM, Ryan DH, Bray GA. Fast-food consumption among US adults and children: dietary and nutrient intake profile. *J Am Diet Assoc*. 2003;103(10):1332–1338.
21. Bowman SA, Gortmaker SL, Ebbeling CB, Pereira MA, Ludwig DS. Effects of fast-food consumption on energy intake and diet quality among children in a national household survey. *Pediatrics*. 2004;113(1):112–118.
22. Bowman SA, Vinyard BT. Fast food consumption of US adults: Impact on energy and nutri-

ent intakes and overweight status. *J Am Coll Nutr*. 2004;23(2):163–168.
23. Moore LV, Roux AVD, Nettleton JA, Jacobs DR, Franco M. Fast-food consumption, diet quality, and neighborhood exposure to fast food the multi-ethnic study of atherosclerosis. *Am J Epidemiol*. 2009;170:29–36.
24. Thompson OM, Ballew C, Resnicow K, Must A, Bandini LG, Cyr H, Dietz WH. Food purchased away from home as a predictor of change in BMI z-score among girls. *Inter J Obes*. 2004;28:282–289.
25. Smiciklas-Wright H, Mitchell DC, Mickle SJ, Goldman JD, Cook A. Foods commonly eaten in the United States, 1989–1991 and 1994–1996: are portion sizes changing? *J Am Diet Assoc*. 2003;103:41–47.
26. Young LR, Nestle M. The contribution of expanding portion sizes to the US obesity epidemic. *Am J Pub Health*. 2002;92:246–249.
27. Nielsen SJ, Popkin BM. Patterns and trends in food portion sizes, 1977–1998. *JAMA*. 2003;289(4):450–453.
28. Young LR, Nestle M. The contribution of expanding portion sizes to the US obesity epidemic. *Am J Pub Health*. 2002;92:246–249.
29. Rolls BJ, Roe LS, Kral TVE, Meengs JS, Wall DE. Increasing the portion size of a packaged snack increases energy intake in men and women. *Appetite*. 2004;42(1):63–69.
30. Young LR, Nestle MS. Portion sizes in dietary assessment: issues and policy implication. *Nutr Rev*. 1995;53:149–158.
31. Ello-Martin JA, Roe LS, Menngs JS, Wall DE, Rolls BJ. Increasing the portion size of a unit food increases energy intake. *Appetite*. 2002;39:74.
32. Young LR, Nestle M. Variation in perceptions of a "medium" food portion: implications for dietary guidance. *J Am Diet Assoc*. 1998;98:458–459.
33. Rolls BJ, Morris EL, Roe LS. Portion size of food affects energy intake in normal-weight and overweight men and women. *Am J Clin Nutr*. 2002;76:1207–1213.
34. Rolls BJ, Roe LS, Meengs JS, Wall DE. Increasing the portion size of a sandwich increases energy intake. *J Am Diet Assoc*. 2004;104:367–372.
35. Rolls BJ, Roe LS, Kral TVE, Menngs JS, Wall DE. Increasing the portion size of a packaged snack increases energy intake in men and women. *Appetite*. 2004;42(1):63–69.
36. Wansink B, Park SB. At the movies: how external cues and perceived taste impact consumption volume. *J Database Marketing*. 1996;60:1–14.
37. Wansink B, Just DR, Payne CR. Mindless eating and healthy heuristics for the irrational. *Am Econom Rev*. 2009;99:165–169.
38. Rols BJ. The supersizing of America: Portion size and the obesity epidemic. *Nutr Today*. 2003;38:42–53.
39. Wansink B. Can package size accelerate usage volume? *J Marketing*. 1996;60:1–14.
40. Wansink, B, Kim J. Bad popcorn in big buckets: portion size can influence intake as much as taste. *J Nutr Educ Behav*. 2005;37:242–245.
41. Savage JS, Fisher JO, Birch LL. Parental influence on eating behavior: conception to adolescence. *J Law Med Ethics*. 2007;35:2–34.
42. Fisher JO, Rolls BJ, Birch LL. Children's bite size and intake of an entrée are greater with large portions than with age-appropriate or self-selected portions. *Am J Clin Nutr*. 2003;77:1164–1170.
43. McConahy KL, Smiciklas-Wright H, Mitchell DC, Picciano MF. Portion size of common foods predict energy intake among preschool-aged children. *J Am Diet Assoc*. 2004;104:975–979.
44. Strazzullo P, E'Elia L, Kandala NB, Cappuccio FP. Salt intake, stroke, and cardiovascular disease: meta analysis of prospective studies. *BMJ*. 2009;339:b4567.
45. Mohan S, Campbell NRC, Willis K. Effective population-wide public health interventions to promote sodium reduction. *CMAJ*. 2009;181(9):605–609.
46. Lawes CM, Vander Hoom S, Rodgers A. International Society of Hypertension. Global burden of blood-pressure-related disease, 2001. *Lancet*. 2008;371:1513–1518.
47. Chang HY, Hu YW, Yue CS, et al. Effect of potassium-enriched salt on cardiovascular mortality and medical expenses of elderly men. *Am J Clin Nutr*. 2006;83(6):1289–1296.
48. Cook NR, Cutler JA, Obarzanek E, et al. Long-term effects of dietary sodium reduction on cardiovascular disease outcomes: observational follow-up of the trials of hypertension prevention (TOHP). *BMJ*. 2007;334(7599):885–893.
49. de Wardener HE, MacGregor GA. Harmful effects of dietary salt in addition to hypertension. *J Hum Hypertens*. 2002;16:213–223.
50. Fields LE, Burt VL, Cutler JA, Hughes J, Roccella EJ, Sorlie P. The burden of adult hypertension in the United States 1999 to 2000: a rising tide. *Hypertension*. 2004;44(4):398–404.
51. Chobanian AV, Bakris GL, Black HR, et al. The Seventh Report of the Joint National Committee on Prevention, Detection, Evaluation, and Treatment of High Blood Pressure. *JAMA*. 2003;289(19):2560–2571.
52. Vasan RS, Beiser A, Seshadri S. Residual lifetime risk for developing hypertension in middle-aged women and men. *JAMA*. 2002;287:1003–1010.
53. Centers for Disease Control and Prevention. High blood pressure, high blood pressure facts. 2011. http://cdc.gov/bloodpressure/facts.htm. Accessed August 26, 2011.
54. Jacobson MF. Salt, the forgotten killer. Center for Science in the Public Interest. 2005, updated 2009. http://www.cspinet.org/salt/saltreport.pdf. Accessed March 12, 2010.

55. Mates RD, Donnelly D. Relative contributions of dietary sodium sources. *J Am Coll Nutr*. 1991;10(4):383–393.
56. US Department of Agriculture and US Department of Health and Human Services. *Dietary Guidelines for Americans, 2010*. 7th ed. Washington, DC: US Government Printing Office, 2010.
57. National Cancer Institute. Sources of Sodium in the Diets of the U.S. Population Ages 2 Years and Older, NHANES 2005–2006. Risk Factor Monitoring and Methods, Cancer Control and Population Sciences. http://riskfactor.cancer.gov/diet/foodsources/sodium/table1a.html. Accessed April 10, 2011.
58. Friedman RR. Menu labeling in chain restaurants, opportunities for public policy. Rudd Report, Rudd Center for Food Policy and Obesity. 2008. http://www.yaleruddcenter.org/resources/upload/docs/what/reports/RuddMenuLabelingReport2008.pdf. Accessed March 14, 2010.
59. Roberto CA, Agnew H, Brownell KD. An observational study of consumers' accessing of nutrition information in chain restaurants. *Am J Public Health*. 2009;99(5):820–821.
60. Bassett MT, Dumanovsky T, Huang C, et al. Purchasing behavior and calorie information at fast-food chains in New York City, 2007. *Am J Pub Health*. 2008;98(8):1457–1459.
61. Burton S, Creyer EH, Kees J, Huggins K. Attacking the obesity epidemic: The potential health benefits of providing nutrition information in restaurants. *Am J Pub Health*. 2006;96(9):1669–1675.
62. Wansink B, Chandon P. Meal size, not body size, explains errors in estimating the calorie contents of meals. *Ann Int Med*. 2006;145:326–332.
63. Chandon P, Wansink B. The biasing health halos of fast-food restaurant health claims: lower calorie estimates and higher side-dish consumption intentions. *J Consum Res*. 2007;34:301–314.
64. Young LR, Nestle M. Portion sizes and obesity: Responses of fast-food companies. *J Pub Health Policy*. 2007;28:238–248.
65. Backstrand J, Wootan MG, Young LR, Hurley J. *Fat Chance*. Washington, DC: Center for Science in the Public Interest, 1997.
66. Kuo T, Jarosz CJ, Simon P, Fielding JE. Menu labeling as a potential strategy for combating the obesity epidemic: a health impact assessment. *Am J Public Health*. 2009;99(9):1680–1686.
67. Boutelle KN, Birnbaum AS, Lytle LA, Murray DM, Story M. Association between perceived family meal environment and parent intake of fruit, vegetables, and fat. *J Nutr Ed Behav*. 2003;35(1):24–29.
68. Gillman MW, Rifas-Shiman SL, Frazier AL, Rockett HRH, Camargo CA, Fired AE, Berkey CS, Colditz GA. Family dinner and diet quality among older children and adolescents. *Archives of Fam Med*. 2000;9:235–240.
69. Neumark-Sztainer D, Hannan PJ, Story M, Croll J, Perry C. Family meal patterns: associations with sociodemographic characteristics and improved dietary intake among adolescents. *J Am Diet Assoc*. 2003;103:317–322.
70. Burgess-Champoux TL, Larson N, Neumark-Sztainer D, Hannan PJ, Story M. Are family meal patterns associated with overall diet quality during the transition from early to middle adolescence? *J Nutr Ed Behav*. 2009;41:79–86.
71. Taveras EM, Rifas-Shiman SL, Berkey CS, et al. Family dinner and adolescent overweight. *Obes Res*. 2005;13:900–906.
72. Eisenberg ME, Olson RE, Neumark-Sztainer D, Story M, Bearinger LH. Correlations between family meals and psychosocial well-being among adolescents. *Arch Pediatr Adolesc Med*. 2004;158:792–796.
73. Ma Y, Bertone ER, Stanek EJ, Reed GW, Herbert JR, Cohen NL, Meriam PA, Ockene IS. Association between eating patterns and obesity in a free-living US adult population. *Am J Epidemiol*. 2003;158(1):88–92.
74. Stroebele N, Ogden LG, Hill JO. Do calorie-controlled portion sizes of snacks reduce energy intake? *Appetite*. 2009;52(3):793–796.
75. Roach J. Are plastic grocery bags sacking the environment? National Geographic News. 2003. http://news.natiaonlgeographic.com/news/pf/80107147.html. Accessed March 4, 2010.

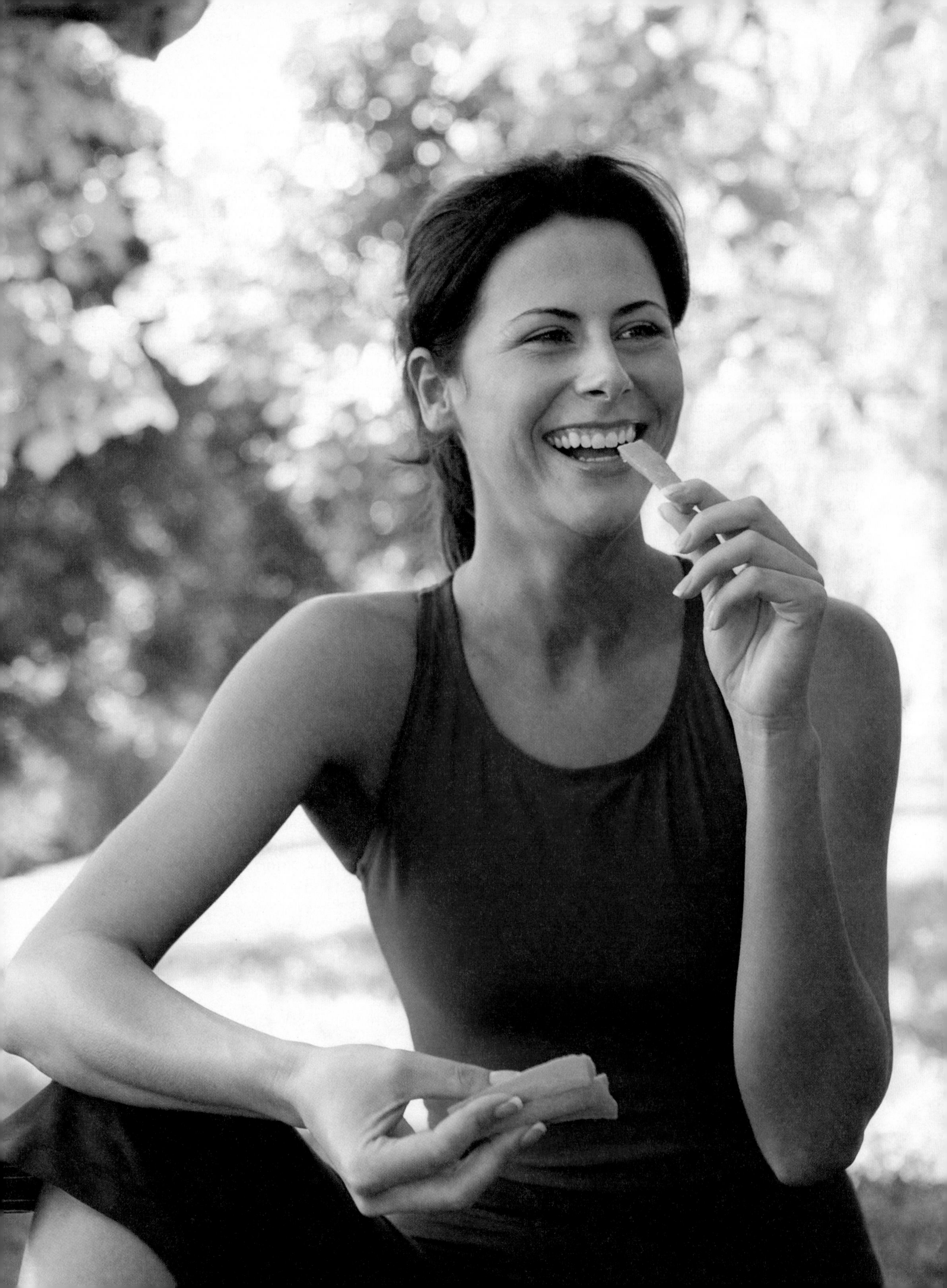

Chapter 4

Digestion and Absorption: How Your Body Uses the Food You Eat

Key Messages

- Digestion is the process by which the body breaks down food into smaller units.
- Absorption is the process of moving energy and nutrients into the body.
- Your body's gastrointestinal tract and supporting organs are efficient in digesting and absorbing nutrients from a wide variety of foods.
- Many common digestive problems can be prevented or treated with a healthy diet, proper water intake, and physical activity.

You eat food to obtain the energy and the nutrients you need for optimal health. How does that turkey sandwich on whole-wheat bread go from a sandwich to nutrients and energy? This is where your body's digestive system comes in. Digestion is the process by which the body breaks down food into smaller and smaller units until they can be absorbed and used for energy and other functions in the body. Your body has the ability to digest and absorb energy and nutrients from a wide variety of foods. The process of digesting and absorbing food is something your body does automatically, no matter what combination of foods you may send its way.

This chapter will examine the fascinating process of digestion and absorption, from when you first smell food to when the nutrients from that food are absorbed. It also presents some common problems that can occur in the digestive system and describes how to prevent them.

Story

Sarah just started college and is away from home and on her own for the first time. She has always relied on her mom to stock the refrigerator with healthy foods and to have dinner ready each night. Now that she has to fend for herself for all her meals she is noticing that the foods she is eating don't always make her feel the best. She always had regular bowel movements, but now she sometimes goes two or three days without having one. Her diet is pretty much the same every week. She frequents the local pizza-by-the-slice restaurant for lunch, because she can eat there for just a few dollars. Dinner is usually a sandwich while studying or something she can make quickly, such as pasta with sauce from a jar or can. She likes most foods but has limited time and money. What suggestions do you have for Sarah to get her digestive system back on track?

Before You Eat: Your Body's First Response to Food

Before you even take the first bite, your senses help you determine if you want to eat a food. You first eat with your eyes, which is why you prefer to eat foods that look appealing. Your sense of smell and taste also attracts you to foods you are likely to consume. Try holding your nose while you eat a familiar food. If your eyes are closed, you will have trouble identifying what you ate.

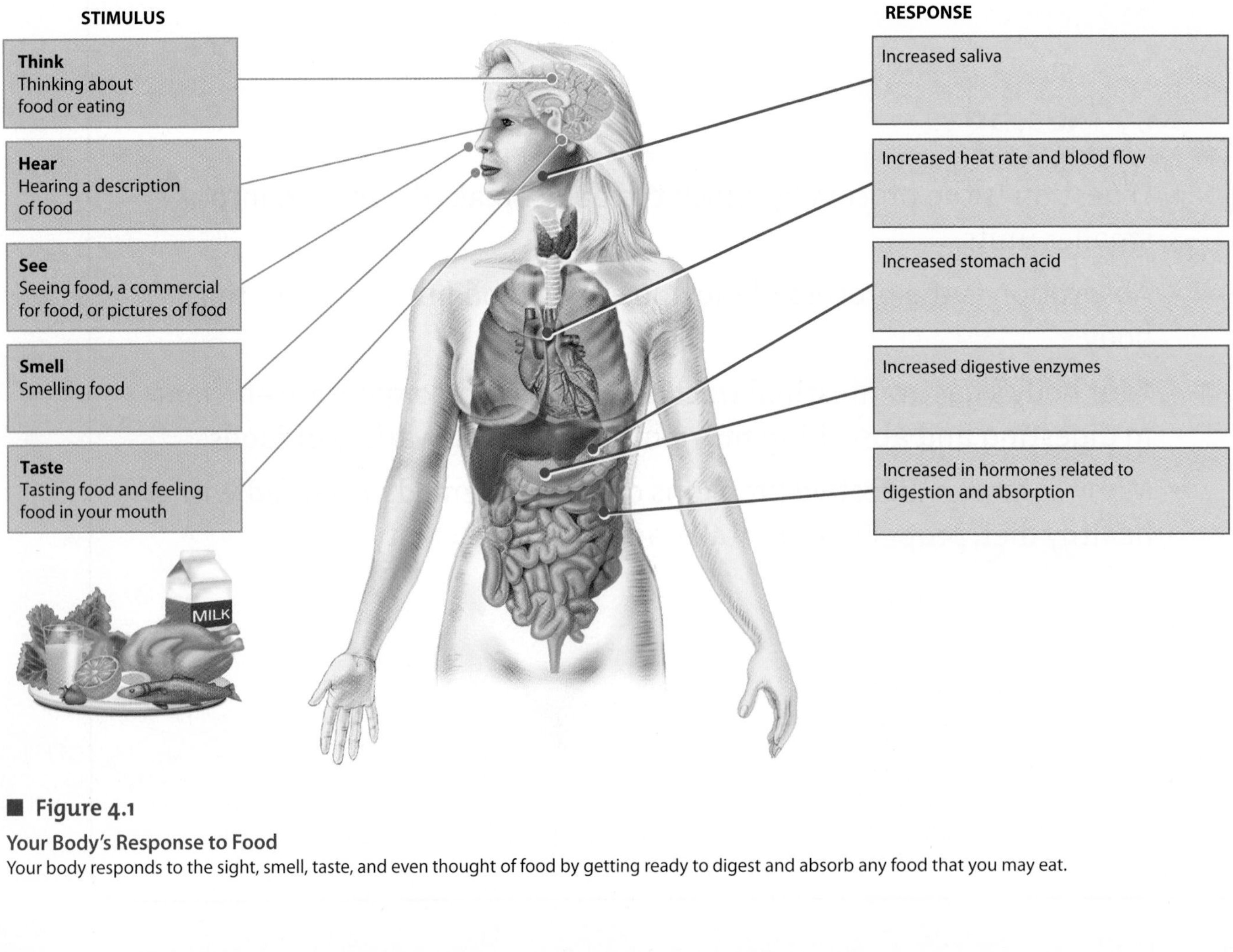

■ **Figure 4.1**

Your Body's Response to Food

Your body responds to the sight, smell, taste, and even thought of food by getting ready to digest and absorb any food that you may eat.

You may be familiar with the story of Pavlov's dog. Pavlov was a scientist who examined psychological responses to external stimuli. Every time he rang a bell he gave his dog food. Soon, his dog began to salivate when it heard the bell, before the food was even provided. The dog was responding to the thought that food would soon be available. Humans also respond to external stimuli when it comes to food.[1] You walk through an airport and smell the baking cinnamon buns, and you start to salivate. You didn't think you were hungry, but after reading a cooking magazine you need a snack. You see beautiful food in a commercial for a restaurant, and your heart beats faster. Your early response to food stimulates the body to be ready to digest the food that may be coming (**Figure 4.1**).

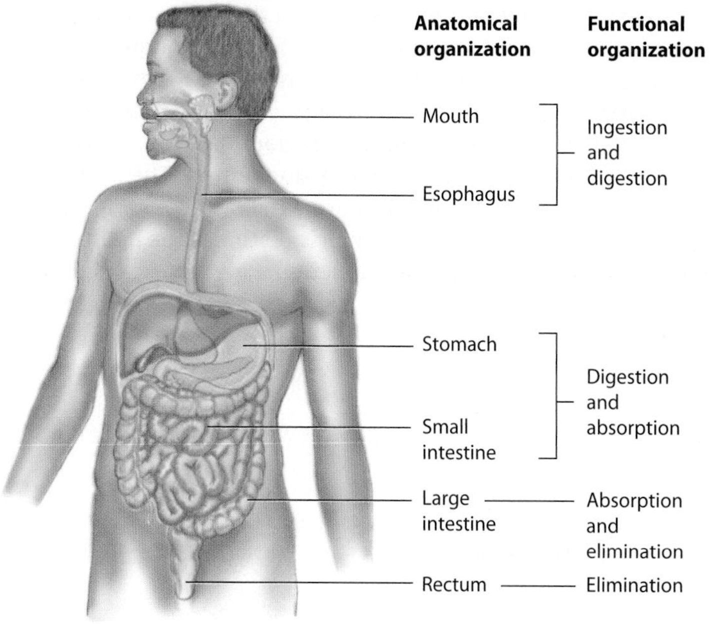

■ **Figure 4.2**
The Gastrointestinal Tract

Your Body: Built to Digest and Absorb

You begin to salivate as you sit down to dinner with the smell of tomato sauce in the air. You see a beautiful plate of pasta with red sauce, and you are ready to dig in. Your digestive system is built to break down the nutrients in your meal and absorb them into your body. The digestive process starts in the mouth and continues along the **gastrointestinal (GI) tract**. The GI tract works with assisting organs to complete the digestion and absorption of food.

Gastrointestinal Tract

The components of the GI tract can be categorized based on their function in the digestive process: ingestion, digestion, absorption, or elimination of food and waste products (**Figure 4.2**).

Inside the GI tract is a lining called the mucosa. The GI tract also contains longitudinal muscles and circular muscles that help to mix and move food. Food travels through the lumen, or the interior, of the GI tract (**Figure 4.3**).

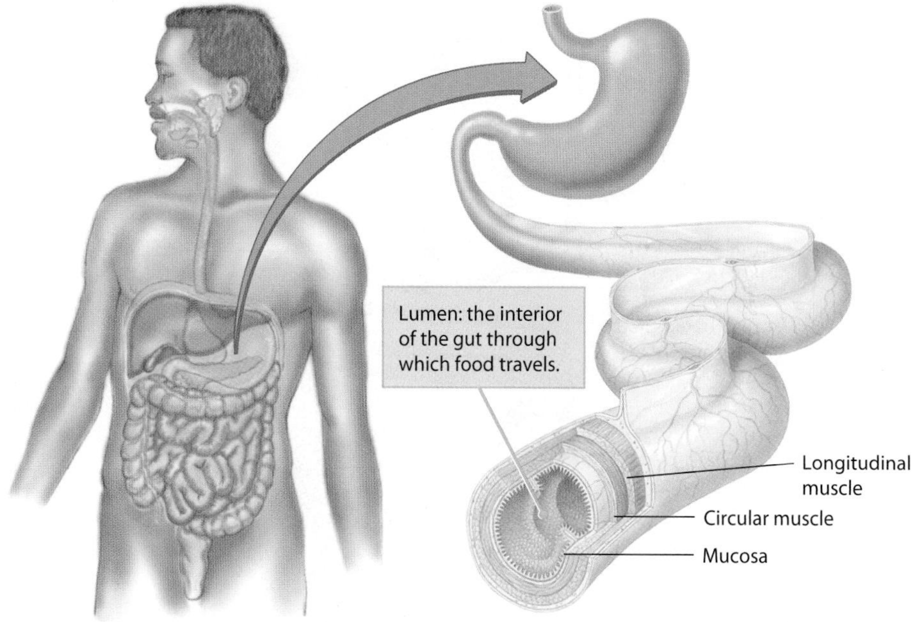

■ **Figure 4.3**
The Wall of the Gastrointestinal Tract

Where one part of the GI tract meets another, such as where the esophagus meets the stomach and where the stomach meets the small intestine, the muscles are thicker and form sphincters. Sphincters keep the contents of the GI tract from flowing in the wrong direction.

The mouth is the first part of the GI tract. It receives food, which is the first step in the digestive process. The esophagus moves food from the mouth to the stomach. The stomach is a saclike organ that acts as a holding tank

TERMS

gastrointestinal (GI) tract A long hollow tube that starts at your mouth and ends at your anus. The organs that comprise the GI tract are the mouth, esophagus, stomach, small intestine, large intestine (also called the colon), rectum, and anus.

for food and liquid as it moves through the GI tract. It has the capacity to hold around a quart of food and liquid.

The small intestine is approximately 10 feet long and is the longest portion of the GI tract (**Figure 4.4**). The small intestine is divided into three regions. The first 10–12 inches of the small intestine is the duodenum. The duodenum is followed by the jejunum, which is about 4 feet long. The final portion of the small intestine is the ileum, which is approximately 5 feet in length.

The small intestine is structured to provide for maximum digestion and absorption of nutrients. The interior of the small intestine has folds, which increases the surface area available for nutrient absorption. In addition, the surface of the small intestine is covered with villi, which increase absorption even more. Villi are fingerlike projections that are approximately 1 millimeter in length. On the surface of the villi are microvilli. Each cell on the villi can contain as many as 1,000 microvilli (**Figure 4.5**). Together—the folds of the small intestine, the villi, and the microvilli—increase the surface area and the absorptive capacity of the small intestine over 30-fold.

The large intestine (colon) has three parts. The first part of the colon is the ascending colon, followed by the transverse colon, the descending colon, and the sigmoid colon. At the base of the colon are the rectum and, finally, the anal canal (**Figure 4.6**).

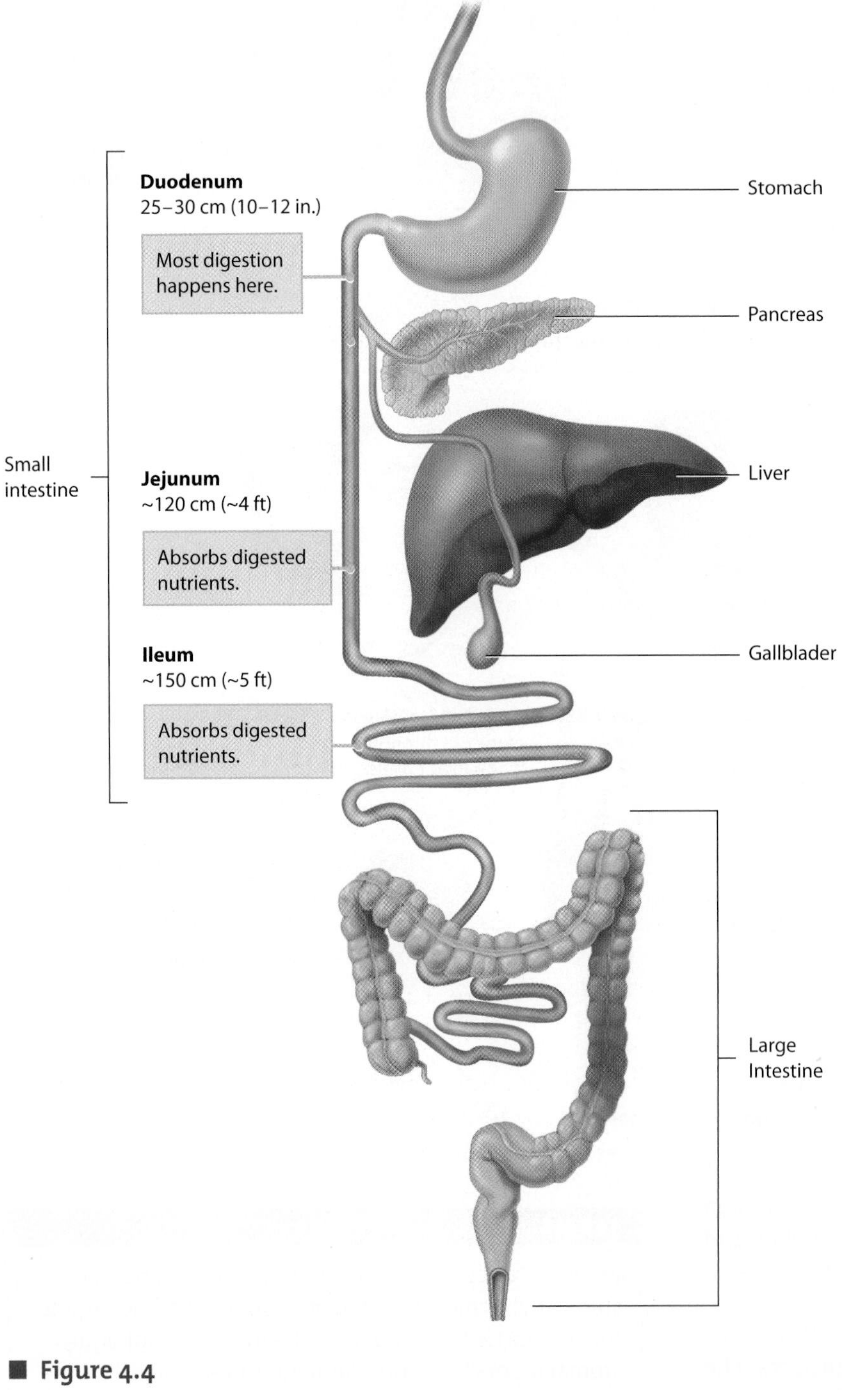

■ **Figure 4.4**

Small Intestine

The small intestine is 10 feet long and runs from the stomach to the large intestine.

Assisting Organs and Glands

A number of assisting organs and glands aid in the digestive process, including the salivary glands, the liver, the gallbladder, and the pancreas.

Salivary Glands You have three sets of salivary glands in and around your mouth and throat. They secrete saliva into your mouth through tubes called salivary ducts. As you chew, food is mixed with saliva. Saliva moistens food as you eat so that you can swallow it more easily. Saliva also allows you to taste foods, because it is difficult to distinguish flavors if food is dry. Saliva also contains enzymes that begin the digestive process.

Liver Your liver performs many functions, including detoxifying the blood, metabolizing drugs, storing glycogen, and producing hormones and components of blood. The liver's specialized tissues regulate a wide variety of biochemical reactions. A function it performs that is critical to digestion and absorption is the production of bile. Bile is a dark-green to yellow-brown fluid that aids in the digestive process. Bile acts as an emulsifier and breaks large fat globules into smaller components. Approximately a quart of bile is produced each day.

Gallbladder Bile, which is produced in the liver, is stored in the gallbladder. As bile is stored in the gallbladder, it becomes more concentrated, increasing its effect

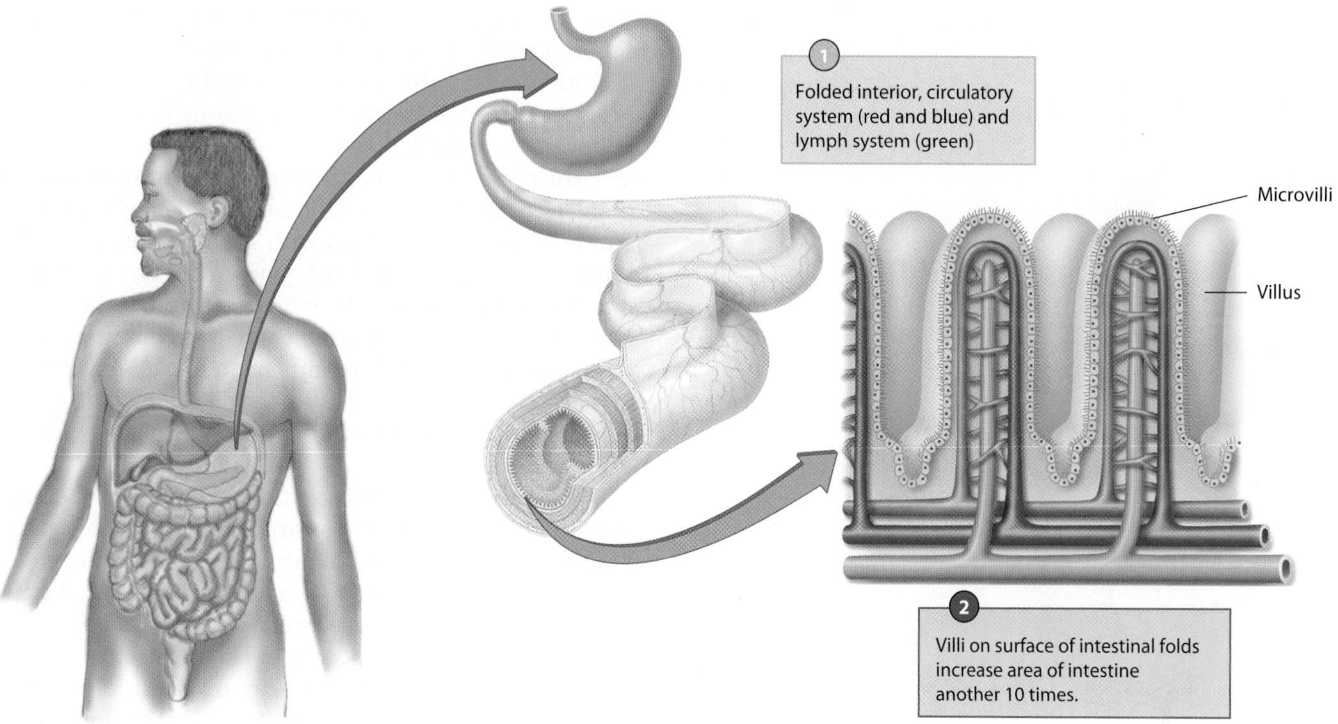

■ **Figure 4.5**

Villi and Microvilli

The small intestine has a folded interior, villi, and microvilli, which increase the surface area available to absorb nutrients.

on dietary fat. As fat enters the small intestine, hormones signal the release of bile from the gallbladder. Bile travels through the common bile duct to the small intestine.

Pancreas The pancreas is an endocrine gland that is only about 6 inches long. What it lacks in size it makes up for in function, and it is a vital part of the digestive process. It produces several important hormones, including insulin and glucagon. It also produces digestive enzymes that help break down food during the digestive process.

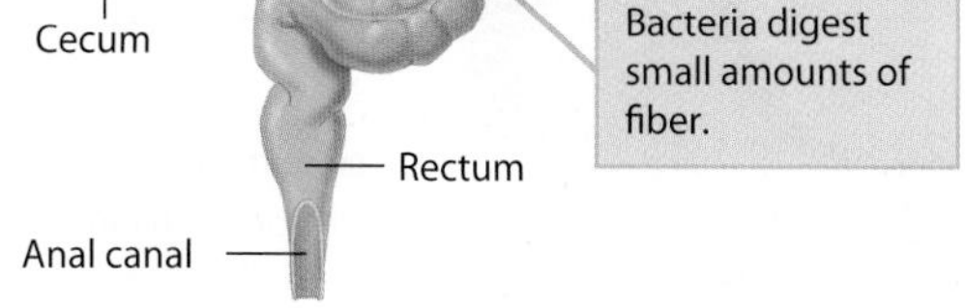

■ **Figure 4.6**

Large Intestine

The large intestine begins with the ascending colon and ends with the anal canal.

Overview of Digestion and Absorption

You now are familiar with the organs and glands that help you to digest food. Let's put it all together and see what happens to the food you eat, from the first bite to when waste products from that meal are eliminated.

The first step of digestion is when you first put food in your mouth. This starts the physical breakdown of food. As you chew, food is broken down into smaller parts. The chemical breakdown of food also begins in the mouth. Enzymes and other substances start the chemical breakdown of food. **Enzymes** are proteins that speed up chemical reactions. The digestive enzymes break the nutrients into compounds that are small enough to be absorbed. Saliva in the mouth contains enzymes that partially break down carbohydrates and fats.

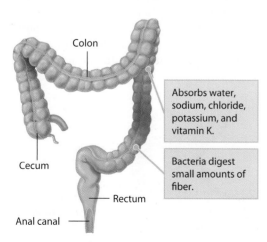

TERMS

enzymes Proteins that speed up chemical reactions. Enzymes are found throughout the body and are especially important in digestion.

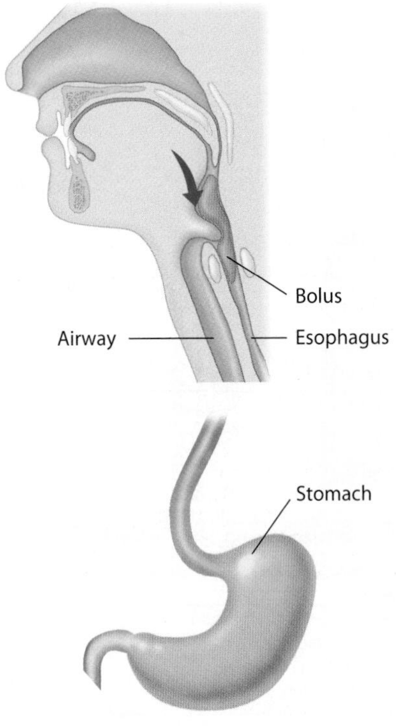

Figure 4.7

Swallowing

Food passes through the epiglottis, which closes during swallowing, and travels through the esophagus to the stomach.

As you continue to chew, saliva mixes with the food and forms a bolus. The bolus, a mixture of food and saliva, is then swallowed and passes the epiglottis, the flap of tissue at the back of your throat that closes off your air passages when you swallow to prevent choking. After the bolus passes the epiglottis, it travels through the esophagus to the stomach (**Figure 4.7**). The bolus enters the stomach through the esophageal sphincter. The esophageal sphincter must close quickly to keep the acid that is in the stomach from entering the esophagus.

The stomach produces gastric juice, which is a mixture of mucus, acid, pepsin, gastric lipase, gastrin, and intrinsic factor. The acid in gastric juice is hydrochloric acid. It makes the stomach contents very acidic, around 1.8 on the pH scale. To give you an idea of how strong stomach acid is, lemon juice has a pH of 2, vinegar has a pH of 3, and battery acid has a pH of 0. So, your stomach is more acidic than lemon juice or vinegar and almost as acidic as battery acid. Your stomach secretes mucus that coats the lining of the stomach to protect itself from the strong acid in gastric juice. The acid in gastric juice has several roles. The acidic environment kills many disease-causing bacteria that may be ingested. It also works to begin the digestion of proteins. Acid in the stomach begins to unfold the proteins so that enzymes later in the digestive process can more easily digest them.

The other components of gastric juice have important roles as well. Pepsin breaks apart long protein chains into smaller pieces. Gastric lipase has a minor role in the digestion of fat. Gastrin stimulates the stomach to secrete gastric juice and aids in motility. Intrinsic factor is a specialized chemical that your body needs to be able to absorb vitamin B_{12}.

The stomach is a very muscular organ with longitudinal, circular, and diagonal muscles. The muscles in the stomach work to mix food with gastric juice, producing a mass of partially digested food called chyme (**Figure 4.8**). The chyme leaves the stomach through the pyloric sphincter, which connects the stomach to the small intestine. Approximately 30% of carbohydrates, 10% of proteins, and less than 10% of fats have been digested when chyme leaves the stomach. Virtually no absorption takes place in the stomach.

More digestion and absorption take place in the small intestine than in any other part of the digestive system. Both physical and chemical digestion occurs in the small intestine. The movement of the muscles of the small intestine is called peristalsis. Peristalsis moves food along the GI tract and continues the process of physically breaking food apart. The small intestine breaks apart large pieces of chyme by back and forth muscular contractions called segmentation (**Figure 4.9**).

The pancreas produces secretin, a hormone that works to neutralize the acid that comes from the stomach. This is important because many of the enzymes that aid in digestion do not function efficiently in an acidic environment. The pancreas and intestinal wall secrete digestive enzymes, and the gallbladder secretes bile into the small intestine. All of these chemicals work together to further break down carbohydrates, proteins, and fats into smaller and smaller components. Other nutrients, such as vitamins and minerals, can be absorbed as is and do not require further digestion.

Now that the nutrients have been broken down into smaller units, they can be absorbed into the body. Just as most of the digestion occurs in the small intestine, most of the absorption occurs here as well. The villi and microvilli of the small intestine allow for efficient absorption of nutrients. Each villus acts as a gateway, passing nutrients into the bloodstream or into the lymph sys-

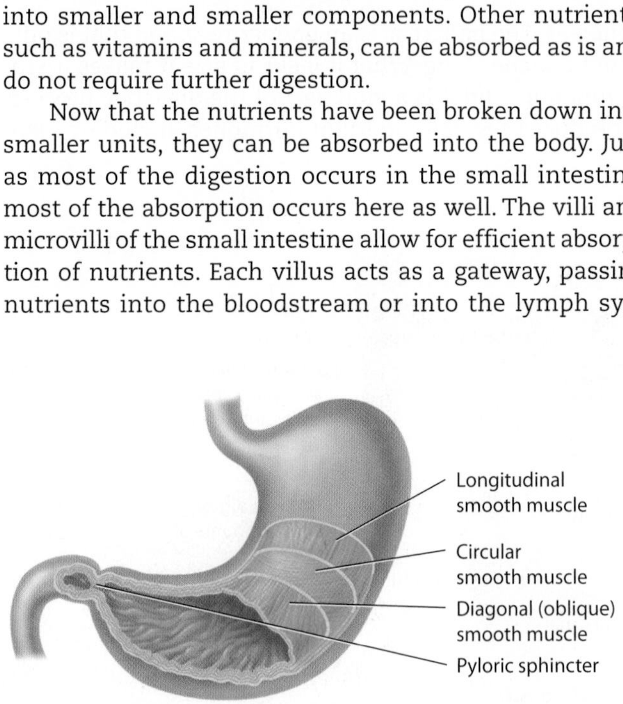

Figure 4.8

Muscles in the Stomach Mix Food with Gastric Juice

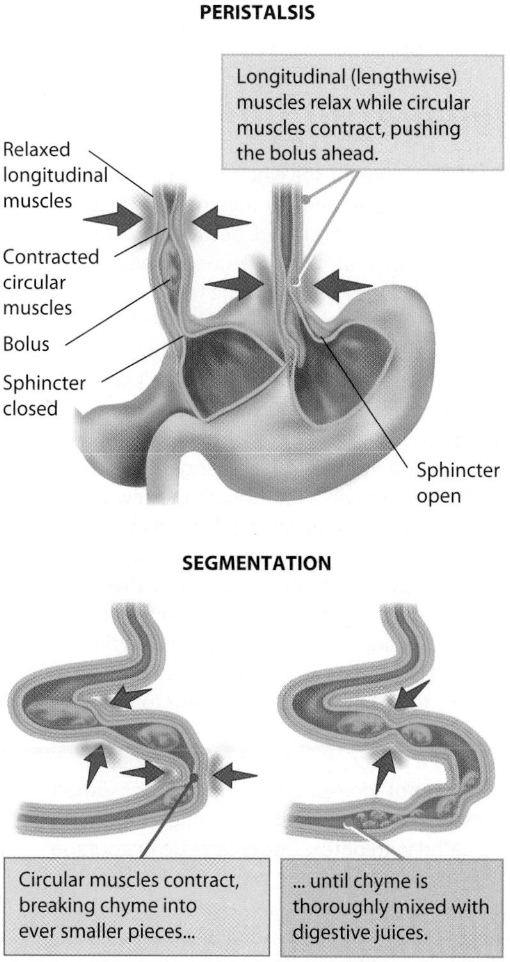
PERISTALSIS
Longitudinal (lengthwise) muscles relax while circular muscles contract, pushing the bolus ahead.
Relaxed longitudinal muscles
Contracted circular muscles
Bolus
Sphincter closed
Sphincter open
SEGMENTATION
Circular muscles contract, breaking chyme into ever smaller pieces...
... until chyme is thoroughly mixed with digestive juices.

Figure 4.9

Peristalsis and Segmentation

Peristalsis and segmentation help move food through the GI tract and break food apart.

tem. The blood in your body is carried by the **circulatory system**, a network of arteries and veins that supply oxygen and nutrients to tissues throughout the body. Blood carries nutrients from the small intestine to the rest of the body. The **lymph system** is a network of vessels that drain lymph. Lymph is a clear fluid that is formed in the spaces between cells. Lymph vessels in the small intestine carry most of the products of fat digestion. The lymph system takes nutrients to the liver for further processing.

TERMS

circulatory system An organ system that connects all the cells in the body. Through the blood, it transports water, oxygen, and nutrients to all the cells of the body and carries away waste.

lymph system Part of the immune system; it is composed of a network of lymphatic vessels that carry lymph (a clear fluid) toward the heart.

After its 3- to 10-hour journey through the small intestine, the chyme is now ready to enter the large intestine. Because most of the digestion and absorption of nutrients has already occurred, the chyme is now mostly indigestible fiber and water. The large intestine performs peristalsis just like the small intestine, but at a much slower rate. It usually takes 18–24 hours for matter to travel the length of the large intestine. As chyme moves through the large intestine it comes into contact with bacteria that digest some fiber. Other than this small amount of digestion, no other digestion occurs in the large intestine. Similarly, little nutrient absorption occurs. The main function of the large intestine is to remove water from the chyme. Water, sodium, potassium, and chloride are absorbed. What remains is the semisolid mass that is excreted as feces. Feces passes into the rectum where strong muscles hold it in the body. When you are ready to have a bowel movement, the rectal muscles relax and the anal sphincter opens to allow feces to pass out of the anal canal.

Common Digestive Problems

Even if you are healthy and eat an overall healthy diet, you will most likely experience digestive problems from time to time. Many common digestive problems such as occasional heartburn or constipation are easily corrected with a slight change in dietary habits. You can avoid most digestive problems and keep your digestive system working properly by eating a healthy diet, being physically active, and maintaining a healthy weight. These strategies will also decrease your risk of serious issues related to your digestive system such as diverticulitis or colon cancer.

Heartburn

You had a bowl of chili for lunch. The jalapenos you topped it off with tasted good, but now your chest is on fire. Heartburn, or acid indigestion, occurs when the sphincter between the esophagus and stomach relaxes and allows stomach acid to flow into the esophagus. When that stomach acid touches the lining of the esophagus, it cases a burning sensation in the chest or throat. Many common foods can trigger a bout of heartburn, including tomato-based foods, citrus fruits, fatty foods, fried foods, carbonated drinks, caffeine, alcohol, spicy foods, garlic, onions, and mint flavorings. Everyone is different; what causes immediate heartburn in one person may have no effect in another. Eating too quickly or consuming large meals can also cause heartburn in some people. Smoking also increases the chance of getting heartburn on a regular basis. Overweight and obesity contribute to heartburn and may make it more frequent or more severe. Eating just before bed can also increase the chance of heartburn.

Learning what triggers heartburn and avoiding those foods can help you control occasional heartburn. Frequent heartburn, more than twice a week, may indicate gastroesophageal reflux disease (GERD). Left untreated, GERD can

Which Side Are You On?

Detox Diets: Cleansing the Body or a Potential Health Threat?

Hundreds of websites and books promote various detoxification (detox) routines. Many celebrities extol the benefits of detoxing. Detox diets promise everything from weight loss, sharper memory, better health, lower cholesterol, and fewer headaches to a better general overall sense of well-being. Is this true? Do we need to detox on a regular basis for good health?

Advocates for detox diets fear that your body is constantly overloaded with toxins from pollution, cigarette smoke, pesticides, a poor diet, food additives, alcohol, drugs, and caffeine. The theory of detox is that these toxins build up in your system and cause health problems such as weight gain, headaches, dull skin, bloating, fatigue, lowered immunity, and overall poor health.

A variety of popular detox diets and routines have been proposed. Some routines suggest the use of laxatives or herbal supplements while following a regular diet. Others prescribe a diet that is restrictive and usually very low in calories. Detox diets vary widely, but fruits, vegetables, beans, nuts, seeds, herbal teas, and water are usually allowed. Foods that are usually on the "do not consume" list during a detox diet are wheat, dairy, meat, fish, eggs, caffeine, alcohol, salt, sugar, and processed foods. One of the more famous detox diets is also the most restrictive; the Master Cleanse used by several A-list celebrities consists only of lemon, water, maple syrup, and cayenne.

Like other fad diets, detox diets promise a quick fix for weight loss and years of consumption of unhealthy foods and unhealthy lifestyle choices. However, scientific evidence does not support the use of detox diets. Your body is equipped with a very sophisticated waste-elimination system. Your liver, kidneys, GI tract, lungs, and skin do a great job of eliminating toxins. There is no evidence that detox diets or any other detox routine aids the body in elimination of toxins in any way.

Any benefits that you might see when on a detox diet can be explained. Fewer headaches and improvement in the skin may be the result of being fully hydrated, because all detox routines encourage the consumption of large volumes of water. Feeling less bloated may be due to the fact that limited food is consumed and laxatives or herbal supplements may increase elimination. Certainly, you may lose weight on a detox diet, especially with those that are most restrictive. Just as certain is that the weight loss is primarily water and will be regained very quickly.

Some detox diets and routines can be dangerous. Severe restriction of calories and nutrients for more than a few days is not recommended. It should not be attempted at all by pregnant women, children, teenagers, seniors, or people with heart disease or other chronic conditions. Use of laxatives can cause dehydration. Colonic irrigation, which is suggested by some detox plans, is risky and can cause bowel perforation or infection. In addition, detox diets and routines may provide a false sense of security that they are advantageous for good health. Several days to detox and then right back to bad habits of eating poorly is not a prescription for overall well-being.

If the detox diet is not too restrictive and only consumed for a few days, it may offer some benefits, although not the ones usually associated with detox. Detox diets do encourage consumption of fruits, vegetables, and water. In turn, they discourage processed foods, caffeine, and alcohol. A moderate detox diet can help you to be more mindful of what you are eating. A quick fix for weight loss and overall health is not what you will get with detox. However, a few days of a moderate plan may help jumpstart a new eating plan and help you be mindful of food choices. There is no shortcut to lifelong habits of good eating, physical activity, moderate alcohol use, and abstention from tobacco.

damage the lining of the esophagus, causing bleeding and scarring. People with GERD also have an increased risk of esophageal cancer. GERD should be treated by a healthcare provider who may prescribe medications in addition to lifestyle changes, such as quitting smoking, losing weight, eating smaller meals, or avoiding certain foods.

Constipation

Constipation is a condition where bowel movements are infrequent or incomplete. With constipation, stools are hard, dry, small in size, and difficult to eliminate. Constipation may make it painful to have a bowel movement and can cause bloating and a sensation of a full bowel.

Some people think they are constipated if they do not have a bowel movement every day. What is normal for you will vary, but bowel movements can be as frequent as three times a day to as few as three times a week. Constipation is one of the most common gastrointestinal complaints in the United States and is most common in women, adults older than age 65, and pregnant women.[2] Almost everyone will experience constipation at some time; it is usually temporary and not cause for great concern.

Constipation is easy to prevent once you know the most common causes. To understand the possible causes of constipation, you need to understand how the colon works. Water is removed from food as it moves along the colon. The colon forms waste, or stool, from what is left. Muscles in the colon move the stool toward the rectum. The stool is solid by the time it reaches the rectum because most of the water has been absorbed. Constipation occurs when too much of the water is absorbed or the muscle contractions of the colon are slow, causing the stool to pass too slowly. As a result, stools become hard, dry, and difficult to pass.

The most common cause of constipation is a diet that is low in fiber and high in fat. A diet that is low in fruits, vegetables, whole grains, and beans is likely to cause at least occasional constipation. Fiber creates bulk in the colon and helps prevent hard, dry stools that can be difficult to pass. Along with enough fiber to create bulk in the colon, you need enough fluid. Even moderate dehydration can cause constipation. Making sure you get enough water will add fluid to the colon and bulk to stools, making bowel movements softer and easier to pass.

Physical inactivity can lead to constipation. This is one reason why constipation is common in older people. Making sure you get enough physical activity is a good choice for many reasons, including a healthy colon.

Another factor in preventing constipation is to give yourself enough time to have a bowel movement. If you ignore the urge to have a bowel movement, the feeling may eventually pass. As the stool sits in the colon, water continues to be absorbed, making the stool hard to pass. If you continually put off the need to have a bowel movement, you can become constipated.

Some medications can cause constipation. Pain medications (especially narcotics), antacids, blood pressure medications, antidepressants, iron supplements, and others can cause constipation. If you are on a medication that is known to cause constipation, check with your doctor to see what he or she recommends. You will also need to be mindful of getting enough fiber and plenty of fluids.

Occasional constipation is best treated by a change in diet, fluid consumption, and physical activity. Over-the-counter laxatives can be harsh and can become habit forming if taken too frequently. A healthcare provider should determine if you need a laxative and what form is best for you.

Sometimes constipation can lead to complications. Hemorrhoids, caused by straining to have a bowel movement, and anal fissures, tears in the skin around the anus, are both caused by hard dry stools. They may cause rectal bleeding that appears as bright red streaks on the surface of the stool. Straining can also cause a small amount of intestinal lining to push out of the anal opening; this is called anal prolapse. Chronic constipation may also lead to an impacted colon when the stool is so hard that the normal pushing action of the colon is not enough to expel the stool. A healthcare provider should treat all of these complications of constipation.

Diarrhea

Diarrhea is loose, watery stools. It is caused by food moving too fast through the large intestine for water to be absorbed. Diarrhea that lasts a few days is usually related to a bacterial or viral infection. Bacterial infections can be from contaminated food or water. Many viral infections, including norovirus, can cause diarrhea.

If you visit a foreign country, you may be at risk for traveler's diarrhea from drinking water or foods that contain bacteria, viruses, or parasites. Natives of the country may have no problem with the same food or water, because they have built up a tolerance to these pathogens over time.

Diarrhea can cause dehydration and electrolyte imbalance. For diarrhea that lasts three or fewer days, replacement of lost fluid is the only treatment necessary. Sports drinks or specialty drinks for diarrhea treatment can help replace lost electrolytes. A diet of bland foods such as toast, broth, or crackers is recommended until the diarrhea completely subsides. Avoid spicy foods, high-fat foods, and foods high in fiber for a few days. Bouts of diarrhea that last longer than three days may be the sign of a more serious problem. Prolonged diarrhea should be treated by a healthcare professional.

Irritable Bowel Syndrome

Irritable bowel syndrome (IBS) is a common disorder that can cause a great deal of discomfort and distress. IBS is not a disease; it is a functional disorder whereby the bowel or colon does not work properly. Sufferers of IBS experience cramping, bloating, gas, diarrhea, and/or constipation. Because it is a syndrome, it has a group of symptoms. There is no definitive way to diagnosis IBS; it is usually diagnosed after all other possible infections or diseases are ruled out. Even thought IBS is painful and causes discomfort, it does not cause permanent harm to the intestines and does not lead to serious diseases of the colon, such as cancer.

It is not known what causes IBS. However, people with IBS appear to have nerves and muscles in the bowel that are extra sensitive. IBS sufferers seem to have a colon that responds strongly to stimuli that would not bother most other people. In people with IBS, the muscles may overreact after a meal, causing diarrhea. Others with IBS have cramps and abdominal pain and constipation.

There is no cure for IBS, but there are things that people can do to relieve its symptoms. Treatment may involve diet changes, medication, and/or stress relief. Some foods or drinks may make IBS worse. Food triggers vary from person to person. Common food triggers for people with IBS include high-fat foods, milk products, chocolate, alcohol, caffeine-containing drinks, or carbonated drinks. Avoiding trigger foods may help alleviate IBS symptoms. High-fiber foods may also help alleviate some symptoms of IBS, especially constipation. Eating small meals can help some people with IBS. Several medications are available that can help with IBS, such as those that treat constipation and antispasmodics that can help control colon spasms. Because IBS can be made worse by stress, stress relief is often prescribed. Meditation, exercise, or counseling may help keep stress in check.

Diverticulosis and Diverticulitis

Diverticulosis is a condition where weak spots in the colon bulge outward, creating pouches called diverticula. The condition becomes more common with age, with about half of people over age 60 having diverticulosis. If the diverticula become inflamed or irritated, the condition is called diverticulitis. Not everyone who has diverticula develops diverticulitis. Only about 10–25% of people with diverticula ever develop diverticulitis. Diverticulosis and diverticulitis together are called diverticular disease.[3]

The most common symptom of diverticular disease is abdominal pain. It also causes pain and tenderness in the lower-left side of the abdomen. The pain can be severe and can come on suddenly or it can be mild and become worse over time. Cramping, nausea, vomiting, fever, chills, or a change in bowel habits can also accompany diverticulitis. Diverticular disease can lead to bleeding, infections, or even blockage of the colon. Diverticulitis requires treatment from a healthcare provider to prevent the condition from progressing.

The exact cause of diverticular disease is not known. The dominant theory is that it is caused by a low-fiber diet. The disease was first noticed in the United States in the early 1900s, which is the same time that processed foods were introduced into the U.S. diet. Consumption of processed foods has dramatically reduced intake of fiber. Low-fiber diets can cause constipation, which may cause straining when passing stool. Straining may cause increased pressure in the colon, which may result in the formation of diverticula. A diet high in fiber may help prevent diverticular disease as well as reduce the symptoms in those who have already developed it. Those with diverticular disease may be warned by healthcare providers to avoid nuts; popcorn; seeds; and vegetables with edible seeds, such as tomatoes and cucumbers, for fear that food particles could irritate the diverticula. However, the evidence does not support this as a treatment measure.[4]

Gas

Everyone has gas. Most people produce about 1–4 pints a day and pass gas about 14 times a day. Gas is eliminated by burping or passing gas through the rectum. Gas is made up primarily of odorless vapors. The unpleasant odor of flatulence (gas) comes from bacteria in the large intestine that release small amounts of sulfur-containing gasses. Even though everyone has gas, it still can be uncomfortable and embarrassing.

Gas in the digestive tract comes from two sources: swallowed air and the normal breakdown of certain undigested foods by bacteria in the large intestine. You commonly swallow small amounts of air when eating and drinking. Eating fast, chewing gum, smoking, or wearing loose dentures can cause more air to be taken in. Burping removes most of the swallowed air from the system. Swallowed air that is not expelled moves along the digestive tract, where it can be partially absorbed or released through the rectum. Other sources of gas are from the breakdown of undigested foods. Some components of food cannot be broken down by the body, such as fiber. This undigested food moves into the large intestine where harmless bacteria break it down. This causes the production of gas, which is then expelled through the rectum.

Several types of foods commonly cause gas. The most common component of food that causes gas is raffinose, a complex carbohydrate that is found in large amounts in beans, cabbage, broccoli, other vegetables, and whole grains. Fiber also can cause gas. High-fiber foods include whole grains, beans, fruits, and vegetables.

There are several ways to reduce the discomfort of gas. Finding out what causes gas in your body is the first step. What causes gas in someone else may not cause gas in you. Adjust your diet accordingly, if possible. Unfortunately, some of the foods that can cause gas are the foods that you should be eating for good health. Try introducing gas-causing foods into your diet slowly and in smaller quantities to see if you can enjoy the offending food over time. Over-the-counter medications are available that can be used to aid the digestion of foods such as beans, broccoli, or cabbage. Eat slowly; this will decrease the amount of air that you swallow and decrease some of the gas in your digestive tract.

Ulcers

You may think that the best way to avoid an ulcer is to live a laid back life without stress. Although a low-stress life is a good idea for many reasons, it may not help you avoid an ulcer. Ulcers are sores that develop on the lining of the stomach (gastric ulcers), the upper part of the small intestine (duodenal ulcers), or the esophagus (esophageal ulcers). Ulcers are common, with more than half a million cases diagnosed in the United States each year.[5] Many people think that spicy foods, stress, smoking, and alcohol cause ulcers. Although all of these can make an ulcer worse, they are not the cause of ulcers. Most ulcers are caused by the bacterium *Helicobacter pylori*. Nonsteroidal anti-inflammatory drugs (NSAIDs), such as aspirin and ibuprofen, are another common cause.[6]

H. pylori causes more than half of all ulcers.[6] The bacterium damages the mucous coating that protects the stomach and duodenum, which allows stomach acid to get through to the lining beneath, which can cause an ulcer to form. It is not clear how *H. pylori* is contracted or spread. Some possibilities are that it is spread through contaminated food or water or by contact with the feces or vomit of an infected person. It is also unclear why many people who have *H. pylori* in their systems never develop an ulcer.

The most common symptom of an ulcer is abdominal pain. The pain can be located anywhere in the abdomen between the navel and the breastbone. It can be a dull burning pain that occurs when the stomach is empty. The pain may be relieved by eating foods or by taking antacids. Other symptoms may include weight loss, poor appetite, bloating, burping, nausea, and vomiting. Some people may only have mild symptoms or no symptoms at all. Some symptoms of an ulcer warrant immediate attention by a healthcare provider; these include sharp, sudden, and severe stomach pain; bloody or black stools; bloody vomit; or vomit that looks like coffee grounds.

If symptoms of an ulcer are present, a healthcare provider may first ask about NSAID use. If this is not a possible cause for the symptoms, a test to see if *H. pylori* is present can be done. Other, more invasive tests can also be performed, such as an endoscopy or an upper gastrointestinal series. These both include the use of a thin, lighted tube with a tiny camera that is inserted into the patient's mouth and down the throat to the stomach. This allows for the physician to examine the stomach and duodenum for problems.

Treatment of ulcers caused by *H. pylori* includes medications that kill the bacteria, reduce stomach acid, and protect the stomach and duodenal lining. If the ulcer is caused by NSAIDs, the patient will be advised to stop taking these medications or to reduce their frequency and/or dosage. Ulcers caused by NSAIDs usually heal once the medication is stopped.

Celiac Disease

Celiac disease is a digestive disease that damages the small intestine. People with celiac disease cannot tolerate gluten, a protein found in wheat, rye, and barley. When people with celiac disease consume gluten, their immune system responds by damaging the villi in the intestine. This can ultimately interfere with the absorption of nutrients. Symptoms of celiac disease include abdominal pain, chronic diarrhea, vomiting, constipation, fat in the stool, and weight loss.

Celiac disease was once thought to be rare. However, prevalence of celiac disease has increased sharply in recent years due to better recognition of the disease. It occurs in approximates 1% of the general population.[7] No single test can definitively diagnose celiac disease; a series of tests may be needed to rule out other diagnoses and to ultimately diagnosis celiac disease.[8] The only scientifically proven treatment for celiac disease is strict, lifelong adherence to a gluten-free diet.[9]

Should You Go Gluten Free? Gluten is a protein found in wheat, rye, and barley. Gluten is predominately found in breads, cereals, pasta, and baked goods. However, small amounts of gluten, usually from wheat, are found in seasonings, sauces, marinades, soy sauce, soups, and salad dressings. Even oats, unless labeled gluten free, may contain small amounts of wheat from contamination during the growing and processing stages of production. Eating a gluten-free diet is very challenging. However, the introduction of more high-quality, gluten-free foods at stores has made going gluten-free easier than in the past.

A gluten-free diet is essential for someone who has been diagnosed with celiac disease. However, gluten-free diets are gaining in popularity at a rate much higher than the diagnosis of celiac disease. Only 1% of the population has celiac disease, yet there are many more people interested in consuming a gluten-free diet. Food manufacturers are responding, and the increase in the number of gluten-free items in the marketplace—from bread to beer—is staggering. Is a gluten-free diet a good idea for people besides those who suffer from celiac disease? Some say that gluten intolerance occurs on a continuum. Although you may not have celiac disease, you may have some gluten intolerance or sensitivity that causes symptoms ranging from bloating to rashes. Controversy exists over whether many of the people going gluten free have any real trouble with gluten. Those on a gluten-free diet may feel better because the diet includes fewer highly processed foods and fast foods and more fruits and vegetables.

If you don't have celiac disease or gluten intolerance, there is no reason to go on a gluten-free diet. Many of the foods that would be eliminated in your diet provide important nutrients. Gluten-free specialty foods are expensive and may be higher in fat and calories than their gluten-containing counterparts.

Colorectal Cancer

Colorectal cancer is cancer of the colon or the rectum. Colorectal cancer is the second leading cause of cancer

Personal Health Check

Screening for Colorectal Cancer

Although the exact cause of colorectal cancer is not known, we do know that the earlier it is caught the better a person's chance for a full recovery. It is recommended that screenings for colon cancer begin at age 50 and continue through age 75.[21] A number of different screening methods are available. Testing your stool for blood is the most noninvasive method of testing. Another test for colon cancer is the flexible sigmoidoscopy. With this test, a thin, flexible, lighted tube is inserted into the rectum so that a physician can check for polyps or cancer in the lower third of the colon. A colonoscopy is similar to a flexible sigmoidoscopy, but it enables the physician to view the entire colon.

If you are older than age 50, you should check with your physician about the right time to begin screening. Not quite to 50 yet? Then mark your calendar to start screenings when you hit the half-century mark. In the meantime, eat a healthy diet, maintain an ideal weight, engage in regular physical activity, and don't smoke to decrease your risk of colorectal cancer.

Special Report

Food Allergies

A **food allergy** is an abnormal immune system response in which the body produces an antibody to a food. These antibodies are proteins that work against a particular food and enter your bloodstream after the food is digested. From there, the antibodies go to target organs, such as the skin or nose, and cause an allergic reaction. If you consume a food to which you are allergic, your body's immune system reacts to that food, resulting in side effects such as sneezing, a rash, or, in severe cases, anaphylactic shock. Allergic reactions to foods can take place within a few minutes to as long as an hour after ingesting the offending food. Persons with food allergies must be very careful not to consume the offending food. Severe food allergies can be very dangerous and can even cause death if not treated immediately.

The most common foods that cause allergic reactions are milk, eggs, peanuts, tree nuts, soy, fish, shellfish, and wheat. These eight foods account for almost all food allergies. Mild food allergies can be treated with an antihistamine or a bronchodilator. Severe reactions, including difficulty breathing or anaphylactic shock, require treatment with epinephrine. There is no cure for food allergies; the best method for managing food allergies is by way of strict avoidance of any food that triggers a reaction.[22]

True food allergies are somewhat rare, affecting only a small percentage of the population. Only about 2% of the adult population and 4–8% of children have food allergies.[23,24] Adults usually keep their allergies for life; however, some children may outgrow their food allergy. Allergies to milk, egg, or soy are more likely to be outgrown than an allergy to peanuts.

Diagnosis of a food allergy is a multistep process. The healthcare provider will first rule out any other health problems, starting with a detailed history about the person's reaction to certain foods. Some healthcare providers will get a diet history to get more details about the pattern of food consumption that may be causing a problem. Sometimes an elimination diet is prescribed, whereby certain foods are removed from the diet to see if symptoms subside. If the history or elimination diet suggests a specific food allergy, a scratch test may be performed. With a scratch test, an extract of the food is placed on the skin and then the skin is scratched with a needle. Swelling or redness may be a sign of an allergic reaction. A blood test can be done in the case of extreme allergies and the possibility of anaphylactic reactions. A blood test may be able to measure the presence of a food-specific antibody in the blood.

More common than food allergies, and often mislabeled as food allergies, are food intolerances and/or food aversions. A **food intolerance** is a reaction to a specific food that does not involve the immune system. An example of this would be lactose intolerance in those who lack the enzyme lactase, which breaks down milk proteins. Even more common are **food aversions**, which are foods that you would prefer not to consume. These may be foods that you know do not agree with you or that you simply do not like; if so, you have an aversion to that food, not a food allergy.

deaths in the United States.[10] The exact cause of colorectal cancer is not known. However, a number of factors can increase a person's risk for developing colorectal cancer. The incidence of colorectal cancer increases with age. Most colorectal cancer occurs in people older than age 50. Colorectal polyps also increase the risk of colorectal cancer. Most polyps are benign and can easily be removed; removing polyps may reduce the risk of colorectal cancer. A family history of colorectal cancer also increases a person's risk, as does a personal history of cancer. There are some risks for colorectal cancer that you can do something about. Smoking is significantly associated with the incidence of colorectal cancer.[11] Overweight and obesity increase your risk of colorectal cancer, as does being physically inactive.[12,13] Diet also has an impact on a your risk for colorectal cancer. Eating a diet that is high in red meat or processed meat increases the risk of colorectal cancer.[14]

A great deal of speculation and scientific inquiry has examined the relationship between a diet that is high in fiber and/or fruits and vegetables and the prevention of colorectal cancer. The theory is that that fiber creates a bulkier stool that may dilute carcinogens in the colon and may decrease the transit time of waste through the colon, reducing the amount of time carcinogens spend in the colon. Although some evidence suggests that a diet high in fiber and fruits and vegetables reduces the risk of colorectal cancer, it is far from conclusive.[12,15–20] Some evidence suggests that a very low intake of fruit and vegetables is associated with an increased risk of colorectal cancer.[12,20]

TERMS

food allergy An abnormal immune response that occurs when the immune system produces antibodies and histamines in response to a specific food.

food intolerance A nonallergic, negative reaction to a food.

food aversions Dislike of a particular food.

How Policy and Environment Affect My Choices

Food Allergy Labeling and Consumer Protection Act

If you have a food allergy, what you eat can be a matter of life or death. You need to know—without a shadow of a doubt—that the food you are about to eat does not contain the food that could land you in the hospital. Effective January 1, 2006, the Food Allergy Labeling and Consumer Protection Act works to provide consumers with allergen information on food labels. It mandates that the labels of foods containing major food allergens (i.e., milk, eggs, fish, shellfish, peanuts, tree nuts, wheat, and soy) declare the allergen in plain language on the label. The allergen must be listed in the ingredient list in recognizable terms or with a parenthetical statement; for example, "albumin (egg)." Food manufacturers may also place "contains" on the label, followed by the name of the major food allergen; for example, "contains wheat." Manufacturers also must list the specific nut (e.g., almond, walnut, cashew) or seafood (e.g., tuna, salmon, shrimp, lobster) that is present. Major food allergens must be listed if they are present in any amount, even if it is only a trace amount in colorings, flavorings, or spice blends. This labeling law makes it a little easier to avoid eating a potentially harmful food.

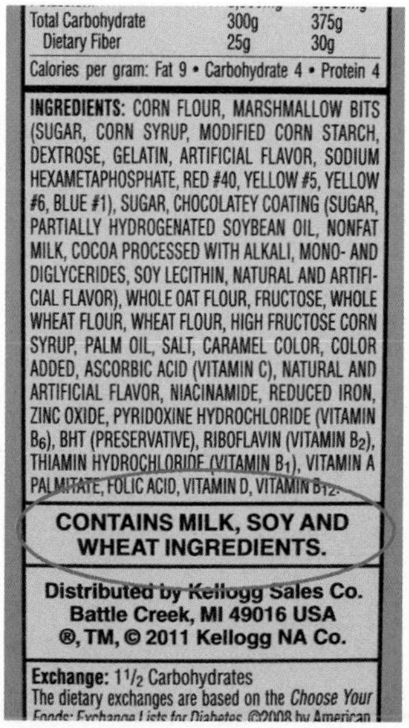
Total Carbohydrate 300g 375g
Dietary Fiber 25g 30g
Calories per gram: Fat 9 • Carbohydrate 4 • Protein 4
INGREDIENTS: CORN FLOUR, MARSHMALLOW BITS (SUGAR, CORN SYRUP, MODIFIED CORN STARCH, DEXTROSE, GELATIN, ARTIFICIAL FLAVOR, SODIUM HEXAMETAPHOSPHATE, RED #40, YELLOW #5, YELLOW #6, BLUE #1), SUGAR, CHOCOLATEY COATING (SUGAR, PARTIALLY HYDROGENATED SOYBEAN OIL, NONFAT MILK, COCOA PROCESSED WITH ALKALI, MONO- AND DIGLYCERIDES, SOY LECITHIN, NATURAL AND ARTIFICIAL FLAVOR), WHOLE OAT FLOUR, FRUCTOSE, WHOLE WHEAT FLOUR, WHEAT FLOUR, HIGH FRUCTOSE CORN SYRUP, PALM OIL, SALT, CARAMEL COLOR, COLOR ADDED, ASCORBIC ACID (VITAMIN C), NATURAL AND ARTIFICIAL FLAVOR, NIACINAMIDE, REDUCED IRON, ZINC OXIDE, PYRIDOXINE HYDROCHLORIDE (VITAMIN B6), BHT (PRESERVATIVE), RIBOFLAVIN (VITAMIN B2), THIAMIN HYDROCHLORIDE (VITAMIN B1), VITAMIN A PALMITATE, FOLIC ACID, VITAMIN D, VITAMIN B12.
CONTAINS MILK, SOY AND WHEAT INGREDIENTS.
Distributed by Kellogg Sales Co.
Battle Creek, MI 49016 USA
®, TM, © 2011 Kellogg NA Co.
Exchange: 1 1/2 Carbohydrates
The dietary exchanges are based on the Choose Your

Common Food Allergens Must Be Identified on the Label

Ready to Make a Change

Digestion and absorption is something your body does automatically; it is not something you have to think about or control. You can, however, take actions to keep your digestive system at optimal health. An overall healthy diet will keep your digestive system running smoothly, ensure proper elimination of wastes, and help you avoid some common digestive problems. If you have digestive problems, see your healthcare provider. He or she can make suggestions on how you may be able to alter your diet for better digestive health. If you have a healthy digestive system, including healthy elimination habits, keep up the good work and continue to eat healthy, drink plenty of fluids, and stay physically active.

Myth Versus Fact

Myth: Ulcers are caused by stress or eating too many spicy foods.

Fact: Spicy foods may make an ulcer worse, as can high stress levels. Ulcers, however, are usually caused by the bacterium *H. pylori* or overuse of NSAIDs.

Myth: The best way to treat constipation is to take a mild over-the-counter laxative.

Fact: It is best to try to avoid constipation in the first place. Consume a high-fiber, low-fat diet and drink plenty of fluids. If you do get occasional constipation, simple changes in your diet and fluid intake can often relieve the symptoms. Laxatives should be a last resort, because they can become habit-forming.

Myth: Smoking a cigarette can help relieve heartburn.

Fact: Cigarette smoking may contribute to heartburn. Heartburn occurs when the sphincter between the esophagus and the stomach relaxes, allowing acid from the stomach to splash back into the esophagus. Smoking can cause the sphincter between the esophagus and stomach to relax.

Myth: Bowel regularity means having a bowel movement every day.

Fact: The frequency of bowel movements varies in healthy people, ranging from three a day to three a week. What is normal for you may be too frequent or too few for someone else.

Myth: Detox diets get rid of all the toxins that build up in your body.

Fact: The scientific evidence does not support the use of detox diets. Your body is equipped with a very sophisticated system to get rid of waste. A short detox diet that includes lots of fruits and vegetables may be a way to jump-start a healthy diet and make you more mindful of what you are eating; however, no detox diet is a substitute for lifelong healthy eating habits.

Myth: Most of the digestion of food occurs in the stomach.

Fact: The real workhorse of the digestive system is the small intestine. More digestion and absorption occur there than in the stomach or the large intestine.

Myth: If you don't feel well after you eat a certain food, you probably have a food allergy.

Fact: True food allergies are relatively rare and must be diagnosed by a healthcare professional. What are more common are food intolerances. We all have foods that don't agree with us; these are usually food intolerances, not food allergies.

Back to the Story

Sarah was used to eating a healthy diet thanks to her mom making sure that the refrigerator was stocked with smart options. Now that she is on her own she relies heavily on processed foods that are low in fiber. Her diet is also lacking in fruits and vegetables. One easy step that Sarah can take is to make sure that she purchases fruits and vegetables to have on hand. She can grab a piece of fruit to take with her to class for a snack or to go with her lunch. She may want to try packing a lunch so that she doesn't always have to rely on pizza. It does not have to be complicated—yogurt with fruit, turkey sandwich on whole-wheat bread, or a pita stuffed with vegetables and cheese. The pizza may be cheap, but, so is a simple lunch that she makes herself. She needs to incorporate some variety into the evening meal. Quick, healthy, affordable options include an omelet with cheese and vegetables, soup and sandwich, or chicken grilled on a countertop grill. When she does have pasta with sauce from a jar or can, she may want to add a salad or try whole-wheat pasta for added fiber. Sarah also needs to make sure she is getting enough water so that her sluggish digestive system has enough fluid to function properly. What other suggestions do you have for Sarah to help get her digestive system back on track?

References

1. Mattes RD. Physiologic responses to sensory stimulation by food: nutritional implications. *J Am Diet Assoc.* 1997;97:406–410.
2. National Digestive Diseases Information Clearinghouse. Constipation. NIH Publication No. 07–2754. July 2007. http://digestive.niddk.nih.gov/ddiseases/pubs/constipation/index.htm. Accessed June 28, 2010.
3. Bogardus ST. What do we know about diverticular disease? A brief overview. *J Clin Gastroenterology.* 2006;40:S108–S111.
4. National Digestive Diseases Information Clearinghouse. Diverticulosis and diverticulitis. NIH Publication No. 08–1163. July 2008. http://digestive.niddk.nih.gov/ddiseases/pubs/diverticulosis/index.htm. Accessed June 28, 2010.
5. Ramakrishnan K, Salinas RC. Peptic ulcer disease. *Am Fam Phy.* 2007;76(7):1005–1012.
6. National Digestive Diseases Information Clearinghouse. *H. pylori* and peptic ulcers. NIH Publication No. 10-4225. April 2010. http://digestive.niddk.nih.gov/ddiseases/pubs/hpylori/index.htm. Accessed June 28, 2010.
7. Fasano A, Berti I, Gerarduzzi T, et al. Prevalence of celiac disease in at-risk and not-at-risk groups in the United States: a large multicenter study. *Arch Intern Med.* 2003;163:286–292.
8. National Institutes of Health. Statement. NIH Consensus Development Conference on Celiac Disease, June 28–30, 2004. *Gastroenterology.* 2005;128(suppl 1):S1–S9.
9. Niewinski MM. Advances in celiac disease and gluten-free diet. *J Am Diet Assoc.* 2008;108(4):661–672.
10. Centers for Disease Control and Prevention. Colorectal cancer screening. CDC Publication #99-6949. Revised June 2009.
11. Botteri E, Iodice S, Bagnardi V, Raimondi S, Lowenfels AB, Maisonneuve P. Smoking and colorectal cancer a meta-analysis. *JAMA.* 2008;300(23):2765–2778.
12. Key TJ, Schatzkin A, Willett WC, Allen NE, Spencer EA, Travis RC. Diet, nutrition, and the prevention of cancer. *Pub Health Nutr.* 2004;7:187–200.
13. Larsson SC, Wolk A. Obesity and colon and rectal cancer risk: a meta-analysis of prospective studies. *Am J Clin Nutr.* 2007;86(3):556–565.
14. Chao A, Thun JM, Connell CJ, et al. Meat consumption and risk of colon cancer. *JAMA.* 2005;293:172–182.
15. World Cancer Research Fund, American Institute for Cancer Research Expert Panel. *Food, Nutrition, and the Prevention of Cancer: A Global Perspective.* Washington, DC: American Institute for Cancer Research, 1997.
16. Fruit and vegetables. *IARC Handbooks of Cancer Prevention.* Vol 8. Lyon, France: International Agency for Research on Cancer, 2003.
17. Beresford SA, Johnson KC, Ritenbaugh C, et al. Low-fat dietary pattern and risk of colorectal cancer: the Women's Health Initiative Randomized Controlled Dietary Modification Trial. *JAMA.* 2006;295:643–654.
18. McCullough ML, Robertson AS, Chao A, et al. A prospective study of whole grains, fruits, vegetables, and colon cancer risk. *Cancer Causes Control.* 2003;14:959–970.
19. Terry P, Giovannucci E, Michels KB, et al. Fruit, vegetables, dietary fiber, and risk of colorectal cancer. *J Natl Cancer Inst.* 2001;93:525–533.
20. Park Y, Subar AF, Kipnis V, et al. Fruit and vegetable intakes and risk of colorectal cancer in the NIH–AARP diet and health study. *Am J Epidemiology.* 2007;166(2):170–180.
21. US Preventative Services Task Force. Screenings for colorectal cancer: US Preventative Services Task Force recommendation statement. *Ann Int Med.* 2008;149:627–637.
22. National Institute of Allergy and Infectious Disease. *Food allergy: an overview.* Bethesda, MD: July 2007. NIH Publication No. 07-5518. www.niaid.nih.gov/topics/foodAllergy/Documents/foodAllergy.pdf. Accessed June 30, 2010.
23. Branum AM, Lukacs SL. Food allergy among US children: trends in prevalence and hospitalizations. NCHS data brief, no 10. Hyattsville, MD: National Center for Health Statistics, 2008. http://www.cdc.gov/nchs/data/databriefs/db10.pdf. Accessed April 21, 2011.
24. Report on the Expert Panel on Food Allergy Research, June 30 and July 1, 2003, National Institute of Allergy and Infectious Diseases, National Institutes of Health. http://www.niaid.nih.gov/about/organization/dait/documents/june30_2003.pdf. Accessed April 20, 2011.

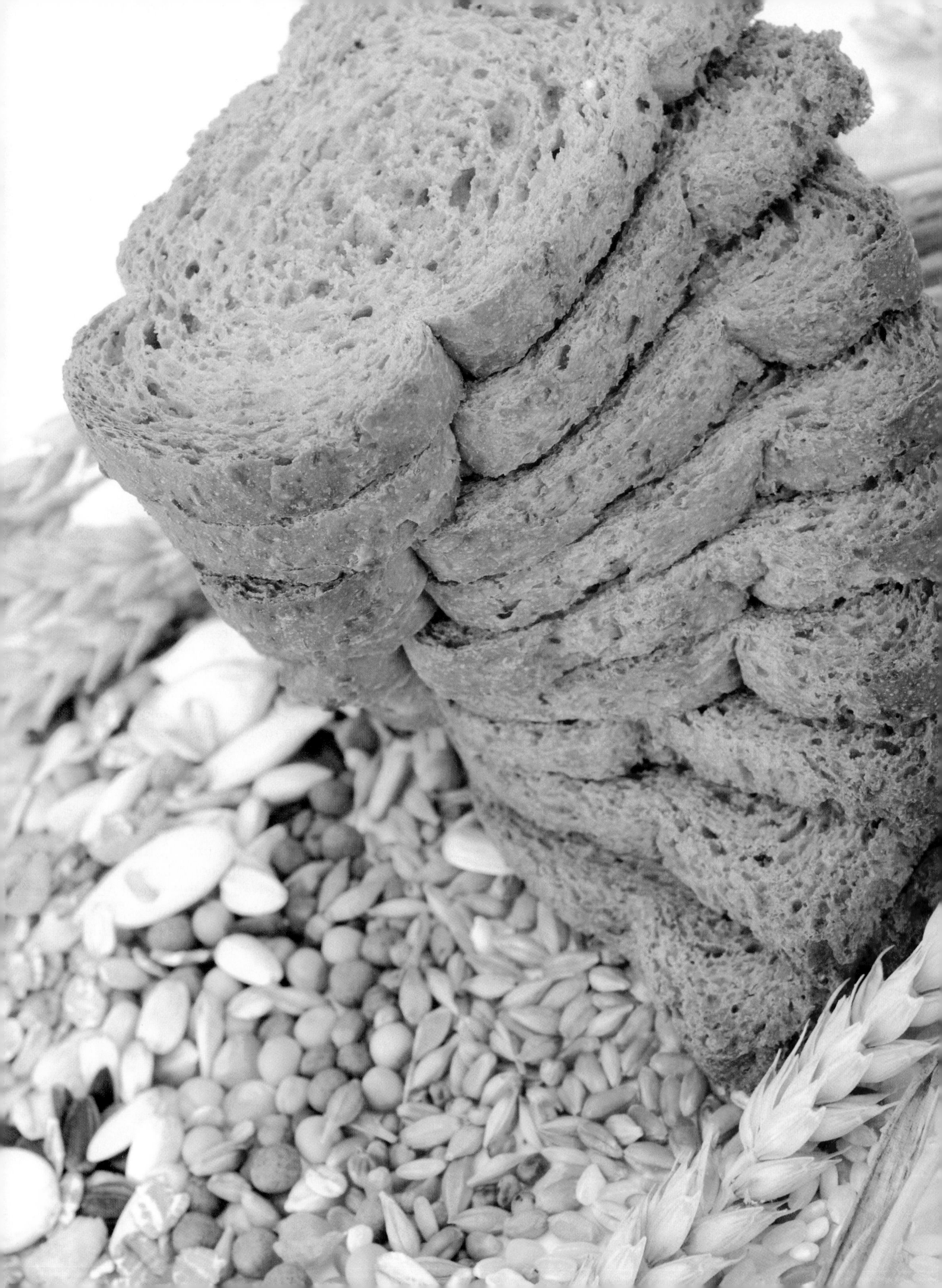

Chapter 5

Carbohydrates: Skip the Simple, Add More Complex

Key Messages

- Carbohydrates provide energy for the body.
- Carbohydrates are categorized as simple or complex.
- Adequate fiber intake is important for overall health.
- Simple sugars should be consumed in moderation.
- Whole grains should be chosen over refined grain.

Few nutrients have been as vilified and misunderstood as carbohydrates. You have probably heard, "Don't eat that, it has too many carbs!" Pasta, potatoes, bread, and rice have been labeled by many dieters as forbidden foods, destined to end up around their waist or on their thighs, when, in fact, too many calories are the culprit, not too many carbohydrates alone. Another popular misconception about carbohydrates is that sugar makes you hyper and causes diabetes. Moms are often overheard saying, "Don't give them any sugar; I want them to sleep tonight." Carbohydrates, both simple and complex, are an important part of your diet and provide most of the energy you need each day. Carbohydrate-rich foods such as whole grains, fruits, vegetables, and legumes also provide protection against chronic diseases. So how did something so good for us get such a bad rap? This chapter will discuss the good and not so good carbohydrates and help you navigate through a sea of misinformation to choose carbohydrates wisely.

Story

Rachel is 21 years old. Her diet consists almost completely of fast food and convenience foods from the deli or grocery store. A typical breakfast is a toaster pastry, a biscuit from a fast-food restaurant, or the occasional bagel and cream cheese. Lunch is pizza or hamburger and fries. Dinner usually consists of takeout from the Mexican restaurant around the corner, a sandwich from the deli, a frozen dinner, or a pizza. Rachel just learned about the importance of fiber and whole grains in a healthy diet. What can Rachel do to significantly increase her fiber intake?

Functions of Carbohydrates

Carbohydrates are the primary source of energy for the body and provide 4 calories per gram. The brain, the nervous system, and the red blood cells can only use carbohydrates for energy. If carbohydrates are not available, your body can use protein or fat for energy, but it prefers to use carbohydrates. Using carbohydrates for energy spares proteins, which are needed to build and repair body tissue. When fats are used for energy in the absence of carbohydrates, **ketone bodies** are produced, which can result in **ketosis**. Adequate carbohydrate consumption provides the body with energy so that it doesn't have to use protein or fat. The body also stores small amounts of carbohydrate in the form of **glycogen** in the liver and in the muscles.

Fiber, a component of some carbohydrate-rich foods, provides bulk to the diet and can make you feel full after a meal. Fiber also contributes to digestive tract health and supports normal bowel function. Adequate fiber in the diet can lower blood cholesterol, reducing the risk of heart disease and other chronic diseases. Finally, fiber can slow the absorption of sugar into the bloodstream.

Table 5.1

Functions of Carbohydrates in the Body

Provide energy.
Spare proteins.
Supply fiber:
• Provide a feeling of fullness.
• Contribute to digestive tract health.
• Support normal bowel function.
• Lower blood cholesterol.
• Slow absorption of sugar.

Types of Carbohydrates

The two types of carbohydrates are simple and complex. **Simple carbohydrates** include natural and added sugars. The sugars found in fruits, vegetables, milk, honey, corn syrup, and table sugar are all simple carbohydrates. **Complex carbohydrates** are starches and fiber. Grains such as rice, corn, and wheat all contain high amounts of starch. Fiber is found in fruits, vegetables, whole grains, and legumes.

Simple Carbohydrates

The two different types of simple carbohydrates are monosaccharides and disaccharides. Monosaccharides are single ("mono") sugar molecules. Common monosaccharides include glucose, fructose, and galactose. **Glucose** supplies energy to the cells. Glucose is the only fuel that can be used by the brain. It is not found in food as glucose, but

TERMS

ketone bodies Molecules formed from breakdown of fats; occurs when there is not enough carbohydrate available.

ketosis Presence of high levels of ketones in the urine; caused when fats are broken down for energy in absence of carbohydrates; can cause dehydration and acidify the blood.

glycogen Storage form of carbohydrate in the body composed of chains of glucose; stored in the liver and muscle.

simple carbohydrates Sugars composed of one sugar molecule (monosaccharides) or two sugar molecules (disaccharides).

complex carbohydrates Long chains of sugars (oligosaccharides or polysaccharides) arranged as starch or fiber.

glucose A monosaccharide and source of energy in the body.

joins together with other monosaccharides to give food a sweet taste. The word glucose comes from the Greek word *glukus*, which means "sweet"; the "-ose" suffix indicates that this is a sugar. **Fructose**, which is found in fruits, vegetables, and honey, is the sweetest of all the natural sugars. **Galactose** rarely occurs in food as galactose, but is joined with another monosaccharide. Galactose is less sweet than either glucose or fructose.

Disaccharides are sugars that are made up of two ("di") sugar molecules. Sucrose, lactose, and maltose are common disaccharides. Sucrose is made up of one molecule of glucose and one molecule of fructose. Sucrose is found in fruits, vegetables, honey, and maple syrup. Sucrose is extracted from sugar cane or beets to make table sugar. Lactose is made up of one molecule of glucose and one of galactose. Also called milk sugar, lactose gives milk its slightly sweet taste. Maltose is made up of two molecules of glucose. Maltose is not found in large amounts in foods; it occurs most often once longer chains of monosaccharides are broken down. Maltose, or malt sugar, can be produced by fermenting grains such as wheat or barley and is part of the brewing process in making beer.

Glucose + Fructose = Sucrose (table sugar)
Glucose + Galactose = Lactose (milk sugar)
Glucose + Glucose = Maltose (malt sugar)

Complex Carbohydrates

Starch and fiber are complex carbohydrates. Complex carbohydrates are chains of two or more monosaccharide molecules. If the chain is relatively short, say, 3–10 monosaccharide molecules, it is called an *oligosaccharide*. If the chain is longer, it is a *polysaccharide*. Polysaccharides can contain hundreds or thousands of monosaccharide units in either straight chains or branched chains.

Starches are monosaccharides that are linked together with bonds that can be digested by the human body, and thus are digestible complex carbohydrates. Fibers are monosaccharides that are linked together with bonds that cannot be digested by the human body, and thus are nondigestible carbohydrates.

TERMS

fructose A monosaccharide found in fruits and honey.

galactose A monosaccharide similar to glucose, usually found joined with other monosaccharides.

starch The major form of carbohydrate stored in plants; it is composed of long chains of glucose molecules.

fiber Carbohydrate found in plants that is not digestible by humans.

Starch Plants produce starch through photosynthesis and use it for energy to support growth and reproduction. **Starch** is found in two basic forms: amylase, which is a straight-chain polysaccharide, and amylopectin, which is a branched-chain polysaccharide (**Figure 5.1**). The starch in some fruits and some vegetables is converted to sugar as they ripen (**Figure 5.2**).

Foods high in starch include grains (e.g., wheat, corn, barley, oats), legumes (e.g., peas and beans), and root vegetables (e.g., potatoes, yams, beets, carrots). The body easily digests the long chains of glucose that comprise starch.

Fiber **Fiber**, like starch, is made up of chains of monosaccharide molecules. The difference is that the glucose molecules are bonded in such a way that the human body cannot digest them, and they pass through the body without being broken apart. Most fibers are polysaccharides, with the exception of the oligosaccharides raffinose and stachyose. These oligosaccharides are found in beans, peas, and lentils. Although your body cannot break the

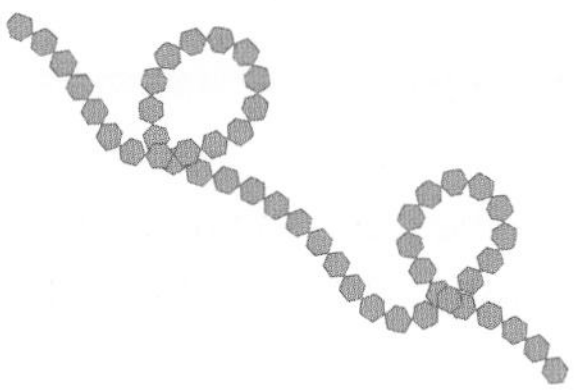

Starch
(amylose)

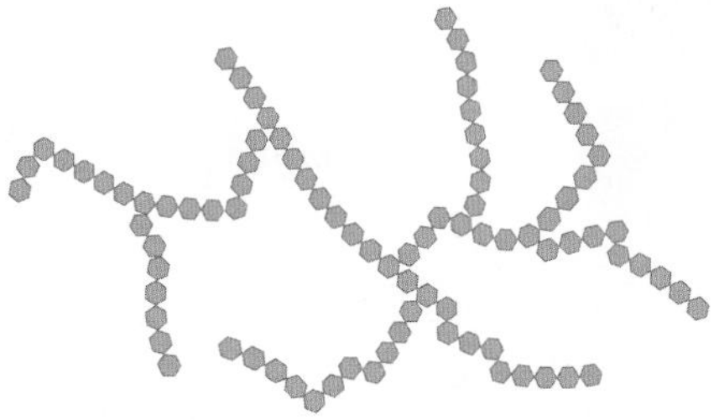

Starch
(amylopectin)

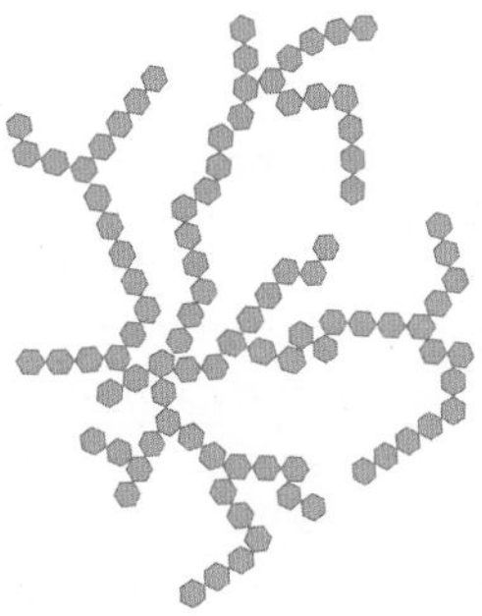

Glycogen

■ **Figure 5.1**
Amylose and Amylopectin

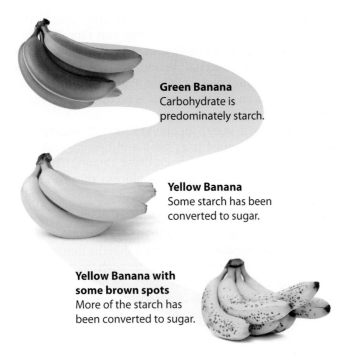

■ **Figure 5.2**
As Fruit Ripens, Starch Is Converted to Sugar

bonds of these oligosaccharides, the bacteria in your intestines can. The bacteria in your intestines break down some of the raffinose and stachyose, which results in the formation of gas.

Fiber is only found in plants and can be categorized as **soluble fiber** or **insoluble fiber**. Soluble fiber dissolves or swells in water. Soluble fibers include the pectins, gums, mucilages, and beta-glucans found in fruits, vegetables, legumes, and oats. Insoluble fiber does not dissolve in water. Insoluble fibers include cellulose and hemicelluloses, which are found in bran, vegetables, seeds, and whole grains.

Pectins are polysaccharides found in the cell walls of fruit. Gums are fibers found between the cell walls in plants. Mucilages are gel-forming fibers that hold plant cells together. They can be used to thicken or add texture to food. Psyllium is a mucilage that is used in the laxative Metamucil. Beta-glucans are branched-chain polysaccharides found in the cell walls of oats and barley. Cellulose is a straight polysaccharide chain of hundreds of glucose units that adds rigidity to plant cell walls. Cellulose is found in grains, fruits, vegetables, nuts, and legumes. Hemicelluloses are similar to cellulose but have a less complex structure. They can be more easily fermented than cellulose. The bran layer of grains is high in hemicelluloses.

Digestion and Absorption of Carbohydrates

We consume many different forms of carbohydrates—simple sugars, starch, fiber. Regardless of the type of carbohydrate that you consume, your body ultimately needs

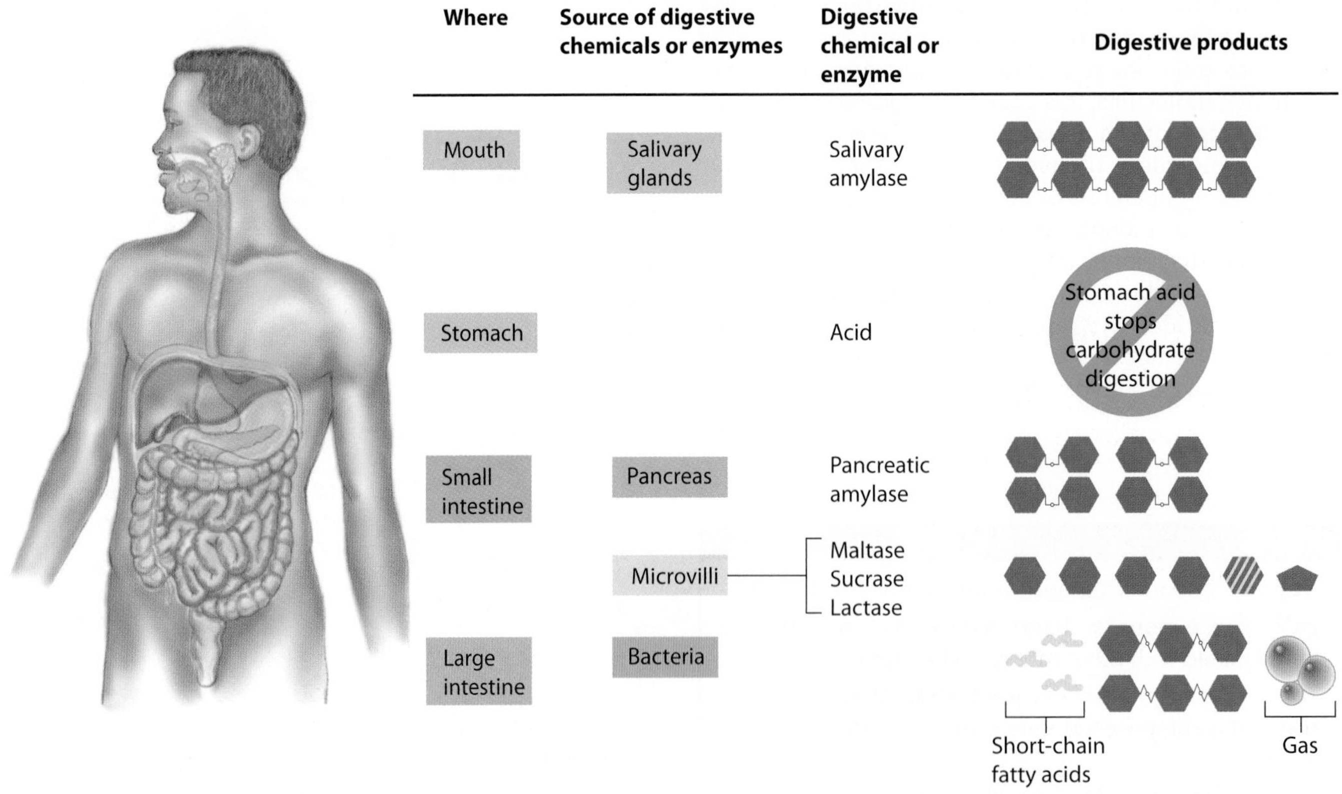

■ **Figure 5.3**
Overview of Carbohydrate Digestion

it to be in the form of glucose. An overview of carbohydrate digestion is provided in **Figure 5.3**.

Carbohydrate digestion begins in the mouth. As you chew, the enzyme salivary amylase is mixed with the food and chemical digestion begins. Salivary amylase breaks down long chains of starch into shorter polysaccharide chains and the disaccharide maltose. No disaccharides are broken down in the mouth. Because food only remains in the mouth a short time, only a small amount of digestion occurs. When the food reaches the stomach, carbohydrate digestion stops. The acid in the stomach causes salivary amylase to become inactive.

Most carbohydrate digestion occurs in the small intestine. Pancreatic amylase, secreted by the pancreas, picks up where salivary amylase left off. Pancreatic amylase continues to break down long starch chains into smaller units until all the polysaccharides are broken down into disaccharides. The microvilli of the small intestine have enzymes that can break apart the disaccharides into monosaccharides. Maltase breaks maltose into two glucose molecules. Sucrase breaks sucrose into glucose and fructose. Lactase breaks lactose into glucose and galactose. Once broken down, the monosaccharides can then be absorbed into the body. Once the monosaccharides are absorbed by the microvilli, they travel to the liver. The liver converts fructose and galactose to glucose.

To this point, no fiber has been digested. The body lacks the enzymes needed to break down fiber; it enters the large intestine virtually intact. Bacteria that are naturally present in the large intestine partially ferment some forms of fiber, such as the oligosaccharides raffinose and stachyose, resulting in the production of gas. Some types of fiber, such as cellulose or psyllium, pass through the large intestine without being fermented at all, thus producing no gas.

Carbohydrates in Your Body

All of the carbohydrates you consume, no matter what form they take on the plate, ultimately become glucose in the body. The liver converts all of the monosaccharides to glucose. Glucose can be used for immediate energy or stored as glycogen or fat (**Figure 5.4**).

Glucose is the primary fuel for the body and is the preferred energy source of the brain and the red blood cells. Glucose can be used in the liver for energy or released into the bloodstream to be used by other parts of the body for fuel.

Once the body's immediate energy needs are met, excess glucose can be stored as glycogen. Glycogen is a long chain of hundreds of glucose molecules. It can easily be broken down to glucose to be used for energy. Glycogen can be stored in very limited amounts in the liver and muscles. Depending on a person's activity level, the body stores enough glycogen to last for about one day.

Once the body's energy needs are met and the maximum amount of glycogen is stored in the liver and muscles, excess glucose is converted to fatty acids and stored in adipose tissue.

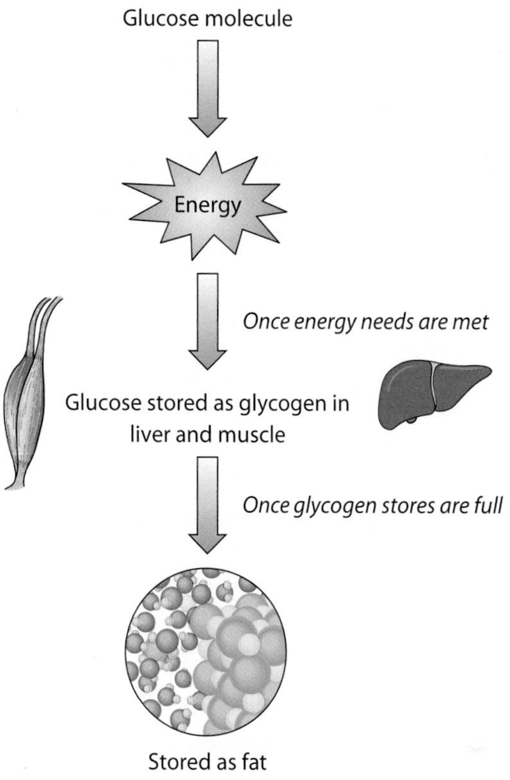

■ **Figure 5.4**

How Your Body Uses Glucose

Glucose is used for immediate energy needs; once those needs are met it is stored as glycogen. Once the body's glycogen stores are full, additional glucose is stored as fat.

Regulating Blood Glucose

It is important for the body to maintain a fairly constant level of glucose in the blood. The amount of glucose in the blood is called the **blood glucose level**, or blood sugar level. The cells need a constant supply of glucose to provide the energy they need to function. Low blood glucose levels can cause weakness or lightheadedness (**hypoglycemia**). High

TERMS

soluble fiber Fiber that dissolves or swells in water; includes pectins, gums, mucilages, and beta-glucans found in fruits, vegetables, legumes, and oats.

insoluble fiber Fiber that does not dissolve in water; includes cellulose and hemicelluloses found in bran, vegetables, seeds, and whole grains.

blood glucose level The amount of glucose present in the blood. Glucose is carried in the bloodstream to provide energy to all the cells.

hypoglycemia A condition that occurs when blood glucose levels are lower than normal.

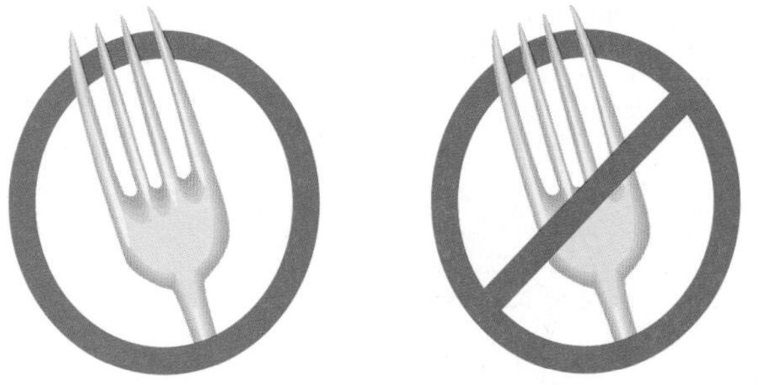

Eat a meal.
- Blood glucose goes up.
- Insulin secreted.
  - Insulin unlocks cells so glucose can enter.
  - Insulin stimulates production and storage of glucose and glycogen.
  - Insulin stimulates storage of glucose as fat.
- Blood glucose goes back to normal.

Lack of food.
- Blood glucose drops.
- Glucagon secreted.
  - Glucagon stimulates breakdown of glycogen to release glucose into blood.
  - Glucagon stimulates breakdown of fat and protein to release glucose into blood.

Figure 5.5
Regulation of Blood Glucose

blood glucose levels can cause fatigue or blurred vision (**hyperglycemia**).

Your body is well equipped to keep blood glucose in a safe range (**Figure 5.5**). The pancreas is responsible for producing hormones that control blood glucose levels. When glucose is absorbed into the bloodstream following digestion and absorption of carbohydrates, the pancreas secretes **insulin**. Insulin has several effects on the body. It attaches to cells and allows glucose to pass into the cell. Insulin is said to be like a key in a lock, unlocking the cell and allowing glucose to enter. Insulin also signals the liver and muscles to store glycogen. If there is more glucose than can be stored as glycogen, insulin signals the liver to convert glucose to fatty acids to be stored in fat cells. As the glucose is cleared from the blood and used for energy or stored as glycogen or fat, blood glucose levels return to normal.

When you have not eaten for a period of time, such as between meals, overnight, or during periods of high-energy needs, the pancreas secretes glucagon. **Glucagon** has the opposite effect of insulin. It signals the breakdown of glycogen to glucose so glucose can enter the bloodstream to provide a ready supply of energy for the cells. In the continued absence of glucose from food, glucagon will stimulate the breakdown of fat and protein to release glucose into the bloodstream.

Low Blood Glucose: Hypoglycemia Hypoglycemia simply means low ("hypo") blood sugar ("glycemia"). As just described, your body has a sophisticated mechanism to keep blood glucose within a normal range. Even when you have not eaten, glucagon signals the release of glucose from glycogen and the release of energy from muscle and fat. Usually this occurs without incident. Sometimes, however, blood glucose may drop rapidly or below what is normal for your body. When this happens, you may experience symptoms of hypoglycemia, such as dizziness, fatigue, or weakness. That shaky feeling you may get when you have not eaten for a while is slight hypoglycemia. These symptoms can occur if you don't eat regular balanced meals, if you skip meals, or if you participate in vigorous exercise. Most of the time transient hypoglycemia is corrected with eating on a regular schedule.

Hypoglycemia that is a result of a chemical imbalance in the body is relatively rare. Most often it is associated with diabetes. When a diabetic generates too much insulin for the amount of carbohydrate that is consumed, too much glucose will enter the cells, causing blood glucose levels to drop below normal. Other causes of hypoglycemia include the side effects of certain medications, liver disease, kidney disease, or a pancreatic tumor. It you have consistent symptoms of hypoglycemia that are not corrected by eating regular balanced meals, consult your healthcare provider.

Diabetes **Diabetes mellitus** is most often referred to simply as *diabetes*. Diabetes is characterized by hyperglycemia, or high ("hyper") blood sugar ("glycemia"). Diabetes results when no insulin is produced, when not enough insulin is produced, when the insulin produced is not used properly, or a combination of these factors.[1] The three categories of diabetes are type 1 diabetes, type 2 diabetes, and gestational diabetes. **Table 5.2** lists some of the more common symptoms of diabetes.

Type 1 Diabetes **Type 1 diabetes** was formerly referred to as *insulin-dependent diabetes* or *juvenile-onset diabetes*. Type 1 diabetes occurs when the cells in the pancreas that produce insulin are damaged or destroyed. Some individuals will present with this disease very early in childhood, whereas in others the destruction of the cells that produce insulin occurs more slowly, and thus they will not show signs of the disease until later in life. As the disease progresses, little or no insulin is produced. Insulin

TERMS

hyperglycemia A condition that occurs when blood glucose levels are higher than normal.

insulin Hormone secreted by the pancreas that is involved in regulating carbohydrate and fat metabolism. Insulin allows for glucose to enter the cells and signals the liver and muscles to store glycogen.

glucagon A hormone that promotes the breakdown of glycogen to glucose to maintain blood glucose levels.

diabetes mellitus A chronic condition where the uptake of glucose into the cells is impaired, resulting in too much glucose in the blood.

type 1 diabetes A type of diabetes that occurs when the cells in the pancreas that produce insulin are damaged or destroyed; usually diagnosed in childhood or early adulthood.

Table 5.2

Symptoms of Diabetes

Symptom	Cause
Increased thirst	High levels of glucose in the bloodstream pull fluid from the tissues, resulting in increased thirst.
More frequent urination	Increased thirst drives increased fluid consumption, which leads to more frequent urination.
Weight loss	Because glucose is not able to enter cells, calories are excreted in the urine.
Increased hunger	Glucose is present but cannot get into the cells. Without energy, the muscles and organs trigger hunger.
Blurred vision	High blood glucose levels cause fluid to be pulled from the lens of the eye, making it difficult for the eyes to focus.
Fatigue	Lack of energy for the body causes fatigue.
Areas of darkened skin (type 2 diabetes)	Patches of dark skin in the armpits and around the neck are often a sign of insulin resistance.

must then be given by injection or by insulin pump. There is no known way to prevent or cure type 1 diabetes. The primary risk factor for type 1 diabetes is a family history of the disease. Type 1 diabetes accounts for only 5–10% of all types of diabetes.[1]

Type 2 Diabetes **Type 2 diabetes** was formerly referred to as *non-insulin-dependent diabetes* or *adult-onset diabetes*. Individuals with type 2 diabetes may produce insulin, but the cells do not use the insulin properly. Ultimately, the pancreas cannot make enough insulin for the body's needs. There are several risk factors for type 2 diabetes (**Table 5.3**), many of which are within our control. The number one risk factor for type 2 diabetes is overweight and obesity.[2–4] The more adipose tissue, the more resistant cells become to insulin. Overweight individuals are more than twice as likely to develop diabetes as healthy-weight individuals. Obese individuals have three times the risk of diabetes compared to those of normal weight, and for someone who is 100 pounds or more overweight, the risk is six times greater.[3] Some evidence suggests that the increased risk of diabetes with overweight or obesity is even higher, perhaps as high as an 11-fold increase.[4]

Another preventable risk factor is physical inactivity. Being physically active not only helps with weight control, but it also makes cells more responsive to insulin.

A number of risk factors for type 2 diabetes are beyond a person's control. Type 2 diabetes risk increases after the age of 45 and is more prevalent in African Americans, American Indians, and Asian Americans. A family history of type 2 diabetes, especially in a parent or sibling, also increases a person's risk. If a woman develops gestational diabetes when pregnant, her risk of developing type 2 diabetes later in life is increased.

Table 5.3

Risk Factors for Type 2 Diabetes

Overweight or obesity
Physical inactivity
Age over 45
Ethnicity: African American, American Indian, or Asian American
Family history
Gestational diabetes
Pre-diabetes

Finally, pre-diabetes is a risk factor for type 2 diabetes. Pre-diabetes is a condition where blood glucose is higher than normal but not high enough to be classified as diabetes. The majority of people with pre-diabetes will develop diabetes unless preventive measures are taken.[2]

Type 2 diabetes is the most common form of diabetes and accounts for 90–95% of all diabetes cases in the United States.[1] Many people with type 2 diabetes can control their blood glucose by following a healthy meal plan and exercise program, losing excess weight, and taking oral medication. Some people with type 2 diabetes may also need insulin to control their blood glucose.

Gestational Diabetes Gestational diabetes is glucose intolerance during pregnancy. It develops in approximately 4% of all pregnancies in the United States.[1] It is more common in obese women and among African Americans, Hispanic/Latino Americans, and American Indians. To avoid complications in the infant, such as high birth weight, blood glucose must be kept within a normal range by use of medication and/or insulin. Although the diabetes may reverse after the child is born, the woman has a 40–60% chance of developing type 2 diabetes within 5–10 years.[5]

Prevalence of Diabetes

Diabetes affects almost 24 million people in the United States, or about 8% of the U.S. population. Over 5 million cases go undiagnosed each year. The incidence of diabetes has more than doubled in the past 15 years. A total of 1.6 million new cases of diabetes were diagnosed in people ages 20 years or older in 2007. This number is expected to continue to climb if the obesity epidemic continues or worsens. The cost of diabetes is staggering. Diabetes costs society $174 billion a year; $116 billion in direct medical costs and $58 billion in indirect costs, such as time missed from work.[6]

TERMS

type 2 diabetes Form of diabetes usually diagnosed later in life whereby the body does not make enough insulin or the cells do not respond as they should to insulin.

Personal Health Check

Are You at Risk for Diabetes?

American Diabetes Association.

ALERT!DAY

ARE YOU AT RISK?

DIABETES RISK TEST

Calculate Your Chances for Type 2 or Pre-Diabetes

The American Diabetes Association has revised its Diabetes Risk Test according to a new, more accurate statistical model. The updated test includes some new risk factors, and projects risk for pre-diabetes as well as diabetes.

This simple tool can help you determine your risk for having pre-diabetes or diabetes. Using the flow chart, answer the questions until you reach a colored shape. Match that with a risk message shown below.

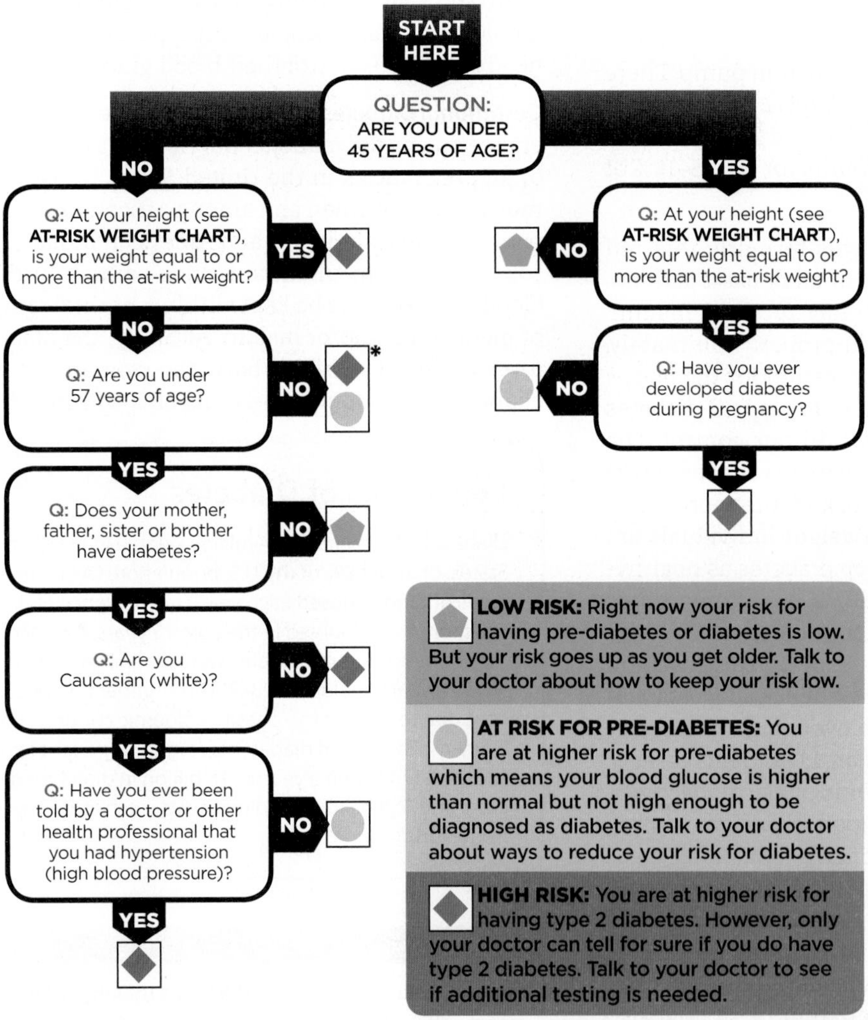
START HERE
QUESTION: ARE YOU UNDER 45 YEARS OF AGE?
NO
YES
Q: At your height (see AT-RISK WEIGHT CHART), is your weight equal to or more than the at-risk weight?
YES
NO
Q: Are you under 57 years of age?
NO
*
YES
Q: Does your mother, father, sister or brother have diabetes?
NO
YES
Q: Are you Caucasian (white)?
NO
YES
Q: Have you ever been told by a doctor or other health professional that you had hypertension (high blood pressure)?
NO
YES
Q: At your height (see AT-RISK WEIGHT CHART), is your weight equal to or more than the at-risk weight?
NO
YES
Q: Have you ever developed diabetes during pregnancy?
NO
YES
LOW RISK: Right now your risk for having pre-diabetes or diabetes is low. But your risk goes up as you get older. Talk to your doctor about how to keep your risk low.
AT RISK FOR PRE-DIABETES: You are at higher risk for pre-diabetes which means your blood glucose is higher than normal but not high enough to be diagnosed as diabetes. Talk to your doctor about ways to reduce your risk for diabetes.
HIGH RISK: You are at higher risk for having type 2 diabetes. However, only your doctor can tell for sure if you do have type 2 diabetes. Talk to your doctor to see if additional testing is needed.

AT-RISK WEIGHT CHART

HEIGHT	WEIGHT
4'10"	148 LBS
4'11"	153 LBS
5'0"	158 LBS
5'1"	164 LBS
5'2"	169 LBS
5'3"	175 LBS
5'4"	180 LBS
5'5"	186 LBS
5'6"	192 LBS
5'7"	198 LBS
5'8"	203 LBS
5'9"	209 LBS
5'10"	216 LBS
5'11"	222 LBS
6'0"	228 LBS
6'1"	235 LBS
6'2"	241 LBS
6'3"	248 LBS
6'4"	254 LBS
6'5"	261 LBS

STOP DIABETES.
1-800-DIABETES
diabetes.org/risktest

*Your risk for diabetes or pre-diabetes depends on additional risk factors including weight, physical activity and blood pressure.

Source: American Diabetes Association, diabetes.org/risktest.

Consequences of Diabetes Control of diabetes through lifestyle changes, medication, insulin, or a combination of these is critical. Glucose that is not absorbed into the cells can circulate in the bloodstream and damage small blood vessels. The complications of diabetes are very serious and can be life threatening. Diabetes is the seventh leading cause of death in the United States. Potential complications of diabetes include:

- **Heart disease and stroke.** Diabetes greatly increases the risk of heart disease and stroke.
- **High blood pressure.** Approximately 75% of people with diabetes have high blood pressure.
- **Blindness.** Diabetes is the number one cause of new blindness.
- **Kidney damage.** Damage to the small blood vessels in the kidney can lead to kidney failure.
- **Nerve damage.** Damage to the blood vessels in the hands and feet can cause poor circulation, resulting in nerve damage and impaired sensation in the hands and feet.
- **Amputation.** Poor blood circulation in the limbs can result in tissue death. In severe cases, this can lead to amputation.

To prevent or delay onset of complications related to diabetes, it is critical to maintain normal, or close to normal, blood glucose levels. This means taking needed medications and insulin and/or modifying lifestyle choices. Controlling blood pressure and blood lipids through medication or change in diet and exercise habits is also important.

Recommended and Actual Carbohydrate Intake

The amount of carbohydrate in your diet should be between 45–65% of calories.[12,13] To calculate the percentage of calories from carbohydrate in your diet, you need to know the number of grams of carbohydrate you consume in a day and the total number of calories you consume (**Figure 5.6**). The specific number of grams of carbohydrate that would be appropriate to consume each day depends on your usual calorie consumption. Someone who needs 2,000 calories per day should consume 225–325 grams of carbohydrate each day.

The source of the carbohydrates is important. Added sugar should be kept to a minimum. *Added sugar* is defined as sugar or syrup that is added to foods during processing or preparation. You should choose and prepare foods and beverages with little added sugar. The specific amount of added sugar you should consume each day depends on your calorie intake and consumption of other discretionary calories in fat and alcohol, as outlined in MyPlate. For example, a person whose calorie needs are 2,000 calories per day and who consumes a moderate amount of fat (approximately 30% of calories from fat) and no alcohol could consume up to 8 teaspoons of sugar per day, which is less than the amount contained in one 12-ounce soft drink. If you use that same example and up the fat intake to 35% of calories, that person should consume no added sugar. The bottom line is that added sugars should be very limited. Added sugars provide calories but no nutritional value.

You should also consume lots of fiber-rich fruits, vegetables, and whole grains. The specific amount of fiber needed each day is based on calorie needs. The recommended dietary fiber intake is 14 grams per 1,000 calories. Men aged 19–50 should consume 38 grams of fiber per day; women aged 19–50 should consume 25 grams of fiber per day.

The average carbohydrate intake in most adults is 49–50% of calories. This is within the range of how much carbohydrate should be consumed; however, when you take a closer look you will see that the type of carbohy-

Children and Diabetes

In the past, diabetes diagnosed in children was predominately type 1 diabetes. In fact, type 2 diabetes used to be called *adult-onset diabetes* because it was most likely to occur in adults older than the age of 45. All of that has changed in the past 20 years. More and more children are being diagnosed with type 2 diabetes.[7–10] Prior to 1990, less than 4% of all new childhood cases of diabetes were type 2 diabetes. That number is now estimated to be between 8–45%.[8] An increase in diabetes in any population is alarming. However, the increase in type 2 diabetes in children is of the utmost concern. Onset of diabetes in childhood places children at risk for other chronic diseases, such as heart disease and stroke, potentially shortening their life expectancy. The primary reason for the increase of type 2 diabetes in children is the increase in overweight and obesity in all age groups. In fact, it is estimated that one in three girls and one in four boys will develop diabetes sometime in their life.[11] These statistics can be turned around if we help children eat healthy, be physically active, and achieve and maintain a healthy weight.

Most of your calories should come from carbohydrates (45–65%). Carbohydrate-rich foods include grains, vegetables, and fruit. Go easy on foods high in simple carbohydrates (or sugar), like candy, soft drinks, or sugary desserts.

How to calculate:

Step 1: Grams of carbohydrates × 4 calories = calories from carbohydrates

Note: the value "4 calories" is a standard unit of measure and does not change. A gram of carbohydrate contains 4 calories.

Step 2: Calories from carbohydrates/total calories × 100 = % calories from carbohydrates

Enter carbohydrates

Total calories

% calories from carbohydrates

■ **Figure 5.6**

How to Calculate Percent (%) Calories from Carbohydrates

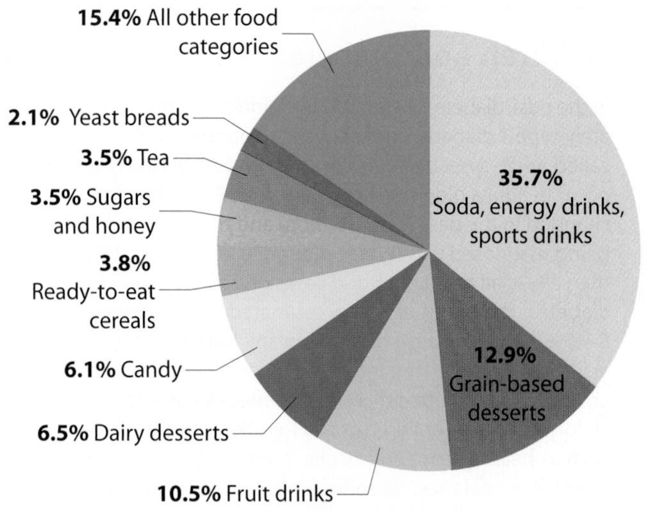

Figure 5.7

Major Sources of Added Sugars in the American Diet

Source: National Cancer Institute. Sources of added sugars in the diets of the U.S. population ages 2 years and older, NHANES 2005–2006. Risk Factor Monitoring and Methods. Cancer Control and Population Sciences. http://riskfactor.cancer.gov/diet/foodsources/added_sugars/table5a.html. Accessed April 9, 2011.

drate consumed by most people is not in line with the recommendations. Consumption of added sugar varies widely in adults, with averages ranging from 10–30 teaspoons per day. Even at the low end of that range, it may be too high, depending on a person's total calorie intake. Certainly, the average added sugar intake is above what would be recommended in a healthy diet. Almost half (49%) of the added sugar that is consumed comes from sugar added to beverages.[14] Other sources of added sugar are baked goods, ice cream, and breakfast cereal (**Figure 5.7**).

In addition to consuming too much added sugar, most people consume too little fiber. The average fiber intake in adults is around 16 grams per day.[12] Men consume slightly more fiber than women, 19 grams versus 13 grams. Both genders, however, fall far short of the recommended 38 grams for men and 25 grams for women. When you examine the two major contributors to fiber in the diet, whole grains and fruits and vegetables, you will see why fiber is lacking. Only 24% of Americans eat five or more servings of fruits and vegetables each day. That means that a large majority (76%) get less than the minimum recommended amount of daily fruits and vegetables.[15] Grains can provide fiber when eaten in the form of whole grain. However, the bulk of the grains eaten by Americans are in the form of refined grains that have most of the fiber removed. On average, Americans consume about one serving of whole grain each day,[16] and only 13% of the grains consumed are in the form of whole grains.[17]

Carbohydrates in Your Diet

The carbohydrates in your diet come primarily from plant sources. Fruits, vegetables, legumes, and grains are all plant sources of carbohydrates, contributing starch, sugar, and fiber in varying amounts. A banana contains mostly starch until it ripens and some of that starch is converted to simple carbohydrates. Whole-grain bread may contain starch and fiber. Most vegetables contain starch and fiber. The amount of starch in vegetables varies greatly; vegetables such as potatoes, peas, and beans are higher in starch than summer squash, tomatoes, and lettuce. The only animal source of carbohydrate is milk, which contains the simple carbohydrate lactose. Sugars and syrups that can be added to foods during processing or preparation also contribute carbohydrate to our diet (**Figure 5.8**).

Choose Carbohydrates Wisely

When we examine what we are eating as a country and compare it to what we should be eating, it is apparent that we should increase fiber by increasing our intake of fruits, vegetables, and whole grains. In addition, we should decrease the amount of added sugar we consume.

Increase Fiber

There are several ways to increase the fiber in your diet. Although there are many fiber supplements on the market, it is best to get the fiber you need from food, not from a pill or powder. Fruits and vegetables are a great way to add fiber to your diet and will be discussed in detail in Chapter 6. The fiber content of a number of common foods is presented in **Table 5.4**.

Along with fruits and vegetables, whole grains are a great way to increase fiber consumption. At least half the grains you consume should be whole grains. More would be better. Most Americans need about six servings of grain a day, so at *least* three should be whole grain.

A whole grain includes the grain's germ, endosperm, and bran (**Figure 5.9**). The **germ** is the part of the grain that grows into a new plant. It is the part of the plant

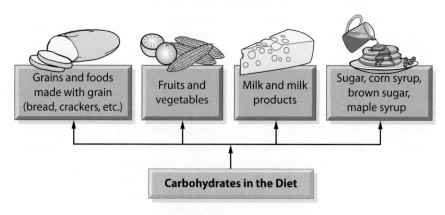

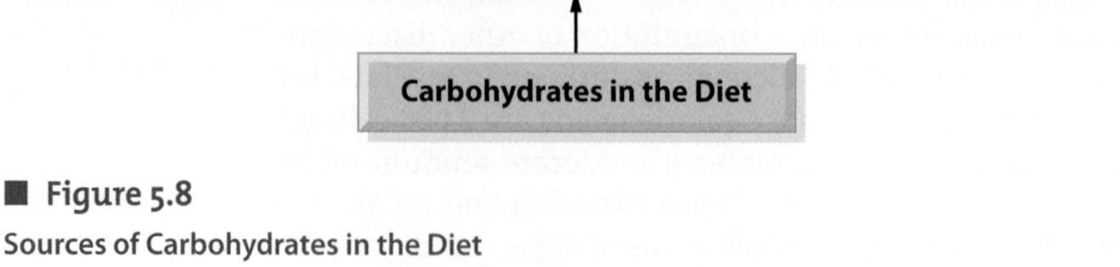

Figure 5.8

Sources of Carbohydrates in the Diet

How Policy and Environment Affect My Choices

The Farm Bill

The types of foods that are grown and processed influence the carbohydrates that are available in the U.S. food supply. What foods are grown is influenced by many factors, including the Farm Bill. The Farm Bill is a massive piece of legislation that is reexamined every five years. The Farm Bill began as a way to help millions of farmers during the Great Depression. Although it may seem hard to believe in a country that prides itself on the right to private property and a free market economy, to a large extent the Farm Bill determines what sorts of foods Americans eat. It also influences how much those foods will cost. The Farm Bill is complex and touches on many aspects of the commercial food system. Here, we will discuss only the aspect of subsidies to farmers.

The Farm Bill determines which crops will receive government subsidies. Five crops receive the bulk of the subsidies: corn, soybeans, wheat, rice, and cotton. The crops receiving the biggest share of subsidies are corn and soybeans, around $25 billion per year. The subsidy of corn and soybeans began in the 1970s. Historically, farmers would hold back crops in years when prices were down or plant less to allow the soil to regenerate. The Farm Bill sought to drive down the price that farmers received for these crops. Farmers were encouraged to plant "fence-row to fence-row" and not to put crops aside and wait for higher prices. The farmers could plant, harvest, and sell regardless of market price, thanks to subsidies from the government. These policies put more corn and soy into the food supply than ever before.

So, how does this influence what we eat in America? Let's use corn as an example. Farmers receive money based on how many bushels of corn they grow. Corn is used to produce high fructose corn sweetener, cornstarch, and other ingredients common in processed foods. Foods that contain these ingredients are generally cheaper than those that do not, thanks to the government subsidy. Corn is so cheap and available that it is in about 25% of the foods in the grocery store.[18]

Another way that subsidies influence your food choices is that corn is used as livestock feed. Cheap, widely available corn feed quickly produces a fat cow, which yields meat that is well marbled and higher in fat than if the cow had been allowed to graze on grass. Fattening a cow on corn instead of grass means that a cow is ready for market in months instead of years.

Why is a fast-food meal of a soft drink and hamburger cheaper than the salad? One reason for the price difference is that the high fructose corn sweetener in the soft drink, the wheat in the bun, and the corn-fed beef in the burger were all influenced by subsidies, which certainly influences their price. The salad, in contrast, contains primarily vegetables that receive little or no help from the Farm Bill.

Many believe that the Farm Bill has inadvertently caused a number of contemporary public health issues, such as obesity and type 2 diabetes, by making unhealthy, high-calorie foods more affordable than healthy fruits and vegetables. What do you think? How could the Farm Bill be changed to promote more healthful foods?

Table 5.4

Fiber Content of Common Foods

Food	Amount	Fiber (g)
Apple	1 medium	4.4
Pear	1 medium	4.0
Banana	1 medium	2.0
Broccoli	1/2 cup	2.6
Corn	1/2 cup	3.0
Carrots	2 medium	3.4
Green beans	1/2 cup	2.7
Beans, black, pinto, etc.	1/2 cup	9.7
Whole wheat bread	1 slice	3.0[1]
Oatmeal	1 cup cooked	4.0
Bran flakes	1 cup	5.0
Popcorn	1 cup	1.0

[1]Fiber content of bread and other baked goods varies greatly depending on the brand.

Source: US Department of Agriculture, Agriculture Research Service. 2008. USDA National Nutrient Database for Standard Reference Release 21. Nutrient Data Laboratory Home Page. http://www.ars.usda.gov/ba/bhnrc/ndl. Accessed April 9, 2011.

that contains the most protein and has a small amount of fat. The **endosperm** is the largest part of the grain and is primarily starch. The outer layer of the grain, the **bran**, is rich in fiber. When a grain is refined, the bran and germ are removed, thus removing most of the fiber and some valuable nutrients. When manufacturers refine grains, they add back the vitamins that are lost but do not add back the fiber. Enriched flour is an example of this process. Wheat kernels start out as whole grains and then end up as enriched flour with virtually no fiber.

Spotting whole grains in the grocery store is easy once you learn a few basic techniques. A great way to start is to look for whole grains in ingredient lists. **Table 5.5** lists some of the various types of whole grains available today.

TERMS

germ The inner part of a whole grain; contains nutrients and fat.

endosperm Starchy portion of a grain.

bran The outer layer of a grain; it is high in fiber.

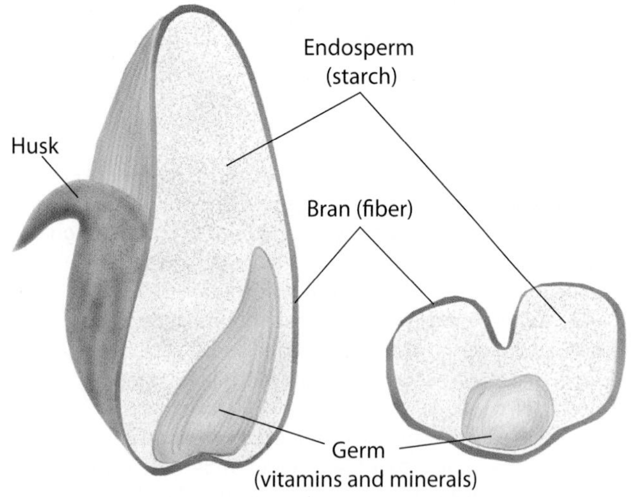

■ **Figure 5.9**

Whole Grains Contain the Endosperm, Germ, and Bran

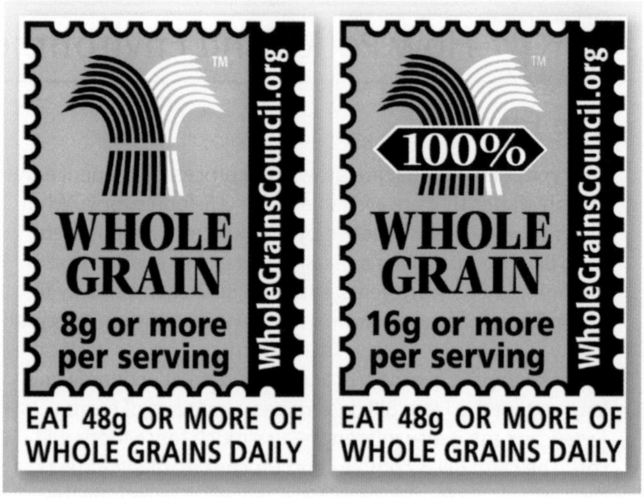
WHOLE GRAIN
8g or more per serving
WholeGrainsCouncil.org
EAT 48g OR MORE OF WHOLE GRAINS DAILY
100%
WHOLE GRAIN
16g or more per serving
WholeGrainsCouncil.org
EAT 48g OR MORE OF WHOLE GRAINS DAILY

■ **Figure 5.10**

Whole Grains Council Labeling System

The Whole Grains Council has a labeling system to help consumers identify whole grains. The Whole Grains Stamp features a stylized sheaf of grain on a golden-yellow background with a bold black border. Although the graphics here illustrates the minimum whole-grain content for qualifying products, actual stamps show a *different* number on each product, reflecting the actual whole-grain content of that particular food. The Whole Grain Stamp tells you exactly the number of grams of whole grain you are getting, while also reminding you to aim for at least 48 grams of whole grain overall each day.

Source: Courtesy of Oldways and the Whole Grain Council. www.wholegrainscouncil.org.

Be careful when you see the words *multigrain*, *100% wheat*, or *made with whole grain*. *Multigrain* just means many grains; the food may contain lots of grains, but they may or may not be whole grains. Similarly, *100% wheat* does not mean that it is 100% whole wheat; it might have a small amount of whole grain mixed with lots of refined grains.

Note that some cookies and baked goods are now being made with whole grains. Although they may be slightly healthier than their non-whole-grain counterparts, it does not mean that whole-grain donuts or whole-grain chocolate chip cookies are health foods that can be consumed everyday. Making these foods with whole grains has done little to change their overall calorie or fat content.

The Whole Grains Council has a labeling system to help consumers identify whole grains (**Figure 5.10**). The Whole Grain Stamp features a stylized sheaf of grain on a golden-yellow background with a bold black border. It tells you exactly the number of grams of whole grain you are getting, while also reminding you to aim for at least 48 grams of whole grain overall each day. Note that this is not 48 grams of dietary fiber; it is 48 grams of whole grain.

One way to increase the fiber in your diet is to choose whole-grain bread. However, the bread aisle in the grocery store is one of the most confusing for shoppers. There are so many choices! How can you know which one is best? Take a look at the two loaves of bread in **Figure 5.11**. They look very similar and cost about the same. They both are brown in color and use the word *wheat* on the label. At first glance, you may think they are both whole-grain products, but take a closer look at the ingredient list. The first ingredient in the bread on the top (**Figure 5.11a**) is whole-wheat flour, while the first ingredient of the bread on the bottom (**Figure 5.11b**) is enriched flour. The bread on the bottom is not a whole-grain food; in fact, it contains no whole grain. The bread on the top is a whole-grain food; whole wheat is the first ingredient and the front label indicates that it is 100% whole-grain wheat.

Table 5.5

Types of Whole Grains

Whole wheat	Buckwheat
Whole-grain corn	Triticale
Popcorn	Bulgur (cracked wheat)
Brown rice	Millet
Whole rye	Quinoa
Whole oats (oatmeal)	Sorghum
Wild rice	Whole-grain barley

Health Benefits of Fiber

Overweight and Obesity Eating whole grains and other high-fiber foods offers a number of nutritional benefits. Most high-fiber foods are low in fat and calories. A big benefit of high-fiber foods is that they help you feel full

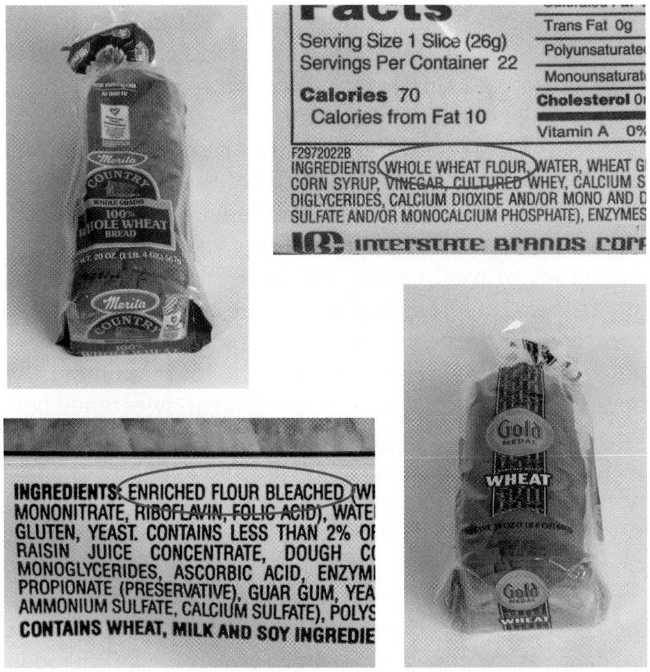

Figure 5.11

Choose a Whole-Grain Bread

(top) Whole-grain bread.
(bottom) Not whole-grain bread.

Try Something New

Increase Your Consumption of Whole Grains

Start slowly, add whole-grain fiber to your diet a little at a time, and consume an adequate amount of water. If you add whole-grain fiber too fast or without adequate fluid, you may experience gastrointestinal distress such as cramps, bloating, gas, or constipation. The following are some easy ways to increase your intake of whole grains:

- Choose oatmeal or another whole-grain cereal to start your day.
- Use brown rice instead of white rice.
- Choose bread made with 100% whole grain.
- Choose unbuttered popcorn as a low-fat snack.
- Substitute whole-grain flour for all-purpose flour in recipes.
- Experiment with new whole grains.

longer.[21,22] High-fiber foods digest more slowly and add bulk to the diet, providing a feeling of fullness. People who consume more whole grains, and thus more fiber, are more likely to have a lower body weight.[16,23–27] A 12-year study found that consuming whole grains increased satiety and made it easier to maintain a healthy weight. Further, those

Oatmeal

Oatmeal is a great quick breakfast that packs a powerful nutritional punch. It is a whole grain, is high in fiber, and can decrease your risk of heart disease.[19,20] However, stay away from flavored or sweetened oatmeal with added sugar. Oatmeal should have just one ingredient—oats. Eat it unsweetened, topped with fruit, or with just a little white or brown sugar. All oatmeal is made from oat groats, which are the whole grain of the oat with only the outer hard husk removed. A number of different types of oatmeal are offered on supermarket shelves:

- **Steel-cut oats (Irish oats):** Made by cutting oat groats into tiny pieces. Steel-cut oats are chewier than traditional oats, are digested more slowly, and may provide longer satiety. This type of oatmeal takes about 30 minutes to cook.
- **Rolled oats (old fashioned):** The most common form of oatmeal. Rolled oats are made by steaming oat groats that are then flattened (rolled) to create oat flakes. Rolled oats cook in about five minutes.
- **Quick cooking oats:** To make this type of oatmeal, rolled oats are pressed into even thinner flakes and cut into small pieces. This type of oatmeal cooks in about one to two minutes.
- **Instant oatmeal:** Oatmeal that has been precooked and dried. To cook, you simply add boiling water. Instant oatmeal is fast, but it does not have the distinctive chewiness of regular oatmeal. Also, many types of instant oatmeal have added sugar.

Try Something New

Try a New Grain

Some of the whole grains in Table 5.5 may not be familiar to you. In the United States, we do not usually consume grains such as millet, bulgur, or quinoa. However, they can add variety, interest, and a healthy dose of whole grain to your diet. One in particular that you may want to try is quinoa, pronounced "keen-wah." Quinoa is a great alternative to rice and has a mild nutty flavor. Quinoa is available in some grocery stores and in many health food stores. It is easy to cook: just use 2 cups of water to 1 cup of quinoa, bring to a boil, cover, and lower the heat. Quinoa cooks fast; only 15 minutes and it will be done. You can use it as-is for a side dish as you would rice or potatoes or you can add it to a recipe. To make a quick salad, cook 1 cup of quinoa and then chill it. Add 2 cups of chopped vegetables, your choice. Good vegetables to choose include mild onions, tomatoes, bell peppers, and carrots. Mix in 1/4 cup of chopped parsley or other herb. Toss with your favorite Italian dressing or oil and vinegar. This salad will keep for several days in the refrigerator and makes a great light lunch.

who consumed more whole grains had a lower chance of becoming overweight over time.[16]

Heart Disease High blood cholesterol is a risk factor for heart disease. Several types of fiber have been shown to decrease blood cholesterol, specifically the bad low-density lipoprotein (LDL) cholesterol.[12,28–30] Fruits and vegetables, legumes, psyllium, oatmeal, and oat bran have all been shown to reduce cholesterol levels. Two of these fibers, oats and psyllium, are so promising that the FDA has authorized a health claim regarding their effects in preventing heart disease.[31] Cereals and other foods containing psyllium, which is found in oats, can now carry a health claim that the food can help reduce cholesterol. It has also been shown that consumption of whole grains can have protective effects against heart disease.[12,32,33] People who eat at least 2.5 servings of whole-grain foods a day are more likely to live a longer life thanks to the protective effect of whole grains against heart disease.[34,35]

Type 2 Diabetes For people with type 2 diabetes, a diet high in fiber and whole grains can delay glucose uptake and improve insulin sensitivity.[29] Current dietary recommendations for those with type 2 diabetes include a diet high in fruits, vegetables, and whole grains.

You can lower your risk of type 2 diabetes by maintaining a healthy weight and engaging in regular physical activity. Fiber also seems to have a protective effect against type 2 diabetes. Scientific evidence suggests that consuming a diet high in fiber, especially whole grains, can lower your risk for type 2 diabetes.[36–38]

Digestive Health Constipation is a common digestive complaint. Constipation is usually characterized by hard, dry stools that are difficult to pass. A combination of a high-fiber diet and adequate fluid intake can help prevent and treat constipation. Consuming a high-fiber diet with plenty of fluid will make stools easier to pass. High fiber intake can also prevent hemorrhoids. Diverticular disease can also be helped or prevented with a high-fiber diet.

Decrease Sugar

We are born liking the taste of sweet foods and drink. Most of us enjoy an occasional dessert or piece of candy. Consuming sugar, in any form, in moderation is not a problem. It is a problem, however, when consumption of sugar is high and takes the place of other healthy foods or causes overall calories to be too high. You should choose and prepare foods and beverages with little added sugars or caloric sweeteners. Sugar is naturally present in foods such as fruit or milk. Added sugar is sugar or syrup that is added to foods at the table, during preparation, or during processing. The body's response to sugar is similar regardless of whether it is natural or added; however, here, we are most concerned with added sugar. Added sugar supplies calories but few other nutrients and may be found in much higher concentration in foods. Individuals who consume foods or beverages high in added sugar tend to consume more calories than those who consume food or beverages low in added sugar.[13]

You can take several steps to decrease the amount of added sugar in your diet. Most of the added sugar in your diet comes from sugar-sweetened beverages. Calories from sugar-sweetened beverages contribute an estimated 7% of total calorie intake.[39,40] People who drink sugar-sweetened beverages take in more calories than those who do not,[41–43] and those who consume more sugar-sweetened beverages also tend to weigh more.[41,43] Several studies point to decreasing sugar-sweetened beverages as a good strategy to decrease calories and manage weight.[41,43,44] Decreasing or cutting out sugar-sweetened beverages altogether will go a long way in decreasing your sugar intake. We will discuss beverages in more detail in Chapter 7.

Sugar-sweetened beverages are not the only place you get added sugar in your diet. Sugar is added to many of the foods we eat, including baked goods, cereals, snack foods, condiments, and sauces. The Nutrition Facts Panel will tell you the total amount of sugar in a food, but it does not discern between natural and added sugar. To see if a food has added sugar, look at the ingredient list for sugar of any type that has been added to the food (**Table 5.6**).

Because ingredients are listed in descending order, you can get a general idea as to how much sugar is in the food. Keep in mind that the food may have more than one type of added sugar.

To decrease the amount of added sugar in your diet:

- Decrease consumption of sugar-sweetened beverages.
- Limit consumption of baked goods and desserts that are high in sugar.
- Read labels carefully to choose foods that are lower in added sugar.
- Choose canned fruit that is packed in water or juice instead of heavy syrup.

Table 5.6

Common Types of Added Sugars

Brown sugar	Invert sugar
Corn sweetener	Lactose
Corn syrup	Maltose
Dextrose	Malt syrup
Fructose	Molasses
Fruit juice concentrates	Raw sugar
Glucose	Sucrose
High-fructose corn syrup	Sugar
Honey	Syrup

Choosing a Healthy Breakfast Cereal or Breakfast Bar

The breakfast cereal aisle contains lots of choices. Making a healthy choice is not always easy. The ones with chocolate in the name or with brightly colored marshmallows are easy to write off as not a great choice. Beyond that, though, how do you choose? Here are some good rules of thumb for choosing either a breakfast cereal or a breakfast bar.

Choose a breakfast cereal that has:

- Less than 200 calories per serving
- Less than 6 grams of sugar per serving
- At least 3 grams of dietary fiber per serving

Choose a breakfast bar that has:

- Less than 200 calories per bar
- Less than 6 grams of sugar per 100 calories
- At least 3 grams of dietary fiber per bar

Sugar and Hyperactivity

One of the most common food myths is that sugar causes hyperactivity or behavior issues. Many mothers have commented on their children's behavior at a birthday party or on Halloween, attributing it to the sugary cake and candy being consumed. Well-meaning aunts and grandmothers have been chastised not to give little Johnny candy or he will be "bouncing off the walls all night." Dan White, who in 1978 murdered San Francisco city supervisor Harvey Milk and mayor George Moscone, blamed his violent act on his high consumption of high-sugar junk food. This became known as the "Twinkie Defense."

Claims that sugar causes behavior problems are unfounded. Many sophisticated studies have examined sugar's affect on behavior; none have found any correlation between sugar and hyperactivity or aggressive behavior.[45,46] In fact, carbohydrates have a calming effect. Consumption of carbohydrate (including sugar) signals the production of the sleep-inducing chemical serotonin. The children at the birthday party or Halloween are most likely reacting with enthusiasm to the event, not the foods that are being served. As to Mr. White, the "Twinkie Defense" did not explain his violent behavior, nor should it have.

Sugar and Dental Health Tooth decay, or dental caries (cavities), is caused by a combination of bacteria and food. Biofilm (formerly referred to as plaque) is a sticky substance that is constantly forming on your teeth. The bacteria contained in biofilm feed on the sugars in the food you eat and create acid. That acid attacks the tooth enamel and over time can result in tooth decay. The longer sugar remains in the mouth, the more likely it is to result in tooth decay. Foods that are high in sugar and stick to the teeth like caramel, jelly beans, and gummy bears are more likely to cause a problem than foods that are easily washed out of the mouth. Even foods like raisins or other dried fruits promote tooth decay if not removed from the teeth. High-sugar beverages can also promote tooth decay, especially if they are consumed frequently throughout the day. Babies should never be put down for a nap or to bed with a bottle. The constant contact of the sugar from milk or juice can cause severe tooth decay on the front and back teeth.

Preventing tooth decay is not difficult. Brushing and flossing are the best defense. Brush at least twice a day; more is better. Brush after meals, if at all possible, especially meals that contain sticky high-sugar foods. Choose a toothpaste that contains fluoride. Fluoride makes the tooth structure more resistant to decay and helps repair decay that has already occurred. Finally, get regular check-ups from a dental-health professional.

Glycemic Index

As you have learned, all carbohydrates are not created equal. The type of carbohydrate content in a food greatly affects how your body metabolizes that food. The glycemic index (GI) is a system that ranks foods according to how they affect blood glucose levels.[47] The GI of a food is a measure of the change in blood glucose after consuming that food. This value is compared to a reference food, usually white bread or glucose. Foods with a high GI show a rapid rise and fall in blood glucose, whereas low GI foods have a slower rise in blood glucose that levels off over several hours. The type of carbohydrate, how the food is prepared or processed, and the absence or presence of fiber and fat all affect the GI of a food. Note that some sugary foods that you would expect to have a high GI, such as ice cream, actually have a moderate GI due to other factors in the foods, in this case fat. Conversely, foods such as potatoes that you might expect to have a low GI because they are low in sugar and high in starch have a relatively high GI.

Many diet books and articles in the popular press promote the use of the GI index as a way to lose weight or prevent chronic disease.[48] Some evidence has indicated that consuming a low GI diet may help in the prevention or treatment of obesity, heart disease, or diabetes.[49–51] However, more recent studies have found strong evidence that the glycemic index and/or glycemic load are not associated with body weight, and thus using the GI index is not necessary when selecting carbohydrate-containing foods and beverages.[13]

Spotlight on Vitamins and Minerals

Enriched flour and whole grains are good sources of many of the B vitamins, specifically thiamin, riboflavin, niacin, and vitamin B_6. The B vitamins are required by the enzymes that are involved in the metabolism of carbohydrates and proteins. Without B vitamins, you

Special Report

The Truth About Low-Carbohydrate Diets

Bacon, sausage, cheese, butter, and steak are all foods that you don't expect to see on the list for a weight-loss diet; that is, unless you read and follow some of the most popular diets of our time, such as the Atkins Diet, Sugar Busters, the Stillman Diet, and others. The diet book section of bookstores is filled with low-carbohydrate diets that promise weight loss without deprivation or hunger. Many of these diets ban starchy foods, such as potatoes, rice, pasta, grains, and bread. Root vegetables, such as beets, carrots, and sweet potatoes, are also forbidden. Fruit should not be consumed at all or at least in very small amounts. What are allowed are high-fat, high-protein foods.

How does eating low carbohydrate, high protein, and high fat promote weight loss? Eating a very low-carbohydrate diet can cause a quick drop in weight. Greatly limiting carbohydrates causes the body to deplete its glycogen stores. As your body converts glycogen to glucose, you lose a great deal of water. Fat is burned for energy in the absence of carbohydrates, but ketones are then produced. Ketones in the body further increase the loss of water. The high-protein and high-fat content of the diet tends to satisfy hunger, but it is also monotonous and acts to decrease appetite. That's what happens in the short term, but what about the long term?

Are low-carbohydrate diets better for weight loss than traditional low-calorie diets? Proponents of low-carb diets point to a 2002 study where low-carb diets beat low-fat ones; low-carb diets had better compliance and more weight loss.[52] Although this made headlines and sent many dieters to the meat counter instead of the produce isle, some health professionals questioned several aspects of the study. The study was short term, looked at a small number of people, and was funded by the Atkins Center for Complementary Medicine.

Since that study, many more have followed. Some results indicate that low-carbohydrate diets are associated with higher weight loss at first, but that over time there is no difference in weight loss between low-carb and low-calorie diets.[53,54] The bulk of the literature supports the fact that even when people are on a low-carb diet, weight loss can be attributed to the fact that calories are also low.[55,56] The bottom line is that overall calories matter most for weight loss, rather than macronutrient composition.[57]

To further debunk the low-carb myth, population data indicate that people who consume more carbohydrates are thinner than those who limit them.[58] A low-carbohydrate diet is associated with a greater chance of being overweight or obese. People who consume a diet that is high in complex carbohydrates, high in fruits and vegetables, and high in vegetable protein have lower body weights.[59]

Although the evidence is clear that calories matter more than macronutrient composition, some people continue to follow low-carb diets. So, are they safe? Long term, low-carbohydrate diets may cause serious complications. If carbohydrate consumption is low over several months, ketones will accumulate, compromising the liver and kidneys. No data support the safety of a low-carbohydrate diet as a lifelong choice. Sticking to a low-carb diet over the long term is very difficult, and most people will not stay on it long enough to experience severe medical problems. Short-term side effects of low-carb diets include constipation, nausea, weakness, and dehydration.

Although you should always look to the scientific literature to answer questions as to what diets are healthy, support good health, and decrease the risk of chronic disease, you also have common wisdom to help guide you. In the case of low-carb diets, consuming steak, bacon, sausage, and pork rinds while shunning fruit, vegetables, and whole grains just does not make good sense.

would not be able to use the energy in the foods you eat. How much thiamin, riboflavin, niacin, and vitamin B_6 you need is based on your daily calorie requirements. Deficiencies of thiamin, riboflavin, niacin, and vitamin B_6 are rare in the developed world.

Pantothenic acid and biotin are other B vitamins that are widespread in the food supply, including whole grains. Like other B vitamins, they are involved in energy metabolism. Deficiencies of either pantothenic acid or biotin are extremely rare.

Whole grains contain two important microminerals: chromium and molybdenum. Chromium is needed in energy metabolism and is required for the use of glucose and fat. Molybdenum is part of the enzymes that allow for the transfer of oxygen between the cells. Deficiency is rare for both of these microminerals.

Ready to Make a Change

Are you ready to make a change, small or large, in the whole grains in your diet? Make the commitment to take the first step. Whether it is a small, medium, or large change, it is a step in the right direction toward a healthier diet.

I commit to a small first step. Change your bread. Switch the bread you usually consume to one that is whole grain. Make sure to read the label carefully to find bread that has whole wheat (not enriched wheat) as the first ingredient.

I am ready to take the next step and make a medium change. Choose oatmeal at least twice a week for breakfast. Oats are a great source of both soluble and insoluble fiber. Choose plain oatmeal, not sweetened or flavored. Add fruit instead of sugar for great taste and added fiber.

I have been making changes for some time and am ready to make a large change with the fiber in my diet. Make at least half of your grains whole grains. When you choose pasta, bread, rice, or other grains, select whole grains whenever possible. Switch white rice to brown rice, regular pasta to whole-wheat pasta, and experiment with other whole grains as side dishes.

Myth Versus Fact

Myth: Sugar is associated with behavior problems in children.

Fact: Carbohydrates actually can make you sleepy, not hyper. It is a common myth that sugar makes children bounce off the walls. However, it may be the circumstance that causes the excitement, not the sugar.

Myth: You are either going to get type 2 diabetes or not; what you eat has nothing to do with it.

Fact: Heredity is one risk factor for developing type 2 diabetes. However, the biggest risk factor for developing type 2 diabetes is overweight and obesity. What you eat and how active you are can play a big role in preventing type 2 diabetes.

Myth: Choose low-carbohydrate foods to manage your weight.

Fact: High-carbohydrate foods such as fruits, vegetables, and whole grains are part of a healthy diet. Choose foods like pasta, refined grains, and potatoes less often and in smaller portions to help you keep your calories in check. Remember it is the calories, not the carbs, that need to be in balance to help manage your weight.

Myth: Fruit is high in sugar and should be consumed in moderation.

Fact: While fruit contains sugar, it is added sugar that should be consumed in moderation. Fruit, especially in its whole fresh form, should be part of your diet.

Myth: The best way to decrease the sugar in my diet is to quit putting sugar in my coffee in the morning.

Fact: Most of the sugar we consume is added to our food by food manufacturers during processing. Sugar-sweetened beverages, cereals, baked goods, and candy all add lots of sugar to your overall diet. While skipping the teaspoon or two you add to your coffee will help, it is not where most of the sugar in your diet comes from.

Myth: Fiber supplements are the best way to stay regular.

Fact: Fiber supplements are one way to add fiber to your diet and help keep bowel function regular. A better way to stay regular is to consume whole grains, fruits, vegetables, beans, and plenty of water.

Myth: Multigrain products are a great way to increase your whole-grain intake.

Fact: Multigrain in the label does not always mean whole grain. The food may contain seven different grains, but if they are not whole grain you may be missing the fiber you need. Read the label carefully to see that you are choosing products that have whole grain on the label and in the ingredient list.

Back to the Story

Now that you know about fiber, where it is found in food, and how to increase your consumption of it, what are some ways that Rachel can increase the fiber content of her diet? First, she could start her day with fruit and whole-grain bread instead of a toaster pastry or biscuit. The biscuit is most likely made with enriched flour and the toaster pastry is not only low in fiber but also high in added sugar. Other good breakfast choices for Rachel would be oatmeal or cereal with milk. For lunch, Rachel could stick with her pizza or burger on occasion, but she should branch out on some days and have a salad with chicken, a turkey sandwich on whole-grain bread, or, better yet, she could bring her lunch from home. This would allow her to have more control over what she is eating as well as save money. Rachel's dinner choices are limited, because she is eating from a restaurant or selecting highly processed foods from the grocery store. Takeout is fine every once in a while, but choosing to cook simple meals with plenty of fruits, vegetables, and whole grains will not only increase the fiber in her diet but help control calories as well. What other suggestions can you make for Rachel?

References

1. American Diabetes Association. Diagnosis and classification of diabetes mellitus. *Diabetes Care*. 2008;31(S1):S55–S60.
2. American Diabetes Association, National Institute of Diabetes and Digestive and Kidney Diseases. Prevention or delay of type 2 diabetes. *Diabetes Care*. 2004; 27(S1):S47–S54.
3. Colditz GA, Willett WC, Stampfer MJ, et al. Weight as a risk factor for clinical diabetes in women. *Am J Epidemiol*. 1990;132:501–513.
4. Carey VJ, Walters EE, Colditz GA, et al. Body fat distribution and risk of non-insulin-dependent diabetes mellitus in women. The Nurses' Health Study. *Am J Epidemiol*. 1997;145:614–619.
5. National Diabetes Information Clearinghouse, A Service of the National Institute of Diabetes and Digestive and Kidney Diseases, NIH. http://diabetes.niddk.nih.gov/dm/pubs/riskfortype2/index.htm. Accessed August 12, 2009.
6. National Institute of Diabetes and Digestive and Kidney Diseases. *National diabetes statistics, 2007 fact sheet*. Bethesda, MD: US Department of Health and Human Services, National Institutes of Health, 2008.
7. Fagot-Campagna A, Narayan KM, Imperatore G. Type II diabetes in children. *Bri Med J*. 2001;322:377–378.
8. Fagot-Campagna A, Saaddine JB, Flegal KM, Beckles GL. Diabetes, impaired fasting glucose, and elevated HBA1c in US adolescents: The Third National Health and Nutrition Examination Survey. *Diabetes Care*. 2001; 24:834–837.
9. Nesmith JD. Type II diabetes mellitus in children and adolescents. *Pediatrics Rev*. 2001;22:147–152.
10. Pinhas-Hamiel O, Dolan LM, Daniels SR, Standiford D, Khoury PR, Zeitler P. Increased incidence of non-insulin-dependent diabetes mellitus among adolescents. *Journal of Pediatrics*, 1996;128:608–615.
11. Venkat Narayan KM, Boyle JP, Thompson TJ, Sorensen SW, Williamson DF. Lifetime risk for diabetes mellitus in the United States. *JAMA*. 2003;290(14):1884–1890.
12. Standing Committee on the Scientific Evaluation of Dietary Reference Intakes, Food and Nutrition Board, Institute of Medicine. *Dietary Reference Intakes for Energy, Carbohydrate, Fiber, Fat, Fatty Acids, Cholesterol, Protein, and Amino Acids*. Washington, DC: National Academies Press, 2005.
13. US Departments of Health and Human Services and US Department of Agriculture. *Dietary Guidelines for Americans, 2010*, 7th ed. Washington, DC: US Government Printing Office, December 2010.
14. National Cancer Institute. Sources of added sugars in the diets of the US population ages 2 years and older, NHANES 2005–2006. Risk Factor Monitoring and Methods. Cancer Control and Population Sciences. http://riskfactor.cancer.gov/diet/foodsources/added_sugars/table5a.html. Accessed April 9, 2011.
15. Centers for Disease Control and Prevention. Behavioral risk factor surveillance system. http://www.cdc.gov/brfss/index.htm. Accessed August 1, 2009.
16. Cleveland LE, Moshfegh AJ, Albertson AM, Goldman JD. Dietary intake of whole grains. *Am College of Nutr*. 2000;19(3):331S–338S.
17. Healthy People 2010 Progress Review: Nutrition and Overweight, January 21, 2004.
18. Pollan M. *The Omnivore's Dilemma*. New York: The Penguin Press, 2006.
19. Ripsin CM, Keenan JM, Jacobs DR Jr, et al. Oat products and lipid lowering. A meta-analysis. *JAMA*. 1992;267:3317–25.
20. Johnston L, Reynolds HR, Patz M, Hunninghake DB, Schultz K, Westereng B. Cholesterol-lowering benefits of a whole grain oat ready-to-eat cereal. *Nutr Clin Care*. 1998;1:6–12.
21. Porikos K, Hagamen S. Is fiber satiating? Effects of a high fiber preload on subsequent food intake of normal-weight and obese young men. *Appetite*. 1986;7: 153–162.
22. Blundell JE, Burley VJ. Satiation, satiety and the action of fibre on food intake. *Int J Obes*. 1987;11:9–25.
23. Liu S, Willett WC, Manson JE, Hu FB, Rosner B, Cloditz G. Relation between changes in intakes of dietary fiber and grain products and changes in weight and development of obesity among middle-aged women. *Am J Clin Nutr*. 2003;78:920–927.
24. Melanson KJ, Angelopoulos TJ, Nguyen VT, et al. Consumption of whole-grain cereals during weight loss: Effects on dietary quality dietary fiber, magnesium, vitamin B-6, and obesity. *J Am Diet Assoc*. 2006;106:1380–1388.
25. Ludwig DS, Pereira MA, Kroenke CH, et al. Dietary fiber, weight gain, and cardiovascular disease risk factors in young adults. *JAMA*. 1999;282:1539–1546.
26. Rolls BJ. Carbohydrates, fats, and satiety. *Am J Clin Nutr*. 1995;61(suppl):960S–967S.
27. Levine AS, Billington CJ. Dietary fiber: does it affect food intake and body weight? In: Fernstrom JD, Miller GD, eds. *Appetite and Body Weight Regulation: Sugar, Fat, and Macronutrient Substitutes*. Boca Raton, FL: CRC Press Inc., 1994:191–200.

28. Marlett JA. Dietary fiber and cardiovascular disease. In: Cho SS, Dreher ML, eds. *Handbook of Dietary Fiber*. New York: Marcel Dekker, 2001:17–30.
29. American Dietetic Association. Health implications of dietary fiber. *J Am Diet Assoc*. 2002;102(7):993–1000.
30. McKeown NM, Meigs JB, Liu S, Wilson WF, Jacques PF. Whole-grain intake is favorably associated with metabolic risk factors for type 2 diabetes and cardiovascular disease in the Framingham Offspring Study. *Am J Clin Nutr*. 2002;76:390–398.
31. US Food and Drug Administration. Health claims: soluble fiber from certain foods and risk of heart disease. *Code of Federal Regulation*. 2001;21:101.81.
32. Jacobs DR, Meyer KA, Kushi LH, Folsom AR. Whole grain intake may reduce the risk of ischemic heart disease death in postmenopausal women: the Iowa Women's Health Study. *Am J Clin Nutr*. 1998;68:248–257.
33. Willet W, Hu FB. Optimal diets for the prevention of coronary heart disease. *JAMA*. 2002;288(20):2569–2578.
34. Mellen PB, Walsh TF, Herrington DM. Whole grain intake and cardiovascular disease: A meta analysis. *Nutr Metab Cardiovasc Dis*. 2008;18(4):283–290.
35. Park Y, Subar AF, Hollenbeck A, Schatzkin A. Dietary fiber intake and mortality in the NIH-AARP diet and health study. *Arch Intern Med*. 2011:18. Published online February 14, 2011. http://www.archinternmed.com. Accessed April 29 2011.
36. Krishnan S, Rosenberg L, Singer M, et al. Glycemic index, glycemic load, and cereal fiber intake and risk of type 2 diabetes in US black women. *Arch Intern Med*. 2007;167(21):2304–2309.
37. Fung TT, Hu FB, Pereira MA, et al. Whole-grain intake and the risk of type 2 diabetes: a prospective study in men. *Am J Clin Nutr*. 2002;76(3):535–540.
38. Schulze MB, Lir S, Rimm EB, Manson JE, Willett WC, Hu FB. Glycemic index, glycemic load, and dietary fiber intake and incidence of type 2 diabetes in younger and middle-aged women. *Am J Clin Nutr*. 2004;80:348–356.
39. Block G. Foods contribute to energy intake in the US: data from NHANES III and NHANES 1999–2000. *J Food Composit Anal*. 2004;17:439–447.
40. Harnack L, Stang J, Story M. Soft drink consumption among US children and adolescents; nutritional consequences. *J Am Diet Assoc*. 1999;99(4):436–441.
41. Centers for Disease Control and Prevention. Does drinking beverages with added sugars increase the risk of overweight? *Research to Practice Series*, no. 3, 2006. http://www.cdc.gov/ nutrition/professionals /researchtopractice/index.html. Accessed April 8, 2009.
42. Malik VS, Schulze MB, Hu FB. Intake of sugar-sweetened beverages and weight gain: a systematic review. *Am J Clin Nutr*. 2006;84:274–288.
43. Vartanian LR, Schwartz MB, Brownell KD. Effects of soft drink consumption on nutrition and health: A systematic review and meta analysis. *Am J Pub Health*. 2007;97:367–675.
44. Ebbeling CB, Feldman HA, Osganian SK, Chomitz VR, Ellenbogen SJ, Ludwig DS. Effects of decreasing sugar-sweetened beverages consumption on body weight in adolescents: A randomized, controlled pilot study. *Pediatrics*. 2006;117(3):673–680.
45. Wolraich ML, Wilson DB, White JW. The effect of sugar on behavior or cognition in children: a meta-analysis. *JAMA*. 1995;274(20):1617–1621.
46. White JW, Wolraich ML. Effect of sugar on behavior and mental performance. *Am J Clin Nutr*. 1995;62;330:301–307.
47. Monro JA, Shaw M. Glycemic impact, glycemic glucose equivalents, glycemic index, and glycemic load: definitions, distinctions, and implications. *Am J Clin Nutr*. 2008;87:237S–243S.
48. Borra ST, Bouchoux A. Effects of science and the media on consumer perceptions about dietary sugars. *J Nutr*. 2009;139:1214S–1218S.
49. Jenkins DJA, Kendall CWC, Augustin LSA, et al. Glycemic index: overview of implications in health and disease. *Am J Clin Nutr*. 2002;76(suppl):266S–273S.
50. McMillan-Price J, Petocz P, Atkinson F, et al. Comparison of four diets of varying glycemic load on weight loss and cardiovascular risk reduction in overweight and obese young adults. *Arch Intern Med*. 2006;166:1466–1475.
51. Ludwig DS. Dietary glycemic index and obesity. *J Nutr*. 2000;130:280S–283S.
52. Yancy WS, Olsen MK, Guyton JR, Bakst RP, Westman EC. A low carbohydrate, ketogenic diet versus a low-fat diet to treat obesity and hyperlipidemia. A randomized controlled trial. *Ann Intern Med*. 2004;140:769–777.
53. Malik VS, Hu FB. Popular weight-loss diets: From evidence to practice. *Nat Clin Pract Cardiovasc Med*. 2007;4:34–41.
54. Foster GD, Wyatt HR, Hill JO, et al. A randomized trial of a low-carbohydrate diet for obesity. *N Eng J Med*. 2003;348:2082–2090.
55. Bravata DM, Snaders L, Huang J, et al. Efficacy and safety of low-carbohydrate diets. *JAMA*. 2003;289:1837–1850.
56. Ness-Abramof R, Apovian CM. Diet modification for treatment and prevention of obesity. *Endocrine*. 2006;29(1):5–9.
57. Sacks FM, Bray GA, Carey VJ, et al. Comparison of weight-loss diets with different compositions of fat, protein, and carbohydrates. *N Engl J Med*. 2009;360:859–873.
58. Merchant AT, Vatanparast H, Barlas S, et al. Carbohydrate intake and overweight and obesity among healthy adults. *J Am Diet Assoc*. 2009;109:1165–1172.
59. Lichtenstein AH, Appel LJ, Brands M, et al. Diet and lifestyle recommendations revision 2006: A scientific statement from the American Heart Association Nutrition Committee. *Circulation*. 2006;114:82–96.

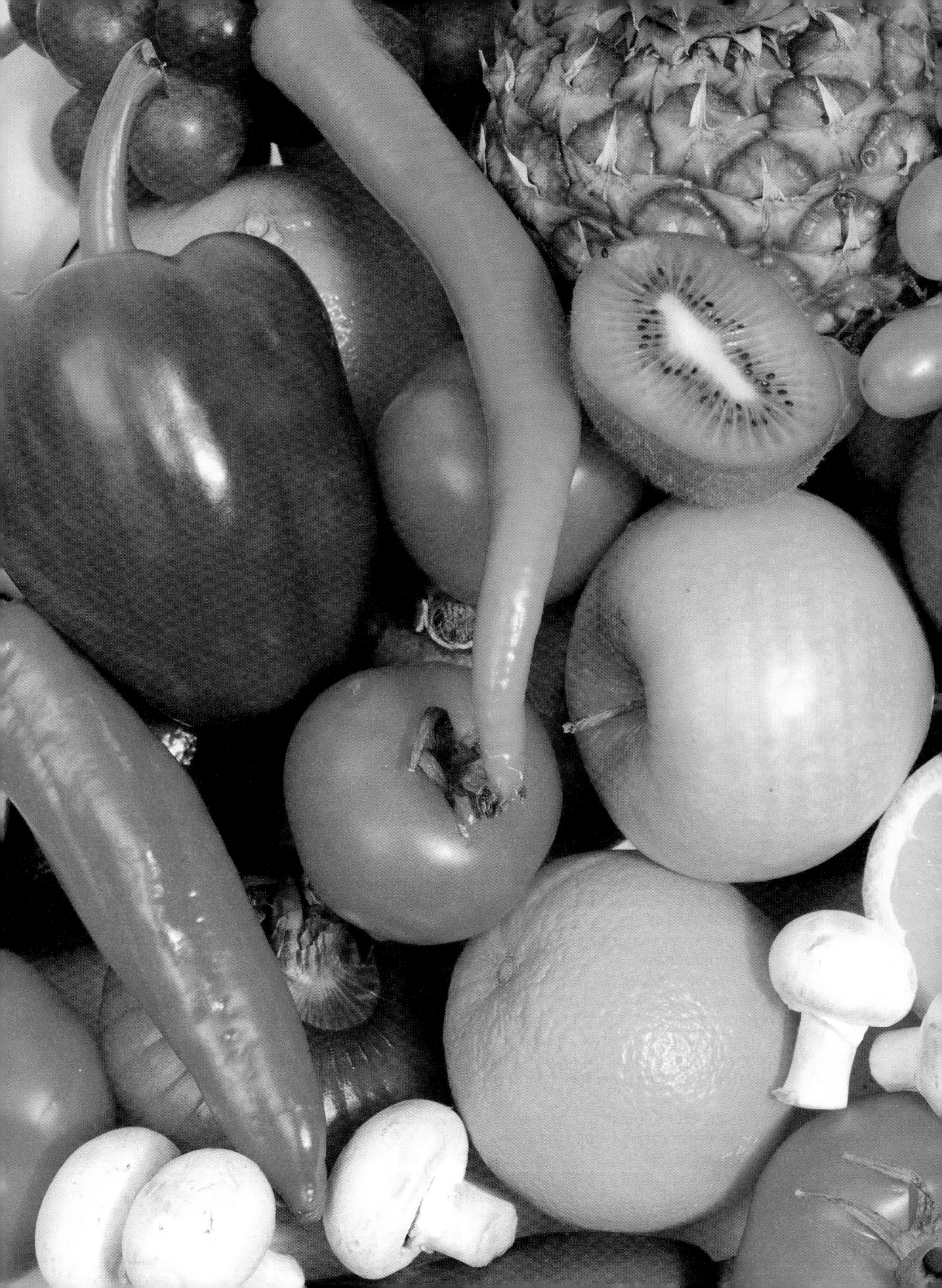

Chapter 6

Fruits and Vegetables: Eat All the Colors

Key Messages

- Most Americans do not get the amount of fruits or vegetables they need each day.
- Fruits and vegetables are high in nutrients and have a protective effect against some chronic diseases.
- Fruits and vegetables, in their natural state, are low in calories and can help with weight management.
- Canned and frozen fruits and vegetables without added sugar or sauce are good alternatives to fresh fruit.

You hear the words *limit*, *moderation*, *less*, and even *don't eat that* when nutrition and what you eat are concerned. But with fruits and vegetables, the words *more* and *supersize* are a good thing. The message for fruits and vegetables is more, more, and more—eat more. Almost everyone should consume more fruits and vegetables for better health. As long as they are not fried or covered in sauce, they are the healthiest foods around. Hot, cold, raw, cooked, canned, frozen, or fresh, take your pick and pick them often. Why are fruits and vegetables so good for us? How can you get more into your diet and stay on your food budget? Is organic best, or is it not worth the extra money? Isn't there a pill you can take if you don't eat enough fruits and vegetables to get the same health benefits? You will learn the answers to these questions and more as you examine the benefits of fruits and vegetables.

Story

Janet is a 25-year-old first-year college student who is working full time to put herself through school. She knows the basics of healthy eating and recognizes that her diet is not what it should be. She sees the messages about eating more fruits and vegetables at the grocery store, on television, and in magazines, but she does not know how she can eat more fruits and vegetables with her tight schedule. She usually skips breakfast since she has to be at work at 7 AM. She takes a class during her lunch break, so she usually grabs something from the vending machine. She often eats takeout or a frozen entrée for dinner while studying or reading. One more piece of information about Janet: She is not a big fan of salads, or any vegetable for that matter. She will eat broccoli from time to time if it is topped with cheese. Janet is ready to take some steps toward a healthy diet. She is skeptical, however, that she can afford or will enjoy eating more fruits and vegetables. What are some ways that Janet can add fruits and vegetables to her diet? Keep in mind her budget and dislike for most vegetables.

Recommended and Actual Intake of Fruits and Vegetables

Increased consumption of fruits and vegetables is recommended for good health.[1] How much is enough? What vegetables and fruits count? The specific amount of fruits and vegetables that you should consume will ultimately depend on your daily calorie needs. A good estimate is two to three servings of vegetables and two servings of fruit (**Table 6.1**). Keep in mind that this is the *minimum*. More is acceptable as long as you don't consume more calories than you need.

Table 6.1

Recommended Intake for Fruits and Vegetables[1]

Category	Recommended Number of Servings	What Counts as a Serving?
Fruits	2 each day	1 cup of fruit 1 piece of whole fruit 1 cup of 100% fruit juice
Vegetables	2–3 each day	1 cup of any vegetable with the exception of raw, green, leafy vegetables 2 cups of salad greens 1 cup of 100% vegetable juice
Deep green vegetables	3 per week	1 cup of deep green vegetables such as kale, spinach, or broccoli 2 cups of raw, green, leafy vegetables such as romaine lettuce or mesclun
Orange vegetables	2 per week	1 cup of orange vegetables such as carrots, sweet potatoes, or winter squash

[1] The amounts given here are estimates. Recommendations vary depending on calorie level.

Source: Data from Choose MyPlate. Available at: www.ChooseMyPlate.gov.

The types of fruits and vegetables you consume is also important. Consume a variety to take advantage of the benefits fruits and vegetables have to offer. Recommendations for vegetable intake suggest no more than three servings per week of starchy vegetables, such as white potatoes or corn. You can include some amount of these vegetables in your diet, but there are many more vegetables that pack much more nutrition than these American staples. You should consume at least three servings of deep green vegetables (**Figure 6.1**) per week and two servings of deep orange vegetables per week (**Figure 6.2**).

Choose whole fruit over fruit juice. Fruit juice is higher in calories than eating a piece of fruit, plus you get the added benefit of the fiber in the whole fruit versus the juice.

What most Americans *should* be eating and what they *are* eating are very different when it comes to fruits and vegetables. Only about 25% of Americans get the recommended amount of fruits and vegetables.[2–5] Some estimates are even lower, suggesting that only 11% of adults consume enough fruits and vegetables.[6,7] According to some estimates, 18% of men and 21% of women consume less than one serving of vegetables each day, and approximately 50% of people consume less than one serving of fruit each day. About half of Americans eat no whole fruit on a daily basis; the fruit they do get is often in the form of juice.[7] In addition, the important dark green and orange vegetables are consumed in less than recommended amounts. Most Americans consume only one serving of dark green vegetables and less than one serving of orange vegetables each week.[4]

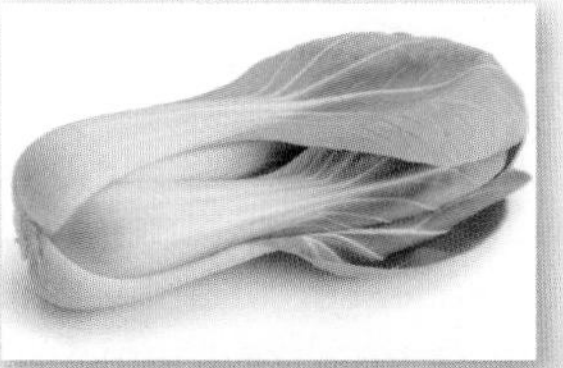

Bok choy—A type of Chinese cabbage that can be stir fried or steamed. It has a taste that is a cross between cabbage and celery. An easy and delicious way to cook bok choy is stir-fry it in a small amount of vegetable oil with a little fresh ginger, crushed red pepper, and soy sauce. Bok choy is readily available in most grocery stores.

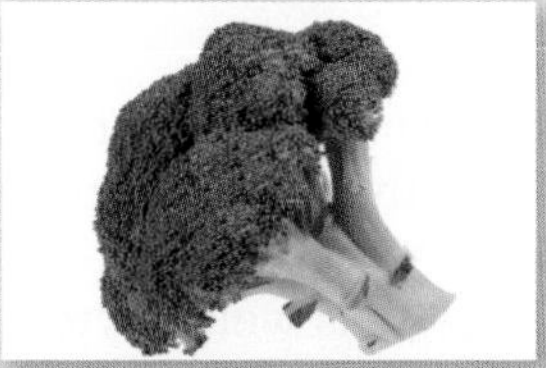

Broccoli—Broccoli is commonly boiled, steamed, stir fried, or microwaved. Skip the cheese sauce and try it plain with just a bit of salt and pepper. Frozen broccoli is great to keep on hand and can be microwaved in just a few minutes. Broccoli is also great raw with a low-fat dip or in salads.

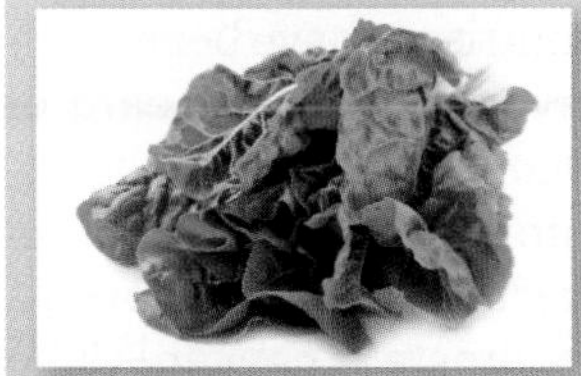

Greens—Collards, kale, mustard greens, turnip greens, or Swiss chard all are considered "greens." Traditionally, greens are boiled or simmered for a long period of time with a piece of ham hock. A healthier alternative is to cook it without meat or with just a small piece of lean meat such as smoked turkey. Vinegar makes a nice condiment that adds no fat or salt.

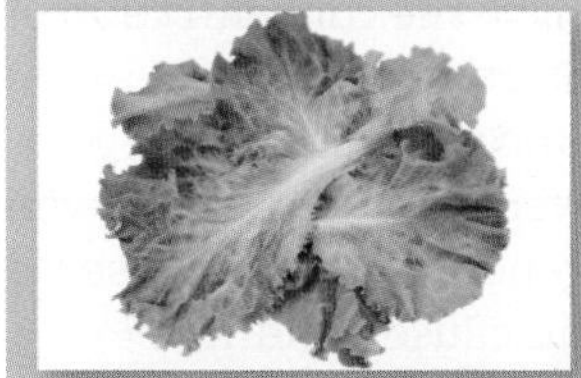

Dark Green Leafy Lettuce—Not all lettuce is created equal. The common iceberg lettuce is not much more than water and has very little nutritional value. Other lettuces, however, that are darker in color, such as mesclun mix, arugula, romaine, green leaf, watercress, and others pack a powerful nutrition punch. Experiment with the many different lettuces on the market; most are available prewashed and ready to go.

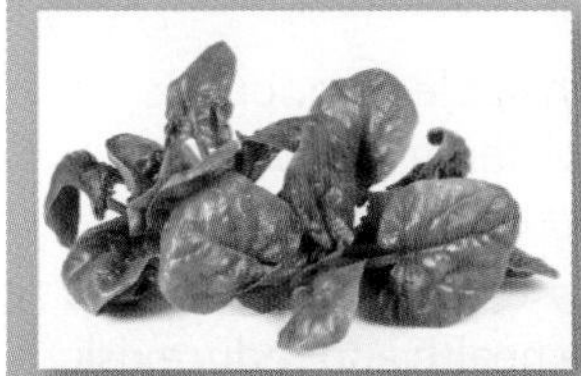

Spinach—One of the most versatile vegetables, spinach is great in salads, on sandwiches, or in omelets. The best way to get spinach into your diet is to sauté it and serve it as a side dish. One bag of prewashed spinach, a stir-fry pan or skillet, a splash of olive oil, a sprinkle of salt, and a dash of pepper and in less than three minutes you have a great tasting, great for you, addition to any meal. Frozen spinach is also a quick easy way to add spinach to your diet.

■ **Figure 6.1**
Deep Green Vegetables

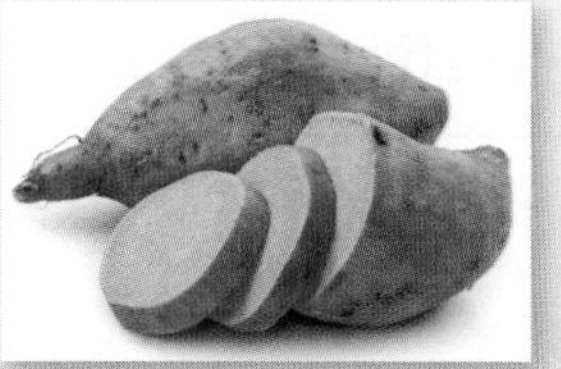

Sweet potatoes—You may only know sweet potatoes as a casserole topped with marshmallows. If so, you are in for a real treat when you really taste a sweet potato. As with a white potato, you can eat a sweet potato roasted, mashed, or raw with a low-fat dip.

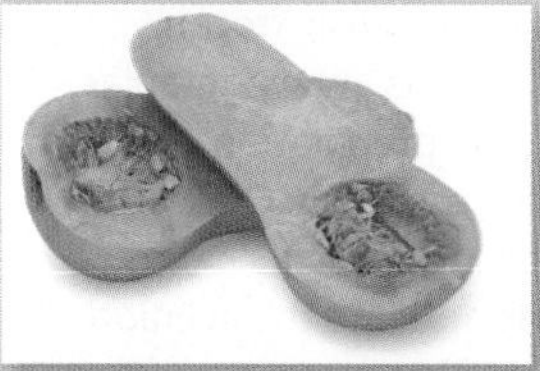

Winter squash—Many types of winter squash can be found in the produce section, including butternut, Hubbard, and acorn. Pumpkin is also in the winter squash family. Winter squash are great in soups, roasted, or baked and mashed.

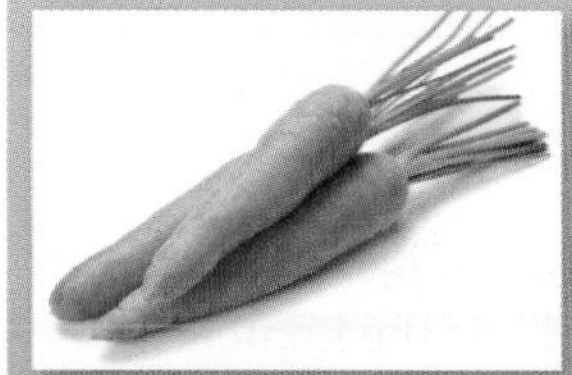

Carrots—Carrots are probably the easiest way to get your orange vegetables each week. You can purchase ready-to-eat baby carrots. Just throw them in a container and take them with you as part of your lunch or afternoon snack. Add carrots to salad or stir-fry or steam them as a side dish.

■ **Figure 6.2**
Orange Vegetables

Why Don't We Eat More Fruits and Vegetables?

Why is fruit and vegetable intake so low for most people? Several different explanations have been offered to explain the overall low consumption. Let's take a look at each so you can learn how to work around these barriers to eat more fruits and vegetables:

- **Food preferences.** You may just not like fruits and vegetables or prefer other foods.[8–10] As a child, you may have disliked certain fruits or vegetables and may have never tried them again. However, tastes change as you grow into adulthood, so trying something again may surprise you. There are many fruits and vegetables from which to choose. Try something new. If you don't like it cooked, try it raw. Try something that you thought you didn't like before. You may even acquire a taste for certain fruits and vegetables that you did not like in the past.
- **Lack of access.** Fruits and vegetables may not be readily available in your community, especially if there is not a full-service grocery store.[11] Convenience stores or drug stores that sell groceries usually do not offer fresh fruits and vegetables.

Personal Health Check

How Is Your Fruit and Vegetable Intake?

We know from national surveys that most of us do not get enough fruits and vegetables on a daily basis. Assess your own fruit and vegetable intake. Keep a fruit and vegetable food diary for three days. Make sure that one of those days is a weekend day. Keep track of all of the fresh, frozen, canned, raw, cooked—any kind of—fruits and vegetables you eat. Keep track of the amount, the preparation method, and any condiments or sauces added. Once you have your diary, add the number of cups of fruits and vegetables you consumed each day and find the average for the three days. How did you do? What are some ways you can increase your consumption if you are below the recommended amounts?

Fast-food restaurants offer only a few choices of fruits and vegetables. Try to limit the number of times you eat fast food or at restaurants each week. This will give you more control over what you eat and give you the opportunity to choose more fruits and vegetables.

- **Lack of advertising.** The food industry spends billions on advertising each year for processed foods; the advertising budget to market fruits and vegetables is much smaller.[12] Lack of funding to communicate what is recommended can lead to confusion about what to eat and how much of it to eat.[13] Even without the big ad budgets, you are now aware of the importance of fruits and vegetables in your daily diet and can work to make any needed improvements.
- **Cost.** Other, less healthy foods are sometimes cheaper than fruits and vegetables, especially if they are snack foods that are made with ingredients such as corn or wheat that are subsidized.[14] Buy fresh fruits and vegetables in season to get the best value. Out of season, try canned or frozen without added sugar or sauces.

Nutrient-Rich Fruits and Vegetables

Fruits and vegetables are powerhouses when it comes to delivering important nutrients and disease-fighting chemicals. Eating fruits and vegetables is almost like taking a vitamin supplement. In fact, they are even better than a supplement. Many of the disease-fighting properties of fruits and vegetables are only available in the natural form, which means that *no pill can take the place of eating plenty of fruits and vegetables.*

Antioxidants

Antioxidants are substances or nutrients in food that can help slow oxidative damage to your body. As your body uses oxygen, free radicals are produced. Pollutants in the air and soil, such as pesticides or cigarette smoke, also cause the production of free radicals. **Free radicals** are dangerous to your body and cause damage to the cells. Over time, free radicals can contribute to diseases such as cancer or heart disease. Fortunately, antioxidants attack free radicals and neutralize them from doing harm to cells and tissues. Fruits and vegetables are rich in the antioxidants vitamin A, vitamin C, vitamin E, and phytonutrients.

Phytonutrients

Phytonutrients are pigments, antioxidants, and other compounds found in plants. They act as the plant's immune system, protecting the plant from disease. When you eat the plant you get some of that benefit as well. Phytonutrients are protective to your body and have disease-preventing properties. Because they are not essential for life, you may hear them referred to as *phytochemicals*.

Hundreds of different phytonutrients have been identified by scientists. Three that you may have heard of in the popular press include lycopene, lutein, and resveratrol. **Lycopene** is found primarily in tomatoes and has been shown to have a protective effect in preventing certain cancers, specifically prostate cancer.[15,16] To increase lycopene in your diet, increase your consumption of tomato products such as tomato sauce and tomato paste. Although raw tomatoes provide other health-promoting compounds, they don't have the concentration of lycopene shown to have the protective effect.

Lutein is a phytonutrient found in green leafy vegetables. It has shown promise in preventing and possibly even treating age-related macular degeneration, an eye disease that causes loss of vision and can cause blindness.[17]

TERMS

antioxidants Substances that neutralize free radicals, thus protecting cells and tissues against damage from oxidation.

free radicals Highly reactive, unstable compounds created by the body as a result of chemical reactions involving oxygen; can damage cells and tissues.

phytonutrients (phytochemicals) Compounds found in plants that may help promote health and reduce risk of some chronic diseases.

lycopene Red pigment found predominantly in tomatoes; has antioxidant properties and may help promote health and protect against heart disease and some forms of cancer.

lutein A yellow pigment found in yellow, orange, and green fruits and vegetables; has antioxidant properties and may protect against macular degeneration.

Eat All the Colors

You may be confused about all the different phytonutrients, antioxidants, and nutrients in different fruits and vegetables. How do you know what to eat to take advantage of all the benefits that fruits and vegetables have to offer? An easy way to remember what to consume is to "eat all the colors." The different pigments in fruits and vegetables have different health benefits. Generally, the darker the color, the more nutrition; for example, dark green lettuce offers more nutrition than iceberg lettuce, and sweet potatoes are more nutritious than white potatoes. Eat a wide variety of fruits and vegetables of all colors, and you will be sure to get the benefits that a variety of fruits and vegetables in your diet will offer.

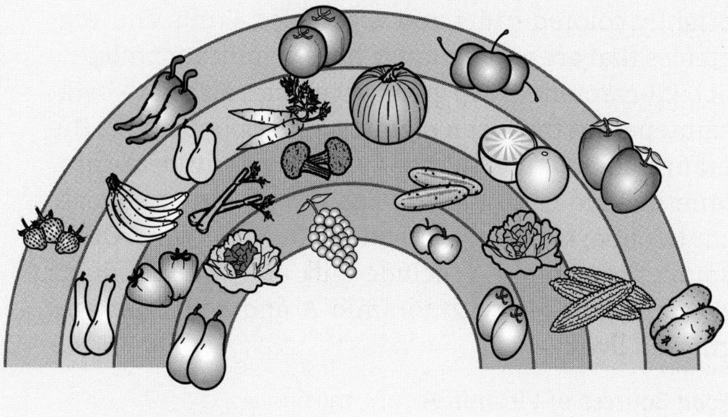

Resveratrol is a phytonutrient that is found in the skin of red grapes and in relatively high concentrations in red wine. The French paradox—the observation that mortality in France is relatively low despite diets that are high in fat—has led some to consider the possibility that consumption of red wine might have some protective health effects.[18] Decreased risk of heart disease has been seen with moderate consumption of red wine; however, the health benefits may be due to other factors in the wine, not resveretrol specifically. There has been little research on resveretrol in humans, and it has not been tested in clinical trials. The animal studies that have been done suggest that very large amounts of resveretrol might be needed to see an effect. More research is needed before recommendations can be made.

Fiber

Undoubtedly, one of the most redeeming qualities of fruits and vegetables is the fiber they contain. Fruits and vegetables are great sources of fiber and contribute much of the fiber you need (**Table 6.2**). The specific amount of fiber needed each day is based on calorie needs. The recommended dietary fiber intake is 14 grams per 1,000 calories.[19] Estimated fiber intake for men is 38 grams per day, for women 25 grams per day. Because most people don't consume enough fruits and vegetables, fiber is, of course, also lacking. For a more detailed discussion of dietary fiber, see Chapter 5.

TERMS

resveratrol An antioxidant found in many plants, it is found in especially high concentrations in the skin of grapes; its ability to protect against heart disease and cancer is still under investigation.

carotenoids Yellow, orange, and red pigments, many of which are precursors of vitamin A; they are found widely in fruits and vegetables.

Spotlight on Vitamins and Minerals

Vitamin A

Vitamin A is essential for healthy vision and is involved in the process that changes incoming light into visual images. Vitamin A is also needed for a healthy immune system, proper bone growth, and healthy reproductive system. Vitamin A also plays an important role in the maintenance and health of skin cells.

The three biologically active forms of vitamin A are retinol, retinal, and retinoic acid. Collectively, they are referred to as *retinoids*. Carotenoids are precursors for vitamin A and are also powerful antioxidants. **Carotenoids** are a class of pigments that range from yellow to red in color. They are what make carrots and sweet potatoes orange and tomatoes red.

Table 6.2

Fiber Content of Common Fruits and Vegetables

Fruit or Vegetable	Serving	Grams of Fiber
Apple	1 medium	4.4
Pear	1 medium	4.0
Banana	1 medium	2.0
Broccoli	1/2 cup	2.6
Corn	1/2 cup	3.0
Carrots	2 medium	3.4
Green beans	1/2 cup	2.7
Beans, black, pinto, etc.	1/2 cup	9.7
Cantaloupe	1 cup, diced	1.4
Orange	1 medium	3.4
Spinach	1 cup, cooked	4.5
Kale	1 cup, cooked	2.6
Collards	1 cup, cooked	5.3

Source: US Department of Agriculture, Agriculture Research Service. 2008. USDA National Nutrient Database for Standard Reference Release 21. Nutrient Data Laboratory Home Page. http://www.ars.usda.gov/ba/bhnrc/ndl.

Beta-carotene is a carotenoid that is found in brightly colored fruits and vegetables. Fruits and vegetables that are bright orange have significant amounts of beta-carotene. Deep green vegetables also have beta-carotene, but the green pigment chlorophyll masks the orange color. Fruits and vegetables high in beta-carotene include carrots, sweet potatoes, winter squash, cantaloupe, spinach, broccoli, and leafy greens. Other sources of vitamin A include milk and dairy products that are fortified with vitamin A and beef liver and chicken liver.

Food Sources of Vitamin A

- Carrots
- Sweet potatoes
- Winter squash
- Cantaloupe
- Spinach
- Broccoli
- Leafy greens
- Milk (fortified with vitamin A)
- Beef liver
- Chicken liver

The body can use preformed vitamin A and beta-carotene to make the active form of vitamin A in the body. The amount of vitamin A in foods is expressed in **retinol activity equivalents (RAE)**, which is a measure of the amount of active vitamin A that your body will get from that food.[20] Vitamin A deficiency is rare because intake is adequate in most people and vitamin A can be stored in large amounts in the liver.

Vitamin C

Vitamin C is needed for the production of collagen, a protein that reinforces connective tissue. Collagen is found in skin, bones, tendons, and teeth. Vitamin C is involved in a healthy immune system and has long been touted as a cure for the common cold. However, studies have consistently shown that vitamin C has little or no effect on curing, or even lessening, the severity of a cold.[21] It is, however, a powerful antioxidant and can help protect the body against free radicals. Vitamin C is found in many different fruits and vegetables. Exceptionally good sources are citrus fruits such as oranges, grapefruit, lemons, and limes.

Food Sources of Vitamin C

- Oranges
- Grapefruit
- Lemons
- Limes
- Strawberries
- Cantaloupe
- Cauliflower
- Broccoli
- Leafy greens
- Pineapple

Scurvy is a deficiency disease caused by too little vitamin C. It is characterized by bleeding gums, as the collagen in gums begins to break down without adequate vitamin C. Left untreated, scurvy is fatal. Vitamin C deficiency is rare in developed countries.

Vitamin E

Vitamin E is a fat-soluble vitamin. Its primary function is to act as an antioxidant. Vitamin E acts as a scavenger, scooping up free radicals that can damage cell membranes. It is often called a vitamin in search of a deficiency disease, because no true deficiency has been seen in humans. Vitamin E is found mostly in vegetable and nut oils, including canola, safflower, and sunflower oils. It is also found in green leafy vegetables, tomatoes, avocados, almonds, and wheat germ.

A growing amount of evidence suggests that higher vitamin E intake may decrease the risk of certain chronic diseases, primarily heart disease. The research to date is inconclusive, thus there is no recommendation for vitamin E supplementation to decrease risk of chronic disease at this time.[22]

Food Sources of Vitamin E

- Sunflower seed oil
- Safflower oil
- Nuts and nut oils such as almond and hazelnut
- Wheat germ
- Green leafy vegetables
- Tomatoes
- Avocados

Potassium

Potassium is essential for the heart to beat properly. Deaths that occur suddenly due to extreme dehydration are usually the result of potassium levels falling quickly. Potassium is found in fruits and vegetables such as bananas, melons, and oranges. Potassium is also found in milk, beans, and fish.

Food Sources of Potassium

- Bananas
- Melons
- Orange juice
- Milk
- Beans
- Fish

Deficiency of potassium is unlikely. However, certain medications, such as diuretics, can increase the risk of potassium deficiency. Too much potassium from supplements can lead to toxicity. For that reason, potassium supplements should never be taken without the advice of a healthcare provider.

Folate

Folate, also called *folic acid* or *folicin*, is important in the synthesis of DNA and red blood cells. A deficiency of folic acid can cause the red blood cells to form incorrectly, resulting in a type of anemia. Folic acid is found in fruits and vegetables. It is found in particularly high amounts in green leafy vegetables and citrus fruits. In fact, green leafy vegetables are so high in folic acid that the name of folic acid is derived from the word *foliage*. Folic acid has a protective effect against the birth defect spina bifida and other neural tube defects character-

TERMS

retinol activity equivalents (RAE) A unit of measure of the amount of vitamin A in a food; 1 RAE = 1 microgram of retinol.

ized by the incomplete closing of the end of the spinal cord. The most critical period for folic acid during pregnancy is the first few weeks, when many women do not yet know they are pregnant. For this reason, all women of childbearing age are advised to consume the recommended level of folic acid plus an additional 400 micrograms in fortified foods or a supplement.[23]

Food Sources of Folate

- Green leafy vegetables
- Citrus fruit
- Pinto beans
- Black beans
- Kidney beans
- Lentils
- Broccoli

Vitamin K

Vitamin K's most well-known function is its role in helping blood to clot. Without vitamin K, a simple cut would bleed uncontrollably. However, vitamin K is also involved in bone health. It is involved in the synthesis of proteins in the body that are responsible for bone mineralization, and it works with vitamin D to help regulate the amount of calcium in the blood.[24] Not getting enough vitamin K is extremely rare because it is found throughout the food supply. Most plant foods, especially green leafy vegetables, are good sources of vitamin K.

Food Sources of Vitamin K

- Green leafy vegetables
- Broccoli
- Cabbage
- Blueberries
- Green beans

Fruits and Vegetables and Health

Consuming adequate amounts of a wide variety of fruits and vegetables is widely accepted as a health behavior that can reduce the risk of several chronic diseases. The combination of nutrients, antioxidants, phytonutrients, and fiber in fruits and vegetables provide multiple health benefits. Specifically, consumption of fruits and vegetables is associated with a reduced risk of certain forms of cancer (see Special Report: Nutrition, Physical Activity, and Cancer Prevention), heart disease, and diabetes and can help a person achieve and maintain a healthy weight.

Heart Disease

Heart disease is the leading cause of death in the United States. Although some of the risks for heart disease are out of your control, such as age, gender, and family history, one thing you can do to protect yourself is consume a healthy diet. When you think about a diet that offers protection against heart disease, a diet low in fat and cholesterol may come to mind. In fact, fruits and vegetables, and lots of them, can also lower your risk.[25–29] The American Heart Association and other national agencies recommend a diet high in fruits and vegetables to reduce the risk of heart disease. A great deal of research has focused on the individual components of fruits and vegetables, such as antioxidants, micronutrients, fiber, and phytonutrients. The evidence suggests that it is the *combination* of these substances in fruits and vegetables that provides the protective effect.[29]

The greatest protective effect seems to come from the consumption of green leafy vegetables and fruits high in vitamin C.[28] However, all fruits and vegetables, with the exception of white potatoes, have at least some protective effect against heart disease.[28] The risk of heart disease decreases as the number of servings of fruits and vegetables increases. As few as four servings of fruits and vegetables a day is associated with at least some decrease in risk; if you consume more, you can expect an even greater benefit. Studies indicate that people who consume the highest amount of fruits and vegetables—10 servings a day or more—get the greatest protection against heart disease.

Diabetes

Adequate intake of fruits and vegetables appears to decrease the risk of developing type 2 diabetes.[30–33] However, the studies are not altogether conclusive, and the protective effect is not as strong as that seen with heart disease and cancer. One interesting finding is that consumption of whole fruits and green leafy vegetables decreases the incidence of type 2 diabetes, but that high fruit juice consumption increases the incidence of type 2 diabetes, most likely because of the lack of fiber and/or high added sugar content in most juices. This finding supports the recommendation to limit juice consumption and to concentrate on whole fruit instead.

Weight Management

The steady rise of overweight and obesity across the country is considered one of the major public health concerns of our time. Can fruits and vegetables help us with this lifelong struggle to achieve and maintain a healthy weight? The simple answer to that question is yes, absolutely.[34] Let's take a closer look as to why fruits and vegetables can be your healthy weight salvation.

Regardless of what types of food you eat, the basic rule of weight loss is that to lose weight you must consume fewer calories than you expend.[35] Oftentimes you stop eating because you are full, not necessarily because you have consumed enough calories. In fact, feeling full is more likely to make you stop eating than the number of calories in a food. Studies have shown that people eat fewer calories when fruits and vegetables are included in their diet.[36–41] Fruits and vegetables are naturally high in water and fiber and low in calories (**Figure 6.3**). These properties of fruits and vegetables provide a feeling of fullness for fewer calories than other foods.

Take a look at **Figure 6.4**. The cinnamon bun on the left is 480 calories, the same number of calories as the entire plate of fruit and vegetables on the right. You could probably eat the cinnamon bun without much problem;

the large plate of fruits and vegetables is another story. More than likely, you would stop eating before you saw the bottom of the plate because you would feel full.

Examine the 100-calorie portions of common snack foods compared to 100-calorie portions of fruits and vegetables (**Figure 6.5**). It is easy to see how you can eat a lot more volume of food if you choose fruits and vegetables. Because you most often stop eating because you are full,

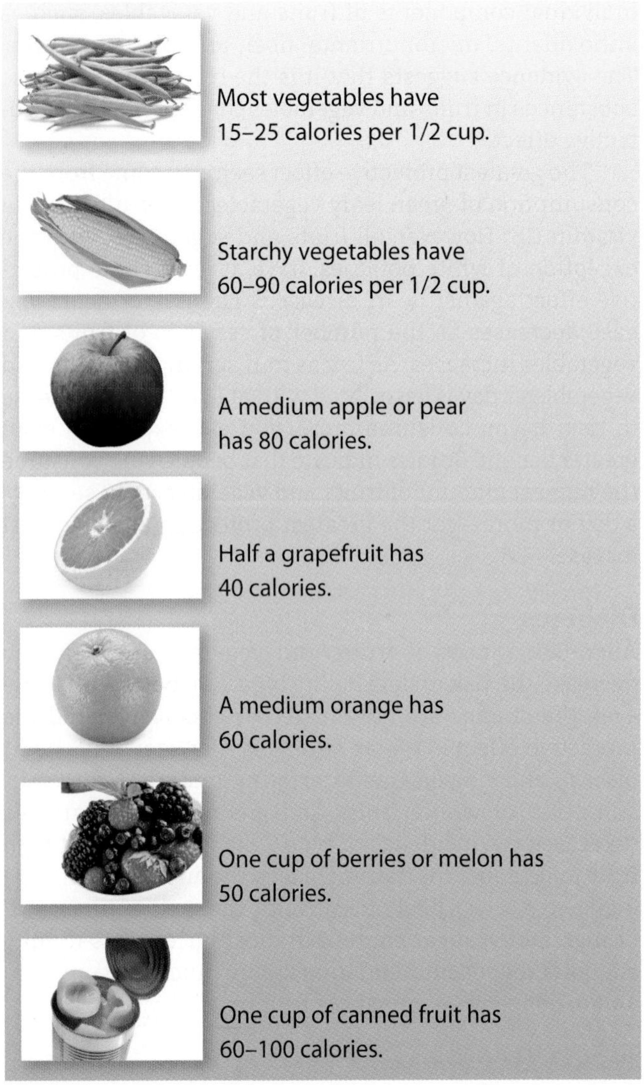

Most vegetables have 15–25 calories per 1/2 cup.
Starchy vegetables have 60–90 calories per 1/2 cup.
A medium apple or pear has 80 calories.
Half a grapefruit has 40 calories.
A medium orange has 60 calories.
One cup of berries or melon has 50 calories.
One cup of canned fruit has 60–100 calories.

■ **Figure 6.3**
Fruits and Vegetables Are Naturally Low in Calories

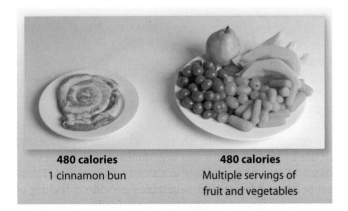

480 calories
1 cinnamon bun
480 calories
Multiple servings of fruit and vegetables

■ **Figure 6.4**
Fruits and Vegetables Are High in Water and Fiber, Low in Calories
It takes a huge plate of fruits and vegetables to equal the calories in just one cinnamon bun.

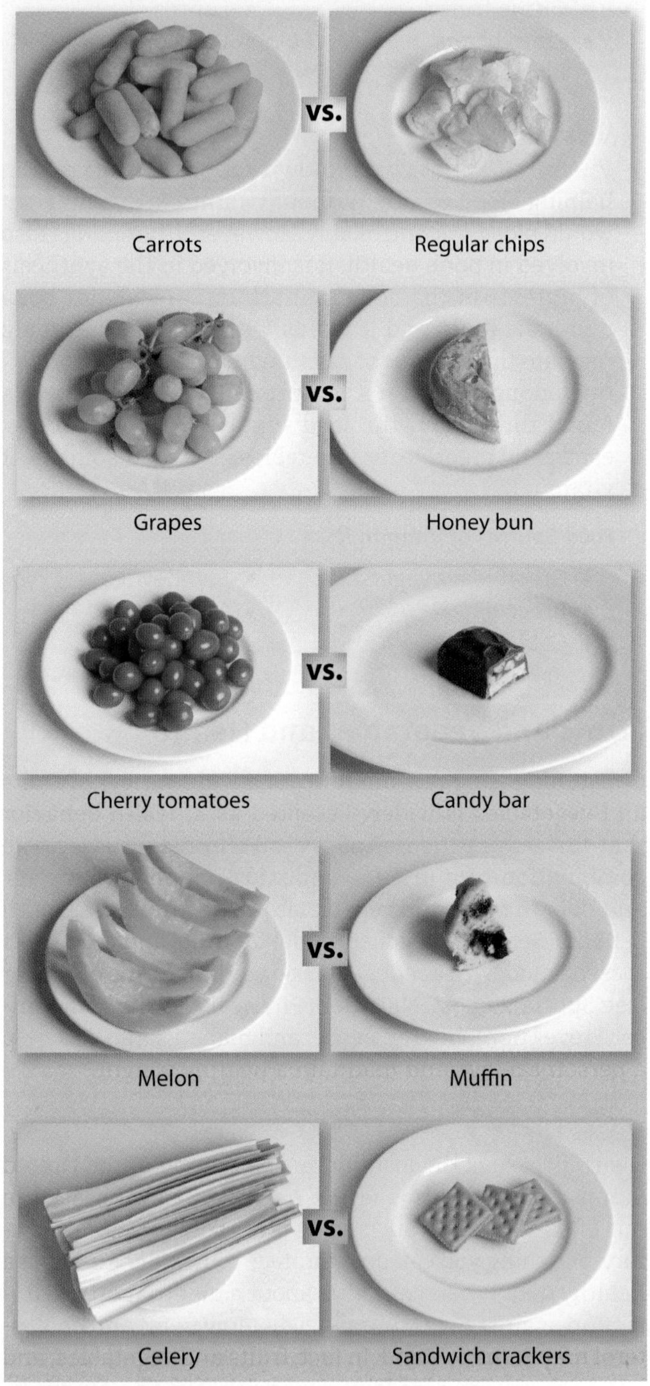

vs.
Carrots
Regular chips
vs.
Grapes
Honey bun
vs.
Cherry tomatoes
Candy bar
vs.
Melon
Muffin
vs.
Celery
Sandwich crackers

■ **Figure 6.5**
100-Calorie Portions of Fruits and Vegetables Compared to Common Snack Options
You get a lot more food when you choose fruits and vegetables.

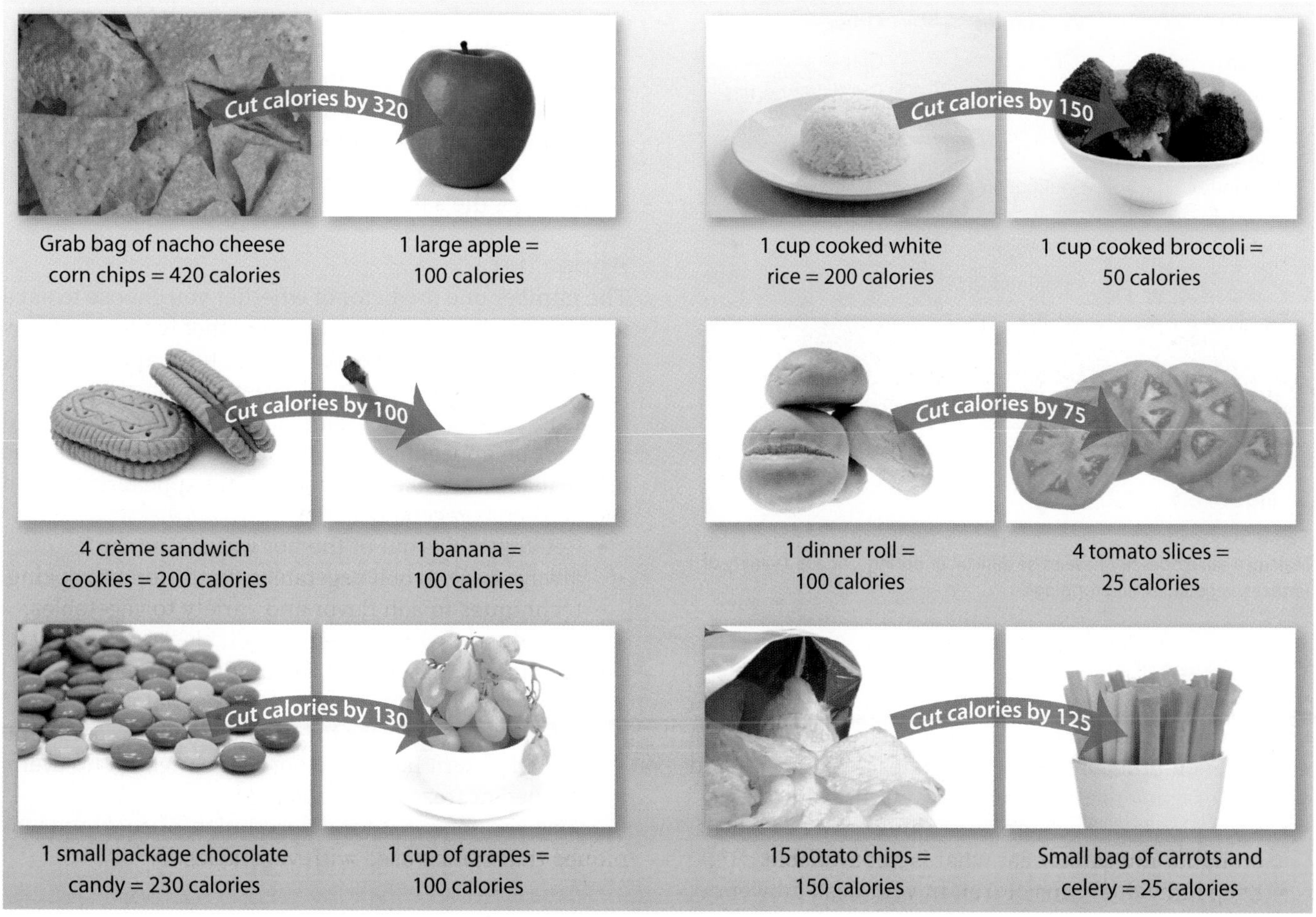

Figure 6.6

Select Fruits and Vegetables Instead of Higher-Calorie Foods to Cut Calories

Energy Density

Energy density is the relationship of calories to the weight of food; that is, the calories per gram of a food item. Water and fiber increase the volume of a food, reducing its energy density. In their natural state, fruits and vegetables have high water and fiber content and are low in calories. Thus, they have low energy density. Foods are categorized as being high, medium, low, and very low with regard to energy density:

- **High energy density:** Foods with high energy density (4.0–9.0 calories per gram) include low-moisture foods, such as crackers and cookies, and high-fat foods, such as butter and bacon.
- **Medium energy density:** Foods with medium energy density (1.5–4.0 calories per gram) include eggs, dried fruit, bagels, whole-wheat bread, and part-skim mozzarella.
- **Low and very low energy density:** Foods with low energy density (0.7–1.5 calories per gram) and very low energy density (0.0–0.6 calories per gram) include tomatoes, melon, broth-based soups, fat-free yogurt, and turkey breast with no skin. Most fruits and vegetables fall into one of these two categories.

filling up on low-calorie fruits and vegetables can decrease overall calorie consumption.

Along with their ability to fill us up with fewer calories, fruits and vegetables can replace higher-calorie foods in your diet (**Figure 6.6**). Substituting lower calorie fruits and vegetables for higher calorie foods has been proven to lower overall calorie intake, thus promoting weight loss[41–46] or protecting against weight gain over time.[47–49]

Fruits and Vegetables: How You Can Increase Your Intake

To increase your intake of fruits and vegetables, you must make them convenient, easy, appealing, and affordable.

TERMS

energy density The number of calories a food contains in a given weight. Foods high in water, such as fruits and vegetables, have lower energy density than foods high in fat and sugar. High-energy-dense foods have a lot of calories in a small package.

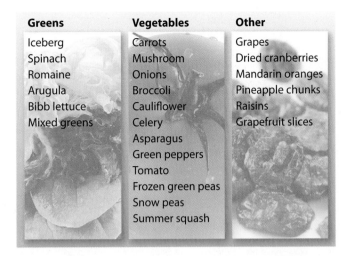

Greens	Vegetables	Other
Iceberg	Carrots	Grapes
Spinach	Mushroom	Dried cranberries
Romaine	Onions	Mandarin oranges
Arugula	Broccoli	Pineapple chunks
Bibb lettuce	Cauliflower	Raisins
Mixed greens	Celery	Grapefruit slices
	Asparagus	
	Green peppers	
	Tomato	
	Frozen green peas	
	Snow peas	
	Summer squash	

■ **Figure 6.7**

Salad Suggestions

Making a salad does not have to be difficult or boring. Choose a variety of lettuces, vegetables, and toppings.

Convenient

You often eat what is easiest or what you see first. If you come into the kitchen for a snack and cookies are on the counter, you probably grab the cookies. Make fruits and vegetables convenient to increase your intake:

- Keep plenty of fresh, frozen, canned, and dried fruit on hand. You cannot eat what is not available.
- Keep individual cans of fruit in your desk drawer or car.
- Make snack bags of fruit and vegetables.
- Keep a bowl of fresh fruit in the kitchen or at eye level in the refrigerator.
- Keep fruit and vegetables front and center so that you are more likely to choose them.

Easy

One of the biggest barriers to increasing your fruit and vegetable consumption is the time they take to prepare. Fruit is usually not the problem. Fruit is the original fast food and is often ready to go with no preparation at all. Vegetables take a little more time but don't have to be a burden to prepare. Consider the following tips:

- Buy prewashed, precut vegetables. They do cost more, so make sure they fit into your food budget.
- Buy bag salad to make salad preparation quick and east. See **Figure 6.7** for some suggestions for making salads.
- Prep vegetables all at once. When you get home from the grocery store, wash and cut up all the vegetables that you purchased. You are more likely to use them if they are ready to use.
- Buy frozen vegetables. Frozen vegetables are as nutritious as fresh. Choose frozen vegetables that do not have added sauces, butter, or cream. You may want to try the frozen vegetables in a microwavable bag for added ease.
- Buy canned vegetables. Canned vegetables are as nutritious as fresh. Keep them in the cabinet at all times for quick heat-and-eat vegetables. If you are concerned about your salt intake, buy low-sodium canned vegetables. If low-sodium isn't available, then rinse canned vegetables in water to wash off some of the salt.

Appealing

The number one predictor of whether you choose to eat a food is taste. You may simply prefer other foods over fruits and vegetables. Most people will grab an apple, orange, pear, or banana. Fruit's natural sweetness makes it appealing as is. Vegetables, however, have a stronger flavor and may not be appealing to some people. Several strategies are available to make vegetables more appealing to even the hard-core vegetable hater:

- Get vegetables out of the hot water. You don't always have to boil vegetables. Try different cooking techniques to add flavor and variety to vegetables. Experiment with different vegetables. Don't know how to cook them? Ask the produce manager or check out the many online sources that can help.
- Add herbs and spices to enhance flavor. Experiment with different herbs and spices to brighten up even canned or frozen vegetables.

Also see **Table 6.3** for a description of cooking techniques that can be used with vegetables.

Try Something New

Create Your Own Stir-Fry Mix

Stir-frying is an easy, quick, and healthy way to cook vegetables. To make stir-fry convenient, try making your own stir-fry mix. Select four or five vegetables; pick your favorites and/or what is on sale that week. Wash and cut the vegetables into bite size pieces and place them in a plastic bag or plastic sealable container. Choose vegetables that all cook in about the same time or keep those that need shorter cooking time, such as mushrooms, separate. Having your stir-fry mix ready to go makes it easy to grab the vegetables you need and have stir-fried vegetables in a matter of minutes. Choose a sauce or just salt and pepper to taste. You don't need a specialty pan to stir-fry vegetables. A skillet works just as well as a wok or stir-fry pan.

Affordable

You may know how important fruits and vegetables are for good health and want to consume more. If you cannot afford to, however, they will not become part of your everyday diet. However, fruits and vegetables don't have to break your food budget. Consider the following budget-friendly suggestions:

Table 6.3

Quick, Easy Vegetable Preparation Techniques

Cooking Method	Technique
Roast	Most vegetables can be roasted. Beets, carrots, asparagus, and onions are all great vegetables to roast: • Toss in a bowl or plastic bag with 1 teaspoon of olive oil. • Put vegetables in a single layer on a baking sheet. • Add salt, pepper, herbs, or spices, as desired. • Roast in a 475-degree oven. Cooking time varies from about 10 minutes for asparagus to 30 minutes for denser vegetables like carrots.
Grill	Use your electric double-sided grill or outdoor grill to grill delicious vegetables: • Choose firm vegetables such as carrots, sweet potatoes, broccoli stalks, onions, zucchini, and yellow squash. • Cut vegetables into uniform, thick slices, about half an inch thick. • Spray the grill with low-fat cooking spray (if you are using an outdoor grill, do this before you turn the grill on). • Put vegetables on the grill in a single layer. • Check after three minutes. It will take seven to eight minutes for most firm vegetables to grill.
Stir-fry	Stir-frying is a quick, easy and delicious way to prepare vegetables. Keep a stir-fry mix on hand. You can cut up your own vegetables for several meals or buy already pre-cut vegetables: • Heat a scant tablespoon of oil in a large skillet or stir-fry pan until it is very hot. • Grab a handful of several vegetables and toss them into the pan. • Denser vegetables, like carrots, need to go in first. High-water-content vegetables, like mushrooms, go in last. • Top with low-sodium soy sauce (optional). • For variety, change the mixture of vegetables you use or top it with different spices or herbs.
Steam	Steaming is a simple, quick way to prepare vegetables: • Use a steamer basket, a regular saucepan with a tight-fitting lid, or a microwave steamer. Add a small amount of water in the bottom. • Once water is steaming, add vegetables to basket or saucepan. Cover. • Don't overcook the vegetables. Steaming only takes a few minutes.

- Look for what's on special. Most grocery stores will have one or more fresh, frozen, or canned vegetables on special each week.
- Use coupons when you can.
- Stock up when canned or frozen vegetables are on special.
- Buy what is in season; you will pay more for vegetables that are out of season.
- Buy local. You may be able to save money by shopping at local farm stands or farmers' markets.
- Grow a garden if you have the space. Even a few pots with tomatoes can provide lots of fresh vegetables for several months.

The fruit and vegetable buying guide in **Table 6.4** provides detailed information on the seasonal availability of different fruits and vegetables as well as tips on choosing and storing them.

Which Side Are You On?

Organic or Conventional?

You are convinced that you need to eat more fruits and vegetables. You go to the grocery store to pick up some apples for your lunch and are faced with the decision of whether to choose **organically grown** or conventionally grown apples. They look very similar, the nutrition information on the bag is similar, but the price is not similar. The organic apples are more expensive. Do organic apples taste better? Are they better for you? Are they better for the environment? Do they contain fewer contaminants? Are they safer? Which apples should you choose? Although there is no black-and-white answer as to whether you should choose organic or conventionally grown produce, there is information that can help you make an informed decision.

Organic Versus Conventional

Organic refers to the methods and conditions under which fresh fruits and vegetables are grown and processed. Organic farming practices are designed to protect the environment by conserving water and the soil and reducing the use of man-made chemicals. **Table 6.5** summarizes the differences between organic and conventional agricultural practices. Organic produce is grown without the use of conventional pesticides, fertilizers made with synthetic ingredients or sewage sludge, bioengineering, or ionizing radiation.

Organic Standards and Certification

The Organic Foods Production Act and the National Organic Program assure consumers that the organic agricultural products they purchase are produced, processed, and certified with consistent national organic standards.[50] Included

TERMS

organically grown foods Food grown by farmers who emphasize the use of renewable resources and the conservation of soil and water to enhance environmental quality for future generations.

Table 6.4

Fruit and Vegetable Buying Guide

Vegetable	Available	How to Choose	How to Store
Beans, green (snap or string)	April–September Year-round in some areas	Select bright-colored and crisp. Avoid bruised or scarred beans. Bulging/leathery beans are old.	Refrigerate, covered up to 5 days
Beets	Year-round, peak season from June–October	Select small-medium beets, large beets are tough and not as sweet.	Trim the beet greens, leaving 1–2 inch stems. Do not cut the long root. Store unwashed in open container in refrigerator for up to one week.
Broccoli	Year-round	Firm stalks with deep green or purplish-green heads that are tightly packed. Avoid heads that are light green or yellowing.	Keep unwashed in covered container in refrigerator for up to 4 days
Cabbage	Year-round	Head should be heavy for its size, leaves should be unwithered, brightly colored.	Refrigerate covered in container up to 5 days
Carrots	Year-round	Choose straight, rigid, bright orange carrots.	Refrigerate in plastic bags up to 2 weeks
Cauliflower	Year-round	Choose solid heavy heads with bright green leaves. Avoid those with yellowed leaves.	Refrigerate in covered container for up to 4 days.
Cucumbers	Year-round, peak season late May–September	Choose firm cucumbers without shriveled or soft spots. Sometimes edible wax is added to prevent moisture loss.	Keep in refrigerator for up to 10 days.
Okra	Year-round, peak season June–September	Choose, small, crisp, bright-colored pods without brown spots or blemishes. Avoid shriveled pods.	Refrigerate, tightly wrapped, up to 3 days
Onions (all varieties)	Vidalia, white, red and pearl onions are available year-round	Select dry bulb onions that are firm, free from blemishes, and not sprouting.	Store in cool, dry, well-ventilated place for several weeks
Peas and Pods	Peas: January–June, peak season March–May. Pea Pods: February–August	Select fresh peas, snow peas, or sugar snap peas that are crisp and brightly colored. Avoid shriveled pods or brown spots.	Store in refrigerator up to 3 days, tightly wrapped
Peppers (hot or sweet)	Year-round	Sweet or hot peppers should be brightly colored and a good shape. Avoid bruised, shriveled, or broken peppers.	Refrigerate in covered container up to 5 days
Potatoes	Year-round	Select firm potatoes with clean, smooth, unblemished skins. Avoid those with green skins, sprouted or are soft, moldy, or shriveled.	Store in a well-ventilated, dark, cool, and slightly humid location for several weeks. Bright light causes green patches that have a bitter flavor. Avoid refrigerating potatoes: cold temperatures cause them to turn sweet and to darken when cooked.
Root vegetables (parsnips, rutabagas, or turnips)	Year-round Parsnips: peak season November–March Rutabagas: peak season September–March Turnips: peak season October–March	Choose vegetables that are smooth-skinned and heavy for their size. Sometimes parsnips, rutabagas, and turnips are covered with a wax coating to extend storage; cut off this coating before cooking.	Refrigerate up to 2 weeks
Squash, winter	Some varieties year-round, peak season September–March	Avoid cracked or bruised squash	Store whole squash in a cool, dry place for up to 2 months. Refrigerate cut squash, wrapped in plastic, up to 4 days
Sweet potatoes and Yams	Year-round, peak season October–January	Choose small to medium, smooth-skinned potatoes that are firm and free of soft spots.	Store in a cool, dry, dark place for up to 1 week
Tomatoes	Year-round, peak season June–September	Pick well-shaped, plump, fairly firm tomatoes.	Store at room temperature up to 3 days. Do not store tomatoes in the refrigerator because they lose flavor.
Zucchini and Summer squash	Some varieties year-round, peak season June–September	Due to its tender skin, it is almost impossible for them to be blemish-free, look for small ones that are firm and free of cuts and soft spots.	Refrigerate squash, tightly wrapped, for up to 5 days; squash fresh from the garden may be stored for up to 2 weeks

Table 6.4

Fruit and Vegetable Buying Guide *(Continued)*

Fruit	Available	How to Choose	How to Store
Apples	Year-round, peak season September–November	Select firm apples free of bruises or soft spots. Select according to use.	Refrigerate up to 6 weeks
Berries	Blackberries: June–Aug. Blueberries: May–Oct. Boysenberries: late June through early August. Raspberries: Year-round, peak season May–Sept. Strawberries: Year-round, peak season May–Sept.	If picking your own, select berries that separate easily from their stems.	Refrigerate berries in a single layer, loosely covered, for up to 2 days. Rinse just before using.
Cantaloupe	Year-round, peak season June–September	Select cantaloupe with a sweet, aromatic scent; a strong smell could indicate over ripeness. It should feel heavy for its size. Avoid wet, dented, bruised, or cracked fruit.	Refrigerate whole melon up to 4 days. Refrigerate cut fruit in a covered container or tightly wrapped for up to 2 days.
Grapefruit	Year-round	Choose fully colored grapefruit with a nicely rounded shape. Juicy grapefruits will be heavy for their size.	Refrigerate for up to 2 weeks
Grapes	Year-round	Select plump grapes without bruises, soft spots, or mold. Bloom (a frosty white cast) is typical and doesn't affect quality.	Refrigerate in a covered container for up to 1 week.
Honeydew melon	Year-round, peak season June–September	Choose honeydew that is smooth skinned and heavy for its size with a sweet, aromatic scent. Avoid wet, dented, bruised, or cracked fruit.	Refrigerate whole melon up to 4 days. Refrigerate cut melon in a covered container or tightly wrapped for up to 3 days.
Lemons	Year-round	Select firm, well-shaped lemons with smooth, yellow skin. Avoid bruised or wrinkled lemons.	Refrigerate for up to 2 weeks.
Limes	Year-round	Select firm, well-shaped, brightly colored limes. Avoid blemished, bruised, or shriveled skin.	Refrigerate for up to 2 weeks.
Oranges	Year-round	Choose oranges that are firm and heavy for their size. Brown specking or a slight greenish tinge on the surface of an orange will not affect the eating quality.	Refrigerate for up to 2 weeks.
Peaches and Nectarines	Peaches: May–Sept. Nectarines: May–Sept., peak season July–Aug.	Select fruit with a golden yellow skin and no green. Ripe fruit should yield slightly to gentle pressure.	Refrigerate for up to 5 days.
Pears	Year-round	Skin color is not always an indicator of ripeness because skin color of some varieties does not change much as the pears ripen. Look for pears without bruises or cuts. Choose a variety according to use.	Refrigerate ripened fruit for several days.
Pineapple	Year-round, peak season March–July	Look for a plump pineapple with a sweet aromatic smell at the stem end. It should be slightly soft to the touch, heavy for its size, and have deep green leaves.	Refrigerate for up to 2 days. Cut pineapple lasts a few more days if placed in a tightly covered container and refrigerated.
Plantains	Year-round	Choose undamaged plantains. Slight bruises are acceptable because the skin is tough enough to protect the fruit. Choose plantains at any stage of ripeness, from green to dark brown or black, depending on intended use.	Black plantains are fully ripe. The starchy fruit must be cooled before eating.
Plums	May–October, peak season June–July	Choose firm, plump, well-shaped fresh plums. They should give slightly when gently pressed. Bloom (light gray cast) on the skin is natural and doesn't affect quality.	Refrigerate for up to 3 days.
Watermelon	May–September, peak season mid-June–late August	Choose watermelon that has a hard, smooth rind and is heavy for its size. Avoid wet, dented, bruised, or cracked fruit.	Watermelon does not ripen after picking. Refrigerate whole melon up to 4 days. Refrigerate cut fruit in a covered container or tightly wrapped for up to 3 days.

Table 6.5

Conventional Versus Organic Farming Practices

Method	Agricultural Techniques Used
Conventional	Chemical fertilizers are used to promote plant growth. Chemical insecticides are used to reduce pests and disease. Chemical herbicides are used to manage weeds.
Organic	Natural fertilizers such as manure or compost are used to promote plant growth. Insects and birds or traps are used to reduce pests and disease. Organic pesticides are used. Crop rotation, hand weeding, mulch, or organic herbicides are used to manage weeds.

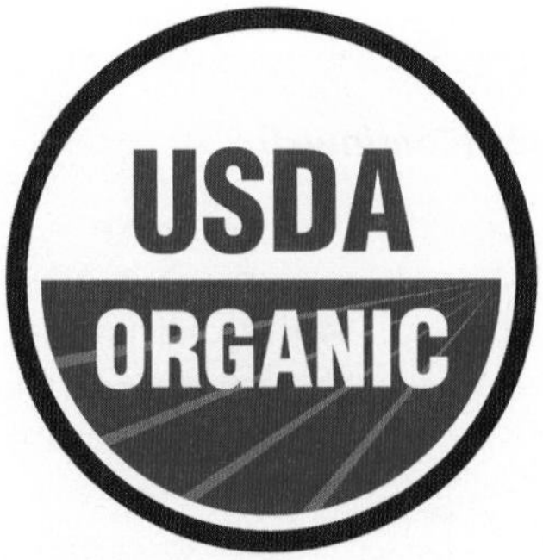

■ **Figure 6.8**

Organic Labeling

This label indicates that at least 95% of this product is organic.

Source: Courtesy of USDA.

in these standards are a list of potentially toxic, naturally occurring pesticides that are approved for use in certified organic production. Before a product can be labeled "organic," a government-approved certifier inspects the farm where the food is grown to make sure the farmer is following all the rules necessary to meet USDA organic standards. Companies that handle or process organic food before it gets to your local supermarket or restaurant must be certified as well.[51]

Organic labels are based on the percentage of organic ingredients in a product (**Figure 6.8**). The following labels are used to help consumers make informed choices when purchasing organic foods:

- **100% Organic**—must contain only organically produced ingredients.
- **Organic**—must consist of at least 95% organically produced ingredients.
- **Made with organic**—products must contain at least 70% organic ingredients. These products cannot use the USDA Organic seal but may list up to three organic ingredients on the front of the package.

Many producers may follow organic practices, preserve the environment, reduce the use, or even refuse to use any nonorganic pesticides but prefer not to become "organically certified" due to the high certification costs.

Points to Consider: Organic Versus Conventionally Grown

There are several points that you the consumer should consider when making the decision to buy organic or conventionally grown produce. Taste, nutrition, pesticide use, food safety issues, and issues related to the environment may all affect your decision.

Taste Some people believe that organic produce tastes better than conventionally grown. Others state that they taste no difference. Taste is highly subjective. Taste may differ depending on the fruit or vegetable; for example, organic carrots may taste better to you than conventionally grown ones, but you may taste no difference in broccoli. The taste of produce can be impacted by many factors, including weather, nutrients, the variety, and postharvest handling—organic or not.

Nutrition Ask 10 nutrition experts about organic produce and the nutrients they provide, and you are likely to get 10 different answers. Answers may range from "organic is a waste of money" to "only eat organic produce." What is the bottom line with respect to organic produce and nutrition? Even with over 100 studies that have examined the nutritional quality of organic versus conventionally grown produce, there is no definitive answer.

Several studies indicate that there is little, if any, nutritional difference between organic and conventionally grown produce.[52–54] However, others have found that organic produce is more nutritious.[55,56] The Organic Center compared over 100 studies that examined organic produce and nutritional quality. Only studies with acceptable or high-quality research designs were included. It examined 135 studies and included 94 in its analysis. Its analysis of existing studies examined antioxidants; vitamins A, C, and E; potassium; phosphorus; nitrates (higher levels are a nutritional disadvantage); and total protein. The differences documented in this analysis justified the statement that "organic produce is, on average, more nutritious."[56]

In the coming years, research will continue on determining the nutritional advantages of organic food. In the meantime, some evidence indicates that organic may

TERMS

community-supported agriculture (CSA) A community of individuals who pledge support to a farm operation; members of a CSA provide monetary support to a farmer and in return receive shares in the farm's production.

Green and Healthy

Buy Local

The average meal in the United States travels 1,300 miles before reaching your plate; produce travels an average of 1,500 miles.[64] A head of lettuce traveling from California to the east coast uses 36 times more fossil fuel energy in transport than it provides in food energy.[65] Supporting local growers helps to reduce fossil fuel consumption, which, in turn, is good for the environment. Sustainable farms conserve soil, keep water sources in our communities clean, and provide wildlife habitat. Keeping farmers on the land also preserves open space and helps our rural communities remain vibrant places to live.

It has been estimated that every $1.00 spent on locally produced foods returns (or circulates) $3.00 to $7.00 within the community.[66,67] Consumers buy produce and other goods from local farmers, who buy farm supplies from local businesses. Those businesses help to keep people in the community employed, and, in turn, they spend their money back in the community. This helps to encourage a thriving community and increases the economic health of the region. In addition, when farmers have direct access to consumers, they are able to keep more of each dollar earned from a sale, because the middle-man is eliminated. This increases profits to producers and keeps their farms competitive with the traditional retail chain stores. Purchasing local produce not only improves the local economy, it can also help you stretch your food dollar and get high-quality fruits and vegetables.

If you do some research, you'll probably find many ways to buy local produce.[68] The right option for you will depend on your budget, the farms in your local area, and the location of outlets that sell local food. The following are some options to explore; check what is available in your area.

Farmers' Markets

Farmers' markets are facilities or sites where several producers gather on a regular basis to sell various fruits, vegetables, and sometimes meat and dairy. Usually, farmers sell directly to the consumer. Farmers' markets may be incorporated; sponsored by a municipality, business, or community organization; or simply a designated gathering place for growers and customers based on tradition. Regardless of the organizational structure, farmers' markets offer growers an opportunity to sell their products directly to consumers while providing consumers access to a variety of local produce in one location. Some cities have mobile mini-markets, smaller versions of farmers' markets that provide on-site sales at worksites or places of worship.

Note that produce vendor markets are set up at a given site and resemble farmers' markets. One or more local produce vendors (generally not a farmer) arrange to sell produce and other goods, which may or may not be locally grown, to consumers. The produce may come from different states or countries, similar to the items available in a grocery store. So, make sure you are buying local. Just ask if the produce is local and where the farm(s) is located.

Community-Supported Agriculture

Community-supported agriculture (CSA) is a direct partnership between a local farmer and individual consumers who commit to a yearly or seasonal membership subscription. You may join a CSA on your own or as part of a setting-supported program (such as a worksite or faith congregation). As a CSA member, you buy shares in a farmer's crop prior to the growing season, and in return you receive a healthy supply of fresh produce (usually weekly) from that farmer throughout the growing season. Farmers may deliver produce to a central pick-up site at a predetermined time. Or, members may come directly to the farm on designated days. Most CSAs inform their members in advance as to which produce items to expect on each delivery day, which helps in making storage decisions and planning menus. Other CSAs allow you to pick the items you want based on your membership level.

Direct produce sales by this advance payment system allows farmers to receive a fair price for their produce and relieves them of much of the burden of marketing during their busy harvest time. You also share in the risks of farming, including unpredictable environmental influences that might affect crop output. There are generally different levels of financial buy-in, which net different amounts of produce at delivery time. Some CSA farms also engage members in assisting with actual work on the farm in exchange for a lower price on their subscription. This shared arrangement creates a sense of personal value, ownership, and responsibility for the farmer, you, and the community. Ultimately, you, as the consumer, benefit. In addition to the fresh produce, you get the privilege of knowing the farmer and how the food was produced.

Buying Club

Cooperative produce delivery, also known as a buying club, is a direct partnership between a local farmer or produce vendor and consumers. You pool your finances with others in order to purchase bulk fruits and vegetables at wholesale prices. Fresh produce is delivered at regular intervals to your site or you go to the vendor and pick up the produce. Check with food/produce distributors, fruit and vegetable wholesalers, and farmers in your area to see what is available for bulk purchase.

Other Options for Local Produce

Other options for obtaining local produce include community and school gardens, tailgate markets, community co-op stores, farm stands, and others.

No matter what the name or how it is set up, all of these approaches operate with the same goals. They take advantage of common spaces where people gather on a regular basis, make it convenient for consumers, and provide a consistent source of high-quality produce for better health. These programs foster local economic stability, contribute to a sustainable environment, and create occasions for education and social gatherings. Also, they give you a measure of control within the global food system and present a unique opportunity to know where your food comes from and how it is produced.

Special Report

Nutrition, Physical Activity, and Cancer Prevention

A 1981 landmark report on prevention of cancer indicated that as many as 35% of cancers could be prevented by lifestyle and dietary changes.[69] Even before this report, healthy eating, physical activity, and healthy lifestyle choices were recommended to protect against cancer. Much research has ensued since early reports of the relationship among diet, lifestyle, and cancer. Currently, the consensus is that 30–40% of cancers are preventable by improvements in diet, regular physical activity, and avoidance of obesity; another one-third could be prevented by abolishing smoking.[69]

Although data are still emerging as to the specific dietary components that may offer the most protection, some definitive recommendations can be made to reduce the risk of certain cancers. For Americans who do not use tobacco, weight control, dietary choice, and physical activity are the most important modifiable determinants of cancer risk.[70] A comprehensive review of all relevant research on food, physical activity, and body composition is offered by the World Cancer Research Fund and its sister organization the American Institute for Cancer Research.[69] They offer scientifically based guidelines with regard to how food, nutrition, and physical activity can be used to reduce the risk of cancer. Their recommendations are consistent with those of the American Cancer Society.[70]

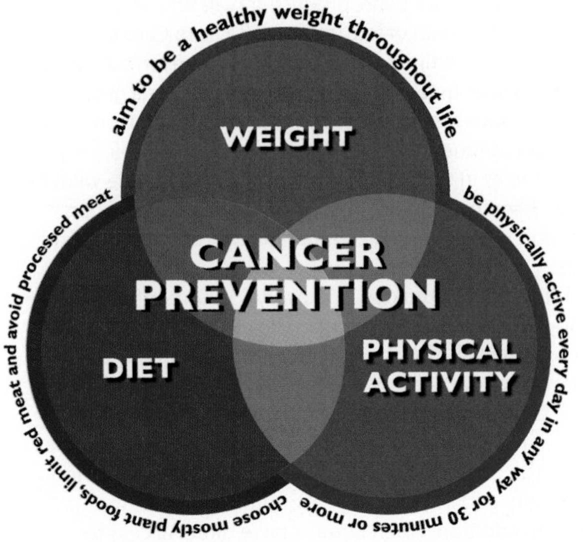

Source: © American Institute for Cancer Research. http://www.aicr.org/reduce-your-cancer-risk/.

Recommendation #1: Body Fatness
Be as lean as possible within the normal range of body weight. Ensure that body weight through childhood and adolescent growth projects toward the lower end of the normal BMI range at age 21. Maintain body weight within normal range and avoid weight gain and increases in waist circumference throughout adulthood. Maintenance of a healthy weight throughout life may be one of the most important ways to protect against cancer. Being overweight increases the risk of several forms of cancer.[71,72]

Recommendation #2: Physical Activity
Make physical activity a part of everyday life. Be moderately physically active, equivalent to brisk walking, for at least 30 minutes every day. As fitness improves, aim for 60 minutes or more of moderate or for 30 minutes or more of vigorous physical activity every day. Limit sedentary habits such as watching television. All forms of physical activity protect against some cancers and can help prevent weight gain.[73–77]

Recommendation #3: Limit Consumption of Foods and Drinks That Promote Weight Gain
Limit consumption of energy-dense foods and avoid sugary drinks. Consume fast food sparingly, if at all. This recommendation is mainly designed to prevent weight gain. Consumption of energy-dense foods, sugary drinks,[78] and fast food[79,80] are all associated with increased risk of overweight and obesity.

Recommendation #4: Plant Foods
Eat mostly foods of plant origin. Eat at least five portions/servings of a variety of nonstarch vegetables and fruits every day. Eat relatively unprocessed grains and/or legumes with every meal. Limit refined starchy foods. People who consume a diet that is high in fruits and vegetables have a lower risk of cancer.[81–83] Although starchy vegetables (potatoes and corn) can be included in a healthy diet and can make up some of the vegetables you consume, the bulk of the vegetables you eat should be nonstarchy vegetables.

provide some nutritional advantages over conventionally grown produce. However, the question remains as to whether slight differences in nutritional quality are worth the cost of buying organic.

Pesticides Experts agree that even small doses of pesticides can cause health problems, especially during fetal development and early childhood. Both organic and conventional agricultural practices use pesticides, but organic production uses pesticides that are of natural origin. You should try to minimize your consumption of pesticides, both those that are organically approved and those used in conventional production. According to USDA pesticide surveillance data, conventionally grown produce in certain instances contains greater pesticide residues than organic produce. However, many of these pesticides are at levels deemed by health authorities to have no adverse impact on short- or long-term health.[56–58] Although some conventionally grown foods do have higher pesticide residues, the FDA limits how much pesticide residue is allowed.

Cruciferous Vegetables

Cruciferous vegetables are those that are in the mustard family. They get their name from their four-petal flowers, which look like a crucifix. Cruciferous vegetables are unique in that they are rich sources of sulfur-containing compounds known as glucosinolates. Some studies indicate that glucosinolates may help protect against cancer.[84–86] Other researchers claim that the protective effects of crucifers may be related to other cancer-fighting compounds in the vegetables. According to the American Institute of Cancer Research, nonstarchy vegetables, such as crucifers, probably protect against some types of cancers.[87] This protective effect is strongest for cancers of the mouth, pharynx, larynx, esophagus, and stomach.

The following crucifers can usually be found in the produce section of your grocery store:

Arugula	Kale
Bok choy	Kohlrabi
Broccoli	Mustard greens
Brussels sprouts	Napa cabbage
Cabbage	Rutabaga
Cauliflower	Radish
Chinese cabbage	Turnips
Collard greens	Wasabi
Horseradish	Watercress

Recommendation #5: Animal Foods

Limit intake of red meat (beef, pork, and lamb) and avoid processed meat. Consume 18 ounces or less of red meat per week. Consume very little, if any, processed meats, such as luncheon meat or cured, smoked, or salted meat, to decrease your risk of cancer.[81,82,88,89] Modest amounts of red meat are acceptable, but be aware that one large steak, like that you might get from a steak house, could easily put you over the recommendation for the week. Decrease the amount and frequency of consumption of red meat and substitute other high-protein foods, such as beans, poultry, and seafood.

Recommendation #6: Alcoholic Drinks

If you consume alcohol, limit consumption to no more than two drinks a day for men and one drink a day for women. A drink is 5 ounces of wine, 12 ounces of beer, or 1.5 ounces of sprits. The evidence for cancer risk is clear: Alcohol consumption increases the risk of cancer.[90] However, some studies have shown that consumption of modest amounts of alcohol can decrease the risk of heart disease. There are no data to suggest that one type of alcohol is better or worse than any other; it is the amount of alcohol that is most important. For reduction of risk of cancer and to gain the benefit that may be seen with alcohol, keep consumption under the recommended amount based on gender.

Recommendation #7: Preservation, Processing, Preparation

Avoid salt-preserved or salty foods. Limit consumption of processed foods with added salt. Strong evidence indicates that foods preserved and processed with salt are a probable cause of stomach cancer. Meats such as ham, bacon, pastrami, and salami are salt-processed meats, as are sausages, bratwursts, and hot dogs. Although an occasional hot dog at a baseball game or from the corner hot dog stand is fine, consumption of these types of meats on a weekly basis increases your risk of cancer.

Recommendation #8: Dietary Supplements

Aim to meet your nutritional needs through your diet. Dietary supplements are not recommended for cancer prevention. The evidence does not support dietary supplements of single nutrients or components of food to protect against cancer. Although some specific nutrients, antioxidants, and phytonutrients have a protective effect against cancer, they are present in foods with hundreds of other chemicals. The best delivery of these potentially beneficial substances is through a healthy diet with plenty of fruits, vegetables, fiber, and whole grains. No magic pill can substitute for a healthy diet.

Special Recommendation: Breastfeeding

Mothers should exclusively breastfeed infants. Aim to breastfeed infants exclusively (no other food or drink) for up to six months and continue with complementary feeding thereafter. Exclusive breastfeeding is protective for both the mother and the child.[91] It also offers a protective effect against childhood obesity.[92]

Special Recommendation: Cancer Survivors

Cancer survivors should follow the recommendations for cancer prevention. All cancer survivors should receive nutritional care from a trained professional and aim to follow the recommendations for diet, healthy weight, and physical activity.

Environment Organic farming practices are designed to minimize the negative impact of food production on the environment. On a per-acre basis, certain organic production practices can put a lower burden on the environment. If you look at the environmental impact per unit of production, however, the picture is slightly different.[55,59,60] Organic farming practices do have a number of environmental benefits, but organic practices can also be less efficient than conventional methods. Increasing productivity while maintaining a low environmental impact is challenging for both organic and conventional farmers. In some cases, organic farming practices have a similar impact on the environment when compared to

TERMS

cruciferous vegetables Members of the mustard family; they are rich sources of sulfur-containing compounds known as glucosinolates that may help protect against cancer.

Will Washing and Peeling Remove Pesticides?

You may wonder if you can rinse the pesticides off. Rinsing reduces, but does not eliminate, pesticides. Removing the peel does remove some pesticides, but you also lose valuable nutrients and fiber if you don't consume the peel.

conventional practices. For example, some studies have found that organic pesticides have a higher environmental impact than synthetic pesticides, often because they have to be used in large doses.[61,62]

Food Safety Several outbreaks of foodborne illness have been linked to fresh produce. Bagged spinach, tomatoes, and jalapenos have all been pulled from the shelves due to contamination with pathogens that cause foodborne illness. Fresh produce, regardless of the production methods used, can become contaminated anywhere from farm to fork. The very factor that provides the most nutrition benefits (fresh and raw) is what leads to the risk for foodborne illness—it's not cooked (and thus pathogens are not killed). Produce can be contaminated by the introduction of pathogens, which can occur during growth, preharvest, harvest, or postharvest. This can occur with organic or conventionally grown produce. Organic produce is no more or less likely to be "safe" with respect to food safety. Recent reviews of fresh produce safety data have shown that overall there is no difference in the end-product contamination potential of organic or conventional produce.[63] Regardless of the production methods used—certified organic, following organic practices, **biodynamic**, or conventional—there is a risk of introducing fecal matter into the agricultural and food-processing systems.

Should You Choose Organic?

Ultimately, the decision to choose organic is up to you, the consumer. You will need to weigh the benefits against the increased cost of organic produce. If purchasing organic produce is not in your food budget, by all means continue to purchase conventionally grown produce. Choose organic only if it fits into your budget. The health benefits of consuming fruits and vegetables are clear. You should not decrease your consumption of fruits and vegetables in order to afford organic produce.

TERMS

biodynamic An organic farming method that treats the farm as an individual organism, emphasizing the interrelationships among soil, plants, and animals.

Ready to Make a Change

Are you ready to make a change, small or large, in your fruit and vegetable consumption? Make the commitment to take the first step. Whether it is a small, medium, or large change, it is a step in the right direction toward a healthier diet.

I commit to a small first step. Add a salad to your lunch or dinner at least three times a week. Include dark green lettuce and other colorful vegetables. Top it off with a low-fat or fat-free dressing.

I am ready to take the next step and make a medium change. Add 1 cup of fruit or vegetable to your diet each day. You could add a banana to your cereal, grab an apple to take with you to school, or buy bagged salad to add to your evening meal. Even 1 cup a day will take you closer to the recommended amount of fruits and vegetables you need.

I have been making changes for some time and am ready to make a large change with the fruits and vegetables in my diet. Aim to get the recommended amount of fruits and vegetables each day. This may mean eating at fast food restaurants less often, preparing more meals and snacks at home or to take with you, and making sure you have fresh, frozen, and canned vegetables on hand for your meals. Experiment with unfamiliar fruits and vegetables and a variety of cooking techniques to keep eating fruits and vegetables interesting.

Myth Versus Fact

Myth: I just don't like vegetables; I take a multivitamin and get all the nutrients I need.

Fact: Taking a multivitamin may feel like a nutritional insurance policy. However, there is no substitute for a healthy diet, especially a diet that is high in vegetables. Vegetables contain nutrients, micronutrients, phytonutrients, antioxidants, and fiber. All of the health-promoting properties of vegetables are just not available in pill form. The multivitamin is OK for backup, but work to include vegetables in your diet to get all the benefits they provide.

Myth: Fresh is the best way to purchase fruits and vegetables.

Fact: Fresh is certainly an option, especially if the fruit or vegetable you purchase is in season. However, frozen and canned offer an economical alternative to fresh produce. Frozen fruits and vegetables are picked at their peak of freshness and flash frozen to preserve their nutrients and color. Choose frozen and canned vegetables that do not have sauce or butter. Choose frozen and canned fruit with no added sugar and that are packed in their own juice.

Myth: I have to go hungry to lose weight.

Fact: Although consumption of fewer calories than you need is required for weight loss, it does not have to mean that you have to go hungry. Fruits and vegetables are high in water and fiber but low in calories. They can help fill you up without putting you over your calorie limit.

Myth: All fruits and vegetables are the same; eat whatever ones you prefer.

Fact: All fruits and vegetables are excellent choices for a healthy diet. However, they are not all created equal. The powerhouses are those that are deep green, orange, red, or yellow. Choose all the colors to get all the health benefits. Choose starchy vegetables, such as white potatoes, less often.

Myth: Drink 100% fruit juice to get the fruit you need each day.

Fact: Fruit juice is not the best way to get the fruit you need each day. It is easy to consume too many calories, and you do not get the fiber in the fruit when you drink it as opposed to eating it. If you drink juice, do so in moderation, only a few ounces a day.

Myth: If you don't like vegetables, just eat more fruit to make up for the difference.

Fact: You need both fruits and vegetables. Variety is key to a healthy diet. You would miss out on many nutrients, antioxidants, and phytochemicals if you only ate fruit. Experiment with different vegetables to find some that you enjoy.

Myth: Fruits and vegetables take too much time to prepare.

Fact: Many preparation shortcuts are available. Fruits are the original fast food; they are often ready to go without any preparation. Try bagged salads, prepared carrots, cut up broccoli, or other washed and cut vegetables to make preparation quick and easy. Frozen vegetables are quick and often come in a bag that can be put directly in the microwave.

Back to the Story

Jane can take a number of steps to improve her diet. As it stands right now, she gets very few fruits and vegetables. In fact, if this is a typical day for Jane, she gets less than one serving of fruits and vegetables per day. First, she needs to consider eating breakfast. Eating breakfast will give her more energy and make her feel better throughout the morning at work. It does not have to be complicated or fancy: an apple with a slice of cheese, a peanut butter and banana sandwich, or other grab-and-go combination of fruit and a high-protein food. She needs to plan for lunch and take something with her. Eating out of the vending machine usually means high calorie, high sugar, and low nutrition; usually, she will not find fruits and vegetables in vending machines. Jane can experiment with bringing her lunch in a small cooler. This will allow her to have control over what she eats during the day instead of being at the mercy of the vending machine. It will also allow for her to pack some fruits and vegetables as part of her lunch. Baby carrots, celery, cucumbers, or other vegetables with low-fat dip add color and fiber to the diet. Jane's repertoire of vegetables that she likes is limited. You have to wonder when was the last time that Jane tried some of the vegetables she claims to not like. Tastes change as you age. Things that you didn't like as a child can become your favorites as an adult. Jane should give vegetables another try and find at least a few vegetables that she can add to her diet. As for dinner, frozen entrees are certainly quick and easy; however, they don't always have very many fruits or vegetables. A number of frozen entrees on the market include stir-fry vegetables or other selections with lots of vegetables. Jane should give them a try. She should also try cooking simple meals at least some of the time and add fresh, frozen, or canned vegetables. What are some other suggestions you have for Jane?

References

1. US Department of Health and Human Services and US Department of Agriculture. *Dietary Guidelines for Americans, 2010*, 7th ed. Washington, DC: US Government Printing Office, December 2010.
2. Serdula MK, Gillespie C, Kettel-Khan L, Farris R, Seymour J, Denny C. Trends in fruit and vegetable consumption among adults in the United States: Behavioral Risk Factor Surveillance System, 1994–2000. *Am J Pub Hlth*. 2004;94:1014–1018.
3. Blanck HM, Gillespie C, Kimmons JE, Seymour JD, Serdula MK. Trends in fruit and vegetable consumption among U.S. men and women, 1994–2005. *Prev Chronic Dis*. 2005;5(2). http://cdc.gov/pcd/issues/2008/apr/07_0049.htm. Accessed November 20, 2009.
4. Cook AJ, Friday JE (2004). Pyramid servings intakes in the United States 1999–2002, 1 Day. [Online]. Beltsville, MD: USDA, Agricultural Research Service, Community Nutrition Research Group, CNRG Table Set 3.0. http://www.ars.usda.gov/sp2UserFiles/Place/12355000/foodlink/ts_3-0.pdf. Accessed April 21, 2011.
5. National Center for Chronic Disease Prevention and Health Promotion, Centers for Disease Control and Prevention. Behavioral Risk Factor Surveillance System, prevalence and trends data, nationwide 2007 fruits and vegetables. http://apps.nccd.cdc.gov/BRFSS/list.asp?cat=FV&yr=2007&qkey=4415&state=All. Accessed November 20, 2009.
6. Guenther PM, Dodd KW, Reedy J, Krebs-Smith SM. Most Americans eat much less than recommended amounts of fruits and vegetables. *J Am Diet Assoc*. 2006;106(9):1371–1379.
7. Casagrande SS, Wang Y, Anderson C, Gary TL. Have Americans increased their fruit and vegetable intake? The trends between 1988 and 2002. *Am J Prev Med*. 2007;32(4):257–263.
8. Shepherd R. Influences on food choice and dietary behavior. *Forum Nutr*. 2005;57:36–43.
9. Van Duyn MA, Kristal AR, Dodd K, et al. Association of awareness, intrapersonal and interpersonal factors, and stage of dietary change with fruit and vegetable consumption: a national survey. *Am J Health Prom*. 2001;16:69–78.
10. Tucker KL, Maras J, Champagne C, et al. A regional food-frequency questionnaire for the US Mississippi Delta. *Pub Hlth Nutr*. 2005;8:87–96.
11. Morland K, Wing S, Diez RA, Poole C. Neighborhood characteristics associated with the location of food stores and food service places. *Am J Prev Med*. 2002;22:23–29.
12. Potter JD, Finnegan JR, Guinard J-X, et al. 5 a Day for Better Health program evaluation report. Bethesda, MD: National Institutes of Health, National Cancer Institute; 2000. http://www.cancercontrol.cancer.gov/5ad_exec.html. Accessed November 20, 2009.
13. Brown D. New dietary guidelines need dietetic interpretation. *J Am Diet Assoc*. 2005;105:1356–1357.
14. Nestle M. *Food Politics: How the Food Industry Influences Nutrition and Health*. Berkeley CA: University of California Press, 2002:130–132.
15. Giovannucci E, Rimm EB, Liu Y, et al. A prospective study of tomato products, lycopene, and prostate cancer risk. *J Natl Cancer Inst*. 2002;94:391–398.
16. Etminan M, Takkouche B, Caamano-Isorna F. The role of tomato products and lycopene in the prevention of prostate cancer: a meta-analysis of observational studies. *Cancer Epidemiol Biomarkers Prev*. 2004;13:340–345.

17. Granado F, Olmedilla B, Blanco I. Nutritional and clinical relevance of lutein in human health. *Br J Nutr*. 2003; 90:487–502.
18. Criqui MH, Ringel BL. Does diet or alcohol explain the French paradox? *Lancet*. 1994;344:8939–8940.
19. Standing Committee on the Scientific Evaluation of Dietary Reference Intakes, Food and Nutrition Board, Institute of Medicine. *Dietary Reference Intakes for Energy, Carbohydrate, Fiber, Fat, Fatty Acids, Cholesterol, Protein, and Amino Acids*. Washington, DC: National Academies Press; 2005.
20. Standing Committee on the Scientific Evaluation of Dietary Reference Intakes, Food and Nutrition Board, Institute of Medicine. *Dietary Reference Intakes for Vitamin A, Vitamin K, Arsenic, Boron, Chromium, Copper, Iodine, Iron, Manganese, Molybdenum, Nickel, Silicon, Vanadium, and Zinc*. Washington, DC: National Academies Press, 2001.
21. Coulehan JL. Ascorbic acid and the common cold: reviewing the evidence. *Postgraduate Medicine*. 1974;86: 153–160.
22. Standing Committee on the Scientific Evaluation of Dietary Reference Intakes, Food and Nutrition Board, Institute of Medicine. *Dietary Reference Intakes for Vitamin C, Vitamin E, Selenium, and Carotenoids*. Washington, DC: National Academies Press, 2000.
23. Standing Committee on the Scientific Evaluation of Dietary Reference Intakes, Food and Nutrition Board, Institute of Medicine. *Dietary Reference Intakes for Thiamin, Riboflavin, Niacin, Vitamin B_6, Folate, Vitamin B_{12}, Pantothenic Acid, Biotin, and Choline*. Washington, DC: National Academies Press, 1998.
24. Standing Committee on the Scientific Evaluation of Dietary Reference Intakes, Food and Nutrition Board, Institute of Medicine. *Dietary Reference Intakes for Vitamin A, Vitamin K, Arsenic, Boron, Chromium, Copper, Iodine, Iron, Manganese, Molybdenum, Nickel, Silicon, Vanadium, and Zinc*. Washington, DC: National Academies Press, 2001.
25. Genkinger JM, Platz EA, Hoffman SC, Comstock GW, Helzlsouer KJ. Fruit, vegetable, and antioxidant intake and all-cause, cancer, and cardiovascular disease mortality in a community-dwelling population in Washington County, Maryland. *Am J Epidemiol*. 2004; 160:1223–1233.
26. He FJ, Nowson CA, MacGregor GA. Fruit and vegetable consumption and stroke: meta-analysis of cohort studies. *Lancet*. 2006;367:320–326.
27. Hung HC, Joshipura KJ, Jiang R, et al. Fruit and vegetable intake and risk of major chronic disease. *J Natl Cancer Inst*. 2004;96:1577–1584.
28. Liu S, Manson JE, Lee IM, et al. Fruit and vegetable intake and risk of cardiovascular disease: the Women's Health Study. *Am J Clin Nutr*. 2000;72:922–928.
29. Joshipura KJ, Hu FB, Manson JE, et al. The effect of fruit and vegetable intake on risk for coronary heart disease. *Ann Intern Med*. 2001;134:1106–1114.
30. Ford ES, Mokdad AH. Fruit and vegetable consumption and diabetes mellitus incidence among U.S. adults. *Prev Med*. 2001;32:33–39.
31. Sargeant LA, Khaw KT, Bingham S, et al. Fruit and vegetable intake and population glycosylated haemoglobin levels: the EPIC-Norfolk Study. *Eur J Clin Nutr*. 2001;55:342–348.
32. Williams DE, Wareham NJ, Cox BD, Byrne CD, Hales CN, Day NE. Frequent salad vegetable consumption is associated with a reduction in the risk of diabetes mellitus. *J Clin Epidemiol*. 1999;52:329–335.
33. Bazzano L, Li TY, Joshipura KJ, Hu FB. Intake of fruit, vegetables, and fruit juices and risk of diabetes in women. *Diabetes Care*. 2008;31:1311–1317.
34. Center for Disease Control and Prevention, National Center for Chronic Disease Prevention and Health Promotion, Division of Nutrition and Physical Activity. Can eating fruits and vegetables help people to manage their weight? Research to Practice Series, No.1. http://www.cdc.gov/nutrition/professionals /researchtopractice/index.html. Accessed November 24, 2009.
35. Duncan KH, Bacon JA, Weinsier RL. The effects of high and low energy density diets on satiety, energy intake, and eating time of obese and nonobese subjects. *Am J Clin Nutr*. 1983;37:763–767.
36. Rolls BJ, Bell EA, Waugh BA. Increasing the volume of a food by incorporating air affects satiety in men. *Am J Clin Nutr*. 2000;72:361–368.
37. Bell EA, Castellanos VH, Pelkman CL, Thorwart ML, Rolls BJ. Energy density of foods affects energy intake in normal-weight women. *Am J Clin Nutr*. 1998;67:412–420.
38. Rolls BJ, Bell EA, Thorwart ML. Water incorporated into a food but not served with a food decreases energy intake in lean women. *Am J Clin Nutr*. 1999;70: 448–455.
39. Yao M, Roberts SB. Dietary energy density and weight regulation. *Nutr Rev*. 2001;59:247–258.
40. Grunwald GK, Seagle HM, Peters JC, Hill JO. Quantifying and separating the effects of macronutrient composition and non-macronutrients on energy density. *Br J Nutr*. 2001;86:265–276.
41. Fitzwater SL, Weinsier RL, Wooldridge NH, et al. Evaluation of long-term weight changes after a multidisciplinary weight control program. *J Am Diet Assoc*. 1991;91:421–4.
42. Epstein LH, Gordy CC, Raynor HA, Beddome M, Kilanowski CK, Paluch R. Increasing fruit and vegetable intake and decreasing fat and sugar intake in families at risk for childhood obesity. *Obesity Res*. 2001;9(3):171–178.
43. Lanza E, Schatzkin A, Daston C, et al. Implementation of a 4-y, high-fiber, high-fruit-and-vegetable, low-fat dietary intervention: results of dietary changes in the Polyp Prevention Trial. *Am J Clin Nutr*. 2001;74:387–401.

44. Singh RB, Rastogi S, Verma R, et al. Randomized controlled trial of cardioprotective diet in patients with recent acute myocardial infarction: results of a one year follow up. *Br Med J*. 1992;304:1015–1019.
45. Singh RB, Rastogi S, Niaz MA, Ghosh S, Singh R, Gupta S. Effect of fat-modified and fruit- and vegetable-enriched diets on blood lipids in the Indian Diet Heart Study. *Am J Cardiol*. 1992;70:869–874.
46. Singh RB, Dubnov G, Niaz MA, et al. Effect of an Indo-Mediterranean diet on progression of coronary artery disease in high risk patients (Indo-Mediterranean Diet Heart Study): a randomized single-blind trial. *Lancet*. 2002;360:1455–1461.
47. He K, Hu FB, Colditz GA, Manson JE, Willett WC, Liu S. Changes in intake of fruits and vegetables in relation to risk of obesity and weight gain among middle-aged women. *Int J Obes Relat Metab Disord*. 2004; 28:1569–1574.
48. Fitzwater SL, Weinsier RL, Wooldridge NH, Birch R, Liu C, Bartolucci AA. Evaluation of long-term weight changes after a multidisciplinary weight control program. *J Am Diet Assoc*. 1991;91:421–424.
49. Rolls BJ, Ello-Martin JA, Tohill BC. What can intervention studies tell us about the relationship between fruit and vegetable consumption and weight management? *Nutr Reviews*. 2004;62(1):1–17.
50. US Department of Agriculture, Agricultural Marketing Service. Organic labeling and marketing. 2008. http://www.ams.usda.gov/nop. Accessed December 11, 2009.
51. US Department of Agriculture. What is organic production? http://www.nal.usda.gov/afsic/pubs/ofp/ofp.shtml. Updated July, 29, 2009. Accessed April 28, 2011.
52. Williamson CS. Is organic food better for our health? *Nutr Bull*. 2007;32(2):104–108.
53. Hoefkens C, Vandekinderen I, DeMeulenaer B, et al. A literature-based comparison of nutrient and contaminant contents between organic and conventional vegetables and potatoes. *Br Food J*. 2009;111(10): 1078–1097.
54. Rossi F, Godani F, Bertuzzi T, Trevisan M, Ferrari F, Gatti S. Health-promoting substances and heavy metal content in tomatoes grown with different farming techniques. *Eur J Nutr*. 2008;47:266–272.
55. Rembialkowska E. Quality of plant products from organic agriculture. *J Sci Food Agricul*. 2007;87:2757–2762.
56. Benbrook C, Zhao, Anez J, Davies N, Andrews P. New evidence confirms the nutritional superiority of plant-based organic foods. The Organic Center. 2008. http://www.organic-center.org/reportfiles/5367_Nutrient_Content_SSR_FINAL_V2.pdf. Accessed December 11, 2009.
57. Woese K, Lange D, Boess C, Bogi KW. A comparison of organically and conventionally grown foods—results of a review of the relevant literature. *J Sci Food Agricul*. 1997;74(3):281–293.
58. Baker BP, Benrook CM, Groth E, Benbrook KL. Pesticide residues in conventional, integrated pest management (IPM)-growth and organic foods: insights from three US data sets. *Food Additives Contaminants*. 2002;19(5):427–446.
59. Van Huylenbroeck B, Mondelaers K, Aertsens J. The added value of organic farming for environment and health: facts and consumer perceptions. *Br Food J*. 2009:111(10).
60. DeBacker E, Aertsens J, Vergucht S, Steurbaut W. Assessing the ecological soundness of organic and conventional agriculture by means of life cycle assessment (LCA): a case study of leek production. *Bri Food J*. 2009;111(10):1028–1061.
61. Organic pesticides not always 'greener' choice, study finds. *ScienceDaily*. June 23, 2010. http://www.sciencedaily.com/releases/2010/06/100622175510.htm. Accessed April 28, 2011.
62. Bahlai CA, Xue Y, McCreary CM, Schaafsma AW, Hallett RH. Choosing organic pesticides over synthetic pesticides may not effectively mitigate environmental risk in soybeans. *PLoS ONE*. 2010:5(6):e11250. http://www.plosone.org/article/info%3Adoi%2F10.1371%2Fjournal.pone.0011250. Accessed April 28, 2011.
63. Diez-Gonzalez F, Mukherjee A. Produce safety in organic vs. conventional crops. In Fan X, Niemira BA, Doona CJ, Feeherry FE, Gravani RB, eds. *Microbial Safety of Fresh Produce*. Ames, IA: Blackwell Publishing, 2009.
64. Pirog R, VanPelt T. How far do your fruits and vegetables travel? Leopold Center for Sustainable Agriculture. 2002. http://www.leopold.iastate.edu/pubs/other/files/food_chart.pdf. Accessed November 16, 2009.
65. Office of Environmental Education, NC Department of Environment and Natural Resources. http://www.eenorthcarolina.org/. Accessed November 16, 2009.
66. Oxfam America. Buy local food and farm toolkit: a guide for community organizers. 2002. http://www.sustainabletable.org/schools/docs/food_farm_toolkit.pdf. Accessed April 21, 2011.
67. Truit T, Collective K. Why the local multiplier effect always counts. *Grassroots Economic Organizing Newsletter*. 2004. http://www.geo.coop/archive. Accessed November 15, 2009.
68. Beth D, Butner F, Creamer N, Dunn C, Lee J, Thomas C. Eat smart North Carolina: bring fresh produce to your setting. 2007. http://www.eatsmartmovemorenc.com/FreshProduce/FreshProduce.html. Accessed April 21, 2011.
69. World Cancer Research Fund/American Institute for Cancer Research. *Food, Nutrition, Physical Activity, and the Prevention of Cancer: a Global Perspective*. Washington DC: AICR, 2007.
70. Kushi KH, Byers T, Doyle C, Bandera EV, McCullough M, Gansler T, Andrews KS, Thun MJ. American Cancer Society guidelines on nutrition and physical activity for cancer prevention: reducing the risk of cancer with

healthy food choices and physical activity. *CA Cancer J Clin*. 2006;56:254–281.

71. Callee EE, Thun MJ. Obesity and cancer. *Oncogene*. 2004;23:6365–6378.
72. Renehan AG, Tyson M, Egger M, Heller RF, Zwahlen M. Body-mass index and incidence of cancer: a systematic review and meta-analysis of prospective observational studies. *Lancet*. 2008;371:569–578.
73. Albanes D, Blair A, Taylor PR. Physical activity and risk of cancer in the NHANES population. *Am J Public Health*. 1989;79:744–750.
74. Paffenbarger RS Jr, Hyde RT, Wing AL. Physical activity and incidence of cancer in diverse populations: a preliminary report. *Am J Clin Nutr*. 1987;45:312–317.
75. Blair SN, Kohl HW 3rd, Paffenbarger RS, Clark DG, Cooper KH, Gibbons LW. Physical fitness and all-cause mortality. A prospective study of healthy men and women. *JAMA*. 1989;262:2395–2401.
76. Hardman AE. Physical activity and cancer risk. *Proceedings of the Nutrition Society*. 2001;60:107–113.
77. Monninkhof EM, Elias SG, Vlems FA, et al. Physical activity and breast cancer: a systematic review. *Epidemiology*. 2007;18(1):137–157.
78. Malik VS, Schulze MB, Hu FB. Intake of sugar-sweetened beverages and weight gain: a systematic review. *Am J Clin Nutr*. 2006;84:274–288.
79. Thompson OM, Ballew C, Resnicow K, et al. Food purchased away from home as a predictor of change in BMI z-score among girls. *Int J Obes*. 2004;28:282–289.
80. French SA, Harnack L, Jeffery RW. Fast food restaurant use among women in the Pound of Prevention study: Dietary, behavioral and demographic correlates. *Int J Obes*. 2000;24:1353–1359.
81. Slattery ML, Boucher KM, Caan BJ, Potter JD, Ma KN. Eating patterns and risk of colon cancer. *Am J Epidemiol*. 1998;148:4–16.
82. Fung T, Hu FB, Fuchs C, et al. Major dietary patterns and the risk of colorectal cancer in women. *Arch Intern Med*. 2003;163:309–314.
83. International Agency for Research on Cancer. *Fruit and Vegetables: IARC Handbook of Cancer Prevention*, Vol 8. Lyon, France: IARC Press, 2003.
84. Liu RH. Potential synergy of phytochemicals in cancer prevention: mechanism of action. *J Nutr*. 2004;134 (12 suppl):3479S–3485S.
85. McNaughton SA, Marks GC. Development of a food composition database for the estimation of dietary intakes of glucosinolates, the biologically active constituents of cruciferous vegetables. *Br J Nutr*. 2003;90(3):687–697.
86. van Poppel G, Verhoeven DT, Verhagen H, Goldbohm RA. Brassica vegetables and cancer prevention. Epidemiology and mechanisms. *Adv Exp Med Biol*. 1999;472:159–168.
87. American Institute for Cancer Research. Foods that fight cancer? Cruciferous vegetables. http://www.aicr.org/site/PageServer?pagename=foodsthatfightcancer_cruciferous_vegetables. Accessed November 25, 2009.
88. Kolonel LN. Fat, meat, and prostate cancer. *Epidemiol Rev*. 2001;23:72–81.
89. Cross AJ, Sinha R. Meat-related mutagens/carcinogens in the etiology of colorectal cancer. *Environ Mol Mutagen*. 2004;44:44–55.
90. Bandera EV, Kushi LH. Alcohol and cancer. In: Heber D, Blackburn GL, Go VLW, et al. (eds). *Nutritional Oncology*, 2nd ed. San Diego: Academic Press, 2006.
91. Collaborative Group on Hormonal Factors in Breast Cancer. Breast cancer and breastfeeding: collaborative reanalysis of individual data from 47 epidemiological studies in 30 countries, including 50302 women with breast cancer and 96973 women without the disease. *Lancet*. 2002;360:187–195.
92. Singhal A, Lanigan J. Breastfeeding, early growth, and later obesity. *Obesity Rev*. 2007;8(suppl 1):51–54.

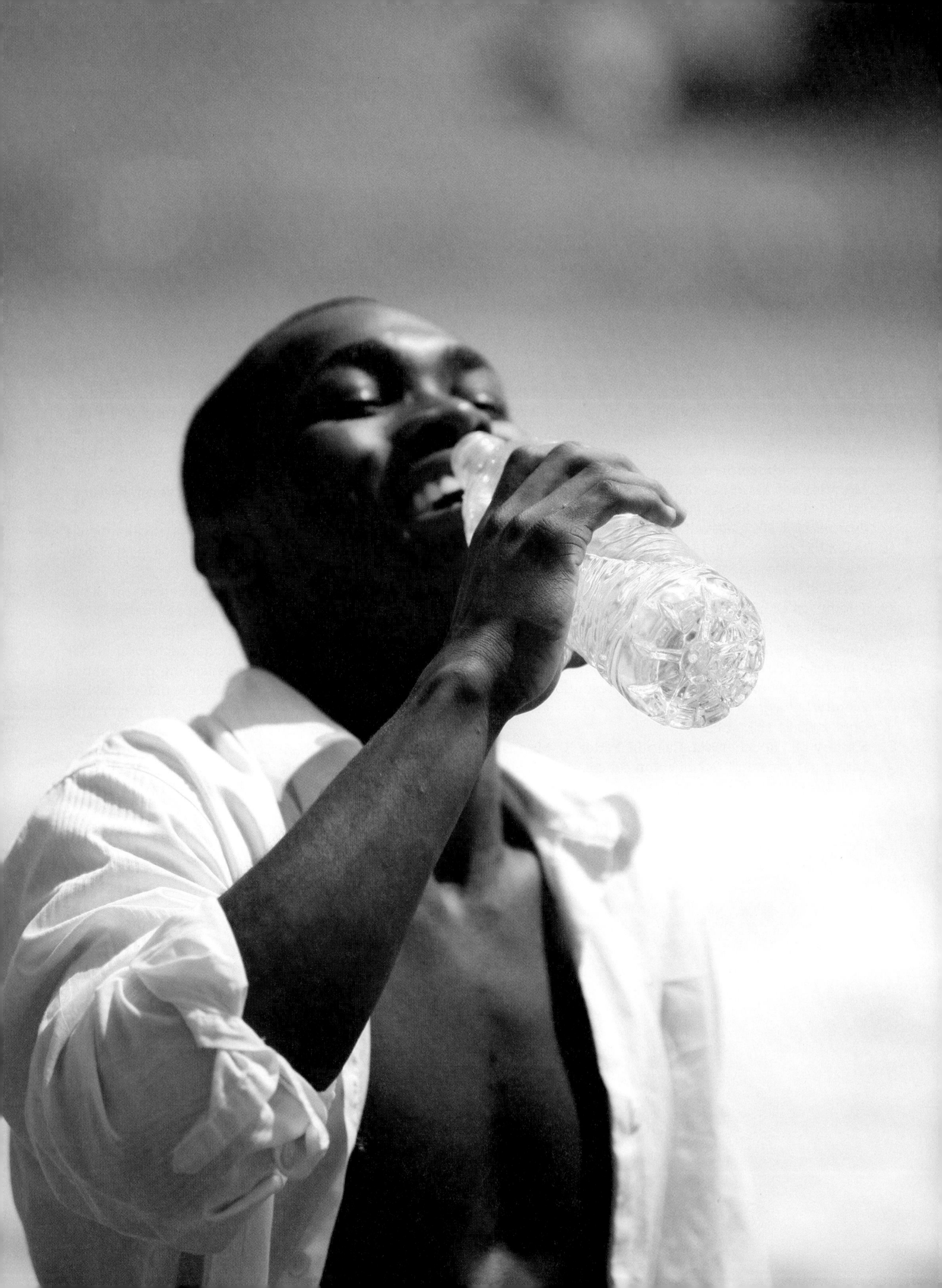

Chapter 7

Beverages: Rethink Your Drink

Key Messages

- Adequate fluid is essential for good health.
- Water should be your number one beverage of choice.
- Beverages can contribute significant calories to your overall diet.
- Your body responds differently to calories from beverages compared to calories from food.
- Changing from calorie-containing beverages to calorie-free beverages is an easy way to decrease total calories.

What comes to mind when you hear the word *beverage* or *drink*? Do you think of water, soft drinks, milk, or coffee? More than likely, you pictured some kind of carbonated soft drink. Carbonated soft drinks are the most popular beverage in America, comprising more than a quarter of all the beverages we consume.[1,2] This is more than twice that of the next closest nonalcoholic beverage, milk (11%). Over the past 25 years, consumption of sweetened beverages—primarily carbonated soft drinks—has increased more than 135%.[3] What effect are all these soft drinks having on health? Over the same period, the bottled water industry has gone from almost nonexistent to becoming a multibillion dollar a year industry. Is bottled water better than tap water? Also emerging on the scene are functional waters that claim to help you focus, stay alert, or have more energy. Are these waters better than plain water? What about juice? Is that a healthy choice? With the tens of thousands of beverage choices out there, what to drink for good health is becoming a more difficult question.

You may often think about the food you eat and how important it is for good health, but you may not have considered how what you drink contributes to overall health. You probably have heard the saying, "you are what you eat." But because about 21% of all of calories come from beverages,[4] you could also say "you are what you drink." That said, it is just as important to drink healthy as it is to eat healthy. This chapter will explore the importance of choosing beverages wisely for good health and to help manage weight. You will examine many common beverage choices and how they affect your health.

Story

Jim is a college sophomore. He starts his day with a cup of coffee from Starbucks. He usually orders a Grande white chocolate mocha. He eats lunch at the cafeteria on campus and has two 14-ounce glasses of Coke from the fountain. In the afternoon before hitting the library, he grabs a 24-ounce Mountain Dew from the snack bar. He drinks a 20-ounce Snapple Lemonade with his dinner. He goes out with friends at night and has three 12-ounce draft beers. Jim is concerned that his weight is creeping up from what it was in his high school days. What do you think about Jim's beverage intake? What changes can he make to decrease calories and make healthier drink choices?

Function of Water in Your Body

Water has been referred to as a life force, an elixir, a chemical, and a nutrient. It is all of these and more. Water is second only to oxygen as being essential for life. The human body can survive for a very long time without food, but without water you would perish in a few short days. Water is the most abundant substance in our bodies. An average woman is about 50% water; an average man is about

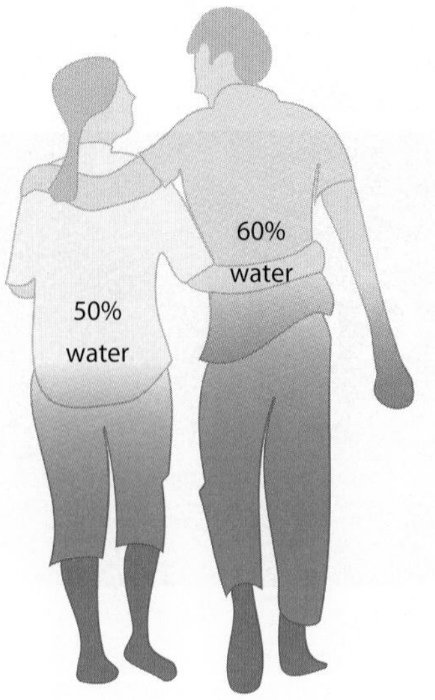

Figure 7.1
Your Body Is at Least Half Water

60% water (**Figure 7.1**).[5] The higher amount of water in a man's body is due to the fact that men generally have greater muscle mass, and muscle contains a large amount of water.

Water performs many functions in the body (**Figure 7.2**). Virtually all metabolic processes occur in water, and it is the major component of all body fluids, including blood, saliva, tears, urine, and amniotic fluid. Water transports nutrients to and waste away from cells. Water is an excellent solvent and allows for the excretion of waste and toxins in urine. Water also lubricates the joints. Synovial fluid, which enables the joints to move freely, is primarily

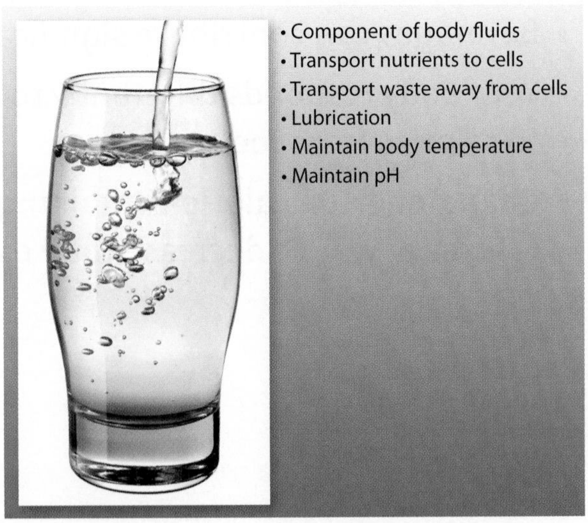

Figure 7.2
Functions of Water

water. Water also lubricates the digestive tract. Imagine trying to swallow without saliva.

Water absorbs heat with relatively little change to its own temperature. Because of this, water is essential to maintaining proper body temperature. Water helps to cool your body when you get hot. Blood vessels rise to the surface of the skin and you begin to produce sweat, which is primarily composed of water. When this sweat evaporates, it cools your body. Water is also involved in keeping your body's acid–base, or pH, balance within the very narrow range needed to support life.

Fluid Balance

The water in your body comes from the consumption of beverages and food and is also a byproduct of several biochemical reactions in the body. You excrete water through urine, feces, sweat, and your breath (**Figure 7.3**).

Fluid balance in the body is critical for good health. Fluid inside the cells is called *intercellular fluid*, and the fluid outside the cells is called *intracellular fluid*. Keeping those two fluid levels constant is important to the body. To do that, you must have enough water and electrolytes. **Electrolytes** are found inside the cell (primarily potassium and phosphorus) and outside the cell (primarily sodium and chloride). The electrolytes generally do not travel across the cell membrane; however, water can travel across the membrane. It is this function of water that enables it to play a major role in fluid balance. Water flows from higher to lower concentration (**Figure 7.4**). For example, if you ate salty potato chips, the sodium in your intracellular fluid would increase. Water would then move from inside the cells to outside the cells to balance the increased extracellular concentration of sodium (**Figure 7.5**). If this continued, and water intake did not increase, the cells would eventually become dehydrated.

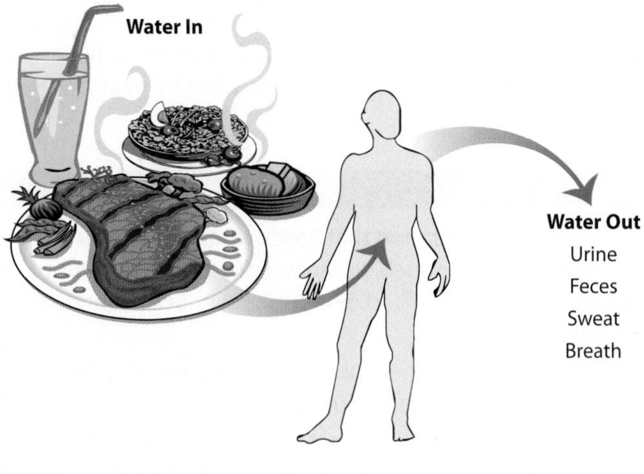

Figure 7.3

Intake and Excretion of Water

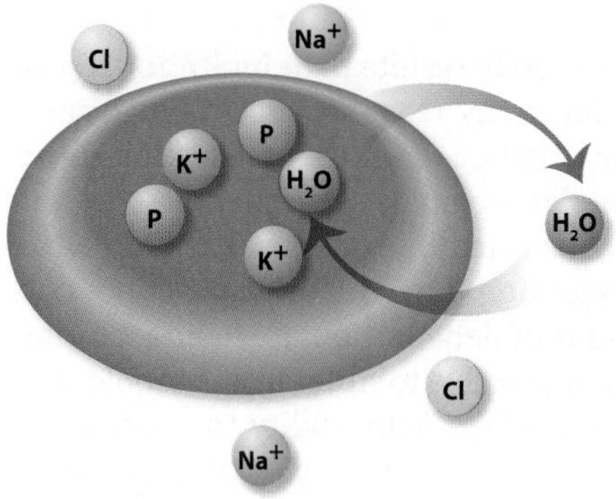

Figure 7.4

Water Movement into and out of Cells

Water moves from higher to lower concentrations. If the concentration of electrolytes is higher in the cell, water will move from outside the cell to inside the cell, and vice versa.

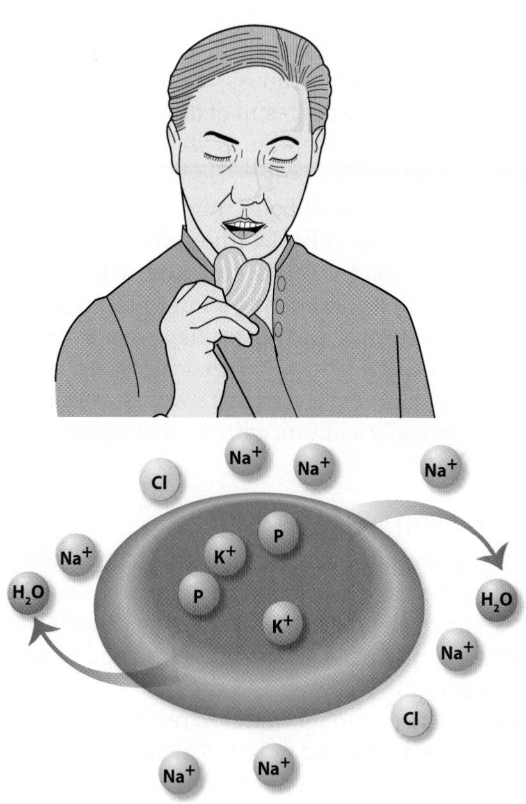

Figure 7.5

Your Body's Reaction to Consumption of Salt

Eating a salty food like chips increases the sodium concentration in the intracellular fluid. This causes water to move from inside the cells to outside the cells to balance the concentration of sodium.

TERMS

electrolytes Substances that separate into charged particles (ions) when dissolved in water; they can conduct an electrical current.

Too Little Water

Too little water in the body results in **dehydration**. Dehydration can occur for many reasons, such as high fever, severe vomiting or diarrhea, or extreme exertion in hot weather without replacing fluids. Alcohol has a **diuretic** effect, and when consumed in excess has the potential to cause mild dehydration if adequate water is not consumed. The first signs of dehydration are headache, dark urine, and fatigue. It is possible to suffer from chronic, mild dehydration. This can affect your ability to concentrate and may impair reaction time. If dehydration continues, it can cause many physiological responses, including nausea, increased body temperature, confusion, and dizziness. In cases of extreme dehydration, kidney failure and death can occur. Treatment for mild dehydration is simply consumption of water. Moderate to severe dehydration may require aggressive electrolyte replacement or hospitalization to receive intravenous fluids.

Too Much Water

Too much water in the body causes water intoxication. Water intoxication is rarely the result of drinking too much water or other fluids. An exception is water intoxication in athletes who exercise for long periods of time in hot weather and lose substantial body fluid. If they replace fluid with plain water not mixed with electrolytes, it can cause a dilution of the body's fluids, and sodium levels can fall to dangerously low levels. Forcing enormous quantities of liquids, as in a fraternity hazing prank, can also cause water intoxication. Signs of water intoxication are headaches followed by seizures. Treatment involves replacing electrolytes, specifically sodium, with food or electrolyte-enhanced water.

Recommended Intake

How much water should you drink each day? Eight glasses, right? For years you have heard that you should be sure to drink eight 8-ounce glasses of water each day. This is one of the most frequently used suggestions for good health. But is it really correct? Well, yes and no.

You need to take in enough water to replace what you lose in sweat, urine, feces, and breath. That exact amount can vary widely from person to person. The amount you need as an individual is based on your age, climate, activity level, and physical condition. Although eight 8-ounce glasses of water a day may be a good rule of thumb, it is not a hard and fast rule.

The Institute of Medicine provides a general recommendation of 91 ounces of water for women and 125 ounces of water for men per day.[5] You get about 80% of your water intake from drinking water and other beverages. The other 20% comes from food (**Table 7.1**).

Using the 80% figure and the recommendations from the Institute of Medicine, simple math suggests that women should be consuming about nine 8-ounce glasses of water and men about 12 and a half 8-ounce glasses of water. Some of this water can come from other beverages, such as tea, coffee, and milk. If you are physically active, especially in hot climates, you may need more water to compensate for sweat loss.[6]

Counting the number of glasses of beverage you consume is one way to make sure you get enough water. However, there are two additional ways you can listen to your body and gauge how much to drink. Most healthy people can adequately meet their daily needs for water by letting thirst be their guide. Be sure to listen to this cue that your body is giving you to drink. Another cue is the color of your urine. If it is dark yellow, you are not drinking enough and may be mildly dehydrated. Your urine should be the color of pale lemonade. Pale urine is a good signal that you are most likely consuming enough water and other beverages.

Table 7.1

Water Content of Common Foods

Food	Percent (%) Water
Watermelon	93
Broccoli	91
Carrots	88
Milk	87
Apple	85
Banana	76
Pasta, cooked	72
Chicken	71
Almonds	7

The Beverage Menu

There are many choices on the beverage menu. You may not think about your drink choice having an impact on your health. However, what you drink is just as important as what you eat. Some beverage choices may contain health-promoting qualities while others are associated with health problems such as overweight and obesity. You most likely have easy access to a wide variety of beverage choices. Choosing wisely can have a big impact on your overall health.

TERMS

dehydration Situation that arises when your body does not have as much water as it needs; can be caused by losing too much fluid, not drinking enough water or fluids, or both.

diuretic Drug or other substance that promotes the formation of urine by the kidneys.

Environmental Protection Agency (EPA) Federal agency founded to protect human health and to safeguard the natural environment, including air, water, and land.

Green and Healthy

Tap Water or Bottled Water?

Water should be your number one beverage of choice. But where that water should come from, the tap or a bottle, is not so clear-cut. The debate over bottled water or tap water includes issues related to water quality, safety, taste, convenience, and, of course, the environment.

Many different types of bottled water are available. The FDA oversees what bottled water can be called and the safety and quality of bottled water. The **Environmental Protection Agency (EPA)** has regulatory oversight for tap water under the Safe Drinking Water Act. Each time the EPA changes or establishes a new standard for drinking water, the FDA either adopts it for bottled water or suggests that the standard is not necessary for bottled water in order to protect the public health. As a result, the standards for bottled water and tap water are very similar.[8] Tap water may have one thing that bottled water doesn't—fluoride. Many municipalities treat their water with fluoride to prevent tooth decay. Oftentimes, fluoride is not added to bottled water or the fluoride has been removed if the water has been purified or distilled. Some bottled water does have fluoride added; if so, this will be indicated on the label. If you drink primarily bottled water without fluoride you should consult your dentist to see if a supplement is in order.

Taste is another factor when answering the question of "bottle or tap?" Water varies from town to town, city to city, and even within a municipality. Water from one location may taste better than that from a different location. If you don't like the taste of your tap water, you probably are not going to drink it. Filtering the water or choosing bottled water may be a better option to encourage you to make water your beverage of choice.

The most prevalent reason that people choose bottled water over tap is convenience. It is easy to grab a bottle of water and go. You can keep it in the car, at your desk at work or school, in your backpack, or in your gym locker.

Finally, what about all the plastic water bottles? Plastic bottles are not environmentally friendly. Several issues are at play here: making the bottles, transporting the bottles, and disposing of the bottles. It takes over 17 million barrels of oil to make the number of water bottles needed in the United States for one year. Then the bottles have to be transported, which means more oil. Finally, only about 15% of bottles get recycled, leaving 85% to sit in the landfill. The Pacific Institute, an independent think tank, estimates that the total amount of energy embedded in the use of one bottle of water can be as high as the equivalent of filling a plastic bottle one quarter full with oil.[8] The Pacific Institute also estimates that it takes about 3 liters of water to make 1 liter of bottled water. This is due to the water used in producing the bottles, transportation, and refrigeration.

So, why demonize bottled water? Why not pick on soda bottles or other plastic containers? The huge increase in the use of bottled water over the last five years is one reason. The other and more compelling reason is that there is an easy alternative: buy a reusable bottle and fill it from the tap. This will save oil, water, and the landfill and keep more money in your wallet.

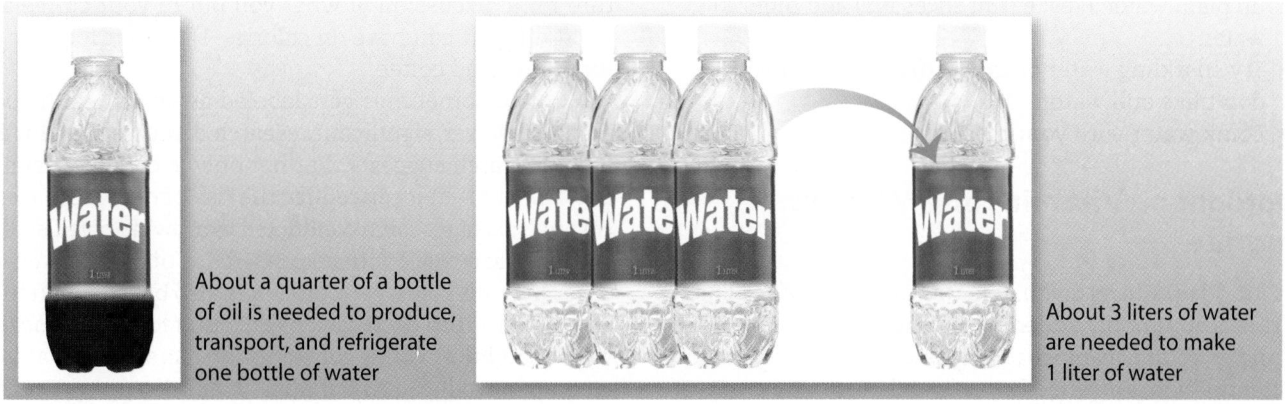
Water
About a quarter of a bottle of oil is needed to produce, transport, and refrigerate one bottle of water
Wate
Wate
Water
Water
About 3 liters of water are needed to make 1 liter of water

Oil and Water Used in Production of Bottled Water

(continues)

FDA-Approved Bottled Water Definitions

Label	Definition
Spring water	Bottled water derived from an underground formation from which water flows naturally to the surface of the earth. Spring water must be collected only at the spring or through a borehole tapping the underground formation feeding the spring.
Purified water	Water that has been produced by distillation, deionization, reverse osmosis, or other suitable processes while meeting the definition of purified water in the United States Pharmacopoeia may be labeled as purified bottled water. Other suitable product names for bottled water treated by one of the above processes may include *distilled water* if it is produced by distillation, *deionized water* if it is produced by deionization, or *reverse osmosis water* if the process used is reverse osmosis.
Mineral water	Bottled water containing not less than 250 parts per million total dissolved solids may be labeled as *mineral water*. Mineral water is distinguished from other types of bottled water by its constant level and relative proportions of mineral and trace elements at the point of emergence from the source. No minerals can be added to this product.
Sparkling bottled water	Water that after treatment, and possible replacement with carbon dioxide, contains the same amount of carbon dioxide that it had as it emerged from the source. Sparkling bottled waters may be labeled as *sparkling drinking water, sparkling mineral water, sparkling spring water*, etc.
Artesian water/artesian well water	Bottled water from a well that taps a confined aquifer (a water-bearing underground layer of rock or sand) in which the water level stands at some height above the top of the aquifer.
Well water	Bottled water from a hole bored, drilled, or otherwise constructed in the ground, which taps the water aquifer.

Source: REPRODUCED FROM FOOD SAFETY MAGAZINE, AUGUST/SEPTEMBER 2002, WITH PERMISSION OF THE PUBLISHERS. © 2002 BY THE TARGET GROUP.

Water

The scientific community is in broad agreement that water should be your number one beverage of choice. Water is sugar free, calorie free, caffeine free, and, if you drink tap water, costs almost nothing. When you are thirsty, the first drink you should turn to is water.

Whether you choose tap water or bottled water is up to you (see the Green and Healthy feature). The following are some tips to help you choose water above other beverages more often:

- Carry water with you in a reusable water bottle.
- Keep water in a jug or pitcher in the refrigerator. Cold water is more appealing than drinking it straight from the tap.
- Add fruit slices or a splash of fruit juice to liven up plain water. Freeze fruit slices and add them to water.
- Try sparkling water or calorie-free seltzer if you don't like still water.
- Drink water with your meals.

Spotlight on Vitamins and Minerals: Fluoride

Fluoride protects against dental caries (cavities). Fluoride is commonly added to community water supplies and is found in most toothpaste. Community water fluoridation is an effective, safe, and inexpensive way to prevent tooth decay. Fluoridation of community water supplies has been credited with reducing tooth decay by 50–60% in the United States since the 1940s. Children and adults who are at low risk of dental decay can stay cavity-free through frequent exposure to small amounts of fluoride. This can be achieved by drinking fluoridated water and using a fluoride toothpaste twice daily. Children and adults at high risk of dental decay may benefit from additional fluoride, such as professionally applied gels and varnishes.[7]

Coffee

Over half of adult Americans drink coffee every day. Millions more drink it on occasion.[9] The recent phenomenon of specialty coffee shops has spawned a whole new generation of coffee drinkers. Whether it is a mocha in the morning or a latte to get you through the afternoon, coffee has become more popular than ever. What effect is this having on your health? Is drinking coffee OK? The answer to that is a qualified yes, depending on what you put in it. Coffee is like the baked potato; plain is OK, even healthy, but add bacon bits, sour cream, and butter and, well, you get the picture. Check out the Try Something New feature for a discussion of what you put in your coffee and what effect it can have on calories. Here, our focus in on unadulterated coffee.

Coffee sometimes gets labeled as an unhealthy beverage. However, significant research disputes that. In fact, most research suggests that not only is coffee consumption OK, but that it can reduce the risk of many diseases.[10] An analysis of research conducted worldwide revealed that coffee is associated with decreased risk of liver cancer and other liver diseases.[11,12] Coffee has also been shown to be associated with a decreased risk of other forms of cancer as well. In addition, coffee consumption has also been associated with a reduced risk of Alzheimer's disease, dementia, gallstones, and Parkinson's disease.[13,14]

A systematic review of the research suggests that coffee consumption is associated with a substantially lower risk of type 2 diabetes.[15] The exact mechanism for producing this effect is unclear. It may be the antioxidants, caffeine, or some other property in coffee, although decaffeinated coffee has also shown some benefit in reducing the risk of type 2 diabetes.

Table 7.2

Common Types of Tea

Type of Tea	Description
Black	Green tea leaves from *Camellia sinensis* that have been oxidized or fermented. This process gives black tea its characteristic reddish color. Black tea is the most common type of tea in the world.
Green	Tea leaves from *Camellia sinensis* that have only been slightly steamed and not fermented.
White	Very young tea leaves picked just after emerging from *Camellia sinensis*. White tea is only slightly steamed and not fermented.
Oolong	A type of black tea that has been slightly fermented and uses larger leaves.
Rooibos	Derived from the rooibous plant (*Aspalathus linearis*), which is native to South Africa. Rooibos is naturally caffeine free and is not really a tea but rather a *tisane*, an infusion made from plant parts.
Herbal	A tisane (infusion) made from the flowers, leaves, seeds, or roots of plants other than *Camellia sinensis*.

The antioxidants in coffee have been linked to decreased risk of cardiovascular disease.[16,17] One to 3 cups of regular or decaffeinated coffee per day has been associated with a decreased risk of death from cardiovascular disease, as well as other inflammatory diseases.

A review of coffee research found that regular coffee consumption provides a small benefit in preventing all causes of death.[18] Taken together, all of this research indicates that coffee consumption is safe and may even provide health benefits.

Tea

Tea is the most commonly consumed beverage in the world, second only to water. Hundreds of different types of teas are available (**Table 7.2**).

Whether it is brewed green tea from Japan, spiced chai tea from India, or iced sweet tea in the United States, tea is a part of almost every culture. Tea has many health benefits, mostly resulting from its high flavonoid content. **Flavonoids**, which are polyphenol compounds, are powerful antioxidants. Flavonoids are found in fruits and vegetables, but tea has the highest flavonoid content of any food or beverage.

Some research suggests that the antioxidant properties in tea can reduce the risk of cardiovascular disease by decreasing inflammation, total cholesterol, and blood pressure.[19,20] Green tea consumption has been shown to be associated with a decrease in mortality from cardiovascular disease. The protective effect was seen with as little as 1 cup per day. More benefits were observed with higher consumption (5 or more cups per day).

Tea has long been thought to help prevent cancer.[19,20] Numerous studies have examined tea's health benefits with regard to cancer. Despite thousands of studies, the potential benefits of tea as protection against or treatment for cancer is unclear.[21] Although some data support this claim, the FDA has yet to deem the data strong enough to allow manufacturers to place a health claim on tea.

A number of scientists are interested in researching tea's potential in addressing obesity. Some researchers theorize that tea, specifically green tea, may boost metabolism and help the body to burn fat more efficiently. Although there have been some promising results,[22–25] other studies have shown no link between green tea and weight loss.[26] Studies that have shown positive results have often used green tea extract, which would be equivalent to 10 cups or more of green tea per day.

Try Something New

Order Something New at Your Favorite Coffee Shop

Break out of your mocha routine at your favorite coffee shop. Although your favorite drink at the coffee shop may sound innocent enough, the calories it contains may surprise you. To cut back on calories:

- Request that your drink be made with fat-free or low-fat milk instead of whole milk.
- Forgo the extra flavoring. The flavored syrups used in coffee shops, such as vanilla or hazelnut, are sweetened with sugar and will add calories to your drink. If you want a flavor added, ask if they have any that are sugar-free.
- Skip the whip. The whipped cream on top of coffee drinks adds calories and fat.
- Get back to basics. Order a plain cup of coffee with fat-free milk and artificial sweetener or drink it black.

Consider the following specialty coffee drinks and their healthier alternatives:

Switch from: Medium mocha made with whole milk and topped with whipped cream—360 calories
To: Small mocha made with skim milk and no whipped cream—170 calories
Calorie savings: 190 calories

Switch from: Medium vanilla latte made with whole milk—280 calories
To: Medium vanilla latte made with skim milk and sugar-free flavoring—130 calories
Calorie savings: 150 calories

Switch from: Grande Vanilla Frappuccino with whipped cream—430 calories
To: Grande Light Vanilla Frappuccino, no whipped cream—190 calories
Calorie savings: 240 calories

TERMS

flavonoids Polyphenol compounds that act as powerful antioxidants; found in fruits and vegetables and in high concentration in tea.

Personal Health Check

Check Your Caffeine Consumption

Caffeine is the drug of choice for many Americans. In fact, 90% of adults consume caffeine daily.[27] Caffeine is a mild central nervous system stimulant. Caffeine is most frequently used to fight drowsiness and enhance alertness. Caffeine or caffeine-containing guarana is found in coffee, tea, soft drinks, energy drinks, chocolate, and prescription and nonprescription drugs.

Caffeine's effects vary greatly from person to person, depending on a person's body size and caffeine tolerance. The more caffeine you are accustomed to consuming, the more it will take for you to feel its effects. Caffeine can help you stay awake, but it cannot replace sleep. Caffeine may help you stay up all night to study for an exam, but your performance on the test may suffer if you are exhausted from a night of no sleep.

Caffeine consumption in moderation is acceptable and may even have health benefits. Most experts recommend no more than 300 milligrams of caffeine per day. Overuse of caffeine can lead to irritability, anxiety, and trouble sleeping. Pregnant women, or women who wish to become pregnant, should consume caffeine only in moderation. Breastfeeding women should avoid caffeine, because it can pass into breast milk.

A habitual caffeine consumer will have withdrawal, usually a headache, if caffeine is not consumed. If you want to reduce your caffeine consumption, cut back gradually. Eliminate one caffeine-containing beverage a day instead of quitting all at once.

Caffeine Content of Common Foods and Beverages

Food or Beverage	Serving Size	Caffeine Content (mg)
Coffee[1]		
Coffee, brewed	8 oz.	102–200
Starbucks, brewed, Grande	16 oz.	320
Dunkin Donuts, brewed	16 oz.	206
Starbucks, latte, Grande	16 oz.	150
Starbucks, espresso	1 oz.	75
Tea[2]		
Tea, brewed	8 oz.	40–120
Snapple, Lemon, Peach, Rasberry (regular or diet)	16 oz.	42
Soft Drinks[3]		
Mountain Dew MDX	12 oz.	71
Jolt Cola	12 oz.	71
Vault	12 oz.	71
Mountain Dew (regular or diet)	12 oz.	54
Coke	12 oz.	35
Diet Coke	12 oz.	47
Pepsi	12 oz.	38
Diet Pepsi	12 oz.	36
Energy Drinks		
Monster	16 oz.	160
Full Throttle	16 oz.	144
Red Bull (regular or sugar free)	8.3 oz.	80
Rock Star	8 oz.	80
Enviga	12 oz.	100
Chocolate		
Dark chocolate	1 oz.	20
Milk chocolate	1 oz.	6
Over-the-Counter Drugs		
NoDoz	1 pill	200
Excedrin Extra Strength	2 pills	130
Vivarin	1 pill	200

Note

[1] Caffeine content of coffee will vary greatly depending on how much coffee is used in the brewing process.

[2] Caffeine content of tea will vary greatly depending on length of time the tea is steeped in hot water.

[3] FDA limits caffeine in cola and pepper drinks to 71 milligrams per 12 ounces.

Although there are conflicting results as to the specific health benefits of tea, the data do support the benefits of consuming tea on a regular basis. The strong antioxidant properties of tea make it a good choice for consumption on a regular basis. Tea comes in a wide variety of flavors and can be consumed hot or cold. The addition of milk or lemon does not affect the positive benefits of tea, so you have that as an option as well. One word of caution, however; sweet tea has as much sugar as most soft drinks. You will be getting plenty of antioxidants, but also a hefty dose of calories. Sweeten your tea lightly or use low- or no-calorie sweeteners.

TERMS

caffeine A compound found naturally in coffee, tea, and chocolate and added to other foods and beverages; it acts as a central nervous system stimulant.

Milk

Milk is an important source of calcium, vitamin D, and high-quality protein and can help maintain bone health and prevent osteoporosis.[28] At 80 calories for an 8-ounce glass of skim milk, this beverage packs a powerful punch when comparing calories to nutrients provided. Most adults benefit from choosing nonfat or skim milk over other choices. For those who cannot or choose not to drink milk, soy-, rice-, or almond-based beverages that also provide calcium and vitamin D can be healthy alternatives. The role of dairy products as they relate to overall health will be discussed in detail in Chapter 9.

Juice

Fruit and/or vegetable juice can be a part of a healthy diet. Make sure to choose 100% juice and not a fruit drink or a fruit-flavored drink; these may contain little or no fruit. A 100% juice counts toward the fruits and vegetables you need each day. Many 100% juices provide vitamins and antioxidants. Citrus juices provide vitamin C, and several brands are enhanced with calcium. Cranberry juice may have a protective effect against urinary tract infections.[29] Tomato juice contains lycopene, a powerful antioxidant that has been found to have a protective effect against some forms of cancer and heart disease.[30]

Juice does have a downside. Although 100% fruit juice sounds like a good alternative to soft drinks, if it is calories you are concerned about, then it is not the best choice. Ounce for ounce, juice contains approximately the same number of calories as soft drinks. Some juices, such as grape juice or pomegranate juice, have even more calories than a sugar-sweetened soft drink. Simply replacing soft drinks with juice, even 100% juice, does not reduce calories. Even though juice is "natural" and the sugar contained in juice is from fruit, your body metabolizes it much the same way as it would a sugar-sweetened beverage.[31]

Consuming small portions of juice on occasion can fit into a healthy diet. Be careful with what are sold as single-serving containers of juice. They may, in fact, have two or more servings and hundreds of calories. The best way to get the fruit you need each day is to eat whole fruit. It is recommended that adults concentrate on eating whole fruit and consume very little fruit juice.[35] This is especially important when you are watching calorie intake (**Figure 7.6**).

You may have heard about acai (AH-sigh-EE) juice. Companies selling acai juice (or pills) indicate that it can help people lose weight, decrease their cholesterol, ameliorate symptoms of arthritis, and improve overall health. The acai berry is a powerful antioxidant; however, there is no evidence that there is anything special about this juice. The health benefits of acai are the same as they are for other similar fruits.[33]

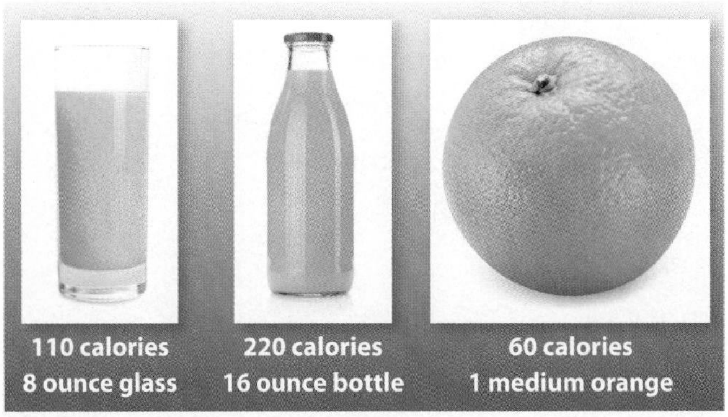
110 calories
8 ounce glass
220 calories
16 ounce bottle
60 calories
1 medium orange

Figure 7.6

Choose Whole Fruit over Fruit Juice

Whole fruit is lower in calories and higher in fiber than fruit juice.

> ### Liquid Versus Solid Calories
>
> A calorie is a calorie; it doesn't matter if that calorie is from Coke or cookies, right? Well, not exactly. Some evidence suggests that the body does not respond to calories in beverages the same way as it does to calories in food. Your body has complex mechanisms in place to detect calorie need and calorie consumption. This mechanism allows for the consumption of calories at a relatively stable rate over time. Liquid calories seem to go undetected, or at least not as readily detected as those from food.[34–38] Research indicates that the body's ability to detect calories in liquid form is not as accurate as its ability to detect calories in solid form. Your body may not register the calories you drink, so you could end up consuming more calories than you need. Even when the food and beverage are similar, as in watermelon versus watermelon juice or coconut versus coconut milk, more calories are consumed when they are consumed in liquid form.[38]
>
> For example, what if you ate 450 calories of jellybeans versus 450 calories of soft drink? Researchers found that the subjects who ate the jellybeans compensated for the calories contained in the jellybeans by consuming fewer calories from other foods. Their bodies recognized the 450 calories in the jellybeans and adjusted consumption of food accordingly. Those drinking their calories did not compensate for the 450 liquid calories. They consumed foods and calories as if the 450 liquid calories did not exist; those calories were essentially invisible to their bodies. It should come as no surprise that these subjects gained weight over the four-week study period.[37]
>
> Liquid calories count toward the calories you need for the day. They may even cause you to consume more calories than you need, because they don't trigger the body's mechanism for recognizing calories. For this reason, and others that will be discussed, choose calorie-free or low-calorie beverages often. Better yet, stick with water.

Soft Drinks: Sugar-Sweetened Beverages

A soft drink is technically any beverage that does not contain alcohol. For the purpose of this chapter, a soft drink is any beverage containing natural or artificial sweeteners. Examples include soda, lemonade, fruit drinks, sports drinks, energy drinks, functional waters, fruitades, or sweet tea. This section will specifically address sugar-sweetened beverages. The term *sugar-sweetened beverage* is used to describe any beverage sweetened with a caloric sweetener. Many forms of sugar can be used as sweetener (**Table 7.3**).

Per capita soft drink consumption has increased almost 500 percent over the past 50 years. Calories from soft drinks contribute an estimated 7% of total calorie intake.[39,40] People who drink sugar-sweetened beverages take in more calories than those who do not,[41–43] and those who consume

Table 7.3

Added Sugars

Sugars are found naturally in foods such as fructose in fruit or juice, or lactose in milk. They are also added to food. Added sugars, known as *caloric sweeteners,* are added to foods at the table or during processing or preparation. They provide calories but few or no nutrients. Some of the names for added sugars are:

Brown sugar	Syrup
Hone	Malt sugar
Corn sweetener	Glucose
High fructose corn sweetener	Molasses
Invert sugar	Fruit juice concentrate
Sugar	Maltose
Dextrose	Raw sugar
Lactose	

more sugar-sweetened beverages tend to weigh more.[38,43] In addition, consumption of sugar-sweetened beverages is associated with a higher risk of type 2 diabetes.[44] Several studies have found that limiting consumption of sugar-sweetened beverages is a good strategy for decreasing calories and managing weight.[41,43,45] Consumption of sugar-sweetened beverages also affects other aspects of people's diets. People who consume sugar-sweetened beverages tend to consume less healthy food overall.[46]

The most popular American beverage is the carbonated soft drink, which accounts for 28% of total beverage consumption. Enough regular soda is produced to supply every American with more than 14 ounces of soda every day.[47] The amount of sugar contained in common soft drinks is staggering (**Figure 7.7**). If you were to consume one 16-ounce Coke per day for one year, that would be equal to 50 pounds of sugar. With no redeeming nutritional value, you have to wonder why Americans consume the volume of soft drinks we do each year. The answer to that question is a complex mix of habit, taste, availability, and preference. Two possible answers to that question warrant further exploration: portion size and advertising.

The portion size of soft drinks continues to increase. When Coke was invented in 1916, the size of the bottle was barely 6 ounces. Today, soft drinks come in 16-, 24-, even 64-ounce sizes; as size increases, obviously so do calories (**Figure 7.8**).[48] In the past, the industry standard for vending machines was a 12-ounce can. Today, vending machines typically serve up 16- or 24-ounce bottles.

Soft drink advertising is a multi-million-dollar industry. Marketing techniques such as television commercials, point-of-sale displays, websites, and product placements in popular television shows and movies attempt to persuade Americans to drink soft drinks more often and in larger quantities.

Enhanced Water

If water should be your beverage of choice, you might think that enhanced water would be even better. With names

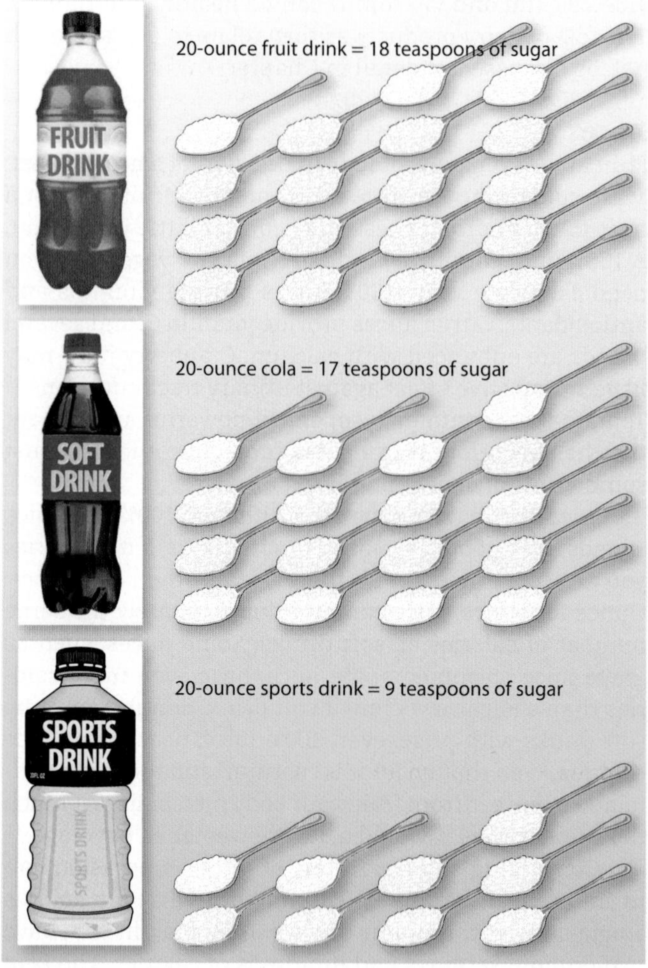
FRUIT DRINK
20-ounce fruit drink = 18 teaspoons of sugar
SOFT DRINK
20-ounce cola = 17 teaspoons of sugar
SPORTS DRINK
20-ounce sports drink = 9 teaspoons of sugar

■ **Figure 7.7**
Sugar Content of Common Soft Drinks

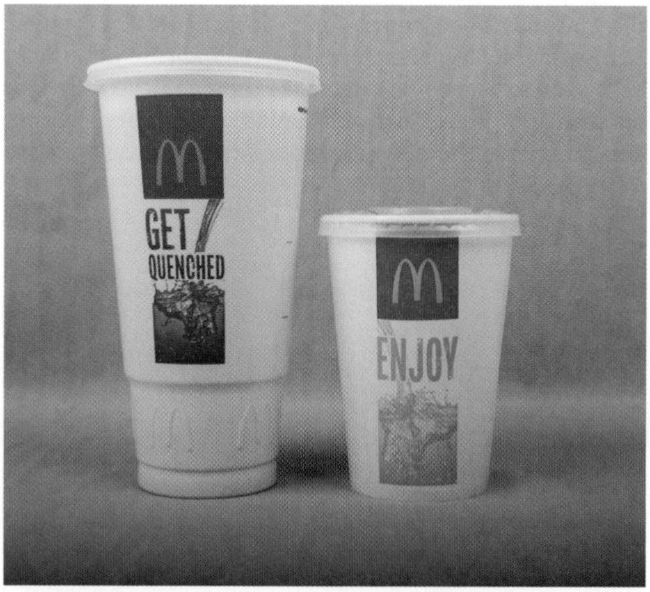
GET QUENCHED
ENJOY

■ **Figure 7.8**
Supersized Soft Drinks Mean Supersized Calories

like B-Relaxed, Defend and Protect, Essential, Endurance, and Life Water, you would think that you could not live without the added benefits such products must have over plain water. Literally hundreds of enhanced waters are on the market, many of which feature claims of doing everything from boosting your immune system to increasing your fiber intake. Many of the enhanced waters, such as Vitamin Water's B-Relaxed and Endurance, contain water-soluble vitamins. Unless you are deficient in one of these vitamins, which is highly unlikely, these drinks provide no benefit. And, certainly, there is no evidence that these waters promote relaxation or improve endurance, as their names imply. Ads for other enhanced waters, such as Snapple's Antioxidant Water or Vitamin Water's XXX (triple antioxidant), suggest that consumption of the product will boost your immune system. They make this claim despite the lack of scientific evidence of any link between antioxidant supplements and disease.[49] A number of enhanced waters contain maltodextrin, a soluble fiber whose benefits are largely unknown. Waters that invigorate, energize, or revive? You bet, if you count a caffeine buzz as energy. Most waters that make energy-boosting claims contain caffeine or the caffeine-containing guarana. Many enhanced waters make a variety of health- or life-enhancing claims, none of which have been substantiated.

Enhanced waters may not be harmful and on occasion may offer variety and a break from plain water; however, there are two potential issues. First, many enhanced waters are sweetened with sugar or high fructose corn sweetener, so they contain calories. For example, a bottle of Vitamin Water has 100–125 calories. Other brands sweetened with caloric sweeteners have similar calorie counts. If you are selecting enhanced waters sweetened with caloric sweeteners in place of plain water, the calories you drink can add up rather quickly. A number of enhanced waters on the market are sweetened with non-caloric or low-calorie sweeteners and have 0–10 calories per serving. These would be a better choice for a lower-calorie option. The second potential issue with enhanced waters is cost; they are more costly than bottled water and certainly more costly than turning on the tap. Your money can be better spent on foods and beverages that have more redeeming nutritional qualities.

As consumers continue to gulp down enhanced waters, companies making these waters will continue to do what they do best: market. Slick marketing campaigns and dazzling in-store displays add up to millions in sales. Unfortunately, what they are too often selling is brightly colored sugar water that does little more than make the grocery store beverage cooler resemble a rainbow.

Energy Drinks

Energy drinks, such as Red Bull or Rock Star, are relative newcomers to the beverage market. They are advertised as a miraculous cure for lack of energy or lack of sleep that will allow you to party like a rock star. With names like Monster, Adrenaline, Whoopass, Full Throttle, and Sprint, they at least sound like they live up to their promise. Most energy drinks contain caffeine or caffeine-containing ingredients. Much like enhanced waters that claim energy-boosting properties, it's more of a caffeine buzz than true energy. Many energy drinks do contain something that will provide energy, or at least calories—sugar. Although there are sugar-free versions of some energy drinks, most contain considerable amounts of sugar. Energy drinks also may contain other ingredients, such as vitamins, amino acids, guarana, and ginseng, to name a few. Very little is known about the effects of the combination of ingredients in many energy drinks; they fall outside the purview of FDA, so their safety is not regulated. Although an occasional energy drink may not be problematic, habitual consumption is unwise, according to most health professionals.

Sports Drinks

Millions of dollars and many keen minds have gone into creating beverages that enhance athletic performance. Early research at the University of Florida gave us Gatorade, named for the school's beloved alligator mascot. Sports drinks contain flavorings, carbohydrates (usually in the form of high fructose corn sweetener), and electro-

How Policy and Environment Affect My Choices

Availability of Sugar-Sweetened Beverages

Our environment has a strong effect on our food and beverage choices. When looking for a beverage, you tend to drink what is available. The environment serves up a menu, and you make a choice. One of the reasons that Americans consume so many soft drinks is that they are available everywhere. Convenience stores, gas stations, dorms, schools, worksites, and most campus buildings will have at least one drink machine. Everywhere you turn you have the opportunity to purchase sugar-sweetened beverages, usually in large quantities for a low price. Health educators working in the area of healthy eating suggest offering healthy options along with the not so healthy ones or, better yet, offering only healthy options. You see this theory in action with the replacement of sugar-sweetened beverages in many schools. Some worksites have replaced some or all of the sugar-sweetened beverages with low- or no-calorie options to support employee wellness. To make a positive change in beverage choices, it must be easy—or at least possible—to make a healthy choice.

lytes. They are formulated to replace fluids, electrolytes, and carbohydrates lost during intense physical activity. The carbohydrates in sports drinks provide energy to working muscles so that activity can continue. The electrolytes—sodium and potassium—keep fluid in your system, limiting its excretion by the kidneys. Sports drinks are flavored, which encourages consumption so the athlete can fully rehydrate. Ample research suggests that athletes participating in competition, workouts, or training for 60 minutes or longer and/or in hot climates or at high altitudes benefit from sports drinks.[50] What about after your nightly workout or afternoon mowing the grass? Do you need sports drinks to stay hydrated?

Since the early days of Gatorade, sports drinks have moved from the locker room to the mainstream. Today, athletes and nonathletes alike drink sports drinks. However, the evidence does not support the use of sports drinks for athletic events or bouts of physical exertion of less than 60 minutes.[50] Sports drinks are not appropriate for those not engaged in athletics or manual labor. At about 100 calories for 16 ounces, sports drinks do have less sugar and calories than other soft drinks; however, they still contain substantial calories and have no redeeming nutritional qualities. For the nonathlete, they are not much better than drinking soft drinks. Several sports drinks on the market are sweetened with artificial sweetener or contain less caloric-sweetener than regular sports drinks. These are good lower-calorie alternatives to the full-sugar version of sports drinks.

Alcoholic Beverages

Ethyl alcohol, or ethanol, is the substance found in beer, wine, and liquor that produces an intoxicating effect. Alcohol is a drug that acts as a central nervous system depressant. Alcohol, like most drugs, is metabolized by the liver. The liver can only metabolize a small amount of alcohol at a time. If alcohol is consumed at a rate or level that the liver cannot metabolize, the remainder stays in the bloodstream and circulates throughout the body. The more alcohol you drink, the greater the effects on the body. Generally, it takes about one hour to metabolize the amount of alcohol in one drink. One drink is 12 ounces of beer, 5 ounces of wine, or 1.5 ounces of spirits (**Figure 7.9**).

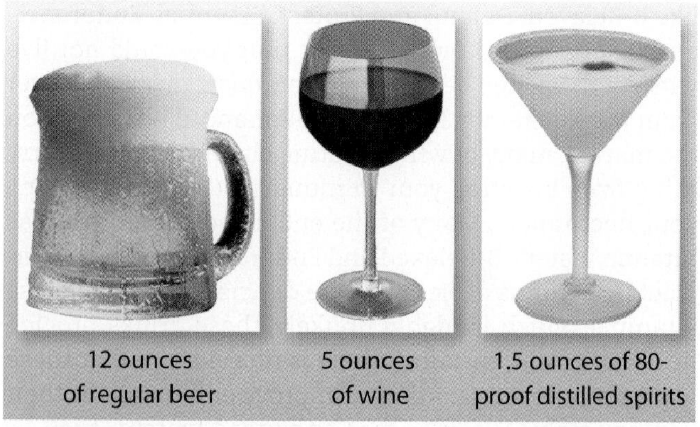
12 ounces
of regular beer
5 ounces
of wine
1.5 ounces of 80-
proof distilled spirits

Figure 7.9
What Is One Drink?

How alcohol affects you is related not only to how much and how fast you drink, but also to your body size, gender, and the amount of food in your stomach:

- **Body size:** Larger people may be able to consume more alcohol without feeling its effects. Higher body weight is associated with higher body water content, which serves to dilute the amount of alcohol in the body.
- **Gender:** Men have a greater capacity for metabolizing alcohol. They have more alcohol dehydrogenase, the liver enzyme that metabolizes alcohol. They also have higher lean body mass than women, and thus a higher percentage of water in their body, making the concentration of alcohol in their body lower than that of a woman of equal size.
- **Food:** Food in the stomach slows the absorption of alcohol. This is especially true with foods that are high in fat. High-fat foods leave the stomach more slowly than other foods, further slowing the absorption of alcohol.

The recommended daily consumption of alcohol by adults is one to two drinks per day for men and one drink per day for women.[32] Moderate alcohol consumption is associated with some health benefits, including lower overall mortality rates and lower rates of heart disease, stroke, type 2 diabetes, and gallstones.[51–58] The potential health benefits of red wine have been the focus of a great deal of research because of the antioxidants it contains. Although this once showed promise, there is not consistent evidence that moderate red wine consumption has additional health benefits over other forms of alcohol.[59–63]

Consumption of alcohol is not without risk. Even moderate consumption is associated with birth defects, specifically fetal alcohol syndrome.[64] Moderate alcohol consumption is also associated with an increased risk of breast cancer.[65,66] Higher alcohol consumption can cause significant health problems, including increased mortality,[67] liver disease,[68] cancer,[65,66,69] and heart disease.[70,71]

Excessive alcohol use can increase the risk of several harmful conditions. Most often these are associated with binge drinking or excessive use of alcohol (**Table 7.4**). Consider the following risks of excessive alcohol consumption:

- Traffic injuries related to drinking and driving[72]
- Unintentional firearm injury[72]
- Injury from falls[72]
- Domestic violence[73]
- Risky sexual behaviors, including unprotected sex[74,75]

Table 7.4

Definitions for Patterns of Alcohol Consumption

Drinking Pattern	Definition
Binge drinking	For women, four or more drinks during a single occasion For men, five or more drinks during a single occasion
Heavy drinking	For women, more than one drink per day, on average For men, more than two drinks per day, on average
Excessive drinking	Heavy drinking, binge drinking, or both

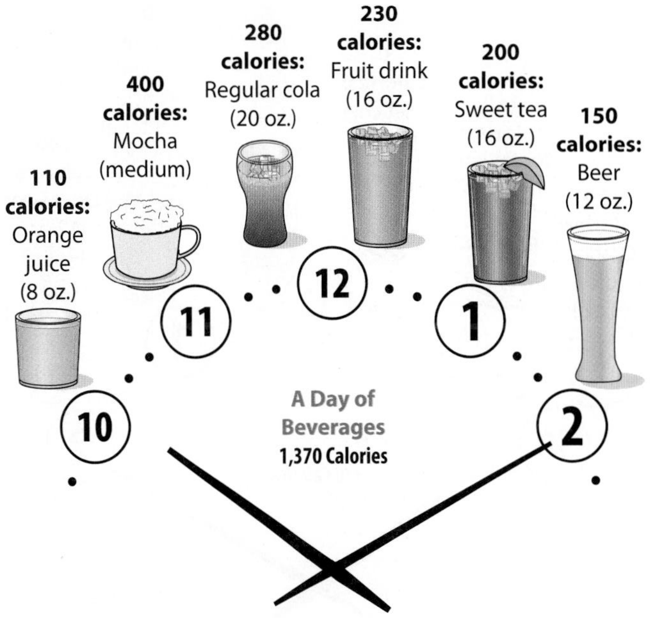

■ **Figure 7.10**
A Day of Beverages

Alcohol is a strong drug and, as such, can cause problems in those who abuse it or who are heavy users. Consumption of alcohol is a problem if it causes trouble in your relationships, school, or social activities. If you are concerned that you, a friend, or a family member might have a drinking problem, consult your personal healthcare provider or campus health services or call the National Drug and Alcohol Treatment Referral Routing Service at 1-800-662-HELP.

Make Good Beverage Choices

Now that you have the facts about many popular beverages, let's examine some strategies to make healthy beverage choices.

Let's say that you start your morning with an 8-ounce glass of orange juice. Between classes at 10 AM you head for the coffee shop and have a medium mocha. At lunch you have a 20-ounce Coke. For a 3 PM pick-me-up, you have a mango Snapple. Dinner is washed down with a large glass of sweet tea. That night you go out with friends and have one 12-ounce beer. This day of beverages adds up to 1,370 calories (**Figure 7.10**)! If you had refills on the tea or another Coke with lunch, it would be even more calories.

Here are some strategies to help you choose healthier beverages:

- Choose water as your number one beverage of choice; it is calorie-free, sugar-free, fat-free, and, if you drink tap water, costs almost nothing.
- Keep water and calorie-free beverages on hand at home and in your car.
- Carry a water bottle with you and refill it throughout the day.
- Jazz up your water by adding slices of lemon, lime, orange, or other fruit.
- Add a splash of juice to regular or sparkling water.
- Choose diet beverages sweetened with low- or no-calorie sweetener.
- Decrease the amount of sugar you add to tea or sweeten tea with no-calorie sweetener.
- Eat whole fruit instead of fruit juice.
- Choose nonfat (skim) milk.
- If you choose to consume alcohol, do so in moderation. Choose lower calorie options such as light beer, wine, or mixed drinks with calorie-free mixer. Avoid specialty drinks that have juice, multiple liquors, and flavored syrups. One margarita can contain more than 200 calories. A pina colada can contain more than 500 calories.

Let's use the strategies above to create a healthier beverage clock (**Figure 7.11**). You may choose to keep the juice in the morning, because it is only 8 ounces. You could substitute a whole orange and save an additional 50 calories. At the coffee shop, you change your order from a mocha to a nonfat latte. Your lunch beverage is now a Diet Coke instead of one that is sugar-sweetened. For your afternoon break, you switch from Snapple to water with lemon. Dinner is now washed down with tea sweetened with calorie-free sweetener (or you could drink it unsweetened). That night with friends, you order a light beer instead of a regular beer. The beverage clock goes from 1,370 to 370! By making some smart choices, you were able to cut 1,000 calories. Consider what changes you would be willing to make in your own beverage clock in the Personal Health Check feature.

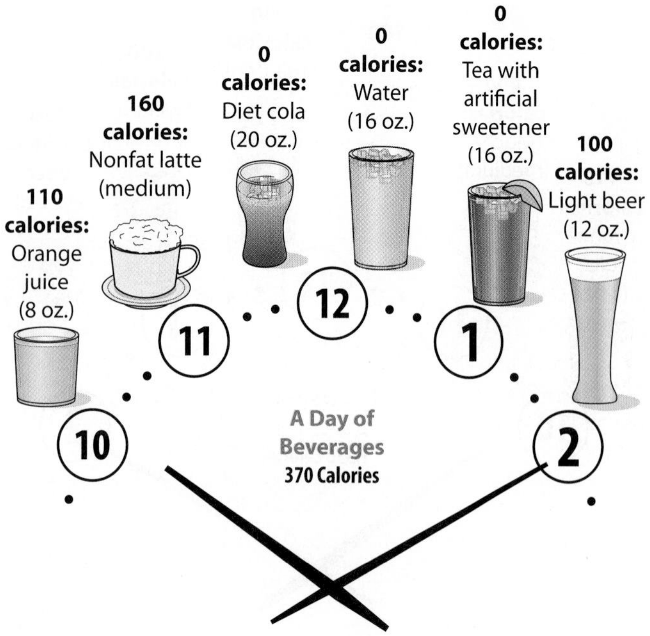

■ **Figure 7.11**

A Day of Beverages with Healthier Choices

Beverage Guidance System

One way to think about beverage selection is to put beverages into different categories. A group of scientists convened a beverage panel that has proposed a beverage guidance system that places beverages into levels based on their health benefits, or lack thereof.[91] The system suggests an optimal pattern of consumption (**Figure 7.12**). The beverage levels are as follows:

Level 1: Water
Level 2: Tea and coffee
Level 3: Low-fat (1.5% or 1%) and skim milk and soy beverages
Level 4: Noncaloric sweetened beverages (diet drinks)
Level 5: Caloric beverages with some nutrients [juice, alcohol, and sports drinks (only for endurance athletes or those performing work in extreme heat)]
Level 6: Sugar-sweetened beverages

The beverage guidance system suggests a consumption pattern where approximately 10% of calories are from beverages. Total beverage intake should be 98 ounces. Water, tea, and coffee, in some combination, should make up 78 ounces of the total for the day, with emphasis on water consumption. Milk consumption should be between 0–16 ounces; noncalorically sweetened beverages 0–32 ounces; fruit juice 0–4 ounces, alcohol 0–1 drinks for women, 0–2 drinks for men; and 0 ounces of sugar-sweetened beverages per day.

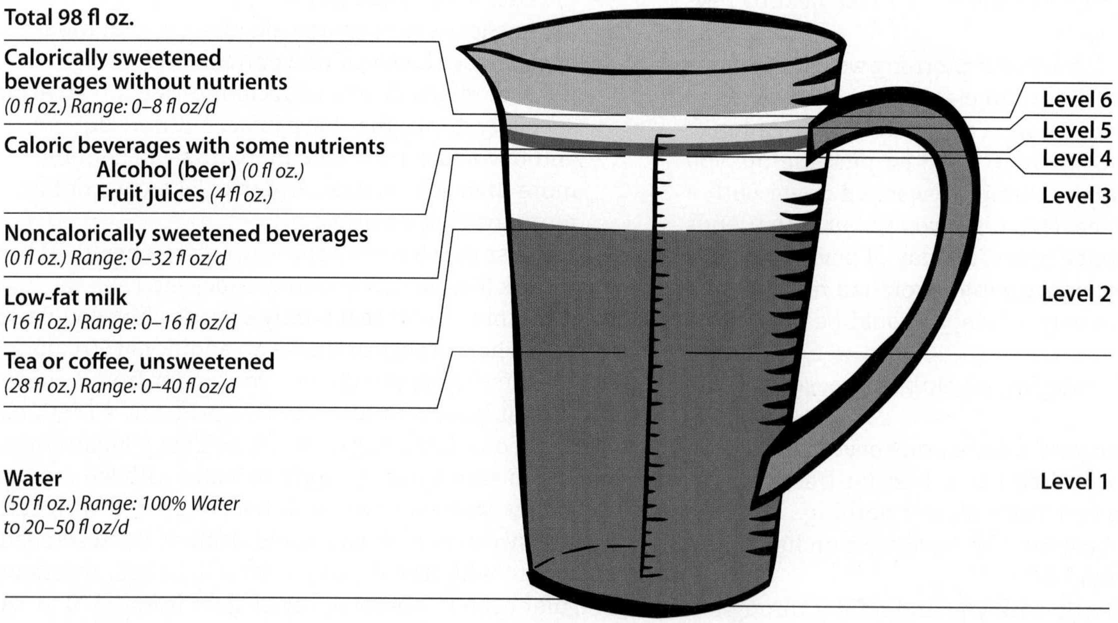

■ **Figure 7.12**

Beverage Guidance System

Source: BM Popkin, LE Armstrong, GM Bray, B Caballero, B Frei, WC Willett. A new proposed guidance system for beverage consumption in the United States. *Am J Clin Nutr.* 2006;83:529–542.

Special Report

Non-Nutritive Sweeteners (Artificial and Natural Low- and No-Calorie Sweeteners)

Aspartame

"The blue stuff," NutraSweet and Equal, are common forms of aspartame. Aspartame was approved in 1981 as a table-top sweetener and for use in gum, breakfast cereal, and other dry products. Use of aspartame in soft drinks was approved in 1983; in 1996 it was approved for use as a general-purpose sweetener in all foods and drinks. Its caloric value is similar to sugar, but the amounts used are so small that is considered calorie free. Aspartame begins to break down and lose its sweetness at high temperatures, thus it is not a good choice for baked products. It also can lose its sweetness over time.

Aspartame was discovered by accident by a chemist searching for a new ulcer drug. Working with amino acids, he found a sweet taste when two amino acids—aspartic acid and phenylalanine—were combined. Because of the high level of phenylalanine, products with aspartame must carry a warning label alerting persons with phenylketonuria. Phenylketonuria is a genetic disorder that affects a person's ability to metabolize phenylalanine.

Saccharine

"The pink stuff," Sweet'N Low, is a common form of saccharine. It was discovered in 1879 and was regarded as safe by the FDA until 1972. At that time, it was removed from the Generally Regarded as Safe (GRAS) list. In 1977, FDA proposed a ban of saccharin due to scientific evidence that it could cause bladder cancer in high doses. The public outcry over a possible ban persuaded Congress to pass the Saccharin Study and Labeling Act. This allowed for more study of the safety of saccharine while the product remained on the market. Products containing saccharine were required to have a label indicating the potential health risk. Further studies did not find an increased risk of cancer associated with saccharine consumption. In 2001, based on a report from the National Toxicology Program, legislation was passed that removed the requirement that foods containing saccharine carry a warning label.[76]

Sucralose

"The yellow stuff," Splenda, is a common form of sucralose. Sucralose is made from sugar but adds no calories to the diet because it is not digested by the body. It is allowed as a general-purpose sweetener and is used in thousands of foods. The soft drink industry quickly latched on to sucralose as a sweetener for diet soft drinks, with most switching from aspartame to sucralose. Sucralose is highly heat stable and thus can be used in baked products. Because sucralose is 200 times sweeter than sugar, bulking agents are added to create a baking ingredient that measures like sugar. This allows the home cook to use sucralose to create baked goods with lower sugar and/or calorie levels. Experimentation is required to adjust recipes for use with sucralose. Sucralose does not attract moisture nor does it fully melt. This may result in a drier baked good than normal, and your crème brûlée topping will not be crispy and brown.

Stevia

There has been much talk about stevia as a natural alternative to artificial sweeteners. Stevia is a plant native to South America. It has been used for centuries as a sweetener in other parts of the world. Proponents of stevia claim that it is a natural, calorie-free substitute for both sugar and artificial sweeteners. Without FDA approval, however, stevia converts had to purchase stevia as dietary supplement. In December 2008, the FDA approved two sweeteners derived from rebaudioside A (reb A), the component of stevia that gives it its sweet taste. The FDA has approved Cargill's Truvia and Merisant's PureVia. These stevia-derived sweeteners are now available in table-top packets and a host of calorie-free and low-calorie soft drinks.

Safety of Sugar Substitutes

You may have heard "artificial sweeteners cause cancer," "artificial sweeteners make you eat more," "you are better off just drinking a soft drink sweetened with sugar than drinking all those chemicals," or "even natural non-nutritive sweeteners are not safe."

People have a lot of questions about artificial and natural calorie-free sweeteners. Whether a substance is allowed to be used in food as an additive is under the purview of the FDA. It must approve a food additive as safe before it can be used and marketed. The FDA evaluates a sweetener's composition and properties, determines how much of the substance is likely to be consumed, and conducts various types of safety studies.[77] Prior to approving a sweetener, the typical amount used by consumers must be within designated acceptable daily intake levels; that is, levels that can be consumed every day over a lifetime.[77] Evaluations of sugar substitutes by other organizations have also found them generally safe to consume.[78–80]

Cancer and Sugar Substitutes

The most common concern is that artificial sweeteners cause cancer. There have been literally thousands of studies and toxicology reports published regarding the safety of artificial sweeteners. Taken together, these studies indicate that there is no association between cancer and consumption of artificial sweeteners.[78,80,81] The American Dietetic Association and the National Cancer Institute both concur that consumption of artificial sweeteners is not associated with an increased risk of cancer. Natural non-nutritive sweeteners have also been studied extensively and have also shown no correlation to cancer.[82–84]

Obesity and Sugar Substitutes

Another concern with artificial sweeteners is that they really don't support weight control and may even make us eat more. Low- and no-calorie sweeteners have the potential to address weight control in that they can be substitutes for higher calorie foods, and thus remove calories from your diet. Whether these sweeteners will be used in this manner is uncertain.[85] The research is inconclusive as to whether no- and low-calorie sweeteners in fact promote weight loss. Some studies have found that consumption of beverages sweetened with non-

(continues)

nutritive sweeteners assist with weight loss.[86–88] Other studies suggest that the relationship is still unclear.[89] There is no evidence that artificial sweeteners increase appetite and cause you to eat more than you would without consumption of artificial sweeteners.[85,90]

One caveat is that consumption of a low- or no-calorie beverage may allow us to give ourselves permission to consume higher calorie foods. Have you ever seen someone order a triple hamburger, large fries, and a Diet Coke? Dumping a diet drink on top of an ultra-high-calorie meal will do little to address weight control.

Overweight and obesity are complicated conditions. No one fix is going to be the magic bullet. Although consumption of beverages sweetened with no- or low-calorie sweeteners can assist in lowering overall calorie intake, it is only one part of the solution.

Which Side Are You On?

High Fructose Corn Sweetener: Just Another Sweetener or a Nutrition Demon?

High fructose corn sweetener (HFCS) is formed by converting corn starch to corn syrup and then to a sweetener with a high fructose content. The sweetener was developed in the 1960s but was not given full approval by the FDA as a Generally Regarded as Safe (GRAS) additive until 1983. Prior to the development and later approval by the FDA of HFCS, sucrose (table sugar) was the predominant sugar added to processed foods. After 1983, HFCS quickly became the sweetener of choice of most food and beverage manufactures. It's similarity to sugar, its versatility, and its lower cost made the additive an easy sell to manufactures with an eye on the bottom line. Today, HFCS is in literally tens of thousands of products on grocery store shelves. You will find HFCS in carbonated soda, fruit drinks, sports drinks, baked goods, breads, sauces, desserts, and snack foods.[92,93] The introduction of HFCS into the American diet coincided with a sharp rise in obesity rates. Researchers hypothesized that HFCS was exerting some effect on metabolism, appetite, or both, thus causing, or at least contributing to, the obesity epidemic.[94,95] Since these early studies, more careful, controlled studies have found that HFCS is metabolized almost identically to table sugar.[96–100] HFCS has also been found to cause a similar insulin response and similar hunger and appetite cues as those found in response to table sugar.[98,99] Taken together, the research indicates that HFCS does not have a unique effect on health any different from sugar or other caloric sweeteners.

Although HFCS has been shown produce similar metabolic effects as sugar, the point remains that it is a cheap, ubiquitous source of calories in the American diet. Although HFCS alone cannot be blamed for the American obesity crisis, it has certainly played a role in creating a food supply that has too many processed foods that are laden with empty calories. In general, the availability of HFCS and added sugar has increased dramatically in the past 30 years. Whether or not HFCS is worse than, better than, or the same as sugar is not really the issue. The issue is that we are consuming more calories than we need as a nation, hence the obesity crisis. Many of those calories are coming from HFCS and other forms of sugar. Less time should be spent demonizing HFCS and more time examining the beverages that Americans are drinking (and foods they are eating) that contain sugar in all forms. You should be mindful of consumption of not only HFCS but of all added sugar and decrease your sugar consumption. Although not a very glitzy message, but one consistent with good health, eat less sugar in all of its forms.

Personal Health Check

Create a Personal Beverage Clock

For the next 24 hours, keep a beverage clock. Write down all the beverages you consume, the amount, the kind, and the time of day. Use the tracker at www.choosemyplate.gov to estimate the number of calories you consume in a day of beverages. Make a list of changes you would be willing to try in the next week to make your beverage clock healthier. Repeat the above exercise and see how you were able to make some positive changes. Remember, you don't have to make all the changes at once. Taking it one beverage at a time is a step in the right direction.

TERMS

high fructose corn sweetener (HFCS) A sweetener made by processing corn syrup to increase the level of fructose; used extensively as a sweetener in processed foods and soft drinks.

Ready to Make a Change

Are you ready to make a change, small or large, in what you drink? Make the commitment to take the first step. Whether it is a small, medium, or large change, it is a step in the right direction toward consuming healthier beverages.

I commit to a small first step. Decrease the number of sugar-sweetened beverages you consume each day and/or decrease the serving size that you usually buy.

I am ready to take the next step and make a medium change. Dump sugar-sweetened beverages altogether from your diet. Substitute low- or no-calorie beverages and water for all soft drinks.

I have been making changes for some time and am ready to make a large change with the beverages I consume. Choose water as your number one beverage of choice throughout the day.

Myth Versus Fact

Myth: You don't have to worry about getting dehydrated in the winter months.

Fact: You can lose substantial body fluids when exercising (or working) in the winter. The relative dryness of the outside air can cause you to lose body fluids. Be sure to drink plenty of fluids to stay hydrated, no matter what the weather.

Myth: Clear soft drinks are healthier than dark-colored soft drinks.

Fact: How the soft drink is sweetened is more important than its color. Is it sugar sweetened or low calorie? Because caffeine can be added to any soft drink, regardless of color, color cannot be a guide for caffeine content. Color is of little consequence unless you plan on spilling it on your shirt.

Myth: Drinking beer causes you to have a beer gut.

Fact: Beer alone is not the cause of excess weight—excess calories are. Beer does contain considerable calories, so knocking back several beers a day can lead to weight gain. However, so can downing several Cokes a day.

Myth: You need eight glasses of water every day.

Fact: Eight glasses of water is a good guide, but it may not be accurate for some individuals. You may need more or less depending on foods you consume, the beverages you consume other than water, and your activity level.

Myth: If you work out an hour each day at the gym, you would benefit from drinking a sports drink after your workout to replace electrolytes.

Fact: Good for you for working out! An hour at the gym is a positive commitment for better health. Although it is far from being a couch potato, it is not at the level that would benefit from a sports drink. Unless you are working out in extreme heat, the electrolytes you lose will easily be replaced with normal food consumption. Be sure to drink plenty of plain water to replace fluids.

Myth: It is better to drink sugar-sweetened beverages than to use artificial sweeteners.

Fact: All of the low- and no-calorie sweeteners on the market have been deemed by the FDA to be safe. If you are going to drink a sweetened beverage, choose a diet drink for calories' sake.

Myth: You cannot count coffee or tea as part of your daily water intake because the caffeine causes you to loose body fluids.

Fact: Although coffee and tea have a mild diuretic effect, it is not strong enough to totally negate the water associated with consumption.

Back to the Story

Now that you know a bit more about beverages, you probably have some suggestions for Jim. His morning trip to Starbucks would be a great place to start. A Grande white chocolate mocha is fine for a sometime treat, but the 470 calories make it a little too heavy for everyday fare. Jim could try the drink without whipped cream and use skim milk to cut back on calories. He could also try switching to a skinny vanilla latte made with skim milk and sugar-free syrup to save even more calories. After his morning coffee, Jim continues with lots of sugar and caffeine. He consumes a total of 72 ounces of sugar-sweetened beverages, all of which have caffeine, with the exception of the Snapple. Jim has a couple of options here. Of course, the healthiest option is to switch out all the soft drinks to water. A step in the right direction would be to substitute water for some of the soft drinks. When he does drink a soft drink, he should switch to sugar-free ones, at least some of the time. As for the beer at night; beer is a college tradition, however, Jim should try to limit it to two in a night to stay within recommendations for good health. What other suggestions can you make for Jim?

References

1. Jacobson MF. Liquid candy: how soft drinks are harming America's health. Center for Science in the Public Interest. 2005. http://cspinet.org/liquidcandy/. Accessed April 19, 2011.
2. USDA Economic Research Service. Food and consumption (per capita) data system. http://www.ers.usda.gov. Updated April 18, 2011. Accessed April 20, 2011.
3. Nielsen SJ, Popkin BM. Changes in beverage intake between 1977 and 2001. *Am J Prev Med*. 2004; 27(3):205–210.
4. Popkin BM, Armstrong L, Bray GM, Caballero B, Frei B, Willett WC. Beverage intake in the United States. Beverage Guidance Panel. http://www.beverageguidancepanel.org. Accessed April 2, 2009.
5. Standing Committee on the Scientific Evaluation of Dietary Reference Intakes, Food and Nutrition Board, Institute of Medicine. *Dietary Reference Intakes for Water, Potassium, Sodium, Chloride, and Sulfate*. Washington, DC: National Academies Press, 2004.
6. Grandjean AC, Reimers KJ, Bennick KE, Haven MC. The effect of caffeinated, non-caffeinated, caloric and noncaloric beverages on hydration. *J Am Coll Nutr*. 2000; 19(5):591–600.
7. American Dental Hygienists' Association. Fluoride facts. 2009. http://www.adha.org/oralhealth/fluoride_facts.htm. Accessed April 19, 2011.
8. Bottled water and energy: a Pacific Institute Fact Sheet. Pacific Institute. 2007. http://www.pacinst.org. Accessed April 1, 2009.
9. Coffee consumption statistics in the United States. Coffee Research Institute. http://www.coffeeresearch.org/market/usa.htm. Accessed April 5, 2009.
10. Higdon JV, Frei B. Coffee and health: a review of recent human research. *Crit Rev Food Sci Nutr*. 2006; 46(2):101–123.
11. Tverdal A, Skurtveit S. Coffee intake and mortality from liver cirrhosis. *Ann Epidemiol*. 2003;13:419–423.
12. Bravi F, Bosetti C, Tavani A, et al. Coffee drinking and hepatocellular carcinoma risk: a meta-analysis. *Hepatology*. 2007;46(2):430–435.
13. Ascherio A, Zhang SM, Hernan MA, et al. Prospective study of caffeine consumption and risk of Parkinson's disease in men and women. *Ann Neurol*. 2001;50:56–63.
14. Leitzmann MF, Willett WC, Rimm EB, et al. A prospective study of coffee consumption and the risk of symptomatic gallstone disease in men. *JAMA*. 1999; 281:2106–2112.
15. vanDam RM, Hu FB. Coffee consumption and risk of type 2 diabetes: a systematic review. *JAMA*. 2005; 294(1):97–104.
16. Andersen LF, Jacobs DR, Carlsen MH, Blomhoff R. Consumption of coffee is associated with risk of death attributed to inflammatory and cardiovascular diseases in Iowa women's health study. *Am J Clin Nutr*. 2006;83:1039–1046.
17. Lopez-Garcia E, vanDam RM, Wilett WC, et al. Coffee consumption and coronary heart disease in men and women, a prospective cohort study. *Circulation*. 2006;113:2045–2053.
18. Lopez-Garcia E, vanDam RM, Li TY, Rodriguez-Artalejo F, Hu FB. The relationship of coffee consumption with mortality. *Ann Int Med*. 2008;148:904–914.
19. Welland D. The latest international research brews up more big benefits for tea. *Environmental Nutr*. 2007; 30(12):1,4.
20. Larsson SC, Wolk AW. Tea consumption and ovarian cancer risk in a population-based cohort. *Arch Intern Med*. 2005;165:2683–2686.
21. Kuriyana S, Shimazu T, Ohmori K, et al. Green tea consumption and mortality due to cardiovascular disease, cancer, and all causes in Japan. *JAMA*. 2006; 296:1255–1265.
22. Venables MC, Hulston CJ, Cox HR, Jeukendrup AE. Green tea extract ingestion, fat oxidation, and glucose tolerance in healthy humans. *Am J Clin Nutr*. 2008; 87:778–784.
23. Kao Y-H, Hiipakka RA, Liao S. Modulation of endocrine systems and food intake by green tea epigallocatechin gallate. *Endocrinology*. 2000;141:980–987.
24. Chantre P, Lairon D. Recent findings of green tea extract AR25 (Exolise) and its activity for the treatment of obesity. *Phytomedicine*. 2002;9:3–8.
25. Dulloo AG, Seydoux J, Girardier L, Chantre P, Vandermander J. Green tea and thermogenesis: interactions between catechin-polyphenols, caffeine and sympathetic activity. *Int J Obes*. 2000;24:252–258.
26. Diepvens K, Kovacs EMR, Nijs IMT, Vogels N, Westerterp-Plantenga MS. Effect of green tea on resting energy expenditure and substrate oxidation during weight loss in overweight females. *Br J Nutr*. 2005;94:1026–1034.
27. Lovett R. Coffee: the demon drink? *New Scientist*. 2005. http://www.newscientist.com/article/mg18725181.700-coffee-the-demon-drink.html. Accessed April 15, 2011.
28. Standing Committee of the Scientific Evaluation of Dietary Reference Intakes. *Dietary Reference Intakes for Calcium, Phosphorus, Magnesium, Vitamin D, and Fluoride*. Washington, DC: National Academies Press, Institute of Medicine, 1997.
29. Kontiokari T, Laitinen J, Jarvi L, Pokka T, Sundqvist K, Uhari M. Dietary factors protecting women from urinary tract infection. *Am J Clin Nutr*. 2003;77:600–604.
30. Porrini M, Riso P, Brusamolino A, Berti C, Guarniere S, Visioli F. Daily intake of a formulated tomato drink affects carotenoid plasma and lymphocyte concentrations and improves cellular antioxidant protection. *Br J Nutr*. 2005;93:93–99.

31. Sigman-Grant M, Morita J. Defining and interpreting intakes of sugars. ILSI Conference: Sugars and Health, 2002; Washington DC. *Am J Clin Nutr*. 2003; 778(suppl):815S–826S.
32. US Department of Health and Human Services and US Department of Agriculture. *Dietary Guidelines for Americans*, 2005, 6th ed. Washington DC. US Government Printing Office, January 2005.
33. US National Library of Medicine, National Institute of Health. Medline Plus: acai. www.nlm.nih.gov/medlineplus/druginfo/natural/1109.html. Updated November 18, 2010. Accessed April 29, 2011.
34. Adriano J. In the drink—how beverages contribute to obesity. *Nutr Action Healthletter*. 2000;7–9.
35. Mourao DM, Bressan J, Campbell WW, Mattes RD. Effects of food form on appetite and energy intake in lean and obese young adults. *Inter J Obesity*. 2007; 31:1688–1695.
36. Wellhoener P, Fruehwald-Schultes B, Kern W, et al. Glucose metabolism rather than insulin is a main determinant of leptin secretion in humans. *J Clin Endo Metab*. 2000;85:1267–1271.
37. DiMeglio DP, Mattes RD. Liquid versus solid carbohydrate: effects on food intake and body weight. *Inter J Obesity*. 2000;24:794–800.
38. Moruao DM, Bressan J, Campbell WW, Mattes RD. Effects of food form on appetite and energy intake in lean and obese young adults. *Inter J Obes*. 2007;31:1688–1695.
39. Block G. Foods contribute to energy intake in the US: data from NHANES III and NHANES 1999–2000. *J Food Comp Anal*. 2004;17:439–447.
40. Harnack L, Stang J, Story M. Soft drink consumption among US children and adolescents; nutritional consequences. *J Am Diet Assoc*. 1999;99(4):436–441.
41. Centers for Disease Control and Prevention. Does drinking beverages with added sugars increase the risk of overweight? *Research to Practice Series*, No. 3. 2006. http://www.cdc.gov/ nutrition/professionals /researchtopractice/index.html. Accessed April 8, 2009.
42. Malik VS, Schulze MB, Hu FB. Intake of sugar-sweetened beverages and weight gain: a systematic review. *Am J Clin Nutr*. 2006;84:274–288.
43. Vartanian LR, Schwartz MB, Brownell KD. Effects of soft drink consumption on nutrition and health: A systematic review and meta analysis. *Am J Pub Health*. 2007;97:367–675.
44. Schulze MB, Manson JE, Ludwig DS, et al. Sugar-sweetened beverages, weight gain, and incidence of type 2 diabetes in young and middle-aged women. *JAMA*. 2004;292:927–934.
45. Ebbeling CB, Feldman HA, Osganian SK, Chomitz VR, Ellenbogen SJ, Ludwig DS. Effects of decreasing sugar-sweetened beverages consumption on body weight in adolescents: a randomized, controlled pilot study. *Pediatrics*. 2006;117(3):673–680.
46. Duffey KJ, Popkin BM. Adults with healthier dietary patterns have healthier beverage patterns. *J Nutr*. 2006;136:2901–2907.
47. Nestle M. Soft drink "pouring rights": marketing empty calories. *Pub Hlth Rep*. 2000;115:308–319.
48. Young, LR, Nestle, M. (2002). The contribution of expanding portion sizes to the US obesity epidemic. *Am J Pub Health*. 92:246–249.
49. Liebman B, Schardt D. The scoop on enhanced waters. *Nutrition Action Healthletter*. June 2008.
50. Sawka MN, Burke LM, Eichner ER, Maughan RJ, Montain SJ, Stacherfield NS. American College of Sports Medicine position stand, exercise and fluid replacement. *Med Sci Sports Exer*. 2007 377–390.
51. Klatsky AL. Drink to your health? *Sci Am*. 2003;288: 74–81.
52. Rimm EB, Klatsky A, Grobbee D, Stampfer MJ. Review of moderate alcohol consumption and reduced risk of coronary heart disease: is the effect due to beer, wine, or spirits. *Br Med J*. 1996;312:731–736.
53. Reynolds K, Lewis B, Nolen JD, Kinney GL, Sathya B, He J. Alcohol consumption and risk of stroke: a meta-analysis. *JAMA*. 2003;289:579–588.
54. Ajani UA, Hennekens CH, Spelsberg A, Manson JE. Alcohol consumption and risk of type 2 diabetes mellitus among US male physicians. *Arch Intern Med*. 2000;160:1025–1030.
55. Conigrave KM, Hu BF, Camargo CA Jr, Stampfer MJ, Willett WC, Rimm EB. A prospective study of drinking patterns in relation to risk of type 2 diabetes among men. *Diabetes*. 2001;50:2390–2395.
56. Leitzmann MF, Giovannucci EL, Stampfer MJ, et al. Prospective study of alcohol consumption patterns in relation to symptomatic gallstone disease in men. *Alcohol Clin Exp Res*. 1999;23:835–841.
57. Leitzmann MF, Tsai CJ, Stampfer MJ, et al. Alcohol consumption in relation to risk of cholecystectomy in women. *Am J Clin Nutr*. 2003;78:339–347.
58. Mukamal KJ, Conigrave KM, Mittleman MA, et al. Roles of drinking pattern and type of alcohol consumed in coronary heart disease in men. *N Engl J Med*. 2003;348:109–118.
59. Adonis S, Rohit A. The cardiovascular implications of alcohol and red wine. *Am J Therapeutics*. 2008;15(3): 265–277.
60. Estruch R, Sacanella E, Badia E, Antunez E, Nicolas JM, Fernandez-Sola J, Rotilio D, de Gaetano G, Rubin E, Urbano-Marquez A. Different effects of red wine and gin consumption on inflammatory biomarkers of atherosclerosis: a prospective randomized crossover trial. Effects of wine on inflammatory markers. *Atherosclerosis*. 2004;175:117–123.
61. Di Castelnuovo A, Rotondo S, Iacoviello L, Donati MB, deGaetano G. Meta-analysis of wine and beer consumption in relation to vascular risk. *Circulation*. 2002;105:2836–2844.

62. Costanzo S, DiCastelnuovo A, Donati MB, Iacoviello L, deGaetano G. Cardiovascular and overall mortality risk in relation to alcohol consumption in patients with cardiovascular disease. *Circulation*. 2010;121:1951–1959.
63. Mayo Clinic. Red wine and resveratrol: good for your heart? September 2011. http://www.mayoclinic.com/health/red-wine/HB00089.
64. American Academy of Pediatrics, Committee on Substance Abuse and Committee on Children with Disabilities. Fetal alcohol syndrome and alcohol-related neurodevelopmental disorders. *Pediatrics*. 2000;106:358–361.
65. Smith-Warner SA, Spiegelman D, Yaun SS, et al. Alcohol and breast cancer in women: a pooled analysis of cohort studies. *JAMA*. 1998;279:535–540.
66. Hamajima N, Hirose K, Tajima K, et al. Alcohol, tobacco and breast cancer—collaborative reanalysis of individual data from 53 epidemiological studies, including 58,515 women with breast cancer and 95,067 women without the disease. *Br J Cancer*. 2002;87:1234–1245.
67. Reynolds K, Lewis B, Nolen JD, Kinney GL, Sathya B, He J. Alcohol consumption and risk of stroke: a meta-analysis. *JAMA*. 2003;289:579–588.
68. Mann RE, Smart RG, Govoni R. The epidemiology of alcoholic liver disease. *Alcohol Res Health*. 2003; 27:209–219.
69. Zhang S, Hunter DJ, Hankinson SE, et al. A prospective study of folate intake and the risk of breast cancer. *JAMA*. 1999;281:1632–1637.
70. Piano MR. Alcoholic cardiomyopathy: incidence, clinical characteristics, and pathophysiology. *Chest*. 2002;121:1638–1650.
71. Ruigomez A, Johansson S, Wallander MA, Rodriguez LA. Incidence of chronic arterial fibrillation in general practice and its treatment pattern. *J Clin Epidemiol*. 2002;55:358–363.
72. Smith GS, Branas CC, Miller TR. Fatal nontraffic injuries involving alcohol: a metaanalysis. *Ann of Emer Med*. 1999;33(6):659–668.
73. Greenfield LA. Alcohol and crime: An analysis of national data on the prevalence of alcohol involvement in crime. Report prepared for the Assistant Attorney General's National Symposium on Alcohol Abuse and Crime. Washington, DC: U.S. Department of Justice, 1998. http://bjs.ojp.usdoj.gov/content/pub/pdf/ac.pdf. Accessed April 20, 2011.
74. Naimi TS, Lipscomb LE, Brewer RD, Colley BG. Binge drinking in the preconception period and the risk of unintended pregnancy: Implications for women and their children. *Pediatrics*. 2003;11(5):1136–1141.
75. Wechsler H, Davenport A, Dowdall G, Moeykens B, Castillo S. Health and behavioral consequences of binge drinking in college. *JAMA*. 1994;272(21):1672–1677.
76. National Toxicology Program. Availability of the report on carcinogens, 9th ed. Federal Register, May 30: Department of Health and Human Services: Public Health Service. 2001.
77. Food and Drug Administration. Artificial sweeteners: no calories ... sweet! *FDA Consumer*. July–August 2006. http://findarticles.com/p/articles/mi_m1370/is_4_40/ai_n26992050/?tag=content;col1. Accessed April 15, 2011.
78. American Dietetic Association. Position of the American Dietetic Association: use of nutritive and nonnutritive sweeteners. *J Am Diet Assoc*. 2004;104:255–275.
79. Kroger M, Meister K, Kava R. Low-calorie sweeteners and other sugar substitutes: a review of the safety issues. *Comp Rev Food Sci Food Safety*. 2006;5(2):35–47.
80. Gallus S, Scotti L, Negri E, et al. Artificial sweeteners and cancer risk in a network of case-control studies. *Annals Oncology*. 2007;18:40–44.
81. National Cancer Institute, US National Institutes of Health. Artificial sweeteners and cancer: questions and answers, National Cancer Institute Fact Sheet. 2006. http://www.cancer.gov/cancertopics/factsheet/Risk/artificial-sweeteners. Accessed April 19, 2011.
82. Kobylewski S, Eckhert CD. Toxicology of rebaudioside A: A review. http://www.wepapers.com/Papers/16164/Toxicology_of_Rebaudioside_A-__A_Review. Accessed April 19, 2011.
83. Brusick DJ. A critical review of the genetic toxicity of steviol and steviol glycosides. *Food Chem Toxicology*. 2008;46(7):S83–S91.
84. Carakostas MC, Curry LL, Boileau AC, Brusick DJ. Overview: the history, technical function and safety of rebaudioside A, a naturally occurring steviol glycoside, for use in food and beverages. *Food Chem Toxicology*. 2008;46(7):S1–S10.
85. Mattes RD, Popkin BM. Nonnutritive sweetener consumption in humans: effects on appetite and food intake and their putative mechanisms. *Am J Clin Nutr*. 2009;89:1–14.
86. Raben A, Vasilaras TH, Moller AC, Astrup A. Sucrose compared with artificial sweeteners: different effects on ad libitum food intake and body weight after 10 wk of supplementation in overweight subjects. *Am J Clin Nutr*. 2002;76:721–729.
87. Blackburn G, Kanders B, Lavin P, Keller S, Whatley J. The effect of aspartame as part of a multidisciplinary weight-control program on short- and long-term control of body weight. *Am J Clin Nutr*. 1997;65:409–418.
88. Drewnowski A. Sweetness, appetite, and energy intake: physiological aspects. In: Corti A, ed. *Low-Calorie Sweeteners: Present and Future*. *World Rev Nutr Diet*. Basel, Switzerland: S. Karger AG, 1999;85:64–76.
89. Vermunt S, Pasman W, Schaafsma G, Kardinaal A. Effects of sugar intake on body weight: a review. *Obes Rev*. 2003;4:91–99.
90. Rolls BJ. Effects of intense sweeteners, food intake, and the body weight: a review. *Am J Clin Nutr*. 1991;55:139–143.
91. Popkin BM, Armstrong LE, Bray GM, Caballero B, Frei B, Willett WC. A new proposed guidance system for

beverage consumption in the United States. *Am J Clin Nutr*. 2006;83:529–542.

92. Fulgoni V. High-fructose corn syrup: everything you wanted to know, but were afraid to ask. *Am J Clin Nutr*. 2008:88(suppl):1715S.
93. Schorin MD. High fructose corn syrups, part 1. *Nutr Today*. 2005;40(6):248–252.
94. Bray GA, Nielsen SJ, Popkin BM. Consumption of high-fructose corn syrup in beverages may play a role in the epidemic of obesity. *Am J Clin Nutr*. 2004;79:537–543.
95. Havel PJ. Dietary fructose: implications for dysregulation of energy homeostasis and lipid/carbohydrate metabolism. *Nutr Rev*. 2005;63:133–57.
96. White JS. Straight talk about high-fructose corn syrup: what it is and what it ain't. *Am J Clin Nutr*. 2008; 88(suppl):1716S–21S.
97. Duffey KJ, Popkin BM. High-fructose corn syrup: is this what's for dinner? *Am J Clin Nutr*. 2008;88(suppl): 1722S–1732S.
98. Stanhope KL, Havel PJ. Endocrine and metabolic effects of consuming beverages sweetened with fructose, glucose, sucrose, or high-fructose corn syrup. *Am J Clin Nutr*. 2008;88(suppl):1733S–1737S.
99. Melanson KJ, Angelopoulos TJ, Nguyen V, Zukley L, Lowndes J, Rippe JM. High-fructose corn syrup, energy intake, and appetite regulation. *Am J Clin Nutr*. 2008;88(suppl):1738S–1744S.
100. Schorin MD. High fructose corn syrups, part 2. *Nutr Today*. 2006;41(2):70–77.

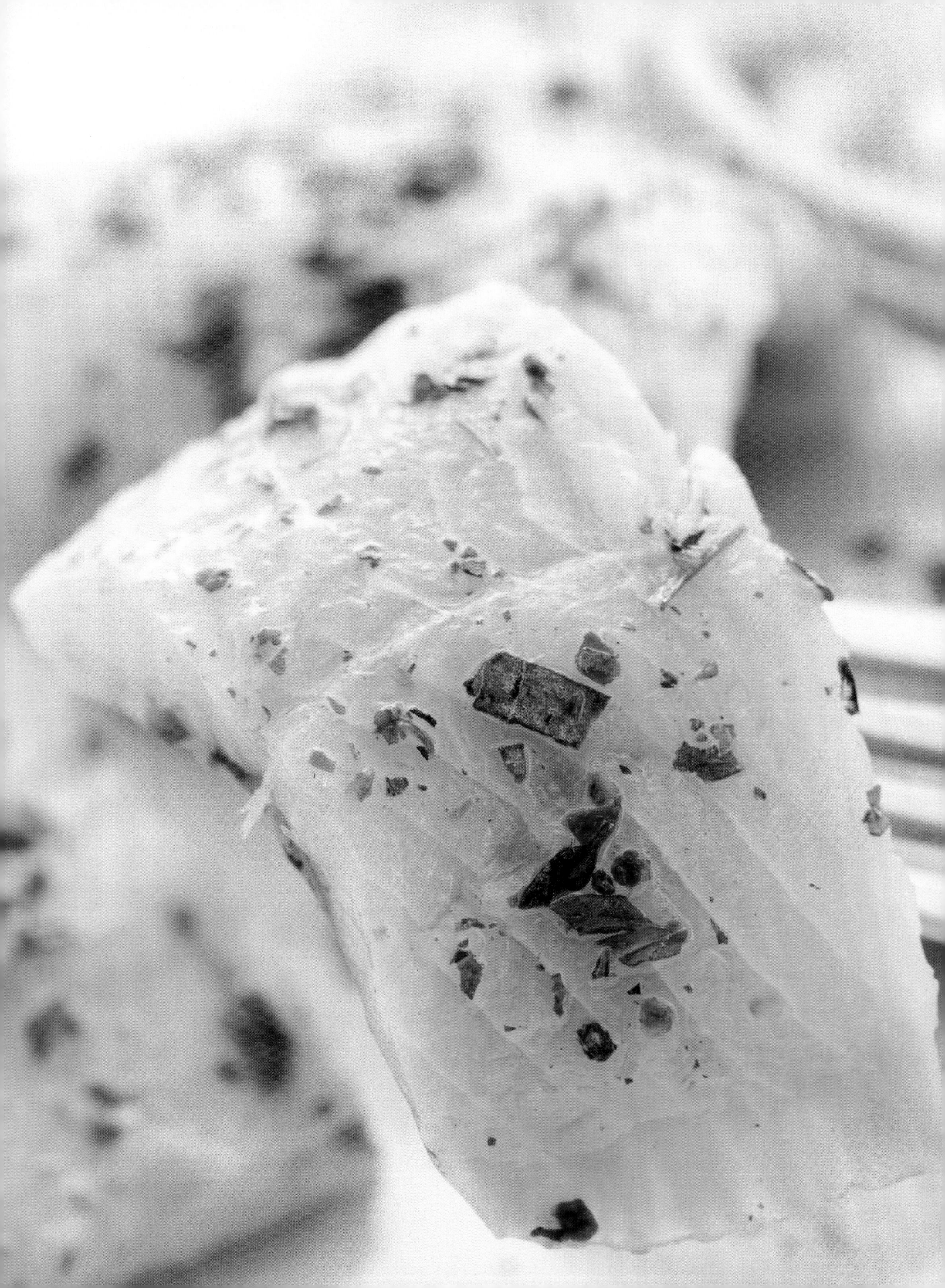

Chapter 8

Protein: More Is Not Always Better

Key Messages

- Protein is fundamental for life and performs many functions in the body.
- Protein from vegetable sources is a healthy alternative to meat.
- Protein should be consumed within recommended guidelines; more is not necessarily better.

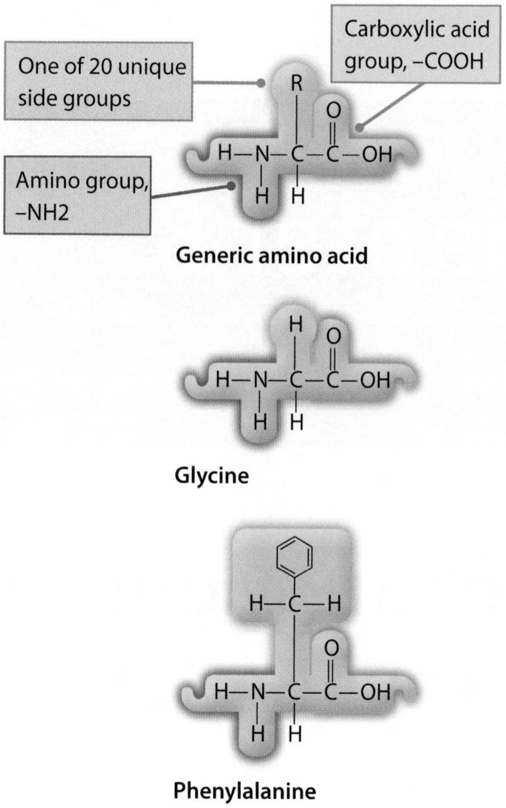

■ **Figure 8.1**
Amino Acid Structure

"Eat your protein to grow up to be big and strong." Many of us heard that while growing up. More recent raves about high-protein diets being the key for weight loss can be found in the popular press. Protein is certainly the most revered of the energy-providing nutrients. Ask most people what their favorite food is and you will most likely get a high-protein answer—steak, lobster, or shrimp. Consumption of high-protein foods is often seen as a sign of wealth, with a big steak signaling that a person is wealthy and successful. When you plan a meal, you may usually think of the high-protein food first and then build the meal around it: steak with baked potato, burger with fries, chicken with green beans, turkey with dressing. The name *protein* even has significance; it is from the Greek word *proteios* meaning "of prime importance." Protein is a vital nutrient and has many important functions.

While you probably think of protein as coming from meat and dairy, what about vegetable sources of protein? Are they healthy? Do you need meat at every meal to get the protein you need? In this chapter, we will discuss the complex functions of protein and explore the many ways to get the protein you need each day.

Story

John is a 20-year-old college student who is tired of being the skinny guy on campus. He sees other guys his age that have big muscles, and he is ready to do what it takes to be bigger and stronger. He starts by joining a local gym. There he is met with not only thousands of pounds of iron, but also hundreds of potions and powders. His membership affords him a discount on all the supplements offered at the gym, so he stocks up. He grabs whey protein powder for protein shakes that he drinks once a day and amino acid tablets that he takes twice a day. His workouts include heavy weight lifting supervised by a personal trainer three times a week. His diet of lots of fast food and late night pizza is somewhat typical for a college student. He frequently skips meals and goes lots of days without eating until dinner. John is drinking the protein shake every day, taking the amino acids, and working out as his trainer instructs. He is seeing some small gains, but is not happy with his progress. What advice can you give John about his diet that may help his progress?

Structure of Proteins

Carbohydrates and fats contain carbon, hydrogen, and oxygen. Protein has these components as well, but it also has nitrogen. It is the nitrogen that makes protein unique as an energy-providing nutrient. Much like carbohydrates are strands of glucose molecules linked together, proteins are strands of **amino acids**. Amino acids are the building blocks of proteins. All amino acids have a similar structure: one hydrogen atom, an acid group, and an amine group attached to a carbon atom (**Figure 8.1**). The word *amine* means "nitrogen containing," thus the amine group contains the nitrogen that makes protein unique.

Amino acids differ depending on the side group. There are 20 different amino acids, all with different side groups. Nine of these amino acids are called *essential amino acids*; your body cannot make them and they must be supplied in the diet (**Table 8.1**). The remaining 11 amino acids are *nonessential*; as long as your body has the materials needed (nitrogen, hydrogen, oxygen, and carbon), they can be produced. In some cases, nonessential amino acids can become essential amino acids. If a nonessential amino acid is made from other amino acids that are not present, it becomes conditionally essential. For example, your body makes cysteine from either methionine or serine. If there is not enough methionine or serine in the diet, then cysteine becomes essential.

Amino acids join together in an almost infinite number of different combinations to form proteins. Amino

TERMS

amino acids Building blocks of proteins; have an acid on one end and a nitrogen-containing amine group on the other.

Table 8.1

Essential, Nonessential, and Conditionally Essential Amino Acids

Essential Amino Acids	Nonessential Amino Acids	Conditionally Essential Amino Acids
Histidine	Alanine	Arginine
Isoleucine	Arginine	Cysteine
Leucine	Asparagine	Glutamine
Lysine	Aspartic acid	Glycine
Methionine	Cysteine	Proline
Threonine	Glutamic acid	Tyrosine
Tryptophan	Glutamine	
Valine	Glycine	
	Proline	
	Serine	
	Tyrosine	

acids are joined together with peptide bonds. Two amino acids joined together is a *dipeptide*; three is a *tripeptide*. Four to 10 combined together is an *oligopeptide*; more than 10 is a *polypeptide*. Most proteins in the body and in the diet are made up of long chains of proteins with hundreds of amino acids joined together. These strands of amino acids are not linear, but fold back on each other, forming a twisted chain or globule.

Functions of Proteins

The body has literally thousands of different proteins. Proteins are found in every cell of your body and make up about 20% of your body weight. Proteins are involved in almost all cell functions; some provide structural support, others are enzymes, hormones, or antibodies (**Figure 8.2**). Protein is involved in fluid balance and acid–base balance and in the transport of substances in and out of cells. Protein provides 4 calories per grams and can be used for energy.

TERMS

keratin The primary protein in hair, nails, and the outer layer of the skin.

collagen The most abundant protein in the body; the primary protein in connective tissue.

Structural Support

Proteins provide structure to bones, skin, hair, and nails. **Keratin** is a strong protein that is a major component of hair, nails, and the outer layer of the skin. Collagen is the main protein of connective tissue. **Collagen** is a very strong protein and is found in ligaments, tendons, bone, and skin. Collagen is responsible the strength and elasticity of the skin. The loss of collagen as you age is responsible for wrinkles. Collagen is also responsible for the elasticity and strength of blood vessels.

Enzymes

Enzymes are proteins that speed up chemical reactions. Enzymes are usually very specific as to what reaction they catalyze. Enzymes help you metabolize food and are uniquely involved in digestion. Enzymes may also help with other aspects of cell metabolism, such as the growth and repair of tissue. Enzymes can help bind two substances or break a substance into smaller components. Exactly how enzymes work is not fully understood. However, it is commonly believed that the surface of the enzyme is uniquely suited to facilitate a specific reaction.

Hormones

Many hormones, such as insulin, are made up of proteins. Hormones act as messengers that are made in one part of

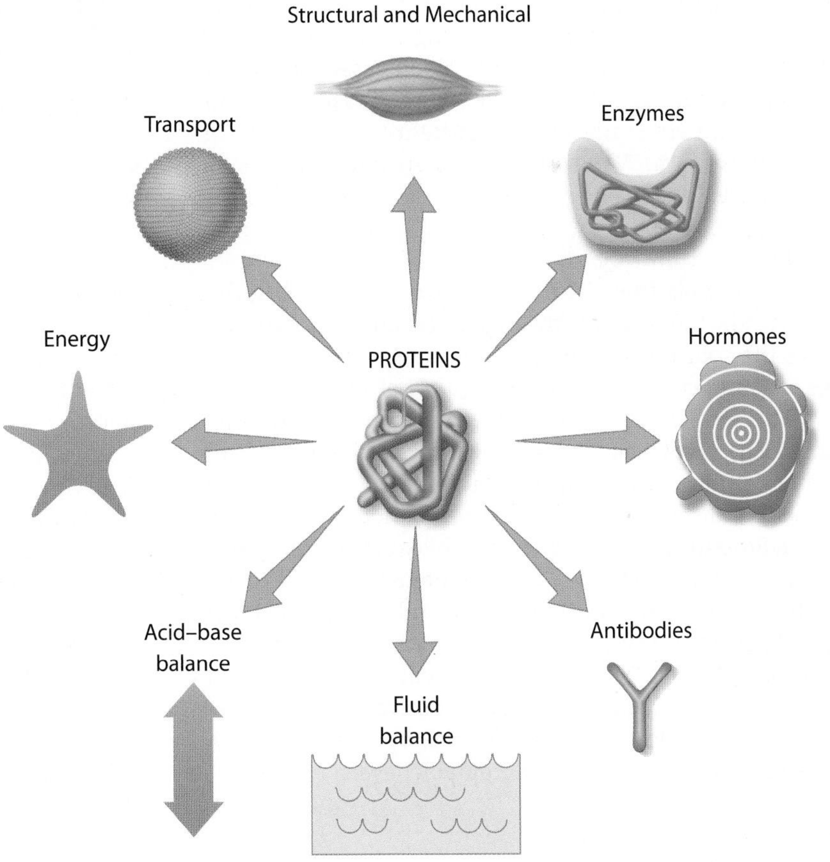

■ **Figure 8.2**
Functions of Proteins in the Body

the body and then carry out important regulatory functions in another part of the body. For example, insulin is released from the pancreas in response to a rise in blood sugar. It travels in the blood working to clear the glucose from the bloodstream.

Antibodies

Antibodies are produced by white blood cells and are used by the immune system to identify, attack, and neutralize the bacteria and viruses that cause infection. There are many different types of antibodies, each with a different antigen-binding site. The antigen-binding site is specific to a certain type of bacteria or virus. When your body is invaded with bacteria or a virus, it quickly makes the specific type of antibody needed to attack the invader. If your diet does not contain enough protein, your body may not be able to make the antibodies it needs, which can compromise your immune system.

Fluid Balance

Proteins help maintain balance between the fluid inside and outside of cells. Cells need a certain amount of water to function properly; too much or too little water will compromise the cell's ability to function. Water can flow in and out of cells; proteins cannot. Proteins, however, can attract water. Proteins in the cell attract water so that an optimal amount of water remains in the cell. The same process occurs in the area outside of the cells. Proteins are also responsible for maintaining a high blood volume. Proteins cannot pass across blood vessel walls and attract water into the blood system. In the case of protein deficiency, there is not enough protein to hold water in the bloodstream. Water moves into surrounding tissue, causing swelling.

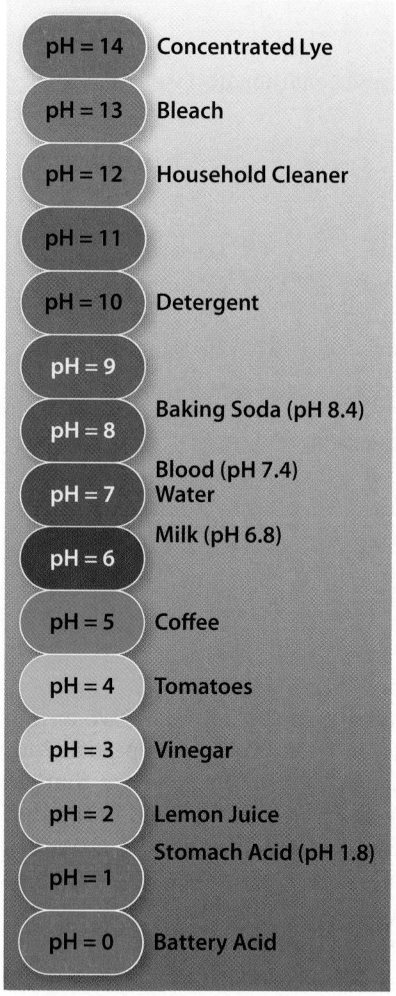

■ **Figure 8.3**
pH Values for Selected Substances

Acid–Base Balance

The **pH** scale is from 0 to 14. The lower the number, the more acidic the solution; the higher the number, the more basic the solution. Battery acid has a pH of 0, water has a pH of 7, and concentrated lye has a pH of 14 (**Figure 8.3**).

The body must maintain its pH within a very narrow range. The pH of blood is 7.4, almost that of water. You can only tolerate small changes in this value. If the pH drops below 6.8 or above 8.0 for even a few hours, death can occur. Proteins help maintain this delicate balance by acting as buffers for acids and bases. Proteins act to make the system more acidic if pH increases and more basic if pH falls. They do this by picking up or donating hydrogen ions. If the body's pH is too high, proteins will donate hydrogen ions to bring the pH back to normal. Conversely, if the system's pH is too low, proteins will pick up extra hydrogen ions to raise the pH back to acceptable levels.

Transportation

Some proteins act as transport proteins and in pumps, moving substances in and out of the cell. Transport proteins may create a channel in the cell membrane to allow certain substances to flow in and out of cells. Other proteins package substances and transport them to other areas of the body. Lipoproteins are an example of this. A protein layer surrounds lipids so they can travel in the blood.

Energy

The body prefers to use carbohydrate or fat for energy and to "spare" protein for other vital functions. That is why adequate carbohydrate intake is said to "spare" protein. If necessary, however, the body can use protein as energy. The protein chain is first broken down into amino acids and then the amine group is removed and excreted. The remaining carbon chain can be converted into glu-

TERMS

antibodies Proteins in the blood that fight infection.

pH A measure of the degree of the acidity or alkalinity of a solution.

cose. If protein is consumed in larger quantities than is needed, a similar process occurs, and the excess energy is stored as fat. Thus, taking protein supplements or eating excess protein is not a way to automatically increase muscle mass—the extra calories from protein are simply converted to fat.

Digestion and Absorption of Proteins

Digestion of proteins begins in the stomach. The acid in the stomach denatures the proteins. **Denaturation** changes the three-dimensional structure of a protein by unfolding its polypeptide chain. Denaturation occurs when proteins come into contact with heat, alkali, extreme agitation, or, in the case of the stomach, acid. When you cook an egg and the egg white goes from clear to opaque, that is due to the proteins being denatured. If you have ever put fish or other seafood in an acidic substance and seen the surface turn opaque, that is due to some of the proteins on the surface of the food beginning to denature.

The stomach produces the proenzyme pepsinogen. The acid of the stomach converts the inactive pepsinogen into the active enzyme pepsin. Pepsin then begins the process of breaking down the amino acid chains into smaller amino acid chains and individual amino acids.

Most protein digestion occurs in the small intestine. Protease further breaks down amino acid chains into individual amino acids. Amino acids and some very small chains of amino acids are absorbed by the small intestine and travel to the liver. There they can travel to other parts of the body, as needed, or be used by the liver to make any number of important substances needed by the body. The body is very efficient at protein digestion and absorption. Very little protein is excreted.

Recommended and Actual Protein Intake

The RDA for protein is 0.8 grams per kilogram of body weight (**Figure 8.4**).[1] The RDA assumes that the protein in your diet is from a variety of sources and that adequate calories are consumed so that protein is not used for energy. Using a reference woman with a body weight of 125 pounds (57 kilograms) the RDA for protein is 46 grams.

Protein RDA

How to calculate:

Convert weight into kg *(pounds ÷ 2.2)* × 0.8 kg = Protein RDA in g

Male	Female
19+ yrs-old, 70 kg (154 lb)	19 + yrs-old, 57 kg (125 lb)
70 kg × 0.8g/kg = 56 g protein	57 kg × 0.8 g/kg = 46 g protein

Figure 8.4

How to Calculate the RDA for Protein

It is suggested that 10–35% of your calories should come from protein.

How to calculate:

Step 1: Grams of protein × 4 calories = calories from protein
Note: the value "4 calories" is a standard unit of measure and does not change. A gram of carbohydrate contains 4 calories.

Step 2: Calories from protein/total calories × 100 = % calories from protein

Grams of protein

Total calories

% calories from protein

Figure 8.5

How to Calculate Percent Calories from Protein

Similarly, for a reference 150-pound man (68 kilograms), the RDA for protein is 54 grams. Thus, for most people, 8–10% of calories in the diet should come from proteins (**Figure 8.5**). Note that actual body weight should not be used to compute an individual's protein requirements when his or her weight falls outside of the healthy range; a healthy weight for height should be used.[1]

Another way to estimate protein needs is the Acceptable Macronutrient Distribution Range (AMDR). The AMDR for protein is 10–35% of calories. This recommendation is slightly higher than the RDA, depending on actual calorie intake.

Current Intake of Protein

Inadequate protein intake is rare in the United States and other industrialized countries. Current protein intake in the United States is, on average, well above the RDA for all age and gender groups. Women consume, on average, 1.15 grams of protein per kilogram of body weight; men consume, on average, 1.38 grams per kilograms of body weight.[2,3]

Too Little Protein

Protein is essential for many critical processes in the body and is a component of every cell. If your body does not have enough protein, you will not have the building blocks needed to repair and build tissue, to regulate fluid, to balance pH, or to complete a host of other essential tasks. Protein deficiency occurs when there is not enough protein in the diet or when there is protein in the diet but not enough calories for energy needs. The body must take care of energy needs first. Thus, if calories are not present in adequate amounts and protein is used for energy, it will not be available for other functions. Protein deficiency is seen primarily in nonindustrialized countries.

TERMS

denaturation Change in the three-dimensional structure of a protein caused by agitation, heat, or acidity.

Protein-energy malnutrition (PEM) is a long-term deficiency of protein, energy, or both. PEM results in wasting of body tissue, impaired body function, and increased susceptibility to infection. The World Health Organization estimates that there are over 180 million malnourished children in developing countries.[4] In south central Asia and eastern Africa, about half of the children have growth retardation due to PEM. Approximately 50% of the 10 million deaths each year in developing countries occur because of malnutrition in children younger than 5 years of age.[4]

The two primary types of PEM are **kwashiorkor** and **marasmus**. Kwashiorkor occurs when there are some calories in the diet, but just not enough protein. Kwashiorkor usually occurs in a child who is weaned from breast milk when a brother or sister comes along. They are put on the family's diet, which in developing countries is often high in carbohydrates but too low in proteins. The inadequate protein intake causes fluid retention, especially in the abdomen and feet. Protein is not available to transport fat from the liver, causing the liver to increase in size. This, coupled with fluid retention in the abdomen, causes the distinct swollen belly common in children suffering from kwashiorkor. Children with kwashiorkor also have poor growth, are weak, and are susceptible to infection.

Marasmus occurs when both protein and calories are deficient in the diet. Children with marasmus have stunted growth and severe wasting of muscles and tissues. As marasmus continues, tissues in the vital organs become compromised. Marasmus causes the victim to be weak and apathetic. Oftentimes children with marasmus do not even cry due to their weakened condition. Although marasmus occurs primarily in children in developing countries, it can occur in adults who experience starvation due to a chronic illness, such as cancer, or an eating disorder.

Too Much Protein

Too much protein is more of an issue in industrialized nations than is protein deficiency. As you have already seen, the average American diet contains ample protein when compared with the recommendations.[1] High protein intake can put strain on the kidneys, because they are responsible for excreting byproducts of protein metabolism, primarily nitrogen. High-protein foods also may be high in fat and/or saturated fat, which is a risk factor for heart disease. High meat consumption is related to a modest increase in death from cardiovascular disease.[5] Some evidence suggests that a high-protein diet, specifically one with high consumption of red meat and processed meat, is associated with an increased risk of colon cancer.[5–7] You have most likely seen the myriad of diet books that suggest that high-protein diets are the best for weight loss (see the section on low-carbohydrate diets in Chapter 5). Excess calories, regardless of their origin, will result in weight gain. The idea that high-protein foods can be consumed without fear of weight gain is simply false. As you have already learned, the body has no problem repackaging protein so that it may be stored as adipose tissue.

> **Personal Health Check**
>
> **How Much Protein Do You Need Each Day?**
>
> Use the formula in Figure 8.4 to calculate the amount of protein you need each day. Record what you eat on a typical day for several days. Use the Food Tracker at ChooseMyPlate.gov to enter your food intake and analyze the amount of protein you are eating. How did you do? Where did most of your protein come from? If you were too low in protein (which is doubtful), how can you make sure you get enough in the future? If you ate too much protein, how can you bring your protein intake in line with recommendations?

Protein and Athletes

Anyone who has gone into a gym or store that specializes in nutrition supplements has seen the huge containers of whey protein and amino acid supplements. The containers feature pictures of bulging muscles and popping veins, giving the illusion that taking these products will produce a bulked-up, ripped body. Ask most body builders or even semi-serious weight lifters if they need more protein than the average Joe or Jane and they more than likely will proclaim "YES!" It is a commonly held belief that athletes need more protein than nonathletes. They are, after all, breaking down and rebuilding lean tissue that is primarily made of protein. It only stands to reason that they need more.

Whether an athlete needs more protein than the 0.8 grams per kilogram of body weight continues to be debated in the scientific literature. The Institute of Medicine's review of the literature for the DRIs indicates that healthy adults who participate in resistance or endurance exercise do *not* need more protein than the RDA.[1] The RDA

> **TERMS**
>
> **protein-energy malnutrition (PEM)** A long-term deficiency of protein, energy, or both. PEM results in wasting of body tissue, impaired body function, and increased susceptibility to infection.
>
> **kwashiorkor** A type of PEM where adequate calories are present in the diet but protein intake is inadequate.
>
> **marasmus** A type of PEM where protein and calories are inadequate in the diet.

is certainly adequate for most people, including those who work out on a regular basis to stay fit and healthy.

But what about the competitive athlete or person who works out at a high level of intensity and/or duration? What about someone who is training for a marathon, lifts weights at a high level of intensity most days of the week, or competes in triathlons on a regular basis? Many scientists, most noted nutrition professionals, and most athletes concur that the protein recommendation of 0.8 grams per kilogram of body weight is not enough for serious athletes. The RDA recommendation may be adequate for good health and to prevent deficiency, but it is not consistent with optimal performance in athletes.[8–12] Recommending protein intake in excess of the RDA to maintain optimal physical performance is commonly done in practice.

Endurance athletes who bike, swim, or run long distances have an increased protein need to assist with recovery from long, intense training sessions or competitive events.[11] The American College of Sports Medicine, the American Dietetic Association, and Dieticians of Canada stated in a joint position statement that endurance athletes need 1.2–1.4 grams of protein per kilogram of body weight.[13] Studies examining the protein intake of endurance athletes indicate that actual protein intake is between 1.2–1.6 grams of protein per kilogram of body weight, which is within the recommended range.[14]

Strength athletes, such as body builders or power lifters, have an increased protein need in order to repair and build lean tissue broken down during strenuous weight-training workouts or competition.[15] The American College of Sports Medicine, the American Dietetic Association, and Dieticians of Canada state that strength athletes need 1.2–1.7 grams of protein per kilogram of body weight.[13] Strength athletes are well known for their high-protein diets and often consume egg whites by the dozen, protein shakes, and amino acid supplements. It is no surprise that when actual protein intake of strength athletes was examined it was found that their actual protein intake was between 2.0–2.5 grams per kilogram body weight and as high as 3.0 grams per kilogram body weight in some athletes, well above what is needed for optimal performance, muscle recovery, and muscle building.[16,17]

The protein needs of both endurance and strength athletes can be met by a healthy diet; protein or amino acid supplements are not needed. In fact, neither protein supplements nor amino acid supplements have been shown to help with athletic performance.[18,19] Athletes should also be sure to get adequate carbohydrate for energy so that the proteins they consume are used to build and repair tissue and are not used for energy. Timing of consumption of protein is also important. To achieve the greatest benefit in muscle recovery and muscle building, a meal or snack containing protein should be consumed within one hour of exercise.

Winning a marathon or a power-lifting contest will not happen just by consuming more protein. More protein will not automatically make your muscles bigger or stronger or make you run faster. Only good genetics, training, and a varied healthy diet can do that.

TERMS

complete protein A protein that contains all of the essential amino acids; proteins from animal sources and soy are complete proteins.

Protein in Your Diet

Protein is found in high concentrations in meat, fish, poultry, milk and milk products, eggs, and legumes (beans) (**Table 8.2**). Grains and vegetables also provide some protein in the diet.

In the United States, most of the protein we eat comes from beef (17%) followed closely by poultry (13.5%) (**Table 8.3**).[20] Only a small amount of protein in the American diet is from vegetable sources such as beans and peas.

Protein from animal sources is **complete protein** in that it contains all nine of the essential amino acids. Pro-

Table 8.2

Protein Content of Common Foods*

Food	Amount	Protein Content (grams)
Dairy foods		
Milk	1 cup	8
Cheese	1 oz.	7
Cottage cheese	1/2 cup	14
Yogurt	1 cup nonfat	13
Eggs	1 large egg	6
Meat		
Pork (lean)	3 oz.	21
Chicken	3 oz.	21
Beef (lean)	3 oz.	21
Fish	3 oz.	21
Vegetables and grains		
Beans	1 cup	16
Tofu	1/2 cup	10
Nuts	1 oz.	6
Oatmeal	1 cup	6
Brown rice	1 cup	4
Whole-wheat bread	1 slice	3

**Note:* Protein content may vary for the different types of the foods listed above (i.e., black beans versus lentils, brands of various breads, different cuts of meat, etc.). This chart provides an estimate of the protein content of common foods.

Source: Data from US Department of Agriculture, Agriculture Research Service. 2008. USDA National Nutrient Database for Standard Reference, Release 21. Nutrient Data Laboratory Home Page. http://www.ars.usda.gov/ba/bhnrc/ndl. Accessed April 10, 2011.

Canned Tuna: A Good, Inexpensive Source of Protein or a Deadly Source of Mercury?

Canned tuna is a staple in many American pantries. A tuna sandwich is a common quick lunch or dinner. Many different types of canned tuna are available. Which one is best? Which one is safe? Canned tuna is either white meat (made from albacore tuna) or light meat (made from a variety of different types of tuna). There are also grades of canned tuna. The grade depends on the size of the chunk. "Solid" or "fancy" is the largest chunk size and is considered the best quality. "Chunk" tuna is slightly smaller pieces, and "flaked" or "grated" is the smallest size chunks. Which grade you buy depends on how you plan to use the tuna. You do not need to spend the extra money on "solid" or "fancy" tuna just to make tuna salad.

All canned tuna is already cooked and is packed in water or oil. Some people prefer oil-packed tuna due to the richer flavor; however, a calorie-saving tip is to choose the water-packed tuna. Even if you drain oil-packed tuna, it has more calories and fat than water-packed tuna.

What about the mercury content of tuna? Canned albacore tuna (white) is listed in an FDA–EPA advisory regarding mercury. It states that you should eat no more than 6 ounces of canned tuna per week. Light tuna is lower in mercury and is not on the list of fish to limit in the diet. Light tuna usually comes from smaller fish that have lower mercury content. For more information about the mercury content of seafood, go to www.montereybayaquarium.org to get its Seafood Watch Pocket Guide. It provides lists of the best seafood to eat and the seafood to avoid in different areas of the United States.

Something else you may see on the label is "dolphin-safe." To have this label, the tuna must be caught in a way that did not kill or seriously injure any dolphins. A number of organizations, such as the Earth Island Institute, closely monitor dolphin safety. Canned tuna that carries that organization's dolphin-safe logo have even stricter guidelines to follow for dolphin safety.

Canned tuna is a low-cost, high-protein food. It is a great food to keep on hand for sandwiches. If you choose white tuna, do so in moderation due to the higher mercury content. Enjoy light tuna more frequently.

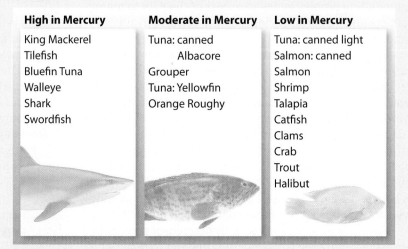

High in Mercury	Moderate in Mercury	Low in Mercury
King Mackerel	Tuna: canned Albacore	Tuna: canned light
Tilefish	Grouper	Salmon: canned
Bluefin Tuna	Tuna: Yellowfin	Salmon
Walleye	Orange Roughy	Shrimp
Shark		Talapia
Swordfish		Catfish
		Clams
		Crab
		Trout
		Halibut

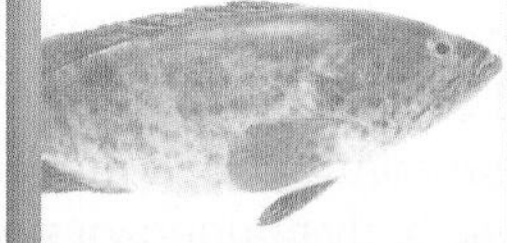
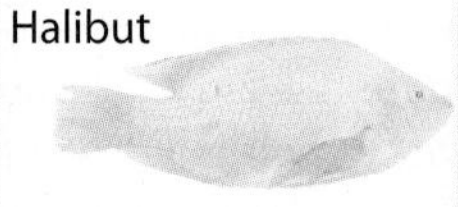

Larger Fish Generally Are Higher in Mercury Than Smaller Fish
Women who might become pregnant, pregnant women, breastfeeding women, and children should not consume fish that are high in mercury and should limit consumption to 12 ounces a week of fish and shellfish that are lower in mercury with only 6 ounces from fish that is moderately high in mercury.

Sources: Data from Food and Drug Administration. Mercury Levels in Commercial Fish and Shellfish (1990–2010). http://www.fda.gov/food/foodsafety/product-specificinformation/seafood/foodbornepathogenscontaminants/methylmercury/ucm115644.htm. Accessed October 2, 2011; US Department of Health and Human Services and Environmental Protection Agency. What You Need to Know About Mercury in Fish and Shellfish. March 2004. Publication EPA-823-R-04-005. http://www.fda.gov/food/foodsafety/product-specificinformation/seafood/foodbornepathogenscontaminants/methylmercury/ucm115662.htm. Accessed October 2, 2011.

tein from plant sources is incomplete protein; it lacks or is low in one or more essential amino acids. Soy is the exception to this rule. It is a plant protein that is also a complete protein. Combining different vegetable proteins can result in a complete protein that provides all of the essential amino acids. Combining beans and grains or beans with seeds results in a more complete protein than if those foods were consumed on their own. If you do not consume animal products, as long as you eat a wide variety of plant proteins your amino acid intake will more than likely be adequate.

Animal Sources of Protein

Meat, poultry, fish, and dairy products all provide dietary protein. When you choose meat, do so in appropriate portions and select low-fat cuts and preparation techniques. We will discuss how to make low-fat choices in Chapter 10. Dairy products are excellent sources of protein. Cheese, cottage cheese, yogurt, and milk all contain the proteins, vitamins, and minerals essential for good health. Choose fat-free or low-fat dairy products so you are not getting too much fat along with your high-quality protein. Eggs are sometimes called the "perfect protein" due to their balanced content of all the essential amino acids. Fish is a great source of low-fat protein and has big health benefits. It is recommended that you consume a minimum of 8 ounces of seafood a week for good health and to reduce the risk of heart disease.[21–23]

Plant Sources of Protein

Although there are several good plant sources of protein, the American diet is generally not high in plant protein.

Table 8.3

Food Sources of Protein Consumed by U.S. Adults

Food Source	Percent (%) of Protein in the Diet
Beef	16.9
Poultry	13.5
Milk	7.5
Yeast bread	7.3
Cheese	6.5
Fish/shellfish (excluding canned tuna)	3.5
Pork	3.0
Eggs	3.0
Pasta	2.5
Ham	2.4
Cakes/cookies/quick breads/ doughnuts	2.0
Dried beans/lentils	2.0

Source: Data from PA Cotton, AF Subar, JE Friday, A Cook. Dietary sources of nutrients among US adults, 1994–1996. *J Am Diet Assoc.* 2004;104(6):921–930.

Beans, peas, and nuts provide protein and other nutrients and fiber. Switching from a typical American diet high in meat and poultry to one that derives proteins from both plants and animals is good for your health and the environment.

Beans and Peas

Legumes, which include beans, peas, and lentils, are an inexpensive source of good-quality protein. In addition to protein, they provide vitamins, minerals, and fiber. The small quantity of fat in beans is healthy unsaturated fat. The *Dietary Guidelines for Americans* suggest that you consume more beans. Research on the health benefits of beans is clear. Studies indicate that consuming beans decreases the risk of heart disease.[28–30] In fact, the FDA now allows a health claim to be used on cans and packages of beans: "Diets including beans may reduce your risk of heart disease and certain cancers." There are many types of beans and peas from which to choose (**Table 8.4**). Most are available in cans or dried. Canned beans are convenient and easy to keep on hand for a quick addition to a meal. Rinsing canned beans can help remove some of the salt added during processing. Dried beans are inexpensive, pennies a serving, and allow you to control the amount of salt added during cooking. You don't have to go totally

TERMS

legumes A category of plants with edible seed pods that split into two halves, such as beans, peas, lentils, and soybeans.

Table 8.4

Types of Beans and Peas and Common Uses

Type of Bean	Common Uses
Black beans (turtle beans) 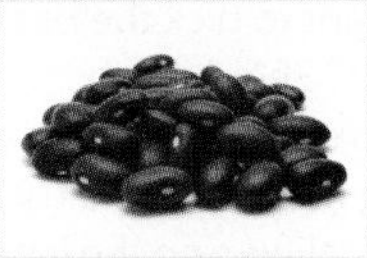	Black beans are popular in Mexican and Southwest cooking. They make great soup and can be used as a side dish with rice, burritos, or tacos.
Black-eyed peas (cow peas) 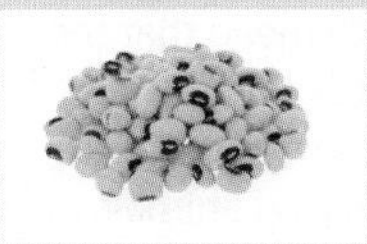	Black-eyed peas are a staple in Southern cooking. They are traditionally served with rice and are often topped with chopped onions. Black-eyed peas are thought to bring good luck when eaten on New Year's Day.
Garbanzo beans (chickpeas) 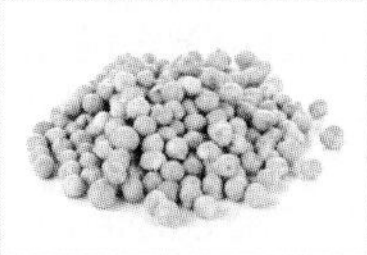	Garbanzo beans are popular in Middle Eastern cooking. They are used to make hummus, a spread that is a mixture of garbanzo beans and tahini (sesame paste). They can also be added to salads or served with rice.
Kidney beans 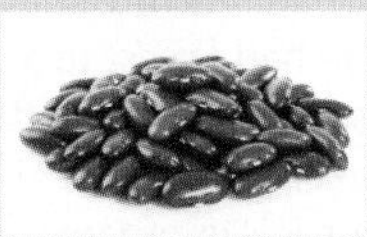	Kidney beans can be light or dark red and get their name from their kidney shape. They are often used in cold salads, in soup or chili, or as a side dish.
Lentils 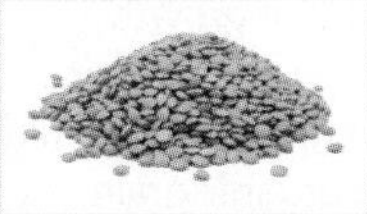	Lentils come in red, brown, and green. They are a small flat pulse that is in the pea family. Lentils cook more quickly than beans and are very versatile. Lentils are wonderful in soup and are great when mixed with curry or other spices.
Lima beans 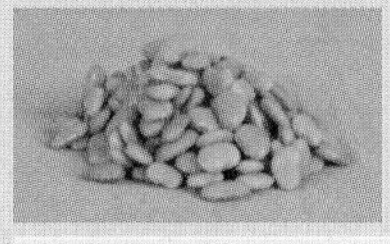	Lima beans have a subtle buttery flavor. They are most often served with just salt and pepper or perhaps a small amount of herb, such as rosemary or basil.
Navy beans 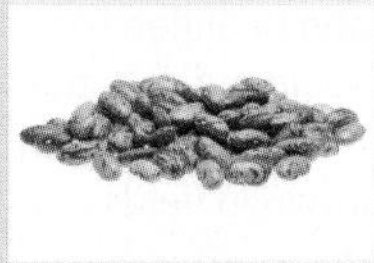	Navy beans have a hearty texture and hold up well in soups and stews. They can be mixed with small amounts of meat, such as ham or pork shank.
Pinto beans 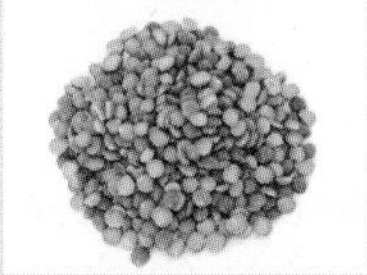	Pinto beans are used extensively in Mexican cooking. They are the beans used in refried beans. A healthy version of refried beans is as simple as mashing cooked pinto beans and topping it with cheese or low-fat sour cream.
Split peas 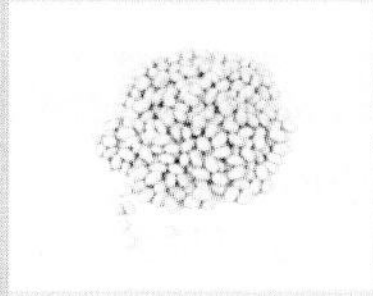	Split peas can be yellow or green. The green variety is most commonly seen in split-pea soup, which is usually flavored with onion and small amounts of ham.

Special Report

Organic, Free Range, Grass Fed: What Does It All Mean?

You are a health conscious shopper and want to pick the best meat and poultry possible. But what is best? Should you choose the one that is lowest in cost or the one labeled organic, free range, or grass fed? Choosing meat and poultry can be confusing with so many different qualifiers on the label. To make the best decision, you first need to understand what all these terms mean.

Pasture-raised beef or pork has come to mean that the animals were raised outdoors in a field instead of a feedlot. However, no federal regulations limit the use of the words *pasture-raised* on the label. Some pasture-raised animals may graze in the pasture for only part of their life and then be finished on a grain feedlot to add flavor to the meat.

The term *free range*, or free roaming, is usually applied to chicken or other poultry. It means that the chicken has been allowed access to the outside for at least some of its life. This can apply to chickens that are raised in coops but that have access to the outside for all or part of the day. The chicken may or may not actually go outside of the coop.

Grass-fed on the label indicates that the animal must have been fed a diet of 100% grass as well as have had access to a pasture during grass-growing season. If it says grass fed on the label, the animal has not been fed any grain at all.

Organically produced meat carries the USDA organic label and certifies that the animal was raised under specific guidelines that prohibit the use of antibiotics or growth hormones and has been fed only organic feed. It does not mean that the animal was pasture raised or grass fed; it could have spent its whole life in a feedlot eating organic grain.

Natural is the vaguest of all labels for meat and poultry. It only means that no artificial ingredients or colors have been added. Some manufacturers use *natural* to mean that the animal has not received antibiotics or hormones. If this is important to you, read the label carefully. Natural does not automatically mean that antibiotics or hormones were not given to the animal.

Meat or poultry may have more than one qualifier. For example, a label of *grass-fed, organic beef* would indicate that the animal was fed grass only, had access to a pasture during grass-growing season, that the grass was grown in fields that were certified organic, and that the animal received no antibiotics or hormones.

Ultimately, what you chose to buy comes down to what is most important to you. Let's examine poultry, beef, and pork buying choices based on five factors: cost, nutrition, taste, animal welfare, and environmental impact.

Poultry

Cost: Free-range chicken can cost three to five times more than conventional chicken.

Nutrition: Free-range chickens that are allowed to roam free are generally leaner than chicken raised in a coop. If they are allowed to scratch for their preferred diet of bugs, worms, and seeds, free-range chicken can be higher in heart-healthy omega-3 fatty acids.

Taste: Opinions vary as to differences in taste between free-range and conventionally raised chicken. Some people think that free-range chicken tastes better.

Animal welfare: Because *free range* on the label does not mean with all certainty that the chicken has been raised according to high animal welfare standards, it is hard to tell if free range is better for the chicken. If you are concerned with poultry welfare, purchase from a local farmer with high animal welfare standards who allows the chickens to roam free, not be in a cage with access to the outside for only a small portion of their life. You could also purchase from a retail outlet that is familiar with the practices of the farm where the chicken is produced.

Environmental impact: Regardless of how the poultry is raised, waste has to be dealt with. Larger farms that tend to use more conventional methods of raising chicken have larger amounts of waste than smaller free-range operations. Often larger farms must transport waste away from the farm, placing an additional strain on the environment.

Beef

Cost: Because of the low cost of the cheaply produced corn feed used in cattle feedlots, conventional beef is much cheaper than grass-fed, pasture-raised beef. The cost of grass-fed, pasture-raised beef can be as much as 50% higher depending on the cut. One way to have your grass-fed beef and stay on a modest budget is to eat smaller servings and eat beef less often.

meatless to use beans. Cook small amounts of meat in bean soup or add small amounts of meat or chicken to rice and beans.

TERMS

organically produced meat Meat produced without the use of antibiotics or growth hormones and fed only organic feed.

Nuts and Seeds

Not too long ago, nuts and seeds were considered taboo because they are high in fat. However, recent research indicates that nuts and seeds are healthy and, in moderation, should be part of a balanced diet. The *Dietary Guidelines for Americans* include a recommendation to include unsalted nuts in your diet.[23] Nuts include almonds, Brazil nuts, macadamia nuts, walnuts, pistachios, pecans, hazelnuts, and peanuts. Although peanuts are actually

Nutrition: Grass-fed, pasture-raised beef is generally leaner and thus lower in calories than conventional beef. It has higher levels of heart-healthy omega-3 fatty acids and is higher in vitamin E.[24–26] Cattle allowed to roam around all day instead of being cooped up in a feedlot have less fat.

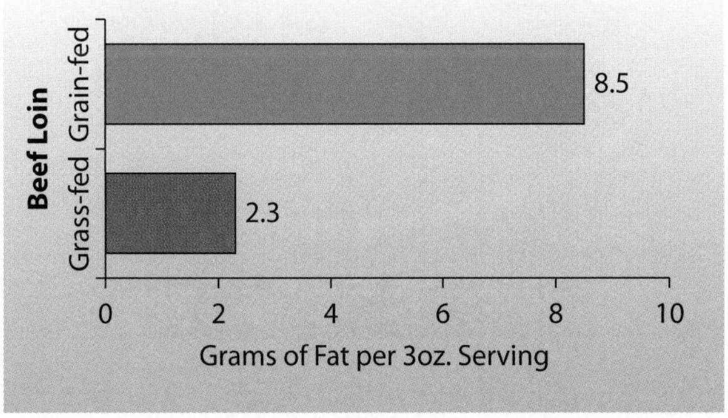

Fat in Grass-Fed Versus Conventionally Raised Beef

Source: Data from DC Rule, KS Broughton, SM Shellito, G Maiorano. Comparison of muscle fatty acid profiles and cholesterol concentrations of bison, beef cattle, elk, and chicken. *J Anim Sci*. 2002;80(5):1202–1211.

Most pasture-raised, grass-fed beef is also produced without hormones or antibiotics, even if there is not the Certified Organic stamp on the label. Many small farms cannot afford the expense of becoming certified but use many practices consistent with that label. Some evidence indicates that meat produced with antibiotics may result in antibiotic resistance in humans.[27] However, this remains a controversial issue.

Taste: If a highly marbled steak is to your liking, grass-fed beef may take some getting used to. The lower fat content of grass-fed beef can lead to beef that can be slightly tougher than conventionally raised beef. Some people, however, prefer the taste of grass-fed beef and say that the lack of melt in your mouth tenderness is more than made up for in flavor.

Animal welfare: There are two issues related to animal welfare with regard to beef. First, the bovine digestive system is much better suited to eating grass than grain. Cows are designed to eat fibrous grasses and other plants, not grains. Cows fed high levels of grain often get sick, which is one reason antibiotic use is high in conventionally raised cattle. Second, a grass-fed, pasture-raised cow roams free and is not confined to a crowded waste-filled feedlot.

Environmental impact: Conventionally raised cattle are fed corn that is produced using incredible amounts of fossil fuel. Vast amounts of waste from the feedlots are concentrated in a small space and must be collected and hauled away. This is expensive and requires fossil fuel for transportation. To save costs, manure is often dumped as close as possible to the feedlot. The land surrounding a feedlot becomes overloaded with nutrients that can end up in the groundwater. Grass-fed, pasture-raised beef feed off of grass that is grown using the energy of the sun. Their waste is spread over a wide area of land and acts as a source of nutrients for the grass. Instead of a waste management problem, you have instant fertilizer.

Pork

Cost: The cost of pasture-raised pork is higher than conventionally raised, especially for some of the more gourmet heritage breeds of pigs.

Nutrition: Most conventionally raised pigs have been bred to be very lean; hence the tag line "the other white meat." Pasture-raised pork is generally higher in fat, but it is also higher in heart-healthy omega-3 fatty acids and vitamin E.

Taste: Pasture-raised pork has a stronger pork flavor thanks to the higher fat content.

Animal welfare: Pigs raised using conventional methods have less opportunity to do things pigs like to do, such as root in the soil and roam around free. Pasture-raised pigs roam free and eat not only what they are given, but also what they may find.

Environmental impact: The story here is similar to beef. Large producers of conventionally raised pork have tons of waste to dispose of. Hog lagoons, pits where waste is disposed, emit methane, a greenhouse gas, and can pollute groundwater. Disposal of hog waste in a way that does as little damage to the environment is an important area of investigation. Promising research is under way on new methods to handle large amounts of hog waste without harming the environment.

a legume (bean); their nutritional composition is more closely related to nuts. Popular seeds include pumpkin, sunflower, and sesame seeds. Nuts and seeds are a good source of protein, fiber, and unsaturated fat. Eating 1 ounce of nuts at least five times a week is associated with a substantially lower risk of heart disease (**Figure 8.6**).[38–42]

A concern about eating nuts and seeds is that they may cause weight gain, because they are relatively high in calories. Interestingly enough, research has found just the opposite. Individuals who consume nuts regularly tend to weigh less than those who rarely eat them. The possible reason for this is that nuts may help suppress hunger or increase satiety because they are high in protein and fat. This does not mean that double handfuls of peanuts will help keep you thin. Portion size is critical with high-calorie foods such as nuts. It does indicate, however, that a once taboo food can be consumed in moderation with some real health benefits.

Try Something New

Beans

Beans are certainly not new. However, they don't make their way into the diet of many Americans on a regular basis. Beans are an inexpensive high-protein, low-fat, high-fiber food that can easily be added to your diet. Beans and rice make a great substitute for meat, bean soup will warm you up on a cold winter day, and bean tacos are great to serve friends while watching the game. Beans are easy to prepare as well. Canned beans are quick and convenient. For a real money saver, try dried beans. For a couple of dollars you get a pound of dried beans that makes about 8 cups of beans. Just soak the beans overnight in the refrigerator. Pour off the water the next morning. Add the beans to a large pot, add water and seasonings, and cook. The cooking time will depend on the type of bean; just check the package for details. If you have a slow cooker (crock pot) it is even easier. Just put the soaked beans in the slow cooker in the morning; add water to cover, plus about 2 inches; incorporate seasonings, such as onion or chili powder; and cook on low for eight hours. When you get home that evening, you'll have beans that are ready to eat. Add a little more water, and you'll have bean soup.

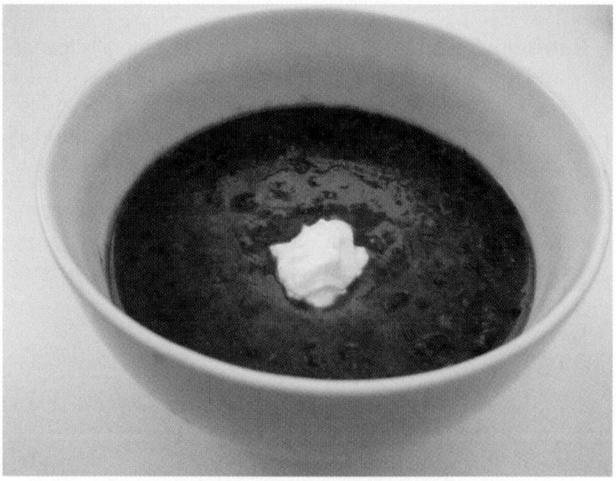

Black Bean Soup

Ingredients

1 tablespoon olive oil
1 medium onion, chopped
1 tablespoon ground cumin or chili powder
2, 14.5-ounce cans black beans, drained
2 cups chicken broth or water
Salt and pepper to taste
Sour cream or cheese for topping (optional)

Instructions

1. Sauté the onion in olive oil in a large pot.
2. After two minutes, add the cumin or chili powder.
3. Add one can of beans and broth or water.
4. Cook for four to five minutes on medium heat, stir occasionally.
5. Remove from heat and use a hand blender to puree ingredients or transfer to a blender and puree.
6. Add the second can of beans to the pot and cook over medium heat three to four minutes or until bubbly.
7. Taste and add salt and pepper as needed.
8. Serve topped with sour cream and/or cheese (optional).

Which Side Are You On?

Soy Protein: Friend or Foe?

Soybeans were once used almost exclusively in the United States for animal feed. Today, soy is used by the food industry as an additive to increase the volume and improve the texture of many processed foods. In addition, over the past 20 years soy consumption has increased in humans in the form of soybeans (edamame), tofu, soymilk, and other products made from soy. This is for good reason. Soybeans are low in saturated fat, high in polyunsaturated fat, high in fiber, low in calories, and high in protein. Soy offers the only plant protein that is similar in quality to that from animal sources. Soy also contains something else of interest—**phytoestrogens**, specifically **isoflavones**. Isoflavones are a class of phytoestrogens and can have estrogen-like effects in the body. The controversy lies in whether these isoflavones provide a protective effect for disease or if they are perhaps dangerous.

A great deal of research has been conducted on the effects of soy on heart disease. In fact, in 1999 the FDA began allowing food companies to claim that foods with soy protein

(continues on page 152)

TERMS

phytoestrogens A group of chemicals found in plants that can have estrogen-like effects in the body.
isoflavones A phytoestrogen found in soy.

Soy-Based Foods

Food	What It Is	How to Use It
Soybeans (edamame) 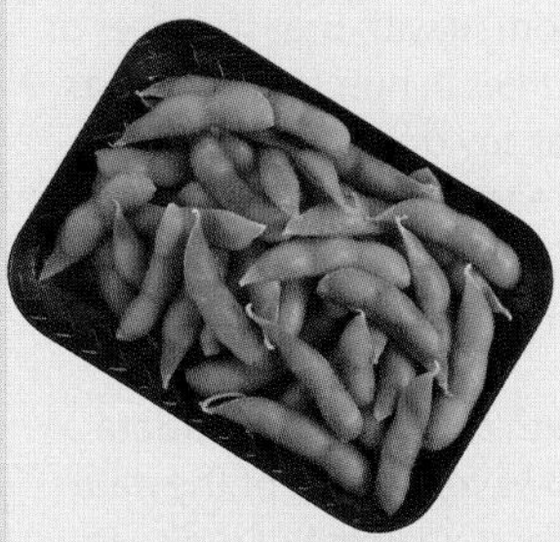	Soybeans that are harvested when still green.	Cook in the pod in boiling salted water for 15 minutes. Serve as-is as a snack or appetizer. Beans can be removed from the pod and used in salads, stir-fry, and casseroles.
Tofu 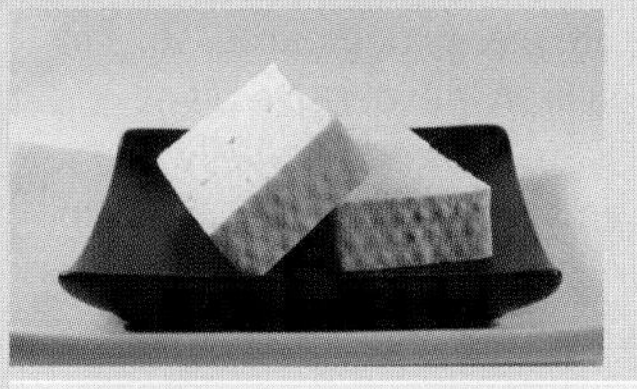	Tofu is made from curdling soymilk, much like cheese is made from cow or goat milk. Tofu is very bland and takes on the flavors it is cooked with. The two basic types of tofu are *silken* and *regular*. Silken tofu is very soft, whereas regular tofu is firm. Regular tofu comes in medium, firm, or extra firm textures.	Silken tofu is used in salad dressings and sauces. Regular tofu can be used in stir-fry, sautéed and used in sandwiches, scrambled like eggs, or cubed and added to soup. There are many delicious recipes that use tofu as a meat substitute.
Soymilk 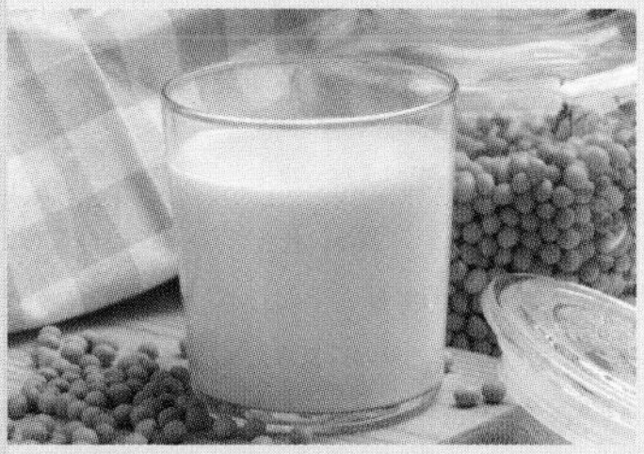	Soymilk is made when soybeans are soaked, ground, and strained. The resulting liquid is soymilk. Soymilk is high in protein and B vitamins. It is usually fortified with calcium. Soymilk can have added sugar and/or flavorings.	Soymilk is used as a substitute for cow's milk.
Miso 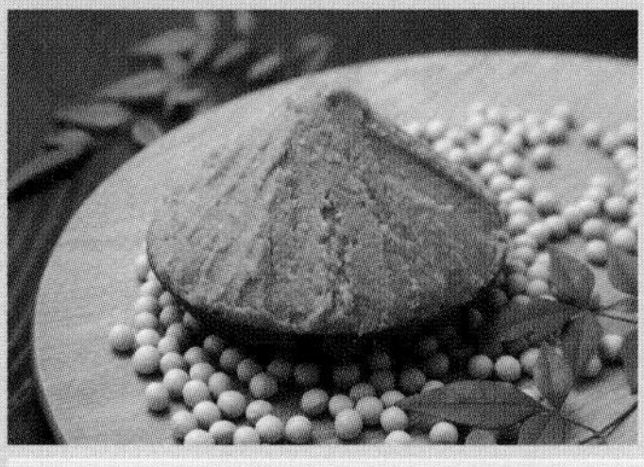	Miso is a paste made from soybeans and a grain (usually rice). Salt and a mold culture is added and the mixture is aged for several years.	Miso is used as a flavoring or condiment in Asian cooking. It is most often used in soups, sauces, and dressings.
Tempeh 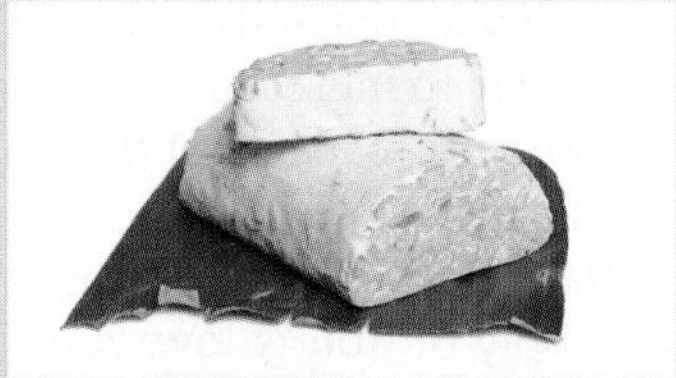	Tempeh is soybeans that have been formed into a cake and fermented.	Tempeh can be sliced, fried or grilled and used as a meat substitute. It can also be added to soups and stews.
Meat alternatives 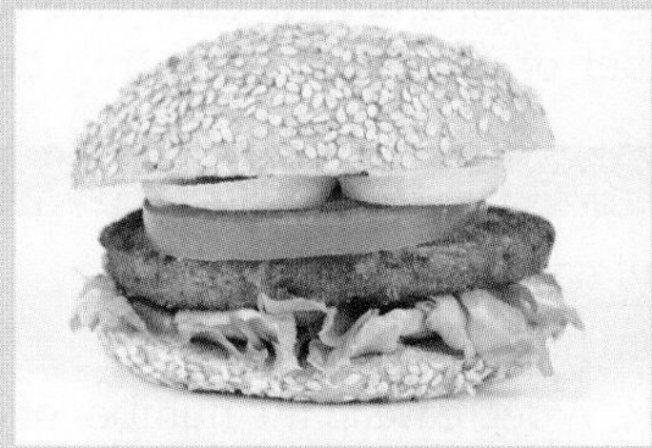	Meat alternatives are products made from soy that closely resemble meat. These products often mimic burgers, bacon, or sausage.	Meat alternatives are used in place of meat.

(continues)

"may reduce the risk of heart disease." This was based on research that indicated that soy protein could lower blood cholesterol levels. Further examination of these studies and new studies on the effects of soy on heart disease have resulted in a different conclusion: Large amounts of soy (1/2 gallon of soy milk or 1.5 pounds of tofu a day) may cause a modest lowering of cholesterol, more realistic consumption of soy has little or no effect.[31] Thus, the FDA no longer allows the claim that soy has a protective effect against heart disease.

Soy has also been suggested as a help for women who are experiencing symptoms of menopause. Many of these symptoms, such as hot flashes, are due to a lack of estrogen in the body. It would only stand to reason that a food that contained an estrogen-like substance would help. Women began drinking soymilk, eating tofu, and making tofu smoothies to alleviate, or at least lessen, some of the symptoms of menopause. The bad news is that overall the research indicates that soy has little effect on hot flashes or other menopause symptoms.[31–33]

The relationship between soy and cancer has also been studied extensively. This connection began with the observation that women in Japan had relatively low breast cancer rates and high soy intake.[34] There is little evidence, however, that soy intake in adult women has a protective effect against breast cancer. Consumption of soy that begins early in life in adolescents does seem to have some protective effect.[35,36]

Based on studies in animals, there is also a concern that soy may in fact increase risk for women with breast cancer or at a high risk for breast cancer. Studies in humans, as well as epidemiological data, suggest that soy does not pose a risk even for women who have had breast cancer.[37] The research continues, and so breast cancer survivors and women at high risk for breast cancer should discuss their dietary needs with their physicians.

So what is the bottom line with soy? Most of the data indicate that eating soy is safe. However, if most of the data say that most of the protective effects against heart disease, symptoms of menopause, and breast cancer are not there, why should you eat soy? There are plenty of great reasons to consume soy in moderation. Soy is an inexpensive plant source of high-quality protein. Eating soy occasionally as a meat substitute provides fiber and protein. Soy is also low in polyunsaturated fat. If you have never tried soybeans, tofu, or other products made from soy, you should!

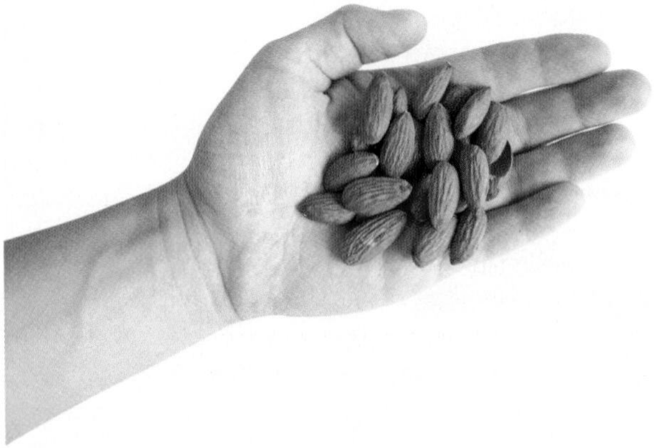

■ Figure 8.6

One Ounce of Nuts

An ounce of almonds is about 20–25 almonds. The number of nuts in an ounce will vary based on the size of the nut. A good way to estimate an ounce of nuts is the number of nuts that will fit into the palm of your hand.

Spotlight on Vitamins and Minerals

Zinc

Zinc is found in foods that are high in protein, especially red meat and seafood. Whole grains contain zinc, but it is not as well absorbed as the zinc in animal products. Zinc is needed for normal growth and proper immune function. Most people in industrialized countries get enough zinc, thus deficiency is rare. You may have seen cold lozenges with zinc that indicate zinc will help lessen the severity or decrease the duration of a cold. Although some people swear by this remedy, there is no concrete evidence that this works.

Iron

Iron is found in food in two forms: **heme iron**, which is found in meat, poultry, and fish, and **nonheme iron**, which is found in plants. Sources of heme iron include beef, poultry, and seafood. Sources of nonheme iron include spinach, beans and peas, whole-grain and enriched grains, and fortified cereals.

Heme iron is better absorbed by the body. Fiber and other substances in plants inhibit iron absorption. However, you can get some of the iron you need from nonheme sources. To increase the absorption of nonheme iron, consume foods high in vitamin C with sources of nonheme iron, such as beans with tomatoes. Consumption of heme iron and nonheme iron together, such as beans with small amounts of meat or spinach with fish, can also increase the absorption of nonheme iron. Another way to increase iron in your diet is to cook in cast-iron pans, especially high-acid foods such as spaghetti sauce.

Iron is essential for the transportation and utilization of oxygen. If your supply of iron is low, you may experience iron-deficiency anemia. **Iron-deficiency anemia** causes fatigue, weakness, and pale color due to a decrease in the number of red blood cells. Iron defi-

TERMS

heme iron Iron from animal sources.

nonheme iron Iron from plant sources.

iron-deficiency anemia A decrease in the number of red cells in the blood caused by too little iron.

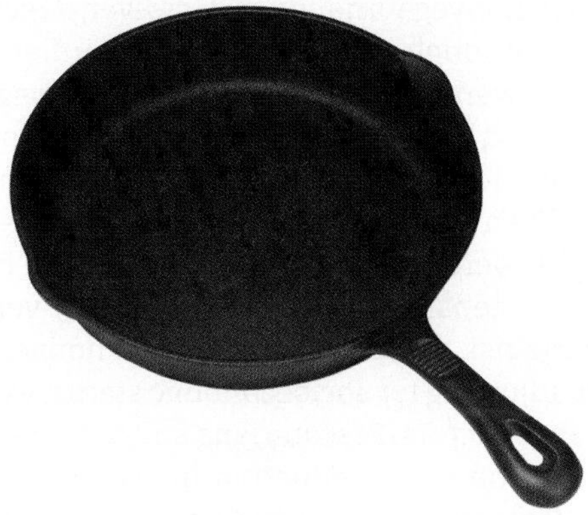

■ Figure 8.7
Cooking in Cast Iron Pans Can Increase Iron Consumption

ciency is the most common nutrient deficiency in the world. It is one of the only nutrient deficiencies that is common in the United States and other industrialized countries.[43,44] Most men and postmenopausal women get the iron they need. Premenopausal women often fall short due to the iron lost each month during menstruation.

Vitamin B_{12}

Vitamin B_{12} differs from the other B vitamins in a number of important ways. First, it is found only in foods of animal origin; plants do not have vitamin B_{12}, but are a good source of other B vitamins. Vitamin B_{12} is found in beef, seafood, and yogurt. Several foods, such as soy milk and breakfast cereals, are fortified with vitamin B_{12}. Second, vitamin B_{12} is stored in the body in large amounts. You may have as much as a two-year supply of vitamin B_{12}; the other B vitamins are not stored in any amount in the body. Vitamin B_{12} is needed for folate to function. Without vitamin B_{12}, folate cannot perform its vital role in blood cell formation and DNA synthesis. Because you can store vitamin B_{12}, deficiency is rare.[44]

Vegetarian Diets

The term *vegetarian* may conjure up a person wearing a tie-dyed T-shirt with faded jeans and Birkenstock sandals. *Granola cruncher*, *tree hugger*, and *animal lover* are all terms used to stereotype vegetarians. However, many people are choosing to go vegetarian for a variety of reasons. No longer relegated to the fringe of society, vegetarian eating is more popular than ever. According to the *Vegetarian Journal*, 2.3% of adults aged 18 and older stated that they "never eat meat, fish, or fowl" and 6.7% stated that they "never eat meat."[45] Other surveys have found higher numbers when the term *vegetarian* is not rigidly defined. Twenty to 25% of adults in the United States stated that they sometimes follow a vegetarian diet or eat four or more meatless meals per week.[46] This indicates an increased interest in at least part-time vegetarianism.

There are several different types of vegetarian diets. A **vegan** is someone who consumes no meat, poultry, fish, eggs, milk, or anything made with animal products. A **lacto-ovo vegetarian** consumes no meat, poultry, or fish, but does consume milk, milk products, and eggs. Someone who is a **pescatarian** is a vegetarian who consumes no meat or poultry but does consume fish. They may or may not consume milk and eggs. Another popular form of vegetarianism is a **semi-vegetarian**. Although there is not a specific definition, semi-vegetarians greatly limit the amount of meat they eat or choose not to eat certain types of meat, such as red meat. Sometimes this type of diet is called *flexitarian*. It is not truly a vegetarian diet, but rather one that seeks to limit meat consumption.

Why would someone choose a diet that restricts the consumption of meat, fish, poultry, and possibly even milk and eggs? There are many reasons a person might choose a vegetarian diet, including religion, ethics, the environment, or health.

Several religions encourage vegetarianism. Buddhists do not eat meat because they have mercy for all living creatures. Hinduism encourages vegetarianism, although not all Hindus are vegetarian. Most Hindus do not eat beef, because they consider the cow to be sacred. The Chinese-based religion of Taoism believes that nature is sacred and, as such, encourages vegetarianism. Seventh-Day Adventists have practiced vegetarianism for more than 130 years. They believe in the holistic nature of humankind and that healthy eating and drinking will preserve the health of the body, mind, and spirit.

Some people choose not to eat meat for ethical reasons. They believe that it is cruel to use animals for food. Others have issues with the way animals that are raised for food are treated, especially those raised in large commercial operations.

There are certainly environmental reasons to choose a plant-based diet. More than one-third of all the fossil

TERMS

vegan Person who consumes no meat, poultry, fish, eggs, milk, or anything made with animal products.

lacto-ovo vegetarian Person who consumes no meat, poultry, or fish but does consume dairy products and eggs.

pescatarian Person who does not consume meat or poultry but does consume fish; may or may not consume dairy products and eggs.

semi-vegetarian Person who limits meat or does not consume red meat; sometimes called a *part-time vegetarian* or a *flexitarian*.

fuels produced in the United States go toward raising animals for food. One calorie of an animal-based food takes 10 times more fossil fuel to produce than 1 calorie of a plant-based food.[47] The United States imports millions of pounds of beef each year from Central America. In addition to the fuel required to transport all that beef, another threat to the environment is the grazing land needed to raise the animals. Often this land comes from the clear-cutting of forests and rainforests. It is estimated that every minute of every day a land area equivalent to seven football fields is cut in the Amazon basin.[48] Cutting forest to make room for cattle is not limited to the rain forest. In the United States, millions of acres have been clear-cut for cattle. If meat consumption continues to grow as our population grows, most likely more trees will be replaced with cattle. The environmental effect of meat production and consumption also affects water usage and water pollution. One pound of beef requires about 25 gallons of water; a pound of soy, 250 gallons; and a pound of wheat, 25 gallons. The manure produced by large-scale animal production can end up in rivers and streams, causing pollution and possibly killing marine life.

Finally, many choose a vegetarian diet for health reasons. Considerable research has evaluated the health effects of vegetarian diets. A well-planned vegetarian diet can have many health benefits. Vegetarians are thinner compared to nonvegetarians.[49–51] However, a recent study found that although all vegetarians, regardless of their specific diet, were lower in weight than nonvegetarians, only vegans had body weights within optimal range.[50] Vegetarians have lower rates of hypertension than nonvegetarians.[52] Even when other factors, such as exercise and body weight, were controlled, vegetarians still had lower rates of hypertension. Vegan and lacto-ovo vegetarians have half the risk of type 2 diabetes than nonvegetarians, even after adjusting for socioeconomic status, weight, and other lifestyle factors. Pescatarians and semi-vegetarians do not have the same reduction in risk as vegans and lacto-ovo vegetarians, but they do show some protection against type 2 diabetes compared to nonvegetarians.[50] Vegetarians enjoy a lower risk of heart disease, largely due to lower cholesterol levels, lower blood pressure, and lower rates of both diabetes and obesity.[49] Overall cancer rates in vegetarians are slightly lower than in nonvegetarians.[7,51] Vegetarians also have lower rates of dementia, diverticular disease, and gallstones.[52]

Dietary Concerns for Vegetarians

A position paper from the American Dietetic Association and Dietitians of Canada states that a well-planned vegetarian diet can be healthful and nutritionally adequate.[52] However, vegetarians must pay particular attention to

Green and Healthy

Can What You Eat Affect the Environment?

If you are concerned about the environment, you may already be recycling, taking the bus, driving a hybrid car, and using your own reusable grocery bags. But have you ever thought about what you choose to eat and how it may affect the environment? Recent research has revealed six major effects that one's choice of diet has on the environment:[55]

1. **Water resources.** Growing crops requires water, growing meat requires even more. It takes significantly more water to raise livestock than it does to grow crops.
2. **Energy consumption.** It takes 2.5–5.0 times the amount of energy to produce a calorie of beef compared to a calorie from plant foods.[56]
3. **Application of chemical fertilizers.** Much of the natural fertility of the soil in the United States has been depleted and has been replaced by chemical fertilizer. The production of fertilizer requires a tremendous amount of energy and often is the single greatest energy input for many crops.
4. **Pesticides.** Increased use of pesticides has raised concerns over groundwater contamination.
5. **Waste generation.** Seven billion heads of livestock generate 130 times more waste than 300 million people. Waste from animals contains high amounts of nitrogen, phosphorous, potassium, and antibiotics; the disposal of this waste can cause serious health and environmental problems.[57]
6. **Land degradation.** Livestock production and its expansion is association with loss of forested land in the United States and other countries.

Diets of people who ate a primarily plant-based diet (lacto-ovo vegetarians) were compared to nonvegetarians for each of these factors. The nonvegetarian diet required 2.9 times more water, 2.5 times more energy, 13 times more fertilizer, and 1.4 times more pesticides than did the vegetarian diet. How can it be that the nonvegetarians used more fertilizer and pesticides, considering that fertilizers and pesticides are placed on plant foods? The largest contributor to the differences in vegetarian and nonvegetarian diets was the consumption of beef. The plant-based feed for the cattle requires fertilizer, energy, and pesticides. So, from an environmental perspective, what you choose to eat can affect the environment.[55]

Does this mean that beef is off the menu if you are concerned about the environment? You don't have to give up beef entirely to be green. Consuming more plant foods and choosing beef less often or in smaller portions is a great step toward making sure your food choices help the environment.

certain nutrients to ensure that they get the nutrients they need.

Protein

The quality of plant proteins varies. It was once thought that different plant proteins needed to be combined in one meal to make sure that all of the essential amino acids were consumed. However, research indicates that a variety of plant proteins eaten over the course of a day can provide all the essential amino acids and adequate protein for healthy adults. Thus, combining protein in one meal is not essential.[53] Lacto-ovo vegetarians and pescatarians get complete protein from milk, milk products, and fish. Most vegetarians, including both vegans and lacto-ovo vegetarians, meet or exceed protein needs.

Iron, Zinc, and Calcium

Vegetarians need to pay special attention to ensuring that their diets are adequate in iron and zinc.[52] Iron is found in whole-grain foods, beans, soy, nuts, and seeds. However, it is nonheme iron, so absorption rate is lower.

Zinc is found in many plant foods. Plant foods that contain zinc also contain fiber, which can decrease the absorption of zinc. Lacto-ovo vegetarians get zinc from dairy products such as yogurt and cheese.

Calcium intake for lacto-ovo vegetarians is not a concern, because dairy products are a significant source of calcium. However, vegans may have a more difficult time getting enough calcium. Although many plant foods, such as beans, soy foods, almonds, broccoli, spinach, and other dark green vegetables, have calcium, fiber and other components of these foods greatly hinder absorption of calcium. Vegans may need to consume calcium supplements and/or choose calcium-fortified soy milk, juice, or cereal.

Vitamins D and B_{12}

Lacto-ovo vegetarians who consume milk fortified with vitamin D do not have to be concerned with getting adequate vitamin D or vitamin B_{12}. Vegans, however, must ensure that they get enough vitamin D and vitamin B_{12}.[54] Plants are not a significant source of vitamin D. Vegans need to pay special attention to get vitamin D in fortified foods. The skin, when exposed to sunlight, can also make vitamin D. Vitamin B_{12} is not present in plant foods. Some foods, such as breakfast cereals, are fortified with vitamin B_{12}. Vegans need to consume plant foods that are fortified with B_{12} or take a B_{12} supplement.

Ready to Make a Change

Are you ready to make a change, small or large, in the protein that you eat? Whether it is a small, medium or large change, it is a step in the right direction toward a healthier diet.

I commit to a small first step. Eat smaller portions of meat. If you usually eat a large burger, switch to a smaller one. If you usually choose the biggest steak from meat counter, go for something a little smaller.

I am ready to take the next step and make a medium change. Replace some of the meat in your diet with seafood. Choose seafood once or twice a week. Aim to get at least 8 ounces of seafood on average per week, more is even better. Choose canned tuna packed in water for lunch or a quick dinner. Check with the seafood counter at your grocery store to see what is on special that week.

I have been making changes for some time and am ready to make a large change with the protein in my diet. Go vegetarian one day a week. You don't have to totally give up meat, just try doing so for one day a week. It is good for you and good for the planet. It is a great way to try new foods and new recipes. Get your friends to join in for "Meatless Mondays" or "Tofu Thursdays."

Myth Versus Fact

Myth: Protein is a good source of energy.

Fact: Protein has 4 calories per gram, just like carbohydrates; however, the body prefers to use carbohydrate and fat for energy and "spare" the protein. Protein is best used by the body for the unique functions it provides, such as building and repairing tissue.

Myth: Soy protein is dangerous and should not be consumed.

Fact: The preponderance of research indicates that soy is not only safe, but healthy. Soy is low in fat, high in fiber, and a good alternative to meat.

Myth: If you work out regularly, your protein needs are higher than the recommendations.

Fact: Competitive athletes may have higher protein requirements, but those working out on a regular basis do not have higher protein requirements. Most Americans, both athletes and nonathletes, get more than the recommended amount of protein.

Myth: Most of the protein in the American diet comes from chicken and fish.

Fact: Beef is the number one source of protein in the American diet.

Myth: Nuts are high in fat and should be avoided.

Fact: Nuts are high in fat but the fat is healthy fat. Nuts also contain fiber and protein. Consuming small portions of unsalted nuts on a regular basis is linked with reduced risk of heart disease. Those who consume nuts on a regular basis are more likely to be a healthy weight.

Myth: If you eat more protein than you need, it will be stored as muscle.

Fact: More calories than you need, regardless of the source, ends up as fat. It is a myth that excess protein automatically goes to creating muscle. If calories are above what you need, even if it is from protein, it is going to be stored as fat.

Myth: What I choose to eat has a little impact on the environment.

Fact: Choosing a diet that has at least some of the protein from plant sources goes a long way in helping the planet.

Back to the Story

Now that you know more about proteins, let's take a closer look at John's diet. His goal is to build muscle and get bigger and stronger. He has joined a gym and is working out with a trainer. Working out properly is certainly a good first step. The old saying is that "muscles are broken down in the gym and built in the kitchen." When you look at the "kitchen" side of the equation, John falls short. He is using amino acid supplements and protein shakes. Amino acid supplements are not needed and have not been proven to be effective at increasing lean body mass. He would be better off spending that money on healthy food. Building muscle and getting fit require more than working out and pouring a protein shake on top of an unhealthy diet. John needs to get his diet in check pronto or he will not see the gains in muscle he could see. John should keep up the workouts but change from fast food to healthier fare of low-fat meat, vegetables, beans, grains, fruit, and low-fat dairy. He should get in a routine of eating regular meals so his body has fuel all day. An occasional protein shake is okay as a meal replacement on a busy day, but it should not be an everyday replacement for good nutrition. Remember, however, that a big factor in how much muscle growth is possible for an individual is related to genetics. With proper workouts and a healthy diet, John will be able to be the best he can be. What other suggestions do you have for John?

References

1. Institute of Medicine, Food and Nutrition Board. *Dietary Reference Intakes for Energy, Carbohydrate, Fiber, Fat, Fatty Acids, Cholesterol, Protein, and Amino Acids*. Washington, DC: National Academies Press, 2005.
2. Moshfegh A, Goldman J, Cleveland L. What we eat in America, NHANES 2001–2002. Usual nutrient intake from foods as compared to dietary reference intakes. US Department of Agriculture, Agricultural Research Service. 2005. http://www.ars.usda.gov/SP2UserFiles/Place/12355000/pdf/usualintaketables2001-02.pdf. Accessed August 25, 2009.
3. Fulgoni VL. Current protein intake in America: analysis of the National Health and Nutrition Examination Survey, 2003–2004. *Am J Clin Nutr*. 2008;87(suppl):1554S–1557S.
4. World Health Organization, Department of Nutrition for Health and Development. Nutrition for health and development: a global agenda for combating malnutrition. World Health Organization. http://whqlibdoc.who.int/hq/2000/WHO_NHD_00.6.pdf. Accessed August 25, 2009.
5. Sinha R, Cross AJ, Graubard BI, Leitzmann MF, Schatzkin A. Meat intake and mortality. *Arch Intern Med*. 2009;169(6):562–571.
6. Willett WC. Diet and cancer: An evolving picture. *JAMA*. 2005;293(2):233–234.
7. Chao A, Thun MJ, Connell CJ, et al. Meat consumption and risk of colorectal cancer. *JAMA*. 2005;293(2):172–182.
8. Dunford M, ed. *Sports Nutrition: A Practice Manual for Professionals*, 4th ed. Chicago: American Dietetic Association, 2006.
9. Phillips SM, Moore DR, Tang J. A critical examination of dietary protein requirements, benefits, and excesses in athletes. *Int J Sports Nutr Exer Metab*. 2007;17:S58–S76.
10. Tipton KD, Witard OC. Protein requirements and recommendations for athletes: relevance of ivory tower arguments for practical recommendations. *Clin Sports Med*. 2007;26:17–36.
11. Burke L, DeakinV, eds. *Clinical Sports Nutrition*. Sydney, Australia: McGraw-Hill, 2006.
12. Phillips SM, Moore DR, Tang JE. A critical examination of dietary protein requirements, benefits, and excesses in athletes. *Inter J Sport Nutr Exer Metab*. 2007;17:S58–S76.
13. American College of Sports Medicine, American Dietetic Association, Dieticians of Canada. Joint position statement, nutrition and athletic performance. *Med Sci Sports Exer*. 2009;41(3):709–731.
14. Tarnopolsky MA. Protein requirements for endurance athletes. *Nutrition*. 2004;20:662–668.
15. Lambert CP, Frank LL, Evans WJ. Macronutrient considerations for the sport of bodybuilding. *Sports Med*. 2004; 34(5):317–327.
16. Kleiner SM, Bazzarre TL, Ainsworth BE. Nutritional status of nationally ranked elite bodybuilders. *Int J Sport Nutr*. 1994;4:54–69.
17. Kleiner SM, Bazzarre TL, Litchford MD. Metabolic profiles, diet, and health practices of championship male and female bodybuilders. *J Am Diet Assoc*. 1990;90:962–967.
18. Ivy JL, Res PT, Sprague RC, Widzer MO. Effect of a carbohydrate–protein supplement on endurance perfor-

mance during exercise of varying intensity. *Int J Sport Nutr Exerc Metab*. 2003;13:382–95.
19. VanEssen M, Gibala MJ. Failure of protein to improve time trial performance when added to a sports drink. *Med Sci Sports Exerc*. 2006;38:1476–1483.
20. Cotton PA, Subar AF, Friday JE, Cook A. Dietary sources of nutrients among US adults, 1994–1996. *J Am Diet Assoc*. 2004;104(6):921–930.
21. Lichtenstein AH, Appel LJ, Brands M, et al. Diet and lifestyle recommendations revision 2006: a scientific statement from the American Heart Association Nutrition Committee. *Circulation*. 2006;114:82–96.
22. He K, Song Y, Daviglus ML, et al. Fish consumption and incidence of stroke a meta-analysis of cohort studies. *Stroke*. 2004;35:1538–1542.
23. US Departments of Health and Human Services and US Department of Agriculture. *Dietary Guidelines for Americans, 2010*, 7th ed. Washington, DC: US Government Printing Office, December 2010.
24. Duckett SK, Neel JPS, Fontenot JP, Clapham WM. Effects of winter stocker growth rate and finishing system on: III. Tissue proximate, fatty acid, vitamin, and cholesterol content. *J Anim Sci*. 2007.85:2691–2698.
25. McCluskey JJ, Wahl TI, Li Q, Wandschneider PR. US grass-fed beef: marketing health benefits. *J Food Dist Res*. 2005; 36(3):1–8.
26. Rule DC, Broughton KS, Shellito SM, Maiorano G. Comparison of muscle fatty acid profiles and cholesterol concentrations of bison, beef cattle, elk, and chicken. *J Anim Sci*. 2002;80(5):1202–1211.
27. World Health Organization. Use of antimicrobials outside human medicine and resultant antimicrobial resistance in humans. Fact Sheet Number 268, January 2001. https://apps.who.int/inf-fs/en/fact268.html. Accessed April 19, 2011.
28. Bazzano LA, He J, Ogden LG, et al. Legume consumption and risk of coronary heart disease in US men and women: NHANES I Epidemiologic Follow-up Study. *Arch Intern Med*. 2001;161(21):2573–2578.
29. Hu FB, Rimm EB, Stampfer MJ, Ascherio A, Spiegelman D, Willett WC. Prospective study of major dietary patterns and risk of coronary heart disease in men. *Am J Clin Nutr*. 2000;72(4):912–921.
30. Fung TT, Willett WC, Stampfer MJ, Manson JE, Hu FB. Dietary patterns and the risk of coronary heart disease in women. *Arch Intern Med*. 2001;161(15):1857–1862.
31. Sacks FM, Lichtenstein A, VanHorn L, Harris W, Dris-Etherton P, Winston M. Soy protein, isoflavones, and cardiovascular health an American Heart Association science advisory for professionals from the nutrition committee. *Circulation*. 2006;113:1034–1044.
32. Kronenberg F, Fugh-Berman A. Complementary and alternative medicine for menopausal symptoms: a review of randomized, controlled trials. *Ann Intern Med*. 2002;137(10):805–813.
33. Krebs EE, Ensrud KE, MacDonald R, Wilt TJ. Phytoestrogens for treatment of menopausal symptoms: a systematic review. *Obestet Gynecol*. 2004;104(4):824–836.
34. Messina M, Nagata C, Wu AH. Estimated Asian adult soy protein and isoflavone intakes. *Nutr Cancer*. 2006;55:1–12.
35. Duffy C, Perez K, Partridge A. Implications of phytoestrogen intake for breast cancer. *CA Cancer J Clin*. 2007;57:260–277.
36. Peeters PH, Keinan-Boker L, van der Schouw YT, Grobbee ED. Phytoestrogens and breast cancer risk. Review of the epidemiological evidence. *Breast Cancer Res Treat*. 2004;77(2):171–183.
37. Messina M, Wu AH. Perspectives on the soy-breast cancer relation. *Am J Clin Nutr*. 2009;89(suppl):1673S–1679S. 2003;77(2):171–183.

38. Kris-Etherton PM, Zhao G, Binkoski AE, Coval SM, Etherton TD. The effects of nuts on coronary heart disease risk. *Nutr Rev*. 2001;59(4):103–111.
39. Hu FB, Stampfer MJ, Manson JE, et al. Frequent nut consumption and risk of coronary heart disease in women: prospective cohort study. *BMJ*. 1998;317(7169):1341–1345.
40. Albert CM, Gaziano JM, Willett WC, Manson JE. Nut consumption and decreased risk of sudden cardiac death in the Physicians' Health Study. *Arch Intern Med*. 2002;162(12):1382–1387.
41. Djousse L, Rudich T, Gaziano JM. Nut consumption and risk of heart failure in the Physicians' Health Study I. *Am J Clin Nutr*. 2008;88(4):930–933.
42. Ellsworth JL, Kushi LH, Folsom AR. Frequent nut intake and risk of death from coronary heart disease and all causes in postmenopausal women: the Iowa Women's Health Study. *Nutr Metab Cardiovasc Dis*. 2001;11(6):372–377.
43. World Health Organization. Micronutrient deficiencies, iron deficiency anemia. http://www.who.int/nutrition/topics/ida/en/. Accessed November 23, 2009.
44. Institute of Medicine, Food and Nutrition Board. *Dietary Reference Intakes Thiamin, Riboflavin, Niacin, Vitamin B6, Folate, Vitamin B12, Pantothenic Acid, Biotin, and Choline*. Washington, DC: National Academies Press, 1998.
45. Stahler C. How many adults are vegetarian? *Vegetarian J*. 2006. http://www.vrg.org/journal/vj2006issue4/vg2006issue4poll.htm. Accessed September 11, 2009.
46. Ginsberg C, Ostrowski A. The market for vegetarian foods. *Vegetarian J*. 2002;4:25–29.
47. Pimentel D, Pimentel M. Sustainability of meat-based and plant-based diets and the environment. *Am J Clin Nutr*. 2003;78(3):660S–663S.
48. Laurance WF, Albernaz AKM, Da Costa C. Is deforestation accelerating in the Brazilian Amazon? *Environmental Conservation*. 2001;28:305–311.
49. Craig WJ. Health effects of vegan diets. *Am J Clin Nutr*. 2009;89(suppl):1627S–1633S.
50. Tonstad S, Butler T, Yan R, Fraser GE. Type of vegetarian diet, body weight, and prevalence of type 2 diabetes. *Diabetes Care*. 2009;32:791–796.
51. Fraser GE. Vegetarian diets: what do we know of their effects on common chronic diseases. *Am J Clin Nutr*. 2009;89(suppl):1607S–1612S.
52. American Dietetic Association. Position of the American Dietetic Association and Dietitians of Canada: vegetarian diets. *J Am Diet Assoc*. 2003;103(6):748–765.
53. Young VR, Pellett PL. Plant proteins in relation to human protein and amino acid nutrition. *Am J Clin Nutr*. 1994;59(suppl):1203S–1212S.
54. Elmadfa I, Singer I. Vitamin B-12 and homocysteine status among vegetarians: a global perspective. *Am J Clin Nutr*. 2009;89(suppl):1693S–1698S.
55. Marlow HJ, Hayes WK, Soret S, Carter RL, Schwab ER, Sabate J. Diet and the environment: does what you eat matter? *Am J Clin Nutr*. 2009;89(suppl):1699S–1703S.
56. Reijnders L, Soret S. Quantification of the environmental impact of different dietary protein choices. *Am J Clin Nutr*. 2003;78(suppl):664S–668S.
57. Delgado C, Rosegrant M, Steinfeld H, Ehui S, Courbois C. Livestock to 2020: the next food revolution. Washington, DC: International Food Policy Research Institute, 2001:27–29.

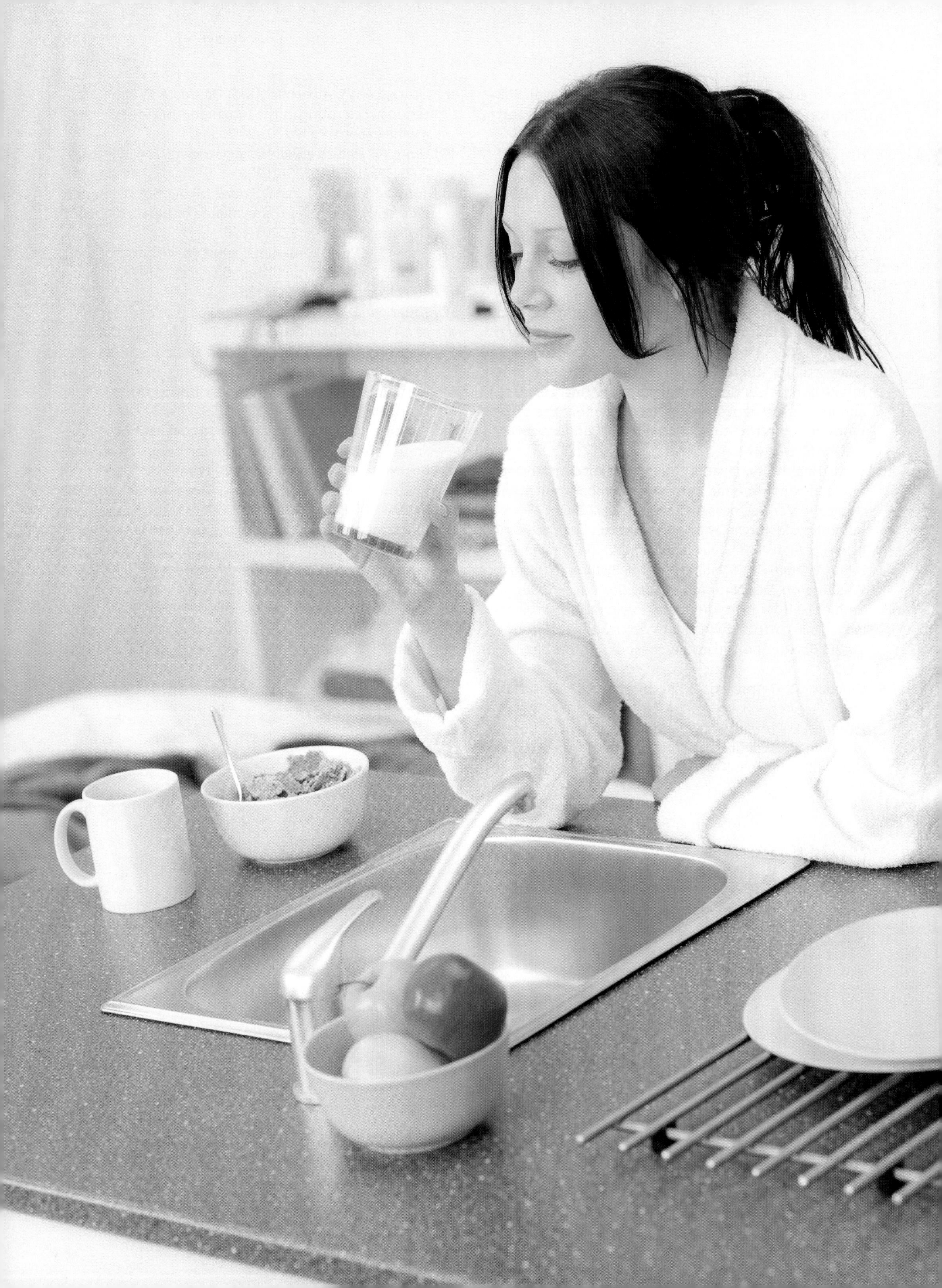

Chapter 9

Milk and Dairy: Not Just for Kids

Key Messages

- Dairy products are an important part of a healthy diet.
- Consumption of dairy products can provide protection against certain chronic diseases.
- Choose dairy products wisely for a healthy diet.
- Dairy products contain many essential nutrients for optimal bone health.

"Drink your milk" is something most of you heard throughout your childhood. Celebrities from Heidi Klum to the cast of *Modern Family* pose with milk mustaches and ask "Got Milk?" (**Figure 9.1**). Milk, yogurt, cheese, and cottage cheese are all heralded by nutrition professionals as products that should be consumed on a daily basis. Why the push to get you to consume milk and other dairy products? Are they really needed for overall health? Can dairy products offer protection against certain chronic diseases? Are some dairy products better than others? Can a dairy-free diet be healthy? Low-fat, fat-free, probiotic, or live cultures—with so many different options, you might be confused about which products to choose. All of these questions will be discussed in detail as we explore dairy products.

Story

Alice is a 19-year-old, first-year college student. Her mom is 51 and has just recently had a bone scan as part of her yearly physical. The test showed that she had osteopenia, which means that her bone mass is below normal. Alice is worried that she may be on the same path, because she and her mother have a similar body shape and size. She is glad that she doesn't have to worry about it for years to come, but it does make her wonder if there is something she can do now to prevent it from happening. Her mom is concerned for her own health as well as Alice's.

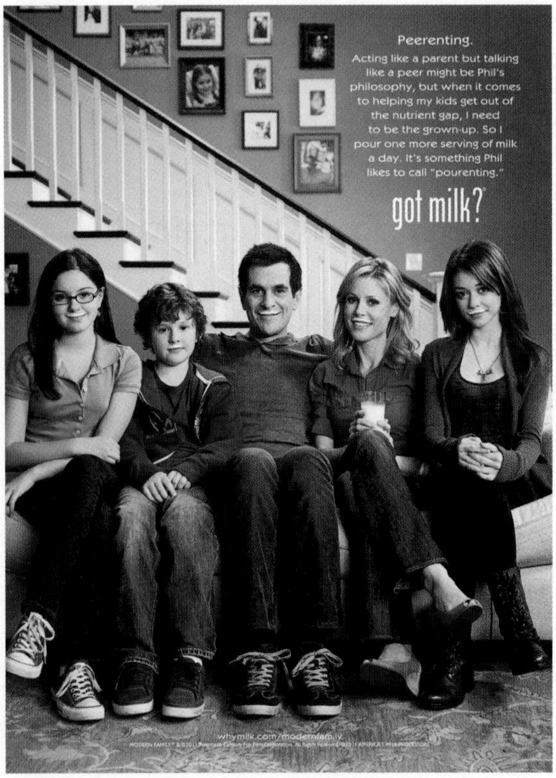

■ **Figure 9.1**

"Got Milk?"

The "Got Milk?" campaign uses celebrities and their famous milk mustaches to encourage milk consumption.

She asks Alice to take a close look at her diet. She asks how much milk Alice drinks. This was an easy answer for Alice, none. How about yogurt? Another easy answer, none. What about cheese? Finally, something she does eat—cheese on pizza about two times per week. Is low bone mass something that Alice needs to worry about now? If so, what can she do to keep from going down the same path as her mom?

Recommended and Actual Intake of Dairy Products

The health benefits of milk and other dairy products have been well documented in the nutrition literature. Adults should consume three servings per day of fat-free or low-fat milk or equivalent dairy products (**Table 9.1**). Milk, yogurt, cheese, and foods made with dairy products all count toward the amount of dairy products you need each day. Because of their similar nutritional value, soy beverages fortified with calcium and vitamins A and D also are considered part of the dairy group.[1]

Most people fall considerably short of the recommended dairy intake. Men over the age of 20 consume an average of 1.8 servings of dairy products per day. Women consume even less; on average, women consume 1.4 servings of dairy per day. Forty-one percent of men and almost half (49%) of women consume less than one serving of dairy a day. Only a few adults, 28% of men and 20% of women, consume the recommended three servings of dairy products each day.[2]

Table 9.1

What Counts as One Serving of Dairy?

Dairy Product	One Serving
Milk	1 cup
Soy milk*	1 cup
Yogurt	1 cup
Cheese	1.5 ounces hard cheese (cheddar, mozzarella, Swiss, Parmesan)
	1/3 cup shredded cheese
	2 ounces processed cheese (American)
	1/2 cup ricotta cheese
	2 cups cottage cheese
Milk-based desserts	1 cup of pudding made with milk
	1 cup of frozen yogurt
	1 1/2 cups ice cream

*Soy beverages fortified with calcium and vitamins A and D are considered part of the milk and dairy group because they are nutritionally similar to milk.

Sources: Modified from US Department of Agriculture. www.mypyramid.gov/pyramid/milk_counts.html#. Accessed April 9, 2011. US Department of Health and Human Services and US Department of Agriculture. *Dietary Guidelines for Americans, 2005*, 7th ed. Washington, DC: US Government Printing Office, December 2010.

Dairy Products and Health

Dairy products provide protein, calcium, magnesium, phosphorus, and other important nutrients.[3,4] In fact, it is very difficult to meet the minimum amounts of calcium and other nutrients important for optimal health without consuming adequate amounts of dairy products. Dairy products are so rich in nutrients that consumption of the recommended servings of dairy products improves overall diet quality.[5,6] In addition, consuming dairy products is important for bone and heart health.

Milk and dairy products are often thought of as "bone builders" because they contain high amounts of the nutrients that are involved in bone health, specifically the minerals calcium and phosphorous and vitamin D. The impact of dairy products on bone health is well documented. A strong relationship exists between intake of dairy products and bone density in both children and adults.[7–10] This chapter's Spotlight outlines the important nutrients found in abundance in dairy products that are critical for overall bone health.

Consumption of dairy products is associated with other health benefits as well. A strong relationship has been found between consumption of dairy products and blood pressure. People who consume adequate amounts of dairy products are more likely to have normal blood pressure levels than those who do not.[11,12] Dairy products also have a protective effect with respect to heart disease. Individuals who consume dairy products, particularly low-fat ones, are less likely to develop heart disease than those who have lower dairy intake.[11–13] However, consumption of dairy products that are high in fat, such as hard cheese, whole milk, and ice cream, can actually increase blood cholesterol, a risk factor for heart disease.[11,13]

In recent years, dairy products have received considerable attention for their role in weight management.[14–19] However, strong evidence indicates that consumption of milk and milk products does not play a special role in weight management.[1] Even without a link between weight loss and consumption of dairy, it is important to keep dairy in your diet even while trying to lose weight. When you cut calories in an attempt to lose unwanted pounds, you may often cut out or decrease consumption of dairy products. Although decreasing calories is certainly needed for weight loss, cutting dairy products may be the wrong way to go. Dairy products provide needed nutrients and should be included in your diet even if you are trying to lose weight. Low-fat dairy products are important for many reasons and should be a part of a healthy weight-loss diet.

Spotlight on Vitamins and Minerals

Calcium

Calcium is the most abundant mineral in the body. It is vital to many of the body's functions. Consumption of adequate calcium is important throughout the life cycle for overall health, especially bone health.

Functions of Calcium

About 99% of the calcium in your body is found in the bones and teeth, where it provides structural support (**Figure 9.2**). The other 1% of the calcium in your body serves important roles in nerve functioning, blood clotting, muscle contraction, and cellular metabolism.

Bone Structure

The structure of your bones is continually changing. During growth, bone formation occurs at a high rate so bones can increase in size and density. Once maximum height is reached, bones continue to add calcium to increase density until peak bone mass is reached. Peak bone mass is usually reached around age 20. In early and middle adulthood, bone loss and formation are usually equal. Later in life, particularly for women, bone loss is higher than bone formation. This increases the risk of fractures and osteoporosis (see the feature on osteoporosis later in this chapter).

Adequate calcium consumption throughout the life span is critical to ensure that peak bone mass is reached and that bone mass is maintained. Bones can continue to grow stronger as a result of stress placed on the bones through weight-bearing exercise or resistance training.

Two types of cells, osteoblasts and osteoclasts, carry out the constant remodeling of bone. Osteoblasts are bone cells that create the matrix that forms the structure of the bone. Osteoclasts are cells that break down the structure of the bone and release calcium into the bloodstream. It is critical for blood levels of calcium to be maintained within a very narrow margin. If calcium levels fall, hormones signal osteoclasts

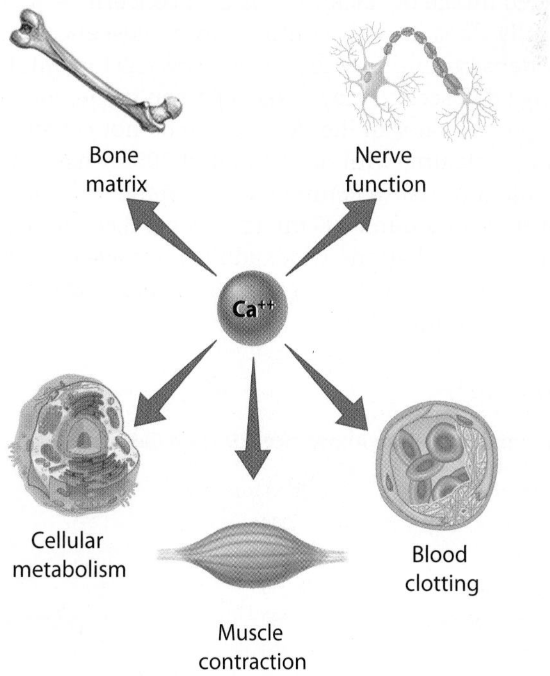

Figure 9.2
Functions of Calcium

to pull calcium from the bones and release it into the bloodstream, even at the expense of weakening bones in the long run.

Other Functions of Calcium

As stated earlier, the 1% of calcium that is not in the bones performs many important functions. Although it is only a small percentage of the calcium in the body, the level of calcium in the blood must be kept constant, even if it means compromising the integrity of bone. Flow of calcium into and out of your muscle cells allows them to contract and relax. Calcium is essential for blood to clot normally and is involved in the production of fibrin, the protein that gives blood clots structure. Calcium is needed for nerve cells to transmit signals. Finally, calcium is involved in general cellular metabolism.

Recommended and Actual Intake of Calcium

Consumption of adequate calcium is important during childhood to promote bone growth, during adolescence and early adulthood to ensure that optimal bone mass is created, and in adulthood to help preserve bone mass. Adequate Intakes (AIs) for calcium are set to minimize the risk of osteoporosis later in life. For adults aged 19–50, the AI for calcium is 1,000 milligrams for both men and women. The AI increases to 1,200 milligrams for both genders for adults aged 50 and older. Postmenopausal women who are not taking estrogen as well as adults over 65 get should consume 1,500 milligrams of calcium per day.[20]

Most people fall short of recommended intake for calcium.[20–22] Adolescents do not meet the recommended intake of calcium. This is of concern because not only does growth continue in adolescence, but bone density continues to increase. Low calcium intake during adolescence may make a person vulnerable to osteoporosis later in life. Adults also do not consume enough calcium, with an estimated 70% consuming less calcium than recommended.[22] Women consume an average of around 800 milligrams per day and men about 1,000 milligrams. Older adults (over age 60) consume even less—800 milligrams in men and 660 milligrams in women.[20,21]

Table 9.2

Recommended Dietary Allowance (RDA) for Calcium

Age	RDA milligrams/day
19–30 years	1,000
31–50 years	1,000
51–70 years (males)	1,000
51–70 years (females)	1,200
> 70 years	1,200

Source: Data from Institute of Medicine, Food and Nutrition Board. *Dietary Reference Intakes for Calcium and Vitamin D.* Washington, DC: National Academies Press, 2010.

Sources of Calcium

Dairy products are the best source of calcium. Fat-free or low-fat milk, yogurt, and fortified soy milk are excellent choices because they contain significant calcium but little or no fat. Cheese is also a good source of calcium, but it should be consumed in moderation due to its high fat content. Although cottage cheese has some calcium, it does not have the high levels found in other dairy products. Ice cream and other frozen dairy desserts contain calcium, but also sugar and fat, thus their consumption should be limited.

Other sources of calcium in the diet include dark-green vegetables, such as broccoli, turnip greens, kale, and collards (**Figure 9.3**). Tofu, if it is processed with calcium carbonate, is also a good source of calcium. Sardines with bones are a good source of calcium, but they are not a common food in the North American diet. Many foods are fortified with calcium, including orange juice, breakfast cereal, soy milk, and bread.

Although it is possible to get the calcium you need without consuming dairy products, it would be very difficult.[3,4] The amount of other foods that would need to be consumed would be extremely high. For example, you would need to eat 2 1/2 cups of broccoli or 1 3/4 cups of kale to get the same amount of calcium in just 1 cup of milk or yogurt. In addition, the AI for calcium assumes that calcium is received from a variety of foods, both dairy foods and other foods. If you don't consume any dairy foods, or consume them infrequently or in small amounts, a calcium supplement may be needed.

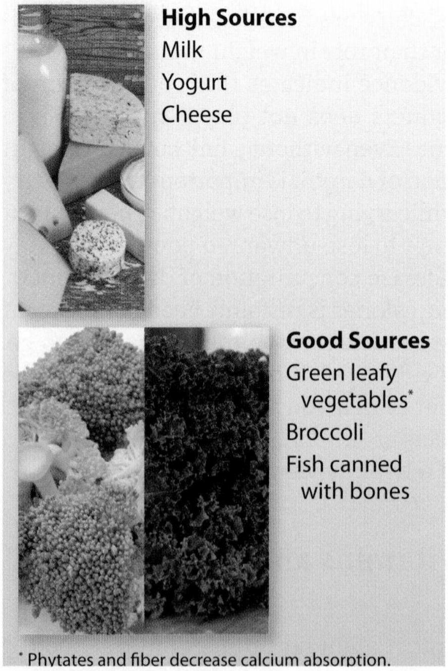
High Sources
Milk
Yogurt
Cheese
Good Sources
Green leafy vegetables*
Broccoli
Fish canned with bones

* Phytates and fiber decrease calcium absorption.

Figure 9.3
Food Sources of Calcium

Absorption of Calcium

Many factors affect the body's ability to absorb calcium. Vitamin D is needed for calcium to be absorbed, and it is added to many calcium supplements and dairy products. Fiber hinders calcium absorption, as do **oxalates** and **phytates**. Oxalates and oxalic acids bind calcium so that it cannot be absorbed from the food. Spinach is high in oxalates, so high in fact that the body can only absorb a very small amount of the calcium in spinach. So even though spinach has a significant amount of calcium, that calcium is not available to the body. Phytates are found in the bran of grains and bind calcium in the stomach so that it cannot be absorbed. Although it is possible to get some of the calcium you need each day from green leafy vegetables, the fiber, oxalates, and phytates in vegetables greatly impede calcium's absorption. Of course, there are many other reasons to increase your consumption of dark-green leafy vegetables in addition to the calcium they contain.

It was once thought that carbonated beverages decreased calcium absorption and weakened bones. No evidence supports this claim, and some evidence even indicates that carbonation actually increases calcium absorption. This does not mean that carbonated soft drinks are good for bone health. If carbonated beverages replace milk in the diet, calcium intake can be compromised. However, the carbonation, in and of itself, is not a problem.[23]

Vitamin D

Vitamin D is most often thought of as a vitamin that is important for bone health. Although this is true, vitamin D is an important nutrient for many different reasons. In the past, it was thought you didn't need to worry about vitamin D because the body produces it when exposed to sunlight; however, today lack of vitamin D is now considered by some to be a major public health threat.

Function of Vitamin D

Vitamin D is essential to healthy bones. Vitamin D increases the absorption of calcium and phosphorus and increases the rate at which the bones calcify or harden. When vitamin D is present, calcium absorption increases as much as threefold.[24–26] Vitamin D deficiency causes **rickets**, a childhood disease that results in softening and weakening of the bones. Low vitamin D can also exacerbate or precipitate osteopenia or osteoporosis in adults. Vitamin D is an important regulator in the body. When calcium levels are low, vitamin D stimulates the release of calcium from the bone into the bloodstream and signals the kidneys to decrease calcium excretion.

Vitamin D has primarily been associated with bone health, but it is now believed to be involved in the health of other organs and tissues in the body. Substantial research and epidemiological inquiry has sought to determine whether vitamin D has a protective effect against certain forms of cancer.[27] The vast majority of the findings indicate that adequate vitamin D has a protective effect against cancers of the colon, pancreas, prostate, ovary, and breast.[27–32] Low levels of vitamin D are associated with as much as a 30–50% increased risk of colon, prostate, and breast cancer, along with a higher mortality rate from these cancers.[28,29] The specific mechanism as to how vitamin D protects against cancer is still under investigation. A possible explanation is that vitamin D acts as a regulator to keep cells from turning into cancer cells and multiplying.[24]

Vitamin D is associated with heart health as well. Low levels of vitamin D and vitamin D deficiency have an adverse effect on cardiovascular health.[33,34] Growing evidence suggests that low vitamin D levels are associated with coronary risk factors and adverse cardiovascular outcomes.[35] Specifically, vitamin D levels are inversely associated with blood pressure.[36–38] Inadequate vitamin D has been linked to many other health concerns, including depression[39,40] and diabetes.[41]

Recommended and Actual Intake of Vitamin D

The AI for vitamin D is 200 International Units (IU) for children and adults up to 50 years of age, 400 IU for adults 51–70 years of age, and 600 IU for adults over 71 years of age.[20]

A growing body of evidence indicates that up to 50% of young adults and children have below optimal levels of vitamin D.[42,43] Ethnic groups with darker skin require proportionally more sun exposure than people with lighter skin; this puts them at a higher risk for low vitamin D levels. In today's modern world, people do not have has much exposure to sunlight due to decreased

Table 9.3

Recommended Dietary Allowance (RDA) for Vitamin D

Age	RDA IU/day
Up to age 70 years	600
> 70 years	800

Source: Data from Institute of Medicine, Food and Nutrition Board. *Dietary Reference Intakes for Calcium and Vitamin D.* Washington, DC: National Academies Press, 2010.

TERMS

oxalates Substances in vegetables, especially spinach, that are capable of forming an insoluble salt with calcium, thus interfering with its absorption.

phytates Substances in vegetables and grains that are capable of forming an insoluble salt with calcium, zinc, iron, and other nutrients, thus interfering with their absorption.

rickets Softening of bones in children or adolescents usually caused by extreme and prolonged vitamin D deficiency.

Personal Health Check

Do You Need a Supplement?

Calcium Supplements

Now that you are thoroughly convinced how important calcium is in the diet, you may be asking, "Do I get enough calcium?" or "Should I take a supplement?" The first step to answering these questions is to examine your diet and assess how much calcium you get now. Use the calcium wheel in the figure below for a rough estimate of how much calcium you get on a regular basis. If you do not consume dairy products on a regular basis or consume them in small amounts, you may need a supplement. Keep in mind that although there are other foods that contain calcium in addition to dairy products, the amount you need to consume to get close to the recommended amounts is very high. This makes it very difficult to get enough calcium without consuming dairy products.

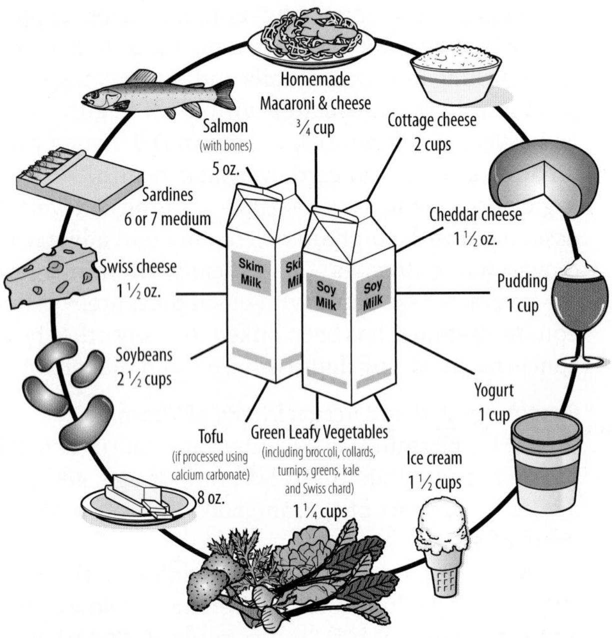

Calcium Wheel

Each portion of food around the outside of the calcium wheel contains about the same amount of calcium as the 1 cup of milk at the center of the wheel. Think about how much of these foods you consume on a regular basis each day. This is a rough estimate of your usual calcium intake.

If you decide that you would like to try a calcium supplement, there are several on the market from which to choose. The most common forms of calcium supplements are calcium carbonate and calcium citrate. Both are absorbed at similar rates. Some people have fewer digestive issues with calcium citrate. The body absorbs calcium carbonate best when consumed with food. Consumption of food has no effect on the absorption of calcium from calcium citrate.[48] Calcium phosphate is also a supplemental form of calcium but is less available and more expensive than either calcium carbonate or calcium citrate. Keep the following in mind when choosing a calcium supplement:

Dose: 500 milligrams of calcium is the maximum dose that should be taken at one time. If you want to take more, break it up over the course of the day.

Vitamin D: Vitamin D will help with calcium absorption. Choose a calcium supplement that also contains vitamin D.

Tolerance: Calcium carbonate can cause side effects such as gas, bloating, or constipation in some people. If these side effects occur, try a different type of calcium supplement or a different brand. Calcium citrate is an alternative that does not cause constipation.

Purity: There are many calcium supplements on the market; choose a familiar brand name with the **United States Pharmacopeia (USP)** symbol on the box or bottle. Don't choose supplements made from unrefined oyster shells, bone meal, or dolomite that don't have the USP symbol. These may contain high levels of lead or other toxic metals.[49]

Price: Calcium supplements vary in price. Chelated calcium supplements have higher absorption rates but are much more expensive. Calcium carbonate tends to be less expensive than calcium citrate. Choose a calcium supplement that can be tolerated by both your budget and your stomach.

Vitamin D Supplements

Adequate vitamin D intake is required to maintain overall health and to reduce the risk of some forms of chronic illness. Many of us don't get enough vitamin D in food or by exposure to the sun. Despite the importance of sun exposure to vitamin D synthesis, it is healthy to limit sun exposure and routinely use sunscreen to decrease risk of skin cancer. An alternative to ensure adequate vitamin D levels is to take a supplement.

Check with your healthcare provider to have a vitamin D screening to see where you are with regard to your vitamin D status. If indicted, your healthcare provider may suggest a vitamin D supplement. Although the AI for vitamin D is 200–600 IU depending on age, most experts recommend 1,000–2,000 IU for optimal vitamin D status.[35,42,47] One word of caution, however; you can get too much vitamin D, which is known as vitamin D toxicity. The upper limit for vitamin D consumption through supplements or fortified foods is 2,000 IU. Exposure to the sun does not cause vitamin D toxicity. Vitamin D toxicity causes the body to deposit calcium in soft tissue, which causes pain. Symptoms of vitamin D toxicity include nausea, vomiting, and loss of appetite.

Table 9.4

Comparison of Calories, Fat, and Saturated Fat in Different Types of Milk

Milk Product	Percent Fat	Calories	Total Fat	Saturated Fat
Whole milk	3.25%	150	8.0 grams	5.0 grams
Low-fat milk	2.00%	120	5.0 grams	3.0 grams
Low-fat milk	1.00%	105	2.5 grams	1.5 grams
Fat-free or skim milk	0.00%	90	0.0 grams	0.0 grams

Source: Data from Institute of Medicine, Food and Nutrition Board. *Dietary Reference Intakes for Calcium and Vitamin D.* Washington, DC: National Academies Press, 2010.

outdoor leisure time activity. In addition, efforts to minimize sun exposure or use topical sunscreen to protect against photo aging and skin cancer decrease the body's ability to produce vitamin D. Sunscreen with a sun protection factor (SPF) of 15 blocks almost all (99%) vitamin D production.[44]

Sources of Vitamin D

Few foods naturally contain vitamin D. The exception is oily fish, such as salmon, mackerel, or cod. Fortified foods provide much of the dietary vitamin D for people the United States and Canada.[45] In the 1930s, vitamin D was added to milk to help combat rickets, then a major public health problem. Today, milk continues to be fortified with vitamin D. One cup of fortified milk contains 100 IU of vitamin D. Several other foods are commonly fortified with vitamin D, including some breakfast cereals, orange juices, and yogurts. Foods made from milk, such as cheese and ice cream, generally are not fortified. The major source of vitamin D is exposure to sunlight.[46] As much as 95% of the body's vitamin D comes from the production of vitamin D by the skin as a result of exposure to the sun.[35]

Phosphorous

Phosphorus, like calcium, is a major component of bone. Phosphorus also plays a key role in energy metabolism and is required to ensure that calcium is absorbed and retained by the bones. Phosphorous is very common in food, so getting enough is almost never a problem. Good sources of phosphorus include yogurt, milk, beans and peas, almonds, chicken, and beef.

Magnesium

Magnesium is found in the bones as well as muscles and other soft tissues. Magnesium is needed for the formation of cartilage and bone and is involved in proper wound healing. Many Americans don't get enough magnesium. However, intake is, in most cases, not low enough to cause health problems.[47] Magnesium is found throughout the food supply. Good sources of magnesium include seeds, nuts, beans and peas, seafood, and dairy products.

TERMS

United States Pharmacopeia (USP)
A nongovernmental, official public standards–setting authority for prescription and over-the-counter medicines and other healthcare products manufactured or sold in the United States.

Choices for Your Daily Dairy

The importance of dairy products is clear; equally clear is that most people don't even get close to enough of what they need. However, it is important to choose lower-fat dairy products so you get all the benefits without the added fat and calories. Let's look at the various types of dairy on the market, examine how you can make healthy choices, and learn strategies for increasing dairy consumption.

Types of Milk

The dairy case offers many different kinds of milk from which to choose. Milk options differ based on fat content, fortification, and added flavors (**Table 9.4**). Addition of vitamin A or D is optional, but if added it must be present in 2,000 International Units (IU) and 400 IU per quart, respectively. State and local governments have established standards for milk. The following are the most common milk products available in North America:

- **Whole milk:** Contains no less than 3.25% milk fat.
- **Reduced-fat/low-fat milk:** Contains 1% or 2% milk fat.
- **Fat-free milk (skim milk):** Contains less than .05% milk fat.
- **Flavored milk:** Flavors such as chocolate, vanilla, or strawberry can be added to any milk with or without sweeteners and colors. Ingredients added to milk must be indicated on the label.

The best choice is fat-free, or skim, milk. Skim milk contains all the benefits of milk, such as calcium, protein, and vitamin D, without the fat. In fact, skim milk has more calcium than whole or low-fat milk. Although 2% or low-fat milk is certainly better than whole milk, it still has more calories, fat, and saturated fat than skim milk.

If you are used to drinking whole or low-fat milk, switching to fat-free milk can be quite a jolt to your taste buds. Make the switch gradually; select the next lowest fat milk to what you are currently drinking. Try that for

Raw Milk and Cheese: A Health Risk?

The French scientist Louis Pasteur developed the process of **pasteurization** to kill disease-causing organisms in milk and cheese. With pasteurization, milk or cheese is heated to a high temperature for a short period of time. This kills any harmful microorganisms that may be in the milk or cheese. However, the rise in temperature is brief enough that it does not change the nutritional quality of milk or cheese. Pasteur developed pasteurization to destroy bacteria that cause tuberculosis. Pasteurization continues today and provides protection from bacteria in milk and products made with milk.

Raw milk and milk products are those that have not been pasteurized. Each year people become seriously ill from consuming raw milk and milk products. Diarrhea, fever, and vomiting are typical symptoms associated with consumption of contaminated raw milk and milk products. Some states outlaw the sale of raw milk and products made with raw milk; however, some states allow it. Check with your state department of agriculture to see where your state falls on raw milk and cheese sales.

Some people actively seek out raw milk and cheese made with raw milk. Queso fresco, a Mexican-style soft cheese, is sometimes sold illegally or brought from other countries. Proponents of raw milk believe it to be nutritionally superior and want to see it legalized across the country. However, the Centers for Disease Control and Prevention, the U.S. Department of Agriculture, and the Department of Health and Human Services disagree and recommend that raw milk and milk products are to be avoided.[1,50] They state that only pasteurized milk and milk products be consumed to guard against illness from disease-causing bacteria that may be found in raw milk and milk products.

How Policy and Environment Affect My Choices

Starbucks

When you think of policy change, you may think of laws passed in Washington D.C. or your state capital. Policy change at that level is certainly important to create environments that are supportive of healthy eating and physical activity; however, don't underestimate the power of smaller policy changes made by individual companies, as was the case with Starbucks.

Prior to the end of 2007, if you walked into a Starbucks and ordered a grande latte, it would have been made with whole milk. A policy in all Starbucks in the United States and Canada changed that. Now, your drink will automatically be made with low-fat (2%) milk. You have always been able to specify that low-fat milk be used in your beverage, but it was not the default milk that it is today. Starbucks has stated that it made the switch based on increased requests from consumers for low-fat milk. The company also tested beverages made with whole milk and low-fat milk and found that customers liked the low-fat drinks better.

Starbucks offers an example of how a policy change by a company can make the healthier choice the default choice. Although you can still specify that you want your drink made with whole milk, if you do as most people do and order your drink without specifying the type of milk you want, you will automatically get a lower-fat option.

What does this change mean for the health of Starbucks customers? If you ordered a grande latte prior to the change without specifying the milk type, it would have been 260 calories. The same order today, with the default low-fat milk, is 190 calories. That is a savings of 70 calories. Although that doesn't sound like much, drink that latte every day for a week and you have a 490-calorie savings. Do this for a year and you have saved the number of calories equal to about 7 pounds.

a while and then go to the next lowest fat level until you get to skim milk. Children older than age 2 should also make the switch to low-fat or skim milk.

Nondairy Products

A variety of nondairy options are also good sources of calcium, including fortified soy milk, rice milk, and almond milk. Soy milk that is fortified with calcium is nutritionally similar to cow's milk. Soy milk is most often sweetened but is also available unsweetened or sweetened with low- or no-calorie sweeteners. Soy milk is naturally low in fat, but fat-free varieties are also available. Milk made from rice or almonds is also available sweetened, unsweetened, or sweetened with low- or no-calorie sweeteners. Most manufacturers of rice and almond milk fortify their products with calcium, vitamin A, and vitamin D, so these nutrients are found in similar amounts compared to cow's milk. The

TERMS

pasteurization A method of treating food by heating it to a certain point to kill disease-causing organisms, but not change the flavor or quality of the food. Milk is pasteurized by heating it to about 145 degrees F for 30 minutes or to 160 degrees F for 15 minutes. This technique is also used with beer, wine, fruit juices, cheese, and egg products.

Which Side Are You On?

Organic or Conventional Milk?

Organic milk is now widely available in most grocery stores across the country. Should you spend the extra money for milk that is certified organic? Is it more nutritious or safer than conventional milk? Controversy surrounds the answers to these questions, and depending on who you talk to organic milk is either a must buy for consumers or a waste of money. Let's take a closer look.

According to the U.S. Department of Agriculture, milk can only be labeled "organic" if the cows have been fed exclusively organic feed, have not been given synthetic hormones, have not been given antibiotics, are kept in pens with adequate space, and are allowed access to the outdoors.

Proponents of organic milk argue that these standards make the milk safer than conventional milk by controlling the antibiotic and hormone levels in the milk. Some people feel that giving cows fewer hormones and antibiotics results in milk that is safer. You can find much information on the Web about the improved safety of organic milk, but note that most of it is not supported by scientific evidence. Milk—conventional and organic—is one of the most tested foods on the grocery store shelf. Studies have found no meaningful difference in hormone or antibiotic content of organic versus conventional milk.[51]

What about nutritional composition? This is an easier one for you, the consumer, to check. A quick look at the nutrition labels on conventional and organic milk will reveal that they are identical with respect to their vitamin, mineral, and protein content. Fat content is also similar based on the type of milk in question.

One difference between organic and conventional milk is price. The higher cost for farms to follow the guidelines required to be certified organic means that organic milk carries a higher price tag.

Safety is similar, and nutrition is similar—why then does the demand for organic milk continue to increase, with an estimated 25% more certified organic cows each year since 2000?[52] Many consumers believe, in spite of evidence to the contrary, that organic milk is a safer and more wholesome product. Consumers also may make the organic choice based on how animals that are certified organic are treated, having access to pasture and less crowded conditions. Another reason to choose organic would be to support organic farming practices that are more environmentally friendly. Ultimately, the decision is up to you as to your choice of milk, organic or conventional. If cost is a factor, conventionally produced milk may be a better choice, because it delivers the same nutritional punch.

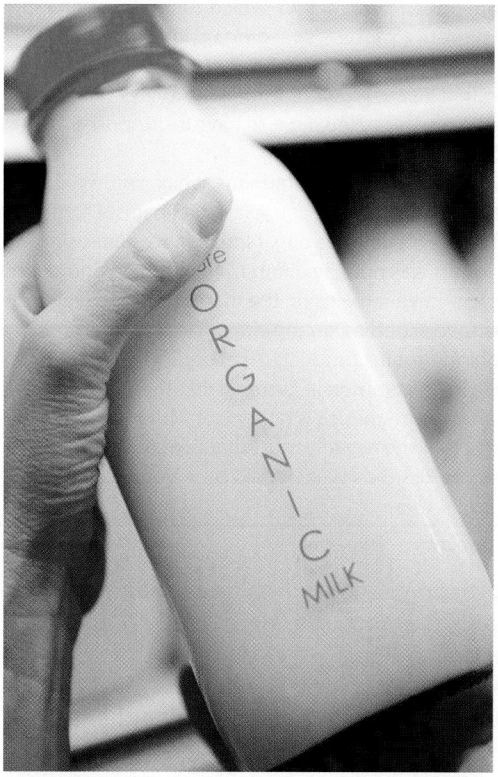

Organic Milk
"Organic" can only be used on the label if the cows have been fed exclusively organic feed, have not been given synthetic hormones, have not been given antibiotics, are kept in pens with adequate space, and are allowed access to the outdoors.

protein content of rice and almond milk, however, is lower than that in cow and soy milk. The taste of soy, rice, and almond milk is mild but different from cow's milk.

Types of Yogurt

The number of yogurts available in the grocery store is staggering. How do you choose the "right" one? Yogurts differ in the sweeteners used and in their fat content. Some have live cultures, and others claim to contain probiotics. Reading all the labels can be time consuming and confusing. Here are some factors to consider when choosing a yogurt:

Fat content: Choose a yogurt with no more than 4 grams of fat per serving. The fat in yogurt is dictated by the kind of milk used; more than 4 grams means whole milk was used to make the yogurt.

Calories: Calories in yogurt are dictated by the kind of milk used and the caloric sweeteners added. Some yogurts have added fruit or other toppings as well. Your calorie limit depends on how often you con-

Probiotics: Yogurt or Medicine?

Probiotics are "good" bacteria, similar to those found in the human intestinal tract. The most common carrier food for probiotics is yogurt. When yogurt is fermented by *Lactobacillus bulgaricus* and *Streptococcus thermophilus*, it becomes a probiotic. If that yogurt is not heated and the bacteria are allowed to stay in the product, the yogurt has live active cultures, or probiotics.

Recently, manufacturers have added other probiotics to yogurt to address specific health concerns. The most popular probiotic-added yogurts on the market are Activia and DanActive by Dannon.

Activia contains *Bifidus regularis*, which some claim can help regulate the digestive process, speeding up intestinal transit time and correcting occasional irregularity.[53–56] Specialists at Dannon modified *Bifidus regularis* so that it survives until it arrives in the colon, thus allowing it to have its proposed beneficial effects.

DanActive contains *L. casei* Immunitas, which some claim can improve immune function.[57–59] A lawsuit against Dannon claimed that the company was engaging in false advertising and that its yogurt was not any different than other yogurts on the market. DanActive remains on the market, but the labeling has been changed slightly. Dannon stands behind its claims about its probiotic yogurt products. Anecdotally, probiotic products have been common in Europe and other parts of the world for years; North America is rather late with regard to probiotics. Whether the use of yogurt that contains additional or different probiotics than what would be in yogurt with live active cultures is worth the extra money is ultimately up to the consumer. If sales of both of these products is any indication, many consumers think the potential benefits outweigh the extra cost.

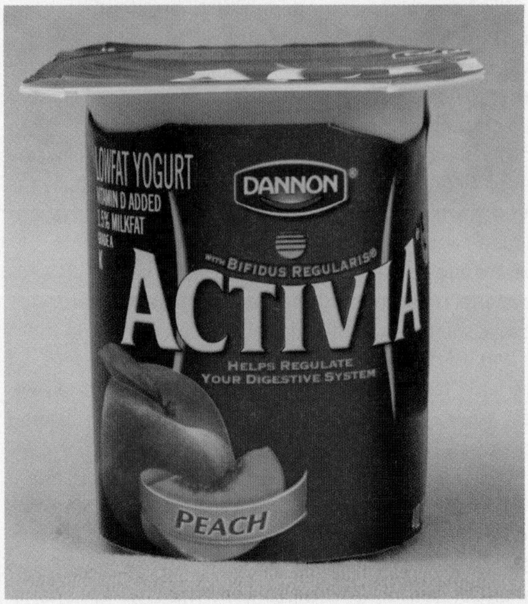

Yogurts on the Market That Contain Probiotics to Address Specific Health Concerns

sume yogurt and your overall calorie needs. A general rule of thumb is to choose a yogurt that is 150 calories per serving or less.

Artificial sweeteners or caloric sweeteners: All yogurts, except plain yogurt, are sweetened with either artificial sweeteners or some form of caloric sweetener such as sugar or high fructose corn sweetener. Some people don't enjoy yogurts sweetened with artificial sweeteners and prefer to consume yogurt sweetened with sugar or another caloric sweetener. Either is fine, as long as calorie level is kept in line.

Live active cultures: All yogurts start off containing *Lactobacillus bulgaricus* and *Streptococcus thermophilus*. These bacteria turn milk into yogurt during fermentation. These bacteria are what give yogurt its tart taste and creamy texture. Some yogurts are heated after fermentation, which can kill bacteria in the yogurt that are beneficial to the digestive system. The health benefits of live cultures include enhanced immune function and health of the digestive tract. Look for **live active cultures** on the label (**Figure 9.4**).

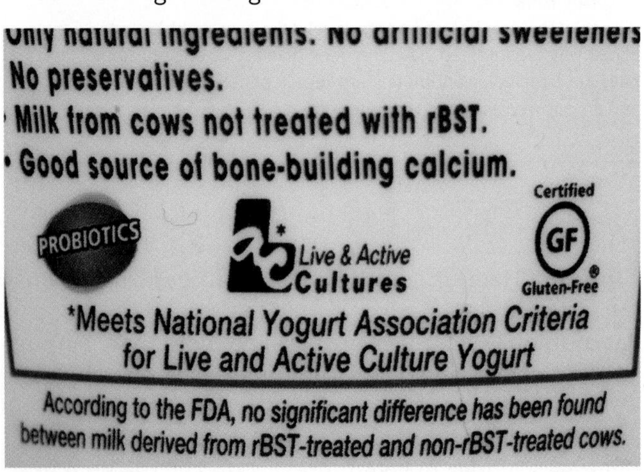
No preservatives.
Milk from cows not treated with rBST.
Good source of bone-building calcium.
Certified
PROBIOTICS
Live & Active Cultures
GF
Gluten-Free
*Meets National Yogurt Association Criteria for Live and Active Culture Yogurt
According to the FDA, no significant difference has been found between milk derived from rBST-treated and non-rBST-treated cows.

■ **Figure 9.4**

Live Active Cultures

Look for the Live & Active Cultures seal or the words "live active culture" on the label of the yogurt you buy.

TERMS

probiotics Microorganisms thought to be beneficial to health; commonly consumed as part of fermented foods such as yogurt.

live active cultures The bacteria *Lactobacillus bulgaricus* and *Streptococcus thermophilus* that convert milk to yogurt during fermentation. These can be killed if the yogurt is heat-treated during processing.

Try Something New

Greek Yogurt

Yogurt has been on supermarket shelves for decades. A relative newcomer to the yogurt aisle, at least in mainstream grocery stores in America, is Greek yogurt. Greek yogurt is made by straining yogurt to remove some of the liquid, or whey. This results in a thicker, creamier product. It is higher in protein and lower in carbohydrate than traditional yogurt. It usually is made with live active cultures, but check the label of the brand you choose to be certain. It comes in full-fat, low-fat, and fat-free varieties. The best thing about Greek yogurt is that even the fat-free version tastes rich and creamy. It is also available in flavors, but be sure to watch that you don't choose a brand with too much added sugar. Greek and traditional yogurts have about the same number of calories when similar products are compared (120 calories for 8 ounces of nonfat plain Greek yogurt versus 100 calories for 8 ounces of nonfat traditional yogurt).

Even if you are not a big fan of regular yogurt you will want to give Greek yogurt a try. Its rich, thick, creamy taste may make you a yogurt convert. If you are already a yogurt fan, try Greek yogurt for a change of pace. The extra protein helps to keep hunger away. You may also want to try Greek yogurt if you are lactose intolerant, because it typically has less lactose than traditional yogurt.

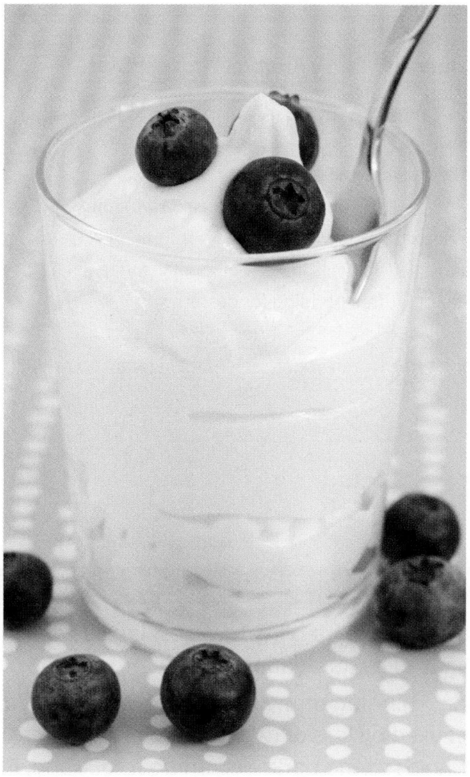

Greek Yogurt Is Thicker and Creamier Than Traditional Yogurt

Green and Healthy

Decrease Your Use of #5 Plastics

Yogurt is a healthy addition to your lunchbox and is great for a quick snack. But what about all of those plastic containers? Can they be recycled? Unfortunately, municipal recycling programs do not accept many yogurt and cottage cheese containers and other polypropylene #5 plastics, so they end up in the landfill. Look for the number on the bottom to see if it is a #5 container. Many companies now offer single-serving packs ready to grab and go, but are they a better choice? Often, they are made of #5 plastic as well.

You have a couple of options to get your dairy and stay green. The first option is to purchase large containers of yogurt and cottage cheese and portion them out into reusable containers for quick grab-and-go additions to lunches or snacks. Reuse the empty large containers to store leftovers, pens, screws, or other household needs. Or, you can find a place in your area that does accept #5 plastics. Many Whole Foods Market stores offer recycling of #5 plastics through a partnership with Preserve's Gimme 5 recycling program supported by Stonyfield Farm, Brita, Tom's of Maine, and Seventh Generation.

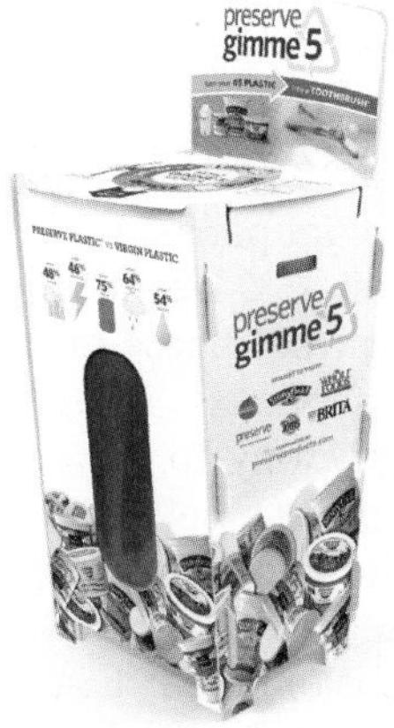

Some Stores Offer Recycling for #5 Plastics

Types of Cheese

Cheese is a food that dates back many centuries. The number of kinds of cheese available on the market today is almost limitless. France and other parts of Europe have a long history of producing a wide variety of cheeses. The famous quote from Charles De Gaulle of "How can you govern a country which has 246 varieties of cheese?" would fall short today, with France claiming over 600 varieties. North America is quickly catching up to our European neighbors with its variety of cheese on the market.

There are also many varieties of processed cheeses on the market. Cheese food has the addition of one or more dairy ingredients, such as cream or buttermilk. Cheese spread has added moisture and other ingredients, such as gum or gelatin, to allow the cheese to be spread more easily. Several types of lower-fat cheeses are also available.

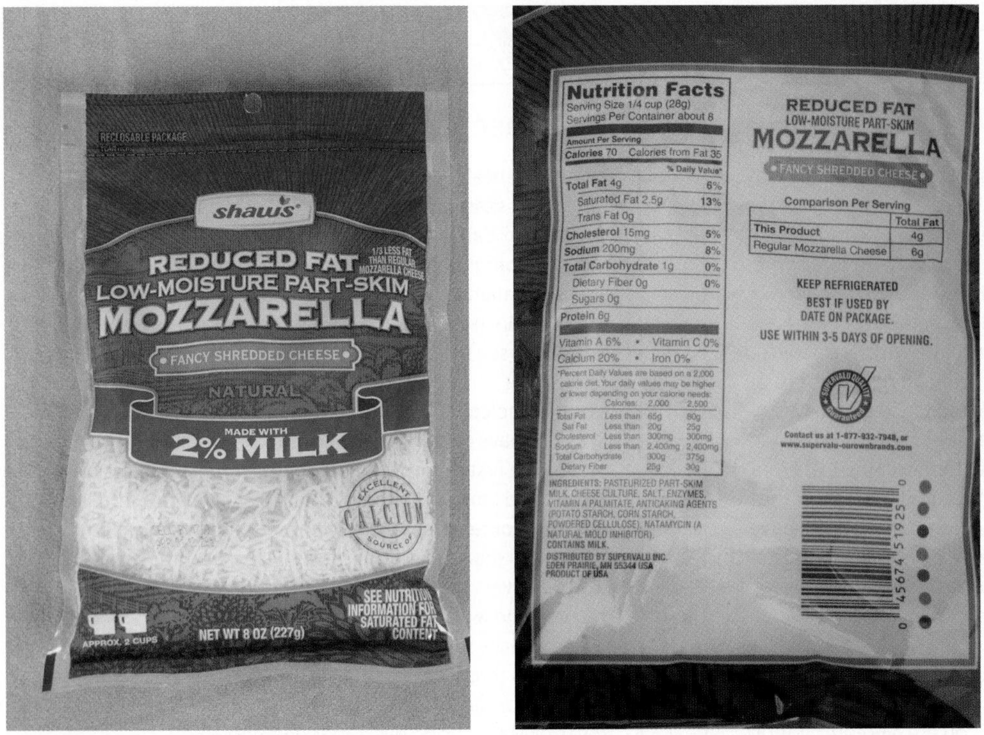

■ **Figure 9.5**

Reduced-Fat Cheese

Reduced-fat cheese must have at least 25% less fat than its full-fat version.

To qualify as a low-fat cheese, the cheese must contain no more than 3 grams of fat per serving. Reduced-fat cheese must contain at least 25% less fat than the full-fat version (**Figure 9.5**). Fat-free cheese must contain less than 0.5 grams of fat per serving.

Cheese is a tasty way to get your dairy. However, with all that taste comes a hefty dose of fat and calories. Although the specific calorie and fat content will depend on the type of cheese, most hard, full-fat cheeses have 150 calories and 12 grams of fat per 1.5 ounces.

You may want to try some of the low-fat cheeses on the market. Many brands now offer cheese made with 2% milk instead of whole milk. Part-skim varieties, such as part-skim mozzarella, that are slightly lower in fat and calories than full-fat cheese are also available. Getting all the dairy you need each day from cheese would make it difficult to stay within calorie and fat limits. Consume cheese in moderation and in smaller quantities. See **Table 9.5** for healthful strategies to increase the amount of dairy in your diet.

Lactose Intolerance

Milk and dairy products are supposed to be good for you, but what if they cause pain, bloating, gas, and diarrhea? If this sounds like you, you could be **lactose intolerant**. Lactose intolerance is the inability or decreased ability to digest lactose. Lactose is the sugar found in milk and products made with milk. Lactose intolerance is caused

Table 9.5

Strategies to Increase Dairy Products in Your Diet

The following are some easy strategies you can take to increase the amount of dairy in your diet:

- Choose fat-free milk as a beverage or snack.
- Eat yogurt with fruit for a quick, healthy breakfast or lunch.
- Add low-fat cheese to sandwiches, baked potatoes, or casseroles.
- Order a latte with fat-free milk instead of regular coffee.
- Choose low-fat or fat-free pudding for dessert.
- Make smoothies with low-fat or fat-free milk or yogurt.
- Try low-fat or fat-free frozen yogurt or ice cream for an occasional sweet treat.

TERMS

lactose intolerant An inability to digest lactose, or milk sugar, caused by inadequate lactase production.

osteoporosis Thinning of the bones with reduction in bone mass caused by loss of calcium and protein from bone, which leads to the bone becoming fragile and, in turn, increasing the risk in fractures.

osteopenia A bone mineral density that is lower than normal but not low enough to be classified as osteoporosis.

Special Report

Osteoporosis

We have all heard stories of someone's grandmother, perhaps even yours, who fell and broke her hip. What may have really happened is that she broke her hip and then fell due to a weakened hipbone. She may have had **osteoporosis**.

Osteoporosis is the most common bone disease in the United States. Osteoporosis is characterized by the loss of bone mass. This leads to brittle or fragile bones that are more likely to fracture. Breaking down the word *osteoporosis* can help us better define this disease. *Osteo* means "bone," and *porosis* means "porous," so osteoporosis literally means "porous bone." Healthy bones are denser and have only small open spaces, whereas osteoporotic bones have much larger open spaces in the their structure. The result is a bone that has less mass, is weaker, and is more easily broken. As the disease progresses, even a minor fall, or even just bending down to pick up a newspaper, can cause a fracture. Osteoporosis can affect any bone in the body; however, the most common sites for fractures related to the disease are the spine, wrist, and hip.

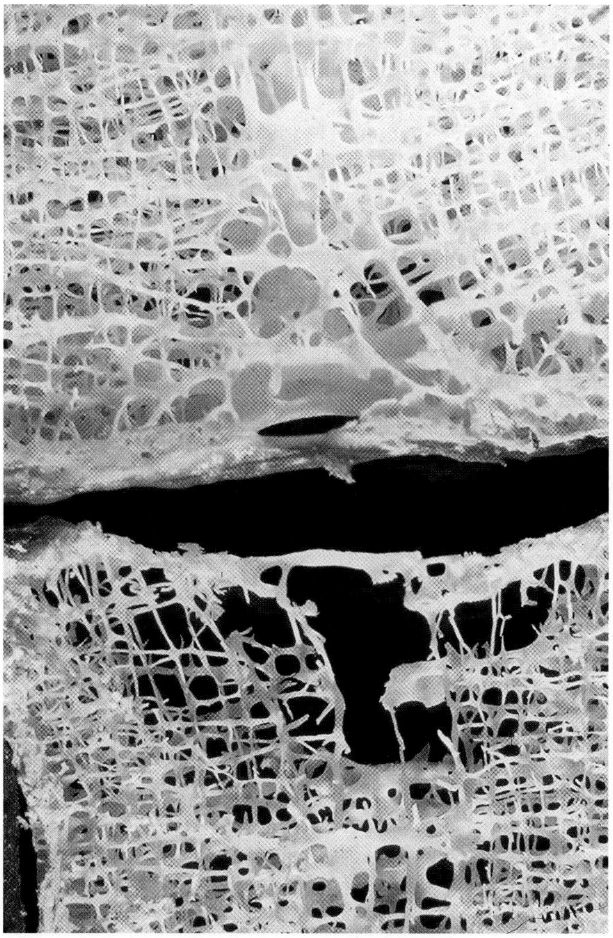

Normal Bone Versus One with Osteoporosis
Normal bone (top) compared to the bone of someone with osteoporosis (bottom). The healthy bone is much denser.

Osteoporosis is a major public health issue. Ten million people in the United States already have the disease, and another 34 million have low bone mass (**osteopenia**) that puts them at increased risk of the disease.[60] Osteoporosis causes 2 million bone fractures each year, which carries a price tag of $17 billion in healthcare costs and lost productivity.[61] It is estimated that by 2020 more than 14 million people in the United States will have osteoporosis.[61] This increase in incidence of the disease will be accompanied by a 50% increase in related costs.

Osteoporosis is usually thought of as a woman's disease. Approximately 80% of people in the United States with osteoporosis are female. Women are at a higher risk than men primarily because they are smaller and have less bone mass to lose. Hormone levels also play a role in bone loss. Estrogen has a protective effect on the bones; as women age and estrogen production decreases, the rate of bone loss can increase.

Women or men who have a small frame (under 130 pounds) are at an increased risk for osteoporosis. Osteoporosis is most common in people over the age of 50. Over half (55%) of people over the age of 50 have osteoporosis.[62] Osteoporosis is more prevalent among Caucasians and Asians; however, other ethnicities, including Hispanics and African Americans, also have high rates of osteoporosis.[64] The risk for osteoporosis is significant for people of all ethnic backgrounds. An inactive lifestyle or diet that is low in calcium and/or vitamin D increases the risk of osteoporosis. In addition, long-term use of steroids, certain anticonvulsants, anticoagulants, and lithium can also increase risk of osteoporosis. Check with your healthcare provider to assess the osteoporosis risk associated with certain medications.

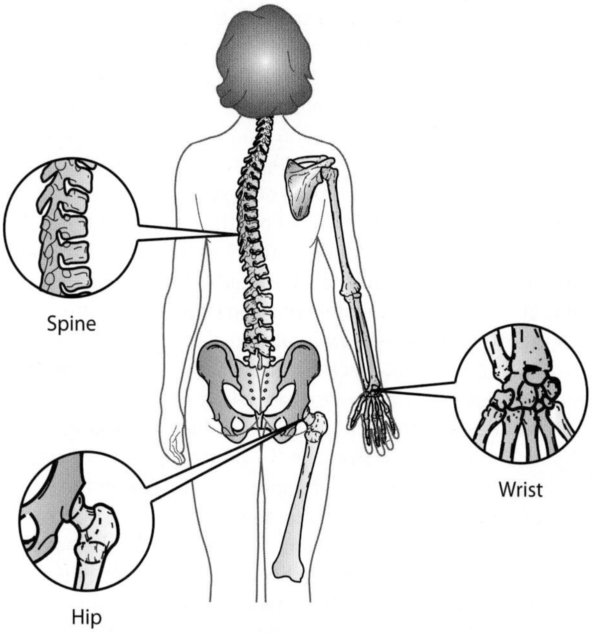

Common Sites for Fractures Caused by Osteoporosis

(continues)

Common Risk Factors for Osteoporosis

Being female
Over 50 years of age
Family history of osteoporosis
Small, thin frame
Caucasian, Asian, or Hispanic race
Low estrogen (including menopause)
Diet low in calcium and/or vitamin D
Inactive lifestyle
Smoking
Excessive alcohol consumption (more than two drinks/day)

Prevention of Osteoporosis

Osteoporosis can often be prevented. Although some of the risk factors of osteoporosis, such as aging, gender, and family history, are beyond your control, you can take steps to decrease your risk of, and in many cases prevent, osteoporosis.

One of the best ways to prevent osteoporosis is to build a high bone mass early in life. All during the life span, the skeleton loses old bone and grows new bone. Children and teens who are still growing add new bone at a higher rate than they are losing old bone. After youth stop growing taller they still add additional bone mass to make the bones denser and stronger until peak bone mass is reached. Peak bone mass usually occurs around age 20. That means the period between childhood and early adulthood is an important time to create a high peak bone mass. A healthy diet that contains optimal calcium, vitamin D, and other nutrients is important throughout life. However, it is critical during adolescence and early adulthood to make sure that the bone-building nutrients are consumed in adequate amounts.

Lifelong healthy eating is also important to keep bone loss to a minimum.[32] Make sure that calcium and vitamin D are consumed in adequate amounts throughout the life span. The first step is to assess what you are consuming now. Based on what you find, you may need to increase consumption of foods rich in calcium and vitamin D and/or talk with your healthcare provider to see if a supplement is needed. Other nutrients are involved in bone health, including magnesium, vitamin K, vitamin B_6, and vitamin B_{12}. A well-balanced diet will ensure that you are getting enough of all of these nutrients for optimal bone health. If you do not get the amount of these nutrients you need from food, a multivitamin may be in order, although it is not a substitute for a healthy diet. Consume a diet that is adequate in protein but don't overdo it. High-protein diets can interfere with calcium absorption.

Bone mass is also affected by how active you are. Weight-bearing and resistance exercise can help maintain strong, healthy bones. Weight-bearing exercises such as walking, jogging, or running put stress on the bones and are associated with helping maintain bone strength.[63–65] The higher the impact of the exercise, the greater the benefit to the bones. Although exercises such as swimming are great for the heart and lungs, they do not promote bone health, because they are not weight bearing. Resistance training, such as weight lifting using free weights or weight machines, is also good for maintaining bone mass.[65] Exercise that uses your body weight for resistance, such as yoga and Pilates, will also help build and maintain strong bones. It is also important to include flexibility and balance exercise in your physical activity routine. Although they may not decrease bone loss, they will help decrease the risk of falls, and thus may decrease the risk of fractures in someone who already has osteopenia or osteoporosis.

Hormone Replacement Therapy

Hormones have an effect on how well bone mass is maintained. In women, the hormone estrogen protects against bone loss. As women approach menopause, estrogen levels begin to drop and then fall sharply after menopause. This drop causes a loss of bone mass. Hormone replacement therapy has been shown to reduce the risk for osteoporosis-related hip fractures and other fractures in postmenopausal women.[66] Replacing hormones by a pill or patch to help slow bone loss is an option for some women. However, there are risks associated with hormone replacement therapy, such as an increased risk of cardiovascular disease, stroke, and some forms of cancer. The risks and benefits of hormone replacement should be discussed with a healthcare provider.

Just as there are things you can do to prevent osteoporosis, namely eat healthy foods and be active, some lifestyle choices increase the risk of osteoporosis. Tobacco use is associated with a higher incidence of osteoporosis.[60,67,68] Smoking decreases calcium absorption and in women can prevent estrogen from having a protective effect on bones.[60,69] So, if you don't smoke, don't start, and if you do smoke, quit for your overall health and the health of your bones. For help in quitting smoking call 1-800-QUITNOW. Alcohol in moderation is fine for bone health. More than two drinks per day, however, is associated with an increased risk of osteoporosis.[60,68,70]

Five Steps to Bone Health and Osteoporosis Prevention

1. **Eat smart.** Get your daily recommended amounts of calcium and vitamin D.
2. **Move more.** Engage in regular weight-bearing and muscle-strengthening exercise.
3. **Maintain a healthy lifestyle.** Avoid smoking and excessive alcohol consumption.
4. **Talk to your healthcare provider.** Talk to your healthcare provider about bone health.
5. **Get tested.** Have a bone density test and take medication, when appropriate.

Source: National Osteoporosis Foundation. National Osteoporosis Foundation five steps to bone health and osteoporosis prevention. http://www.nof.org/aboutosteoporosis/prevention. Accessed April 9, 2011.

Another step to preventing osteoporosis is to talk to your healthcare provider about your specific risk factors. He or she can offer suggestions to help ensure that you do all you can to promote good bone health and suggest testing and medication, if indicated.

Early Detection of Osteoporosis

Several of the risk factors for osteoporosis are beyond your control. Even with a healthy diet and physical activity, osteoporosis can occur. Osteoporosis can be present without any signs or symptoms. Detecting osteoporosis early so treatment can begin and be most effective is important. A bone mineral density (BMD) test analyzes the amount of bone mineral present in the bone being measured. BMD testing can be done on different bones in the body, such as the hip, spine, wrist, or heel. A BMD test is the only way to detect low bone density or to diagnosis osteopenia or osteoporosis. Several different kinds of BMD testing are available; the type recommended by the National Osteoporosis Foundation is dual-energy x-ray absorptiometry (DEXA), which measures the bone density of the spine, hips, or total body.[71]

BMD testing may be done for several reasons. People at risk of osteoporosis should be tested. Also, long-term use of medications known to compromise bone health may indicate that a BMD test be done. Women aged 65 and men aged 70 and older should be screened routinely for osteoporosis. Women under age 65 and men aged 50–70 who have risk factors such as bone fracture caused by normal activity, early menopause, loss of height, or a strong family history of osteoporosis should also be screened.[72] A healthcare provider may suggest that a person be tested for other reasons as well. Tests are repeated every two to five years, depending on the outcome of the test.

The BMD test results are compared to what would be a healthy 30-year-old adult with peak bone density. The result from the BMD test is a number called a T-score. The World Health Organization defines normal bone as having a T-score between +1.0 and −1.0, osteopenia as a T-score between −1.0 and −2.5, and osteoporosis as a T-score of less than −2.5.

The results of a BMD test can help to inform treatment options. No treatment is needed if the score is in the normal range. Osteopenia may indicate that osteoporosis medication is needed if other risk factors are present. A person with a score that indicates very low bone mass or osteoporosis should strongly consider taking osteoporosis medication. Several osteoporosis medications are available that slow bone loss and can even build bone mass. In addition to pharmacological treatment, a healthy diet with optimal levels of calcium and vitamin D and weight-bearing physical activity are important.

by a deficiency of the enzyme lactase. The disaccharide lactose is too large to be absorbed by the intestine and must be broken down by lactase into the two monosaccharides glucose and galactose. Without lactase, lactose passes through the intestine and causes pain, bloating, gas, diarrhea, and/or nausea. Symptoms usually occur 30 minutes to 2 hours after consuming milk or products made with milk. The severity of symptoms depends on the level of lactose intolerance and the amount of milk or milk products consumed.

Lactose intolerance is a relatively common condition and occurs in about 25% of U.S. adults.[20] Some ethnic populations are more prone to lactose intolerance. For example, the incidence of lactose intolerance is higher among African Americans, Hispanic Americans, American Indians, and Asian Americans. An estimated 85% of Asian Americans and 50% of African Americans are lactose intolerant.[20] Although many people self-diagnosis lactose intolerance, symptoms of lactose intolerance are similar to other digestive disorders, such as irritable bowel syndrome. To accurately diagnose lactose intolerance, a healthcare provider can order a hydrogen breath test. This test examines the amount of hydrogen in the breath after ingestion of a beverage high in lactose. Undigested lactose causes high levels of hydrogen in the breath.

Consumption of milk and products made with milk, such as cheese and yogurt, is needed for optimal health. Avoiding milk and dairy products has health consequences, such as increased risk of osteoporosis. If you are lactose intolerant, you can take steps to make sure you get the nutrients you need. Following are several suggestions to stay healthy if you are lactose intolerant:

- **Consume small amounts of dairy.** Most people who are lactose intolerant can tolerate some milk and milk products.
- **Try yogurt.** Often yogurt, especially with active cultures, is better tolerated than milk.
- **Choose lactose-free milk.** Most grocery stores now carry lactose-free milk. This specialty milk has the lactose already broken down to glucose and galactose. It tastes very similar to regular milk and can be consumed by anyone, even if they are not lactose intolerant.
- **Use lactase tablets.** Lactase drops or tablets can be taken just prior to the consumption of a meal that contains lactose.
- **Choose soy, rice, or almond milk.** These contain no lactose. Choose a brand that is fortified with calcium and vitamin D.
- **Consume hard cheeses, such as cheddar or Swiss.** Hard cheeses are low in lactose and high in calcium. Keep in mind that cheese is also high in fat, so moderation is important.
- **Take a supplement, if needed.** Consider taking a supplement to make sure that you get adequate calcium and vitamin D.

Ready to Make a Change

Are you ready to make a change, small or large, in the amount and type of dairy products in your diet? Make the commitment to take the first step. Whether it is a small, medium, or large change, it is a step in the right direction toward a healthier diet.

I commit to a small first step. Change your milk. If you usually drink whole milk, switch to 2%. If 2% is what you usually drink, switch to fat-free milk. You can do this gradually to help your taste buds adjust. Mix half of the milk you are used to drinking with half of the milk you want to start consuming. Eventually you will be drinking low-fat or fat-free milk.

I am ready to take the next step and make a medium change. Try adding some additional dairy products to your diet. Chances are you are not getting three servings a day. Try adding at least one additional serving each day of yogurt, milk, or cheese.

I have been making changes for some time and am ready to make a large change in the dairy products in my diet. One of the best things you can do to improve the nutrient content of your overall diet is to make sure you get three servings of dairy products each day. Commit to three servings on most days of the week. Start your day off with milk as a beverage or on your cereal, add cheese to your sandwich at lunch, and choose pudding or yogurt for dessert after dinner, and you are well on your way to three servings a day of dairy.

Myth Versus Fact

Myth: I get plenty of calcium since I eat lots of green vegetables.

Fact: Green vegetables, particularly dark-green leafy green vegetables like collard greens, do contain calcium. However, it would be close to impossible to eat enough each day to fulfill your calcium requirement. Substances in some vegetables, such as fiber, phytates, and oxalates, make it difficult for the body to absorb calcium. Keep eating green vegetables, because they provide more benefits than just calcium. But, for optimal calcium intake, be sure to include dairy as well.

Myth: Milk and other dairy products are only important during childhood.

Fact: Milk and other dairy products are critical during childhood to promote growth of bones. However, another critical period is adolescence and early adulthood. Bone mass continues to form even after maximum height is reached. Peak bone mass is not be reached until age 20 or even later. A high bone mass will serve you well later in life when bone mass tends to decline. Consumption of foods high in calcium and vitamin D, such as dairy products, is important at all stages of life.

Myth: Low-fat milk is lower in calcium than regular milk.

Fact: Low-fat and fat-free milk are higher in calcium than whole milk. Some of the volume in whole milk is displaced by fat, which has no calcium.

Myth: If you are watching your weight, dairy products should be limited.

Fact: Consuming fewer calories than you use leads to weight loss. However, cutting out dairy products is not the way to go. If you are trying to lose weight or just want to make sure your weight stays in check, choose lower-calorie low-fat or fat-free dairy products and limit high-fat cheeses.

Myth: I don't like milk or yogurt; a good substitute is to choose cheese for all the servings of dairy I need each day.

Fact: Three servings of high-fat cheese would add up to lots of fat and calories. Cheese is fine on occasion and in small amounts. However, consuming the 4.5 ounces a day you would need to get your three servings is too much high-fat cheese on a daily basis. Experiment with different types of yogurt, add milk to cereal, or make smoothies with milk or yogurt.

Back to the Story

Now that you know more about osteopenia, osteoporosis, calcium, and dairy products, you can suggest several steps that Alice can take to protect against following in her mother's footsteps. First, she needs to include milk and dairy products in her diet. Cheese a couple of times a week is nowhere near what is recommended. She almost certainly is not getting the recommended amount of calcium or vitamin D. Consumption of adequate dairy products at this point in her life is critical to build a high peak bone mass. If consuming dairy products is not something she is willing to add to her diet, she may want to consider taking a calcium and/or vitamin D supplement. If she is not physically active, she should add some weight-bearing exercise to her routine to help further with building strong bones. Finally, because she has a family history of osteopenia, she should discuss when she should get a baseline bone scan with her physician. Many of the risk factors for osteopenia/osteoporosis are beyond your control. However, there are several steps Alice can take now and throughout her life to decrease the risk or delay the onset of osteoporosis. What other suggestions do you have for Alice?

References

1. US Department of Health and Human Services and US Department of Agriculture. *Dietary Guidelines for Americans, 2010*, 7th ed. Washington, DC: US Government Printing Office, December 2010.
2. Cook A, Friday J. Pyramid Servings Intakes in the United States, 1999–2002. Beltsville, MD: Agricultural Research Service, US Department of Agriculture, 2005. http://www.ars.usda.gov/sp2UserFiles/Place/12355000/foodlink/ts_3-0.pdf. Accessed November 10, 2009.
3. Heaney RP. Dairy and bone health. *J Am Col Nutr*. 2009;28(1):82S–90S.
4. Heaney RP. Calcium, dairy products and osteoporosis. *J Am Coll Nutr*. 2000;19(2Suppl):83S–99S.
5. Ranganathan R, Nicklas TA, Yang SJ, Berenson GS. The nutritional impact of dairy product consumption on dietary intakes of adults (1995–1996): the Bogalusa Heart Study. *J Am Diet Assoc*. 2005;105:1391–1400.
6. Fulgoni V, Nicholls J, Reed A, et al. Dairy consumption and related nutrient intake in African-American adults and children in the United States: continuing survey of food intakes by individuals 1994–1996, 1998, and the National Health and Nutrition Examination Survey 1999–2000. *J Am Diet Assoc*. 2007;107:256–264.
7. Cheng S, Lyytikainen A, Kroger H, et al. Effects of calcium, dairy product, and vitamin D supplementation on bone mass accrual and body composition in 10–12-y-old girls: a 2-y randomized trial. *Am J Clin Nutr*. 2005;82:1115–1126.
8. Moschonis G, Manios Y. Skeletal site-dependent response of bone mineral density and quantitative ultrasound parameters following a 12-month dietary intervention using dairy products fortified with calcium and vitamin D: the Postmenopausal Health Study. *Br J Nutr*. 2006;96:1140–1148.
9. Manios Y, Moschonis G, Trovas G, Lyritis GP. Changes in biochemical indexes of bone metabolism and bone mineral density after a 12-mo dietary intervention program: the Postmenopausal Health Study. *Am J Clin Nutr*. 2007;86:781–789.
10. Huncharek M, Muscat J, Kupelnick B. Impact of dairy products and dietary calcium on bone-mineral content in children: results of a meta-analysis. *Bone*. 2008;43:312–321.
11. Lamarche B. Review of the effect of dairy products on non-lipid risk factors for cardiovascular disease. *J Am Col Nutr*. 2008;27(6):741S-746S.
12. Kris-Etherton PM, Grieger JA, Hilpert KF, West SG. Milk products, dietary patterns and blood pressure management. *J Am Col Nutr*. 2009;28(1):103S–119S.
13. Elwood PC, Givens DI, Beswick AD, Fehily AM, Pickering JE, Gallacher J. The survival advantage of milk and dairy consumption: an overview of evidence from cohort studies of vascular diseases, diabetes and cancer. *J Am Coll Nutr*. 2008;27(6):723S–734S.
14. VanLoan M. The role of dairy foods and dietary calcium in weight management. *J Am Col Nutr*. 2009;28(1):120S–129S.
15. Pereira MA, Jacobs DR, Van Horn L, Slattery ML, Katashov AI, Ludwig DS: Dairy consumption, obesity, and the insulin resistance syndrome in young adults: the CARDIA study. *JAMA*. 2002;287:2081–2089.
16. Jacqmain M, Doucet E, Despres JP, Bouchard C, Tremblay A. Calcium intake, body composition, and lipoprotein-lipid concentrations in adults. *Am J Clin Nutr*. 2003;77:1448–1452.
17. Zemel MB, Thompson W, Milstead A, Morris K, Campbell P. Calcium and dairy acceleration of weight and fat loss during energy restriction in obese adults. *Obes Res*. 2004;12:582–590.
18. Zemel MB, Richards J, Russell A, Milstead A, Gehardt L, Silva E. Dairy augmentation of total and central fat loss in obese subjects. *Int J Obes*. 2005;29:341–347.
19. Zemel MB, Richards J, Milstead A, Campbell PJ. Effects of calcium and dairy on body composition and weight loss in African American adults. *Obes Res*. 2005;13:1218–1225.
20. Institute of Medicine, Food and Nutrition Board. *Dietary Reference Intakes for Calcium and Vitamin D*. Washington, DC: National Academies Press, 2010.
21. Ervin RB, Wang CY, Wright JD, Kennedy-Stephenson J. Dietary intake of selected minerals for the United States population: 1999–2000. Advanced data from *Vital and Health Statistics*, number 341. Hyattsville, MD: National Center for Health Statistics, 2004.
22. Moshfegh A, Goldman J, Ahuja J, Rhodes D, LaComb R. *What We Eat in America, NHANES 2005–2006: Usual Nutrient Intakes from Food and Water Compared to 1997 Dietary Reference Intakes for Vitamin D, Calcium, Phosphorus, and Magnesium*. Washington, DC: US Department of Agriculture, Agricultural Research Service, 2009.
23. Schroder BG, Griffin IJ, Specker BL, Abrams SA. Absorption of calcium from the carbonated dairy soft drink is greater than that from fat-free milk and calcium-fortified orange juice in women. *Nutr Res*. 2005;25:737–742.
24. Holick MF, Garabedian M. Vitamin D: photobiology, metabolism, mechanism of action, and clinical applications. In: Favus MJ, ed. *Primer on the Metabolic Bone*

Diseases and Disorders of Mineral Metabolism, 6th ed. Washington, DC: American Society for Bone and Mineral Research, 2006:129–137.
25. Bouillon R. Vitamin D: from photosynthesis, metabolism, and action to clinical applications. In: DeGroot LJ, Jameson JL, eds. *Endocrinology*. Philadelphia: W.B. Saunders, 2001:1009–1028.
26. Hruska KA. Hyperphosphatemia and hypophosphatemia. In: Favus MJ, ed. *Primer on the Metabolic Bone Diseases and Disorders of Mineral Metabolism*, 6th ed. Washington, DC: American Society for Bone and Mineral Research, 2006:233–242.
27. Garland CF, Garland FC, Gorham ED, et al. The role of vitamin D in cancer prevention. *Am J Public Health*. 2006;96:252–261.
28. Gorham ED, Garland CF, Garland FC, et al. Vitamin D and prevention of colorectal cancer. *J Steroid Biochem Mol Biol*. 2005;97:179–194.
29. Giovannucci E, Liu Y, Rimm EB, et al. Prospective study of predictors of vitamin D status and cancer incidence and mortality in men. *J Natl Cancer Inst*. 2006;98:451–459.
30. Ahonen MH, Tenkanen L, Teppo L, Hakama M, Tuohimaa P. Prostate cancer risk and prediagnostic serum 25-hydroxyvitamin D levels (Finland). *Cancer Causes Control*. 2000;11:847–852.
31. Feskanich D, Ma J, Fuchs CS, et al. Plasma vitamin D metabolites and risk of colorectal cancer in women. *Cancer Epidemiol Biomarkers Prev*. 2004;13:1502–1508.
32. Holick MF. Calcium plus vitamin D and the risk of colorectal cancer. *N Engl J Med*. 2006;354:2287–2288.
33. Zittermann A. Vitamin D and disease prevention with special reference to cardiovascular disease. *Prog Biophys Mol Biol*. 2006;92:39–48.
34. Melamed ML, Muntner P, Michos ED, et al. Serum 25-hydroxyvitamin D levels and the prevalence of peripheral arterial disease. Results from NHANES 2001–2004. *Art Thromb Vasc Biol*. 2008;28:1179–1185.
35. Lee JH, O'Keefe JH, Bell D, Hensrud DD, Holick MF. Vitamin D deficiency: An important, common, and easily treatable cardiovascular risk factor? *J Am Coll Cardiol*. 2008;52:1949–1956.
36. Rostand SG. Ultraviolet light may contribute to geographic and racial blood pressure differences. *Hypertension*. 1997;30:150–156.
37. Martins D, Wolf M, Pan D, et al. Prevalence of cardiovascular risk factors and the serum levels of 25-hydroxyvitamin D in the United States: data from the Third National Health and Nutrition Examination Survey. *Arch Intern Med*. 2007;167:1159–1165.
38. Scragg R, Sowers M, Bell C. Serum 25-hydroxyvitamin D, ethnicity, and blood pressure in the Third National Health and Nutrition Examination Survey. *Am J Hypertens*. 2007;20:713–719.
39. Gloth FM, Alam W, Hollis B. Viamin D vs. broad spectrum phototherapy in the treatment of seasonal effective disorder. *J Nutr Health Aging*. 1999;3:5–7.
40. Hoogendijk WJG, Limp P, Dik M, Deeg DJH, Beedman ATF, Pennix BWJ. Depression is associated with decreased 25-hydroxyvitamin D and increased parathyroid hormone levels in older adults. *Arch Gen Psychiatry*. 2008;65(5):508–512.
41. Scragg R, Sowers M, Bell C. Serum 25-hydroxyvitamin D, diabetes, and ethnicity in the Third National Health and Nutrition Examination Survey. *Diabetes Care*. 2004;27:2813–2818.
42. Holick MF. Vitamin D deficiency. *N Engl J Med*. 2007;357:266–281.
43. Looker AC, Dawson-Hughes B, Calvo MS, Guner EW, Sahyoun NR. Serum 25-hydroxyvitamin D status of adolescents and adults in two seasonal subpopulations from NHANES III. *Bone*. 2002;30:771–777.
44. Marks R, Foley PA, Jolley D, Knight KR, Harrison J, Thompson SC. The effect of regular sunscreen use on vitamin D levels in an Australian population. Results of a randomized controlled trial. *Arch Dermatol*. 1995;131(4):415–421.
45. Calvo MS, Whiting SJ, Barton CN. Vitamin D fortification in the United States and Canada: current status and data needs. *Am J Clin Nutr*. 2004;80:1710S–1716S.
46. Holick MF. Vitamin D: A millennium perspective. *J Cell Biochem*. 2003;88:296–307.
47. Bischoff-Ferari HA, Giovannucci E, Wilett WC, Dietrich T, Dawson-Hughes B. Estimation of optimal serum concentrations of 25-hydroxyvitamin D for multiple health outcomes. *Am J Clin Nutr*. 2006;84:18–28.
48. Straub DA. Calcium supplementation in clinical practice: a review of forms, doses, and indications. *Nutr Clin Pract*. 2007;22:286–296.
49. National Institutes of Health Osteoporosis and Related Bone Diseases—National Resource Center. Calcium supplements: what to look for. http://www.niams.nih.gov/Health_Info/Bone/Bone_Health/Nutrition/calcium_supp.asp. Updated January 2011. Accessed April 20, 2011.
50. Centers for Disease Control and Prevention. Raw milk and cheeses: Health risks are still black and white. http://www.cdc.gov/healthypets/cheesespotlight/cheese_spotlight.htm. Updated July 28, 2010. Accessed April 20, 2011.
51. Vicini J, Etherton T, Dris-Etherton P, et al. Survey of retail milk composition as affected by label claims regarding ram-management practices. *J Am Diet Assoc*. 2008;108:1198–1203.
52. McBride WD, Greene C. Characteristics, costs, and issues for organic dairy farming. ERR-82, U.S. Department of Agriculture, Economic Research Service, 2009.
53. Picard C, Fioramonti J, Francois A, Robinson T, Neant F, Matuchansky C. Review article: bifidobacteria as probiotic agents—physiological effects and clinical benefits. *Aliment Pharmacol Ther*. 2005;22(6):495–512.
54. Bouvier M, Meance S, Bouley C, Berta JL, Grimaud JC. Effects of consumption of a milk fermented by

the probiotic *Bifidobacterium animalis* DN-173 010 on colonic transit time in healthy humans. *Bioscience and Microflora*. 2001;20(2):43–48.

55. Marteau P, Cullerier E, Meance S, et al. *Bifidobacterium animalis*, strain DN-173 010 shortens the colonic transit time in healthy women. A double-blind randomized controlled study. *Aliment Pharmacol Ther*. 2002;16:587–593.
56. Méance S, Cayuela C, Turchet P, Raimondi A, Lucas C, Antoine JM. A fermented milk with *Bifidobacterium* probiotic strain DN-173 010 shortened oro–fecal gut transit time in elderly. *Microb Ecology Health Dis*. 2001;13:217–222.
57. Pedone CA, Bernabeu AO, Postaire ER, Bouley CF, Reinert P, Danone, CIRDC. The effect of supplementation with milk fermented by *Lactobacillus casei* (strain DN-114 001) on acute diarrhoea in children attending day care centres. *Int J Clin Pract*. 1999;53:179–184.
58. Pedone CA, Arnaud CC, Postaire ER, Bouley CF, Reinert P, Danone, CIRDC. Multicentric study of the effect of milk fermented by Lactobacillus casei on the incidence of diarrhoea. *Int J Clin Pract*. 2000;54:568–571.
59. Turchet P, Laurenzano M, Auboiron S, Antoine JM. Effect of fermented milk containing the probiotic *Lactobacillus casei* DN-114 001 on winter infections in free-living elderly subjects: a randomized, controlled pilot study. *J Nutr Health Aging*. 2003;7:75–77.
60. US Department of Health and Human Services. *Bone Health and Osteoporosis: A Report of the Surgeon General*. Rockville, MD: U.S. Department of Health and Human Services, Office of the Surgeon General, 2004.
61. Burge R, Dawson-Hughes B, Solomon DH, Wong JB, King A, Tosteson A. Incidence and economic burden of osteoporosis-related fractures in the United States, 2005–2025. *J Bone and Mineral Res*. 2007;22(3):465–475.
62. National Osteoporosis Foundation. Osteoporosis fast facts. http://www.nof.org/node/40. Accessed April 20, 2011.
63. Warburton DER, Nicol CW, Bredin SSD. Health benefits of physical activity: the evidence. *CMAJ*. 2006;174(6):801–809.
64. Warburton DE, Gledhill N, Quinney A. The effects of changes in musculoskeletal fitness on health. *Can J Appl Physiol*. 2001;26:161–216.
65. Bonaiuti D, Shea B, Iovine R, Negrini S, Robinson V, Kemper HC, Wells G, Tugwell P, Cranney A. Exercise for preventing and treating osteoporosis in postmenopausal women. *Evid Based Nurs*. 2003;6(2):50–51.
66. National Institutes of Health. Women's Health Initiative. http://www.nhlbi.nih.gov/whi/. Accessed November 4, 2009.
67. US Department of Health and Human Services. *The Health Consequences of Smoking: A Report of the Surgeon General*. Atlanta, GA: U.S. Department of Health and Human Services, Centers for Disease Control and Prevention, National Center for Chronic Disease Prevention and Health Promotion, Office on Smoking and Health, 2004.
68. McGlynn, KA, Gridley G, Mellemkjaer L, et al. Risks of cancer among a cohort of 23,935 men and women with osteoporosis. *Int J Cancer*. 2008.122(8):1879–1184.
69. Tansavatdi K, McClain B, Herrington DM. The effects of smoking on estradiol metabolism. *Minerva Ginecol*. 2004;56(1):105–114.
70. Grisso JA, Kelsey JL, Strom BL, et al. The Northeast Hip Fracture Study Group. Risk factors for hip fracture in black women. *N Engl J Med*. 1994;330(22):1555–1559.
71. National Osteoporosis Foundation. BMD testing, what the numbers mean. http://216.247.61.108/osteoporosis/bmdtest.htm. Accessed April 20, 2011.
72. US National Library of Medicine, National Institutes of Health. Medline Plus. Bone mineral density test. www.nlm.nih.gov/medlineplus/ency/article/007197.htm. Updated December 22, 2010. Accessed May 3, 2011.

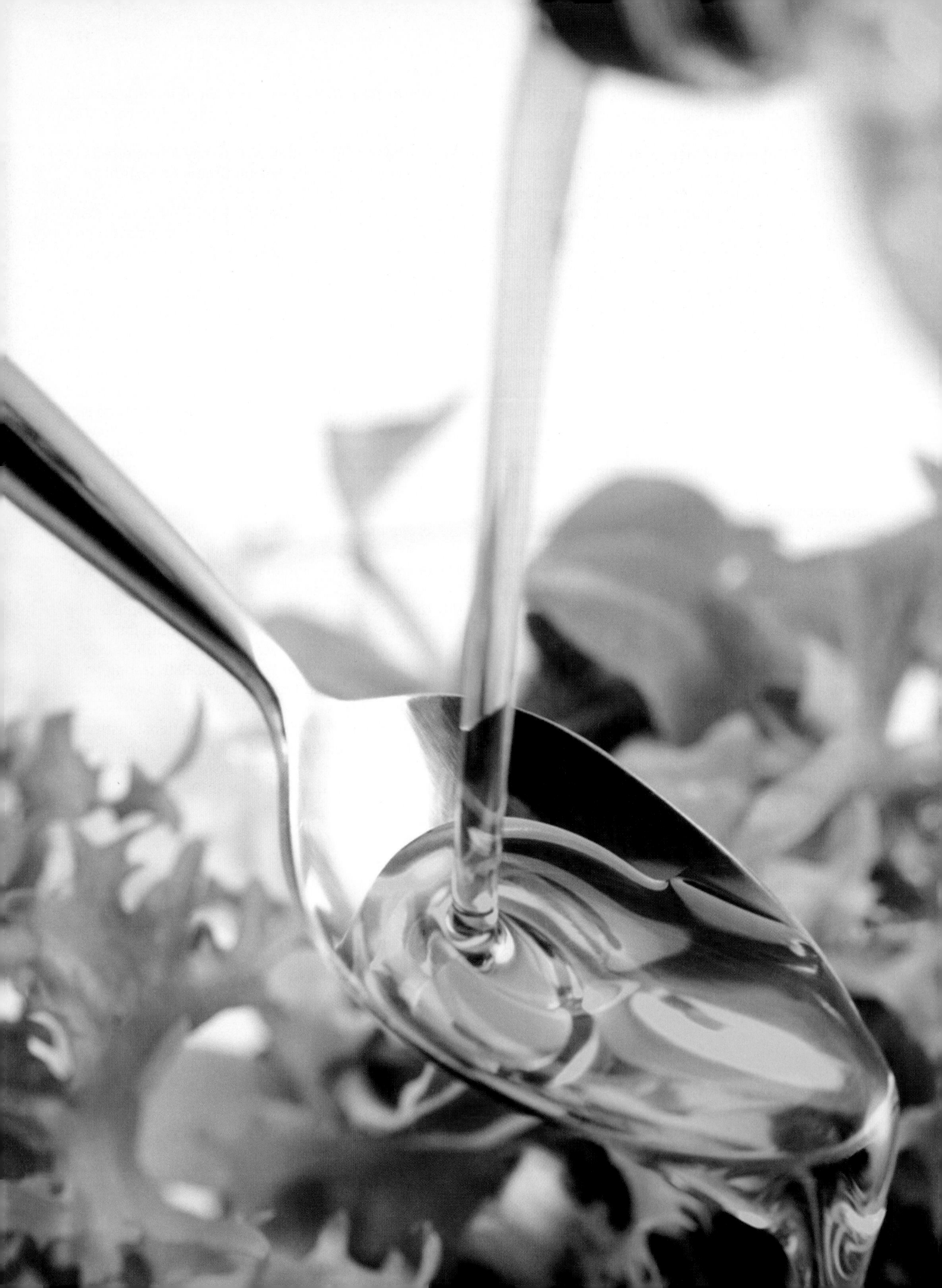

Chapter 10

Fats and Oils: A Little Goes a Long Way

Key Messages

- Fats are a dense form of energy.
- Choose fats wisely for a healthy diet.
- Low fat does not always mean healthy.
- A moderate-fat diet, low in saturated fat, can reduce the risk of heart disease.

"Don't eat butter, it is too high in animal fat; eat margarine instead." "Wait, margarine can have trans fats that are really bad, so better stick with butter." "Don't eat anything with hydrogenated fat in it." "Low-fat diets are the way to lose weight and be healthy." "No, go low-carb, don't worry about fat." Few nutrition messages are more complicated than those about fat. Even the terms are confusing—*polyunsaturated, saturated, hydrogenated*. Perhaps it is because fats are complex and require some careful examination to reveal the whole truth. There are fats in your diet, some good and some bad, and fats in your body, some good and some bad. We will discuss all of these in this chapter.

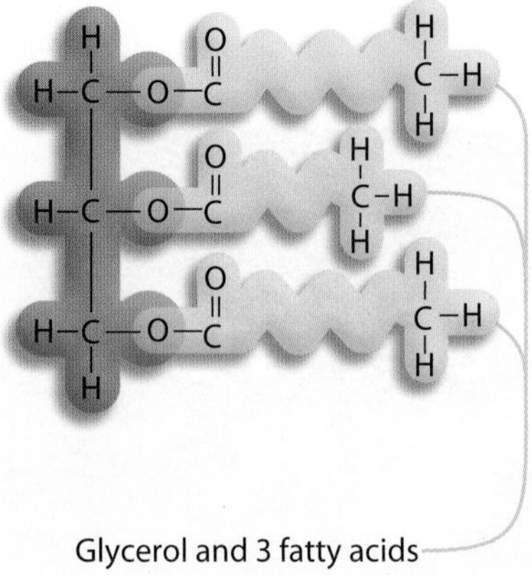

Figure 10.1
A Triglyceride Molecule

Story

Jane is 22 and considers herself to be very healthy. Her father had a heart attack a few months ago at age 52. Jane's grandfather died of a heart attack at age 65. The doctor who treated Jane's dad said there was a strong history of heart disease in Jane's family. Jane was worried that she could be heading for heart disease later in life. She went to her doctor to check out how she was doing. She found out that she is 20 pounds overweight and has borderline high cholesterol. How can this be when she feels fine and has plenty of energy? What can Jane do now to decrease her risk of heart disease later in life?

Functions of Fat

Fat is often demonized as something you should avoid in your diet. With all the negative talk about fat, it may be easy to overlook the fact that it has specific functions in your body and is essential for optimal health (**Table 10.1**). Fat acts as an energy reserve in the body for use between meals or during times of physical activity. The body stores small amounts of carbohydrate and protein. Fat, however, can be stored easily in fat cells throughout the body. Each pound of fat contains 3,500 calories. You can store 20–30 pounds of fat without even being overweight. Fat is a component of every cell membrane in the body. Fat nourishes the skin and hair, keeping your skin supple and your hair shiny. **Subcutaneous fat** acts as insulation, protecting the body from extreme heat and cold. Fat also protects the vital organs by cushioning them from trauma. The pad of fat that covers the kidneys is a good example of this. Fat also carries fat-soluble nutrients, such as the fat-soluble vitamins A, D, E, and K. Because these nutrients are soluble only in fat, their absorption is increased by fat. For example, the vitamin A in carrots is better absorbed if it is eaten in a salad that also contains olive oil.

Table 10.1

Functions of Fat

Provides energy reserves
Serves as the primary component of cell membranes
Nourishes skin and hair
Insulates body from extreme temperatures
Cushions vital organs
Transports fat-soluble vitamins and essential fatty acids

Types of Fats

The three main classes of fats are triglycerides, phospholipids, and sterols.

Triglycerides

About 95% of the fat in your body is triglycerides. A triglyceride is a glycerol molecule with three fatty acids attached (**Figure 10.1**). Triglycerides are further classified based on how the fatty acids are held or bonded together (**Figure 10.2**). A fatty acid is a carbon chain with an acid at one

TERMS

subcutaneous fat Body fat that acts as insulation, protecting the body from extreme heat and cold.

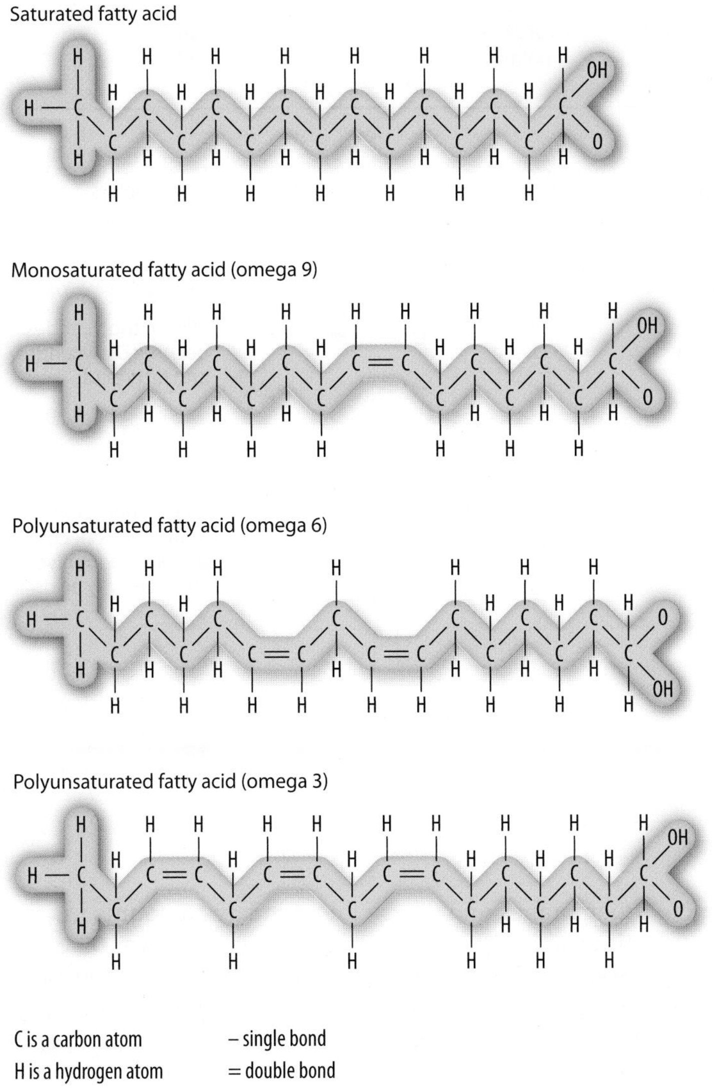

Figure 10.2
Types of Fatty Acids

end with hydrogen atoms attached all along the way to each carbon. A carbon atom has four bonds that must be occupied by another atom. If it is a **saturated fatty acid**, the bonds between all of the carbon atoms will be single bonds, thus the fatty acid is saturated with hydrogen. No more bonds are available for hydrogen. If the fat is unsaturated, one or more of the bonds between the carbon atoms will be double bonds, thus there are not as many hydrogen atoms as in the saturated fatty acid.

Monounsaturated fatty acids have one double bond; **polyunsaturated fatty acids** have two or more double bonds. Polyunsaturated fats are further classified based on where the double bonds occur. Counting from the end of the carbon chain without the acid attached (the omega end), the number of the carbon containing the first double bond will dictate the type of fat. If the first double bond occurs at the third carbon, it is an **omega-3 fatty acid**; if the first double bond occurs at the sixth carbon, it is an **omega-6 fatty acid**.

Phospholipids

Phospholipids are similar to triglycerides in that they have fatty acids and glycerol. Phospholipids have two fatty acids attached to a glycerol backbone, but instead of a third fatty acid that you would see in a triglyceride, they contain a phosphate. The phosphate is soluble in water but the two fatty acids are not. This property of having both water-soluble and fat-soluble properties makes phospholipids good emulsifiers. An emulsifier is a substance that helps fat suspend in water. In your body, phospholipids are essential components of cell membranes. Phospholipids also help in transporting lipids in the blood to where they need to go in the body.

The body can easily make phospholipids, so they are not essential in the diet.

Phospholipids are found naturally in many of the foods you eat. Soybeans, peanuts, and egg yolks

TERMS

saturated fatty acid A fatty acid with the maximum possible number of hydrogen atoms. Saturated fats are usually solid at room temperature and are found in meat, poultry, dairy products, and tropical oils (coconut and palm).

monounsaturated fatty acid A fatty acid with one double bond between two carbon atoms. Monounsaturated fats are found in peanuts, peanut oil, safflower oil, olives, olive oil, canola oil, and avocados and are liquid at room temperature.

TERMS

polyunsaturated fatty acid A fatty acid with two or more double bonds between two carbon atoms. Polyunsaturated fats are found in fatty fish, nuts, most vegetable oils, and soybeans and are liquid at room temperature. There are different types of polyunsaturated fats depending on where the double bonds between the carbon atoms are located.

omega-3 fatty acid A polyunsaturated fatty acid that has the first double bond three carbons from the endmost (omega) carbon in the chain. Omega-3 fatty acids are found in fatty fish and flaxseed.

omega-6 fatty acid A polyunsaturated fatty acid that has the first double bond six carbons from the endmost (omega) carbon in the chain. Omega-6 fatty acids are found in most vegetable oils.

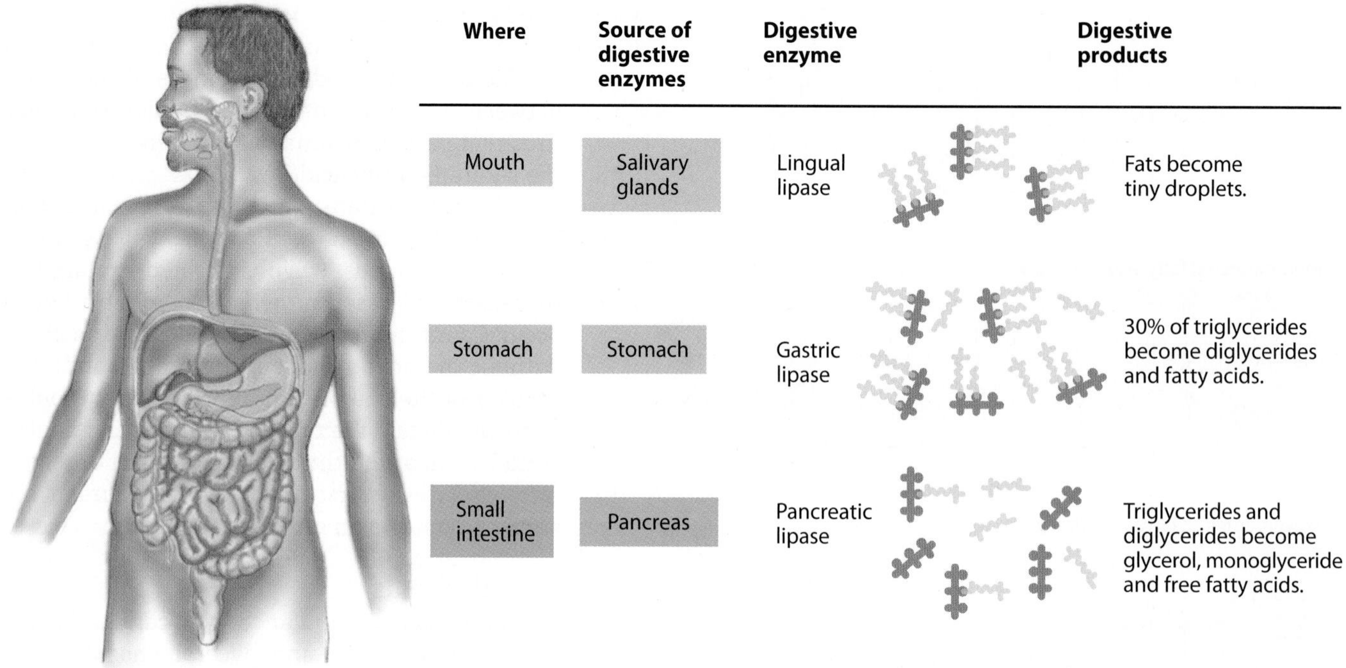

Where
Source of digestive enzymes
Digestive enzyme
Digestive products
Mouth
Salivary glands
Lingual lipase
Fats become tiny droplets.
Stomach
Stomach
Gastric lipase
30% of triglycerides become diglycerides and fatty acids.
Small intestine
Pancreas
Pancreatic lipase
Triglycerides and diglycerides become glycerol, monoglyceride and free fatty acids.

Figure 10.3
Digestion of Fat

all contain phospholipids. The phospholipids in egg yolks allow for the addition of oil and lemon juice to form mayonnaise. The egg yolk acts as an emulsifier, pulling the watery lemon juice and oil together as an emulsion. The food industry uses phospholipids as emulsifiers. One of the most common emulsifiers used by the food industry is lecithin, which is derived from soybeans. Lecithin is used in salad dressings, marinades, chocolate, baked goods, and other products as an emulsifier.

Sterols

Sterols are very different in structure from triglycerides or phospholipids. Both triglycerides and phospholipids have a glycerol backbone and at least two fatty acids. In contrast, sterols are composed of multiple rings, and most have no triglycerides at all. The most common sterol in your body is cholesterol. When you hear the word *cholesterol*, it most likely brings to mind disease, specifically heart disease. However, cholesterol is a very important substance in your body. It is a component of all cell membranes and can be found in large amounts in organ tissues, such as those in the brain and liver. The body uses cholesterol to create bile, which is needed for fat digestion, as well as vitamin D and some hormones. The body can produce all the cholesterol it needs, so it is not required in the diet.

TERMS

lingual lipase An enzyme secreted by the salivary glands that begins the breakdown of fat in the mouth.

gastric lipase An enzyme secreted by the stomach that breaks down triglycerides into diglycerides and fatty acids.

Digestion and Absorption of Fat

The digestion and absorption of fat is unique because the digestive enzymes and blood are watery substances and fat is not water soluble. The body is equipped to handle the digestion and absorption of fat even with its hydrophobic properties. Digestion of fat begins in the mouth as chewing, body heat, and **lingual lipase** begin to break down fat. As it moves into the stomach, **gastric lipase** further breaks down fat, as triglycerides become diglycerides and fatty acids. The bulk of fat digestion occurs in the small intestine (**Figure 10.3**).

When fat enters the small intestine, the hormone **cholecystokinin (CCK)** is secreted. CCK signals your **pancreas** to secrete **pancreatic lipase** so that fat can be further broken down in the small intestine. CCK also signals to your **gallbladder** to release **bile** into the small intestine (**Figure 10.4**). Bile coats fat molecules and keeps them from forming large fat globules that would be hard for your body to absorb. The small fat globules formed by bile and fat are called **micelles**. Micelles ferry fat to the wall of your small

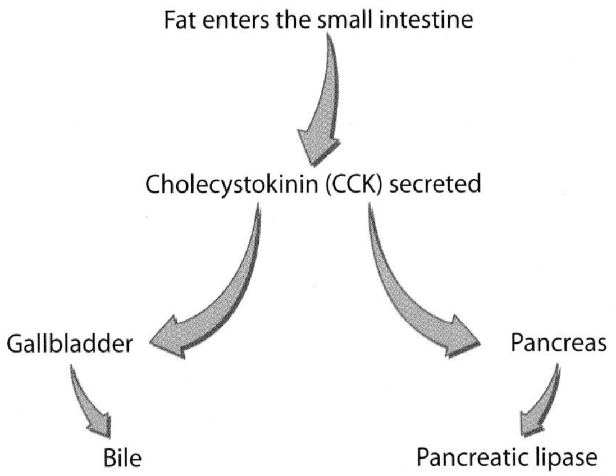

■ **Figure 10.4**

Fat in the Small Intestine Signals the Release of CCK, Bile, and Pancreatic Lipase

intestine so it can be absorbed. Inside the intestinal cells, long-chain fatty acids are repackaged into **chylomicrons**. Short-chain fatty acids, medium-chain fatty acids, and glycerol are absorbed directly into the blood. The bile goes back into your small intestine to form another micelle and bring more fat to the intestinal cells. The chylomicrons travel via your lymph system to the bloodstream, and ultimately to adipose tissue and your liver. Lipoprotein lipase breaks apart the chylomicrons so that the fat can be converted back into a triglyceride and used as energy by the muscles or stored as energy in your adipose tissue (**Figure 10.5**).

Cholesterol is digested and absorbed differently than other fats. Digestion does very little to break down cholesterol. Cholesterol is very poorly absorbed, with only 50% absorbed by the body. Cholesterol absorption declines even further if it is eaten in a meal that contains fruits, vegetables, or whole grains.

TERMS

cholecystokinin (CCK) A hormone produced by the intestine that stimulates the secretion of bile from the gallbladder and pancreatic lipase from the pancreas.

pancreatic lipase An enzyme secreted by the pancreas into the small intestine that breaks down triglycerides and diglycerides into monoglycerides and free fatty acids.

pancreas An organ that produces digestive enzymes and hormones, including insulin.

gallbladder A nonessential organ that stores and concentrates bile from the liver.

bile A mixture of compounds, including bile salts, bile acids, and lecithin, made by the liver and stored and concentrated in the gallbladder. Bile is secreted into the small intestine to help emulsify fats and transport them to the intestinal wall so they can be absorbed.

micelle Monoglycerides and free fatty acids surrounded by bile. Micelles allow for the transport of fat to the intestinal wall.

chylomicrons Large lipoprotein particles that allow fat to travel in the bloodstream. They contain triglycerides and small amounts of cholesterol and phospholipids and have an outer coating of protein.

very-low-density lipoprotein (VLDL) A type of lipoprotein, very high in triglycerides, that releases triglycerides to cells.

low-density lipoprotein (LDL) Often referred to as "bad cholesterol," it transports cholesterol and triglycerides from the liver to other tissues. Remember *L* for *lousy* cholesterol.

high-density lipoprotein (HDL) Often referred to as "good cholesterol," it is high in protein and picks up cholesterol from inside the arteries. Remember *H* for *healthy* cholesterol.

Fat in Your Body

To move in the water-based environment of the bloodstream, the fat must be packaged into lipoproteins. Lipoproteins have a core of fat surrounded by a protein layer. The protein outer layer creates a water-soluble package that allows the fat to travel in the bloodstream. There are several different types of lipoproteins (**Figure 10.6**).

One type of lipoprotein we have already discussed, chylomicrons, are very large lipoproteins that are composed of large amounts of triglycerides and a small amount of cholesterol.

Very-low-density lipoprotein (VLDL) is high in triglycerides. The liver assembles VLDL. As the VLDL circulates in the bloodstream, it is broken down by lipoprotein lipase, providing triglycerides to cells. A diet high in saturated fat will cause the liver to produce more VLDL.

Low-density lipoprotein (LDL) has a high level of cholesterol. LDL attaches to cells on special receptors, providing cholesterol to the cells, which is then used to make cell membranes and hormones.

LDL is sometimes called the "bad cholesterol" because high LDL levels in the blood can increase the risk of heart disease. Over a period of time, high LDL levels can cause cholesterol to build up on the artery walls, which results in the formation of plaque. This plaque makes the walls of the artery thick and narrow. Plaque buildup on the artery walls may interfere with blood flow to the heart and over time cause heart damage or a heart attack. You can remember that LDL is the bad cholesterol by thinking of *L* for *lousy*.

High-density lipoprotein (HDL) is sometimes called the "good cholesterol." You can remember HDL as the good cholesterol by thinking of *H* for *healthy*. In contrast to LDL, HDL protects against cholesterol buildup on the blood vessels. HDL is high in protein and low in cholesterol. It travels the bloodstream and gathers cholesterol

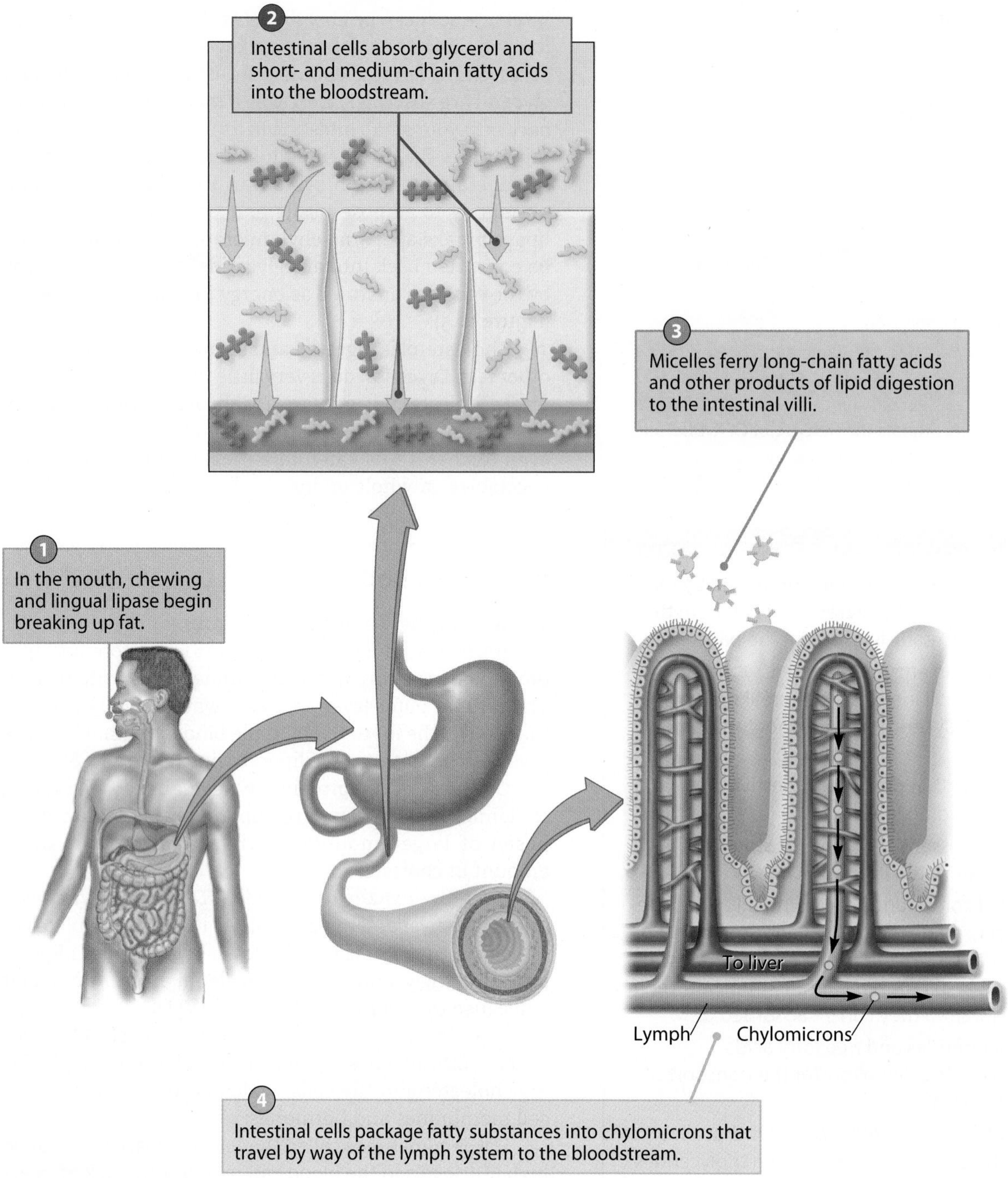
2
Intestinal cells absorb glycerol and short- and medium-chain fatty acids into the bloodstream.
3
Micelles ferry long-chain fatty acids and other products of lipid digestion to the intestinal villi.
1
In the mouth, chewing and lingual lipase begin breaking up fat.
To liver
Lymph
Chylomicrons
4
Intestinal cells package fatty substances into chylomicrons that travel by way of the lymph system to the bloodstream.

■ **Figure 10.5**
Digestion and Absorption of Fat

from dying cells. High HDL levels are associated with a decreased risk of heart disease.

Recommended and Actual Intake of Fat

An Acceptable Macronutrient Distribution Range (AMDR) for fat is between 20–35% of calories.[1,2] To calculate the percent of calories from fat in your diet, you need to know the number of grams of fat you consumed and the number of calories you consumed in a day (**Figure 10.7**). The specific number of grams of fat that would be appropriate to consume each day depends on your usual calorie consumption (**Table 10.2**).

The type of fat that you consume—saturated, monounsaturated, polyunsaturated, or **trans fat**—is more important in influencing the risk of cardiovascular disease than is the total amount of fat in the diet.[2] Saturated fat has been strongly linked to high LDL levels. As saturated fat in the diet goes up, so do LDL levels.[1–11] Because LDL levels are associated with an increased risk of heart disease,

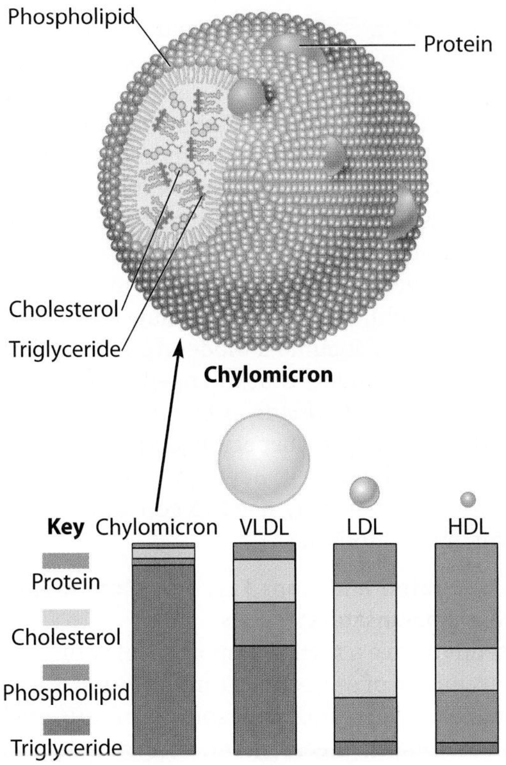

■ **Figure 10.6**

Lipoproteins Vary in Size and Composition

the amount of saturated fat in the diet needs to be monitored carefully. It is recommended that consumption of saturated fat be less than 10% of calories.[1,2] The American Heart Association recommends an even lower threshold of no more than 7% of calories from saturated fat.[4] Thus, most of the fat you eat should come from monounsaturated and polyunsaturated fats. It recommended that you keep trans fat consumption as low as possible.

Dietary cholesterol should be limited to 300 milligrams per day. Dietary cholesterol has been shown to raise LDL cholesterol in some people; however, the effect is reduced when saturated fat is low. The negative effect

It is suggested that 20–35% of your calories should come from fat.

How to calculate:

Step 1: Grams of fat × 9 calories = calories from fat

Note: the value "9 calories" is a standard unit of measure and does not change. A gram of carbohydrate contains 9 calories.

Step 2: Calories from fat/total calories × 100 = % calories from fat

Grams of fat

Total calories

% calories from fat

■ **Figure 10.7**

How to Calculate Percent Calories from Fat

Table 10.2

Recommended Fat Consumption Based on Calorie Intake

Fat consumption should be between 20–35% of calories, with no more than 10% of calories from saturated fat.

Total Calorie Intake	20% of Calories from Fat	35% of Calories from Fat	Maximum Saturated Fat Intake (10% of calories)
1,600	36 grams	62 grams	≤ 18 grams
2,000	44 grams	78 grams	≤ 22 grams
2,200	49 grams	86 grams	≤ 24 grams
2,500	56 grams	97 grams	≤ 28 grams
2,800	62 grams	109 grams	≤ 31 grams

of dietary cholesterol is relatively low compared to the effect of saturated fat.[2]

Current Intake of Fat

Now that you know how much and what kind of fat you should be eating, let's examine what we currently eat as a nation. Over the past 30 years, the number of calories consumed by both men and women has increased significantly. This is of interest, because fat in the diet is characterized as a percentage of calories. Over the same 30-year period, fat consumption has decreased from 36% to 33% of calories.[12–15] Although the percentage of fat has decreased, the actual amount of fat eaten has gone up because of the higher calorie intake. Also, the amount of fat eaten as part of prepared and packaged foods has increased.[15] Saturated fat intake has decreased from an average of 13% to 11%. Again, however, actual intake of saturated fats has gone up, because the total number of calories increased during this period.[12,13] Keep in mind that this is an average intake. A closer look at saturated fat intake reveals that only 42% of Americans consume the recommended less than 10% of calories from saturated fat.[16,17] This means that more than half of all Americans consume more saturated fat than they should. Most of this saturated fat comes from high-fat cheese and meat.[14]

Fat in Your Diet

Fat is a dense source of energy and has more than twice the number of calories per gram than carbohydrates or

TERMS

trans fat A type of fat that is formed when hydrogen is added to a liquid fat to form a solid or semisolid fat. Trans fats are also found naturally in small amounts in dairy and meat. Consumption of trans fats is linked to an increased risk of heart disease.

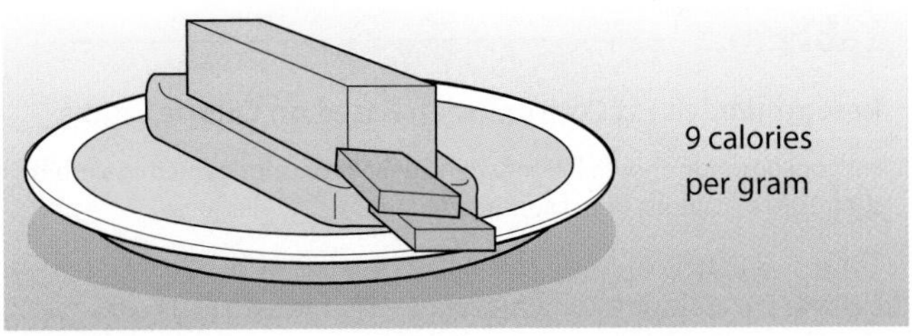

■ **Figure 10.8**

Fat Is a Dense Source of Calories

Fat has 9 calories per gram, whereas carbohydrate and protein have 4 calories per gram.

proteins (**Figure 10.8**). Fat has 9 calories per gram, whereas carbohydrates and proteins have 4 calories per gram. Just a few bites of a high-fat food can deliver a hefty dose of calories. Fat provides satiety in your diet. It is digested more slowly than either proteins or carbohydrates, so it makes you feel full longer. A plain bagel in the morning for breakfast may mean mid-morning hunger because the bagel is primarily carbohydrate. Add some cream cheese to the bagel and your hunger may be delayed for hours longer. Of course, you would be consuming more calories as well.

Fat performs several very important functions in food. First and foremost, it makes our food taste good. Fat is the magic carpet that carries flavor to our taste buds. Adding fat to a sauce or using oil to fry a food accentuates the flavor of the food. Chefs and restaurant cooks are keenly aware of this; it is one reason why eating out can mean a high-fat meal. Fat also helps make baked goods tender and flaky. Biscuits, cakes, and piecrust are all tender because fat coats the flour molecules. This is why low-fat cookies are harder and lower-fat biscuits can be tough. Fat also provides a distinct mouth feel to foods such as sauces, cream soups, and ice cream.

Choose Fat Wisely

A great deal of research has examined fat and its relationship to health. In the 1970s and 1980s, epidemiological studies suggested that a very low fat diet was the pathway to health. Populations in Africa and Asia were healthy and had almost no heart disease while consuming an ultra-low-fat diet.[18–21] Experts concluded that a fat-free diet was the key to a long life free of chronic disease. Continued examination of fat's role in the diet of people in developed countries has revealed that the quality of the fat is as important, or maybe even more important, than the quantity consumed.[1,2] Your diet should be low in saturated and trans fats and higher in monounsaturated and polyunsaturated fats.

Balancing the quantity and quality of fat in your diet is key for overall good health. Choose wisely from each food group so that you consume a moderate-fat diet, but also one that has the good fats that you need (**Table 10.3**). You should think of high-fat foods as being "sometimes" or "rarely" foods. Elimination of specific foods is not necessary to have a healthy diet. If, however, a food is high in fat or saturated fat, you may need to consume it less frequently or in small amounts.

Choose Less Saturated and Trans Fats and More Monounsaturated and Polyunsaturated Fats

Animal fats tend to have a higher proportion of saturated fat (with the exception of seafood). Saturated fats are usually solid at room temperature. Major sources of saturated fat in the diet are butter, cheese, meat, poultry, desserts, and snack foods.[2] Choose lower fat cuts of meat to help keep total fat and saturated fat in line. See **Figures 10.9**

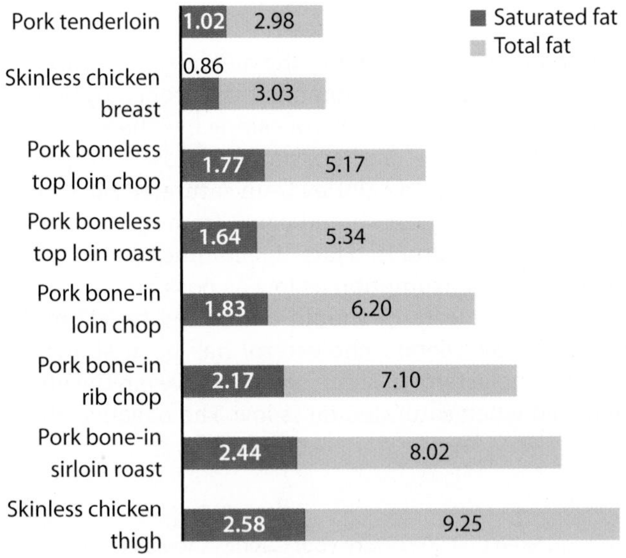

■ **Figure 10.9**

Total Fat and Saturated Fat in Cuts of Pork and Chicken

Source: National Pork Board, http://www.porkandhealth.org/filelibrary/porkandhealth/porkandchickencomparisonhandout.pdf. Accessed April 9, 2011.

> ## Essential Fatty Acids
>
> Your body needs a number of different types of fatty acids. Your body can make most of the different fatty acids you need from carbohydrates, proteins, and fats or they may be present in the diet. **Essential fatty acids**, however, cannot be made by your body and must be present in your diet. The two essential fatty acids are alpha linolenic and linoleic. Both are found in fish and plant oils. They also can be stored by your body, thus deficiencies are rare.

TERMS

essential fatty acids Fatty acids that are needed but cannot be made by the body and must be obtained in the diet.

Table 10.3

Low-Fat Options from Each Food Group

Anytime	Sometimes	Rarely
Meat and beans		
Lean ground beef (90–96% lean)	Ground beef (80–90% lean)	Ground beef (70–85% lean)
Lean cuts of beef (cuts with round or loin in the name; i.e., eye of round or top round)	Moderate-fat cuts of beef (e.g., chuck roast, brisket, flank steak)	High-fat cuts of beef (e.g., ribs, heavily marbled steaks)
Poultry without skin	Poultry with skin	Fried poultry
Fish	Chicken, tuna, or egg salad with low-fat mayo	Fried fish
Canned fish packed in water	Low-fat hot dog	Regular hot dog
Lean pork	Canadian bacon	Bacon
Egg whites	Eggs	Sausage
Beans	Baked beans	Pork BBQ
Veggie (soy or bean) burgers	Nuts	
Tofu	Peanut butter	
	Seeds	
Grains		
Whole-grain cereal	Waffles or pancakes	Pastries
Oatmeal	Low-fat muffin	Doughnut
Grits	Cornbread	Sweet-muffin
Sandwich bread	Stuffing	Biscuit
Pita bread	Pretzels	Hard taco shell
Tortillas	Baked chips	Croissant
Pasta	Granola bar	Hush puppies
Rice	Crackers	Regular chips
Popcorn without butter		Popcorn with butter
Whole-grain, low-fat crackers		Cookies
Vegetables and fruit		
Fresh vegetables or fruit with no added fat	Vegetables or fruit with small amount of added fat, such as butter, dip, cream cheese, etc.	Vegetables or fruit in butter, cream sauce, or cheese sauce
Frozen vegetables or fruit with no added fat	Cole slaw, potato salad, or fruit salad made with low-fat dressing	Fried vegetables, such as French fries, hash browns, onion rings
Canned vegetables or fruit with no added fat	Avocado and guacamole	Cole slaw, potato salad, or fruit salad made with regular dressing
		Fruit pies or cobblers
		Coconut
Milk		
Nonfat milk (skim)	Reduced fat milk (2%)	Whole milk
Low-fat milk (1/2–1%)	Low-fat yogurt	Cheese
Soy milk	Part-skim or reduced-fat cheese	Cheese spread
Nonfat yogurt	Low-fat frozen yogurt or ice cream	Ice cream
Fat-free or low-fat cottage cheese	Low-fat pudding	

* Choose frozen and canned vegetables and fruit with no added sugar. Although sugar does not affect the fat content, it does add calories with no nutritional benefit.

and **10.10** for the total fat and saturated fat content of different meats.

Plant foods have a higher proportion of unsaturated fat (with the exception of coconut oil, palm kernel oil, and palm oil). Monounsaturated and polyunsaturated fats are liquid at room temperature. Foods that are high in monounsaturated fat include safflower oil, canola oil, olives, olive oil, peanut oil, and avocados. Foods high in polyunsaturated fat include soybean oil, corn oil, and sunflower oil.

Full-fat dairy products such as hard cheese and whole milk contain significant amounts of saturated fat. Switch to low-fat or fat-free milk and dairy products to decrease fat and saturated fat in your diet.

The way food is prepared can greatly affect the overall fat content (**Table 10.4**). Replace saturated fats such as butter or lard with healthy monosaturated or polyunsaturated fats. Good choices for cooking oils are olive, safflower, corn, peanut, and canola oil (**Table 10.5**). Remember, even the

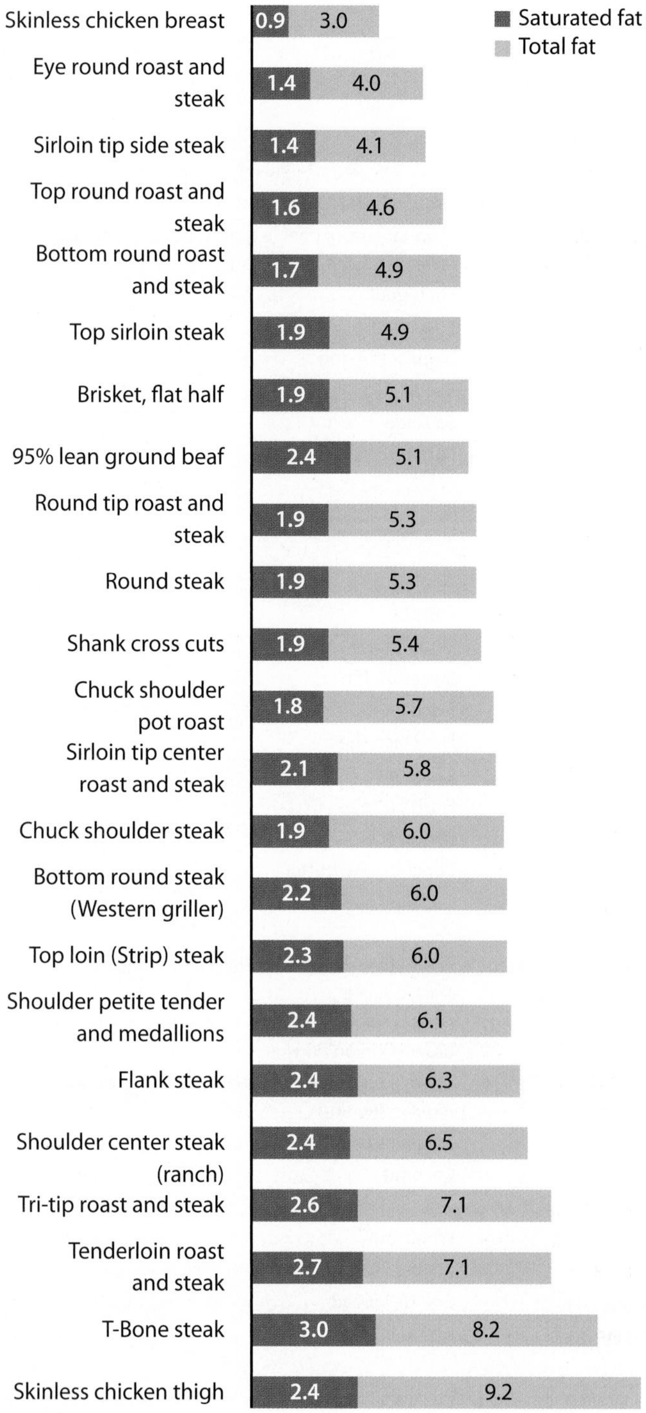

■ **Figure 10.10**

Total Fat and Saturated Fat in Cuts of Beef and Chicken

Source: Cattlemen's Beef Board, http://www.beefboard.org/news/files/29%20Lean%20Cuts.pdf. Accessed June 20, 2009.

healthy oils should be used in moderation due to their high calorie content. Grill, bake, or broil foods, especially meat and fish, instead of frying them. For some foods, you can use nonstick cooking spray instead of oil when pan-frying or sautéing.

Table 10.4

Cooking Tips to Cut the Fat and Keep the Flavor

Choose low-fat cuts of meat
- Select skinless, white meat chicken
- Choose beef or pork with the word *loin* or *round* in the name, such as pork tenderloin or eye of round
- Select beef or pork with minimal visible fat

Use low-fat cooking methods
- Grill, broil, or bake without added fat
- Use a rack when cooking meat to allow the fat to drip away from food
- Stir-fry vegetables and/or meat with cooking spray or a small amount of oil
- Use vinegar and spices or fat-free dressing as marinades
- Add stock, broth, or wine to make a pan sauce instead of butter or cream

Choose low-fat/fat-free seasonings and condiments
- Use herbs and spices instead of high-fat seasonings
- Use low-fat or fat-free dressing for salad

Condiments can add lots of fat and/or saturated fat. Select low-fat or fat-free salad dressing or make your own using olive oil or other monounsaturated or polyunsaturated oils. Choose a bread spread that is made from plant oils. Check the label and choose a spread without hydrogenated or partially hydrogenated oil listed in the ingredient list so that you buy a trans fat–free spread (see the How Policy and Environment Affect My Choices feature).

Eating away from home can mean too much saturated fat (see Chapter 3). Restaurant meals, especially fast food, are often high in saturated fat, which you should not consume on a regular basis. Part of the problem with restaurant food is the sheer size and volume of what is served; also of concern are the saturated or trans fats that may be used in its preparation. Eat out less often, and when you do eat out choose lower-fat options.[22–29]

Can Margarine Really Lower Your Cholesterol?

Several margarines on the market containing plant sterols called stanols make the claim that they can lower blood cholesterol. Consumption of stanols has been shown to lower LDL cholesterol levels.[4] Benecol and Take Control are brands of margarine that contain stanols. Another product on the market, Smart Balance, uses a patented blend of fats developed by Brandeis University. The blend of fats in Smart Balance has been shown to improve the ratio of LDL to HDL cholesterol. So, if you choose well, yes, margarine can help lower your cholesterol. But be sure to make your healthier margarine part of an overall healthy diet.

Table 10.5

Common Fats Used in Cooking

Fat or Oil	Type of Fat	Uses
Butter	Saturated	Butter adds a unique flavor and richness to food. It is best used where its flavor can be enjoyed, such as a spread for bread or to finish a sauce. It is highly saturated, so use it sparingly.
Canola oil	Monounsaturated	The most unsaturated oil in common use. Its mild flavor makes it a versatile oil for salads and cooking.
Coconut oil	Saturated	Can be used to fry or in baking. Coconut milk, which is high in coconut oil, is used to add flavor and richness to curry dishes. It is highly saturated, so use it sparingly.
Corn oil Cottonseed oil Safflower oil Soybean oil Sunflower oil	Polyunsaturated	These polyunsaturated oils have a mild flavor and are good all-purpose salad and cooking oils. They are also often used in making margarine.
Lard	Saturated	Lard is rendered fat from hogs and is very high in saturated fat. Once the most popular cooking fat, lard has largely been replaced by vegetable oils.
Olive oil	Monounsaturated	The pleasing peppery taste of olive oil makes it popular in salad dressing and for a bread topping. It is not recommended for baking due to its strong flavor.
Peanut oil	Monounsaturated	Peanut oil can be heated to a very high temperature without smoking. This characteristic makes it a good choice for stir-fry.
Sesame oil	Polyunsaturated	Sesame oil, especially toasted sesame oil, makes a great flavor addition. Add a small amount toward the end of cooking.

Monitor Cholesterol Intake

Cholesterol is only found in animal foods. Generally speaking, the lower the fat content, the lower the cholesterol content. So, if you are making wise choices from the meat aisle and practicing portion control, chances are your cholesterol intake will be under the 300-milligram recommendation. There is, however, one food that is high in cholesterol and low in fat—eggs. Should you eat eggs or steer clear of them because of their high cholesterol content? Eggs are often considered the "bad guy" because of their relatively high cholesterol content. Eggs do have cholesterol—a whole egg has a little over 200 milligrams. However, eggs also contain protein, vitamins, and healthy unsaturated fat. Research shows that, for most people, cholesterol in food has a much smaller effect on blood cholesterol than does saturated fat in the diet. Consuming up to one egg a day is not associated with an increased risk of heart disease in healthy people and can be part of a healthy diet.[36,37] This does not mean that three-egg, cheese, and bacon omelets should be a regular part of

Fake Fat: Is It Safe?

What about olestra? Is it safe? Olestra was approved by the FDA in 1996 after a firestorm of controversy about its safety. It was approved for use in a small number of products, including potato and tortilla chips. Olestra, which goes by the trade name Olean, is similar to fat in how it tastes and functions in food. It is highly heat stable; in fact, you can fry foods in olestra. It has similar properties to fat yet it is calorie free. The body does not produce enzymes that can break down olestra, so it goes through the digestive tract undigested. Early concerns about olestra included scares of anal leakage, diarrhea, cramping, and malabsorption of fat-soluble vitamins. Procter & Gamble, the maker of olestra, was required to put warning labels on products containing olestra indicating these risks. These warning labels are no longer required, as additional studies have indicated that the claims of severe side effects are rare and that olestra has not been shown to adversely affect fat-soluble vitamin concentrations in the body.[30] The American Dietetic Association,[31] the American Heart Association,[32] and the American Diabetes Association[33] all agree that fat substitutes such as olestra, when used judiciously, may offer people a choice when planning their diet. Olestra has shown promise in short-term studies on its effects on weight loss.[34,35] However, long-term studies are needed to fully determine its health effects.[31]

Try Something New

Choose Low-Fat Dressings

Salads are a great way to add lots of vegetables to your diet. They also can be a low-fat addition; that is, unless you drown them in high-fat dressing. Many low-fat and fat-free dressings are available in restaurants and grocery stores. When you eat out, ask for low-fat or fat-free dressing. At home, try making your own fat-free dressing. Experiment with your own favorites. It will keep for several days in the refrigerator.

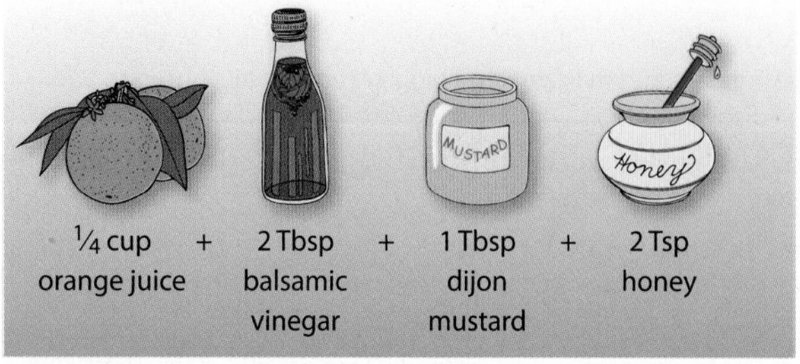
Mustard
Honey
¼ cup orange juice
+
2 Tbsp balsamic vinegar
+
1 Tbsp dijon mustard
+
2 Tsp honey

Make Your Own Oil-Free Dressing
Blend the ingredients together in a small container. It will keep for several days in the refrigerator.

Personal Health Check

Does Low Fat Mean Low Calorie?

To address consumers' desire to have their cake and eat it too, or shall we say have a low-fat diet and still eat their cake, food manufacturers have bombarded the public with low-fat and fat-free options of popular foods. Low-fat or fat-free cookies, dairy products, baked goods, chips, crackers, frozen desserts, and many other foods are available. How manufacturers take these foods from regular to low fat or fat free depends on the type of food. Some foods, such as dairy products, may have some or all of the fat removed without anything being added to the product. Other foods, such as frozen desserts, may have some or all of the fat replaced with a substance that mimics the fat it is replacing.

Let's examine two foods, cookies and mayonnaise, and their low-fat counterparts to see just how much fat and calories you are saving. In some cases, choosing the low-fat option does result in a significant difference in fat and calories. Other times, however, low-fat or fat-free versions of a food are very similar in calories to the regular version. You still need to read the whole label carefully. The bottom line is that you may want to ignore what is on the front of the package and go straight to the Nutrition Facts label and the ingredient list. Fat free, reduced fat, and low fat may sound healthy, but these foods may still be loaded with sugar and calories. Next time you go to the grocery store, check out the low-fat and regular version of foods that you usually purchase. Which one is the best choice for you?

Low-fat cookies

Nutrition Facts
Serving Size 3 Cookies (34g)
Servings Per Container About 15

Amount Per Serving	
Calories 150	Calories from Fat 40
	% Daily Value*
Total Fat 4.5g	7%
Saturated Fat 1g	5%
Trans Fat 0g	
Polyunsaturated Fat 1g	
Monounsaturated Fat 2.5g	
Cholesterol 0mg	0%
Sodium 190mg	8%
Total Carbohydrate 26g	9%
Dietary Fiber 1g	4%
Sugars 14g	
Protein 2g	

Vitamin A 0% • **Vitamin C** 0%
Calcium 0% • **Iron** 10%

*Percent Daily Values are based on a 2,000 calories diet. Your daily values may be higher or lower depending on your calorie needs

	Calories:	2,000	2,500
Total Fat	Less than	65g	80g
Sat Fat	Less than	20g	25g
Cholesterol	Less than	300mg	300mg
Sodium	Less than	2,400mg	2,400mg
Total Carbohydrate		300g	375g
Dietary Fiber		25g	30g

Regular cookies

Nutrition Facts
Serving Size 3 Cookies (34g)
Servings Per Container About 15

Amount Per Serving	
Calories 160	Calories from Fat 60
	% Daily Value*
Total Fat 7g	11%
Saturated Fat 2g	10%
Trans Fat 0g	
Polyunsaturated Fat 1g	
Monounsaturated Fat 3g	
Cholesterol 0mg	0%
Sodium 190mg	8%
Total Carbohydrate 25g	8%
Dietary Fiber 1g	4%
Sugars 14g	
Protein 2g	

Vitamin A 0% • **Vitamin C** 0%
Calcium 0% • **Iron** 10%

*Percent Daily Values are based on a 2,000 calories diet. Your daily values may be higher or lower depending on your calorie needs

	Calories:	2,000	2,500
Total Fat	Less than	65g	80g
Sat Fat	Less than	20g	25g
Cholesterol	Less than	300mg	300mg
Sodium	Less than	2,400mg	2,400mg
Total Carbohydrate		300g	375g
Dietary Fiber		25g	30g

Reduced-fat mayonnaise

Nutrition Facts
Serving Size 1 TBSP (15g)
Servings 36
Calories 45
Fat Cal 35

Amount/Serving	% DV*	Amount/Serving	% DV*
Total Fat 4g	**7%**	**Cholest.** 0mg	**0%**
Sat Fat 0g	**5%**	**Sodium** 0mg	**0%**
Trans Fat 0g		**Total Carb.** 0g	**0%**
Poly Fat 1g		**Protein** 0g	
Mono Fat 0g			

Regular mayonnaise

Nutrition Facts: Serving Size 1 TBSP (15g), Amount Per Serving: **Calories** 90, **Fat Calories** 90, **Total Fat** 0g (0% DV), **Saturated Fat** 1.5g (8% DV), **Trans Fat** 0g, **Polyunsaturated Fat** 1g, **Monounsaturated Fat** 0g, **Cholesterol** 0mg (0% DV), **Sodium** 70mg (3% DV), **Total Carbohydrates** 0g (0% DV), **Sugar** 0g, **Protein** 0g, **Vitamin A** (0% DV), **Vitamin C** (0% DV), **Calcium** (0% DV), **Iron** (0% DV), **Vitamin E** (4% DV)

Are Low-Fat Foods Low in Calories?
The low-fat version of the cookie does have less fat—4.5 versus 7 grams for three cookies. However, the regular and low-fat cookies have almost the same number of calories. Not a big calorie savings.
The lower-fat version of mayonnaise not only has a lower fat content, but also has significantly fewer calories.

How Policy and Environment Affect My Choices

Finding the Trans Fats

Hydrogenation is a process by which hydrogen is bubbled through a liquid fat such as soybean or corn oil. This process breaks some of the double bonds between the carbons and attaches hydrogen to the bonds. The once polyunsaturated oil is now partially hydrogenated. The process of hydrogenation turns the liquid oil into a solid or semisolid spread. The high cost of butter in the 1950s and 1960s led to the commercialization of making liquid vegetable oil solid so that it could be used as a spread. Later, the realization that polyunsaturated fats were heart-healthy made hydrogenated spreads even more popular. An added benefit to these hydrogenated fats was that they added shelf life to processed foods such as crackers, snack foods, and cookies.

Butter and lard were out and margarine was in—that is until we learned more about the types of fats that were being produced by the hydrogenation process. The hydrogenation of oils produces fatty acids with a trans configuration. Trans fats increase LDL cholesterol and decrease HDL cholesterol in the blood, thus increasing the risk of heart disease.[39–48] Trans fats increase the risk of heart disease more than any other single nutrient, with a substantial risk at even low levels of consumption.[39]

To assist consumers in locating trans fats in their foods, the FDA now requires the Nutrition Facts panel to include trans fats in a separate line under saturated fat. As a result of this requirement, many manufacturers have removed some or all of the trans fats from their products.

A word of caution about what's on the label. With consumer interest in consuming "trans fat free" at a peak, manufacturers begun putting the words "contains 0 grams of trans fat per serving" on the label. Does this statement ensure that you are consuming a trans fat–free product? No, it does not, and here is why: If a product has 0.5 grams or less of trans fats per serving, the amount can be rounded down to 0 grams of trans fat per serving, hence the wording of the claim to read "0 grams of trans fat PER SERVING." So, for example, if you had a product that has 0.5 grams of trans fat per tablespoon and you had 3 tablespoons, you would be getting 1.5 grams of trans fat. Hardly trans fat free! The only way to see if a product really is trans fat free is to read the ingredient label. If the product contains an ingredient that is hydrogenated or partially hydrogenated, such as partially hydrogenated soybean oil or hydrogenated cottonseed oil, it is not trans fat free. If the word *hydrogenated* is in the ingredient list, it has at least some trans fat in the product.

Another source of trans fats in the American diet is restaurant food. Restaurants, for the most part, do not have to reveal the type of fat they use in cooking and often use hydrogenated oils. To further protect the public from unhealthy trans fats, New York City and California have banned the use of trans fats in restaurants. Other cities and states are sure to follow as the public becomes savvier about the dangers of trans fats.

The requirement of labeling foods with the amount of trans fat in the product and the ban of use of trans fat in restaurants are examples of how policy change can affect the health of the population. Consumers now have an easy way to know how much trans fats are in the foods they buy. The even bolder step of banning trans fats in restaurants further protects consumers from unknowingly consuming harmful trans fats.

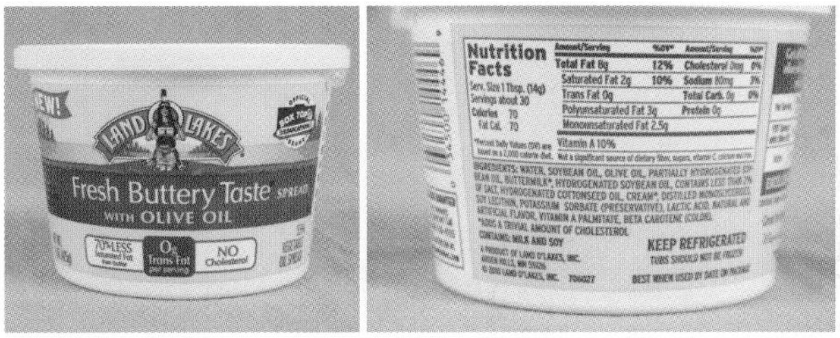

Zero Trans Fat
Zero grams of trans fat per serving does not always mean trans fat free. Look for the word *hydrogenated* in the ingredient list. This indicates that the product has trans fat.

your diet. Choose healthy side dishes such as whole-grain toast, use vegetables as filling for omelets, and limit egg consumption to an average of one per day. Combine one whole egg with two egg whites or choose egg substitute for a breakfast lower in cholesterol. People who have been diagnosed with heart disease or diabetes should limit consumption to three egg yolks per week.[38]

Increase Omega-3 Fatty Acids

It is widely accepted that a low-fat diet is healthy and will decrease your risk of heart disease. Why then, when the diet of the Eskimos of Greenland was studied, did researchers find that they had a diet that was very high in fat but experienced almost no heart disease?[49–51] On further examination, it was found that the Eskimo diet consisted primarily of whale blubber and fish from the cold waters surrounding their home. Their diet was very high in the omega-3 fatty acids docosahexanoic acid (DHA) and eicosapentaenoic acid (EPA). These epidemiological studies spurred further research on how omega-3 fatty acids affect our health. The years of research that have followed suggest that consumption of these marine oils can greatly improve your health, specifically decreasing your risk of heart disease.[52,53] We now have the challenge of incorporating the knowledge that more omega-3 fatty acids are a good idea for our health into an American diet that is historically very low in DHA and EPA.

TERMS

hydrogenation A process by which hydrogen is added to liquid fat to produce a more saturated fat; the result is a trans fat.

Green and Healthy

Farm Raised or Wild Caught: Which Salmon Is King?

You are convinced that you should consume more fish, especially oily fish. You go to the fish market or local grocery store to pick up some salmon for tonight's dinner. At the store you are faced with the choice of farm-raised or wild-caught salmon. Wild caught must be better for you and it must be better for the environment, right? Let's take a closer look at which type of salmon you should choose.

Some news stories have reported that farm-raised salmon are higher in **polychlorinated biphenyls (PCBs)**. PCB levels in both farm-raised and wild-caught salmon vary widely depending on farming practices and where the fish are caught. PCBs are present in both farm-raised and wild-caught salmon; however, neither have levels above what is recommended by the FDA. The benefits outweigh the risk in both farm-raised and wild-caught salmon.[56–58] Another concern with fish is mercury. Both farm-raised and wild-caught salmon consistently rate among the fish with the lowest mercury levels.[59]

Farm-raised and wild-caught salmon both provide similar amounts of healthy omega-3 fatty acids.[60,61] Farm-raised salmon is available year round and can be half the price of wild-caught salmon. Currently, farm-raised salmon accounts for about 50% of worldwide consumption. As more people choose salmon for health or for taste, there could be a danger of waters becoming overfished. Thus, a supply of farm-raised salmon will be necessary to meet consumer demand.[62]

Now that we know the facts, let's get back to your choice at the fish market. Do you choose farm-raised or wild-caught salmon? If the wild-caught salmon looks good and fits your food budget, go for it. The same holds true for the farm-raised salmon. If it looks fresh and is a good value, have the fishmonger wrap it up. You cannot lose by choosing either farm-raised or wild-caught salmon. Both provide heart-healthy omega-3 fatty acids. Throw the salmon on the grill (farm or wild), add a squeeze of lemon and dill, and enjoy your dinner.

For optimal health and to reduce the risk of chronic diseases such as heart disease, the American Heart Association recommends consuming a ratio of 6:1 omega-6 to omega-3 fatty acids.[53] Currently, the American diet has a ratio of about 10:1; that is, we consume a great deal more omega-6 fatty acids than we do omega-3 fatty acids. Further, most of the omega-3 fatty acids that we do get in the American diet are alpha linolenic acid from foods such as soybeans, canola oil, and olive oil. Although your body can create DHA and EPA from alpha linolenic acid, the conversion rate is not very high.[54,55] Most Americans need to improve their ratio of omega-6 fatty acids to omega-3 fatty acids, which will increase the amount of DHA and EPA.

So, how can you improve your ratio of omega-6 fatty acids to omega-3 fatty acids? You can do this by increasing the number of times per week you consume fish high in omega-3 fatty acids. In addition, substituting canola or soybean oil for other vegetable oils will increase the amount of omega-3 in your diet. You can also incorporate foods such as flaxseed or walnuts into your diet. You should also include oils and foods rich in alpha linolenic acid, such as flaxseed and canola oil. Getting the amounts recommended for good health is best achieved through foods (**Figure 10.11**) as opposed to supplements.[2,53]

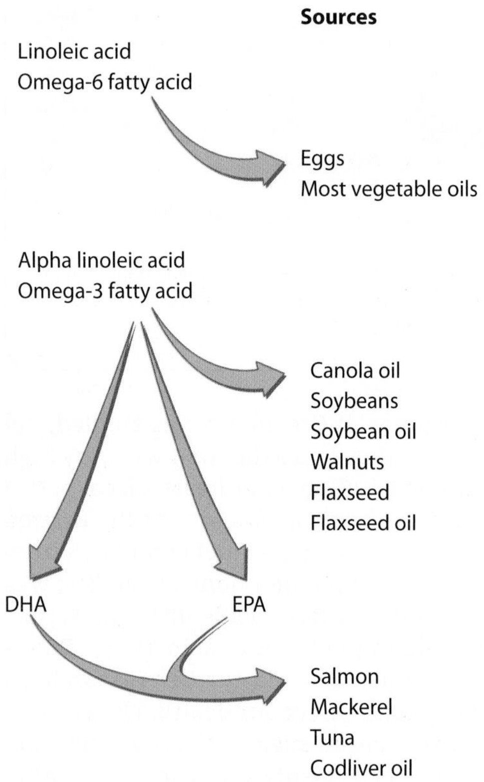

Figure 10.11

Sources of Omega-3 and Omega-6 Fatty Acids

The essential fatty acids linoleic and alpha linolenic acid are omega-3 and omega-6 fatty acids, respectively. DHA and EPA can be made from linolenic acid.

TERMS

polychlorinated biphenyls (PCBs) A chemical once used as a coolant or lubricant. Although no longer produced in the United States, it still exists as an environmental pollutant. It is a known carcinogen.

Special Report

Cardiovascular Disease

Cardiovascular disease (CVD) is the leading cause of death in the United States and Canada for both men and women.[63,64] Even though CVD is often thought to disproportionately affect men, approximately 50% of the deaths from heart disease are women.[63] The two types of CVD that occur most often are heart disease and stroke. Both are caused by atherosclerosis, a build up of fatty plaque in the artery wall. Plaque narrows the arteries and interferes with blood flow. Blockage of an artery that supplies oxygen-rich blood to the heart causes a heart attack. Blockage of an artery to the brain results in a stroke.

Warning Signs for a Heart Attack

Some heart attacks are sudden and intense, but most start slowly, with mild pain or discomfort. Oftentimes, the person affected is unsure of what it wrong and waits too long before getting help. The following are some signs of a heart attack:

- **Chest discomfort.** Most heart attacks involve discomfort in the center of the chest that lasts more than a few minutes or that goes away and comes back. It can feel like uncomfortable pressure, squeezing, fullness, or pain.
- **Discomfort in other areas of the upper body.** Symptoms can include pain or discomfort in one or both arms, the back, neck, jaw, or stomach.
- **Shortness of breath.** May occur with or without chest discomfort.
- **Other signs.** These may include breaking out in a cold sweat, nausea, or lightheadedness.

If you or someone you are with has chest discomfort, especially with one or more of the other signs, do not wait longer than five minutes before calling 9-1-1. Calling 9-1-1 is almost always the fastest way to get lifesaving treatment. Emergency medical services (EMS) staff can begin treatment when they arrive—up to one hour sooner than if someone gets to the hospital by car. EMS personnel are trained to revive someone whose heart has stopped. You will also get treated faster in the hospital if you come by ambulance.

Sources: Data from American Heart Association. Heart attack warning signs. http://www.americanheart.org/presenter.jhtml?identifier=3053. Accessed June 15, 2009; National Institutes of Health, National Heart Lung and Blood Institute. http://www.nhlbi.nih.gov/actintime/haws/haws.htm. Accessed October 6, 2011; and Ornato JP, Hand M. Warning signs of a heart attack. *Circulation* 2001;104:1212–1213.

A great deal of research has focused on identifying risk factors for CVD. Some of the risk of heart attack or stroke is related to factors that cannot be changed. Even though some risk factors cannot be controlled, it is important to be aware of all of the risk factors for CVD. Possessing one or more of the uncontrollable risk factors, as all of us do, makes it even more important to address the risk factors you *can* control:

- **Age.** As age increases, so does the risk of CVD.
- **Family history.** If you have a family member with CVD, you are more likely to have the disease yourself; the closer the relation to you, the higher the risk. African Americans are at a higher risk than Caucasians for CVD due to higher blood pressures, on average.
- **Gender.** Men have a greater risk of heart attack than women and have heart attacks earlier in life. As women reach menopause, their rate of death from heart attack increases. Stroke is more common in men than women; however, more than half of the total deaths from stroke occur in women. Use of birth control pills and pregnancy also put women at risk for stroke.

Several risk factors for CVD can be controlled. The American Heart Association has developed the following diet and lifestyle goals for CVD risk reduction:[4]

Consume an overall healthy diet. An overall healthy diet is associated with a substantial reduction of CVD risk.[3,65–68] The American Heart Association recommends consumption of a variety of fruits, vegetables, and grain products, especially whole grains. It also suggests choosing fat-free and low-fat dairy products, legumes, poultry, and lean meats. Fish, preferably oily fish, should be eaten at least twice a week. Alcohol, if used, should be consumed in moderation.

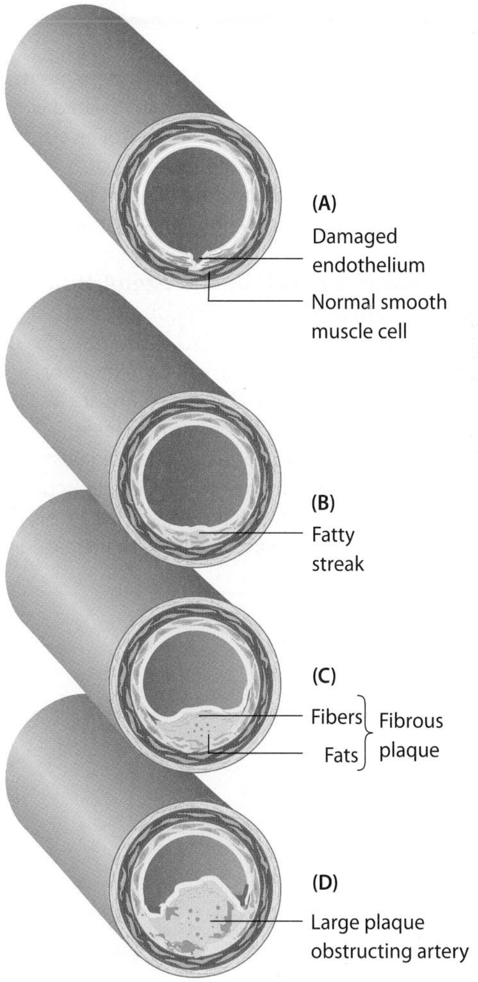

Atherosclerosis
Atherosclerosis is a buildup of plaque in the artery and may cause a blockage which causes heart attack or stroke.

(continues)

Blood Cholesterol and Triglyceride Levels (all units are milligrams/deciliter)

Total cholesterol	Desirable: < 200 Borderline high: 200–239 High: > 240
LDL cholesterol	Optimal: < 100 Near or above optimal: 100–129 Borderline high: 130–159 High: 160–189 Very high: ≥ 190
HDL cholesterol	Increased risk of CVD: < 40 for men and < 50 for women HDL > 60 has a protective effect for CVD
Triglyceride	Normal: < 150 Borderline high: 150–199 High: 200–499 Very high: > 500

Source: Modifield from National Heart, Lung, and Blood Institute. Executive Summary of the Third Report of the National Cholesterol Education Program (NCEP) Expert Panel on Detection, Evaluation, and Treatment of High Blood Cholesterol in Adults (Adult Treatment Panel III). http://www.nhlbi.nih.gov/guidelines/cholesterol/atp3xsum.pdf. Accessed April 9, 2011.

Aim for a healthy body weight. Obesity is an independent risk factor for CVD.[69] In addition, obesity is associated with high LDL cholesterol levels, low HDL cholesterol levels, high blood pressure, and increased prevalence of diabetes. These also are risk factors for CVD. Aim to achieve and maintain a healthy weight throughout life.[70–72]

Aim for recommended levels of LDL cholesterol, HDL cholesterol, and triglycerides. Higher LDL levels are associated with an increased risk of CVD.[73] Saturated fat and trans fat intake are strong dietary determinants of LDL levels. Dietary cholesterol and body weight are also positively related to LDL levels, but to a much lesser extent. HDL cholesterol has a protective effect against CVD.[73] Diet is not a major influence on HDL levels. Regular aerobic exercise is associated with increased HDL levels.[74] Elevated triglyceride levels are associated with increased risk of CVD. High triglyceride levels are associated with overweight and obesity, physical inactivity, smoking, and excessive alcohol consumption.[11]

Aim for normal blood pressure. Normal blood pressure is a systolic blood pressure (top number) of less than 120 mm Hg and a diastolic blood pressure (bottom number) of less than 80 mm Hg. High blood pressure is a strong risk factor for CVD. Even people with only slightly elevated blood pressure would benefit from reducing blood pressure to normal levels. Further, there seems to be no threshold; that is, as blood pressure continues to rise, the risk for CVD continues to increase.[75] Multiple dietary and lifestyle factors affect blood pressure.[76] Physical inactivity is a risk factor for high blood pressure.[77,78] Consumption of an overall healthy diet that is high in fruits and vegetables, low-fat dairy products, whole grains, and lean meats and that is low in fats, red meat, sweets, and sugar-containing beverages is critical to achieving a healthy blood pressure.[67,77,78]

Aim for normal blood glucose levels. Normal fasting blood glucose is ≤ 100 milligrams per deciliter (mg/dL); ≥126 mg/dL is considered diabetic. High levels of blood glucose are associated with higher risk of CVD. Moderately high fasting glucose levels can be addressed by weight loss by being physically active and adopting dietary modifications.[79,80]

Be physically active. Regular physical activity is essential for cardiovascular fitness and for achieving and maintaining a healthy weight.[1,2,81] Regular physical activity also helps improve other CVD risk factors, such as blood pressure, blood glucose, and HDL cholesterol levels.[1,2,4,82] Thirty minutes of moderate activity on most days of the week plus muscle-strengthening activities two times per week is the minimum that is recommended by the Centers for Disease Control and Prevention.[83] More physical activity will provide additional health benefits.

Avoid use of and exposure to tobacco products. There is a preponderance of evidence that use of tobacco and exposure to secondhand smoke increases the risk of CVD.[84–87] If you use tobacco products, see your physician for ways you can quit. Avoid exposure to secondhand smoke.

Ready to Make a Change

Are you ready to make a change, small or large, in the amount and type of fat in your diet? Make the commitment to take the first step. Whether it is a small, medium, or large change, it is a step in the right direction toward a healthier diet.

I commit to a small first step. Change your spread. Make your bread spread of choice one that is from a plant oil and has no trans fats. No hydrogenated oils should be in the ingredient list. Save butter for every once in a while or on special occasions.

I am ready to take the next step and make a medium change. Choose heart-healthy oils for cooking and for salad dressing. Olive oil, soybean oil, and canola oil are all good choices. Make your own dressing so you can control the amount of oil you use. Traditional vinaigrette has three parts oil to one part vinegar; try using half vinegar and half oil to lower the overall fat content. When you eat at a restaurant, ask for low-fat dressing or use balsamic vinegar with just a splash of olive oil.

I have been making changes for some time and am ready to make a large change with the fat in my diet. If you already have a diet that is moderate in fat and you choose monosaturated and polyunsaturated fats instead of saturated fats, take the next step and include two servings of fish per week in your diet. Choose a variety of fish, preferably a fish with a high omega-3 fat content, such as salmon.

Myth Versus Fact

Myth: Trans fats are no worse than other fats.

Fact: Manufactured trans fats have been linked to an increased risk of heart disease. It is recommended that consumption of trans fats from hydrogenated oils be as low as possible. The vast majority of trans fats come from manufactured products that contain hydrogenated oils.

Myth: A low-fat diet will ensure that I am not fat.

Fact: More calories than you need, regardless of where they come from, leads to weight gain. Fat does have more calories per gram than either proteins or carbohydrates, so it is easy to consume more calories if your diet is high in fat. Going low fat, however, does not automatically keep your calories in line with what you need. Balance calories with activity to achieve and maintain a healthy weight.

Myth: The best snack is one that is fat free.

Fact: Fruits and vegetables that are naturally low fat or fat free make great snacks. A small handful of almonds, which are relatively high in fat, is also a great snack to grab on the go. Snacks should fit into your overall calories for the day. They don't have to be fat free.

Myth: I should always choose the low-fat or fat-free version of a food.

Fact: Low fat or fat free is not always the best bet. Read the label carefully to see what they have used to replace some or all of the fat in the food. Many low-fat or fat-free foods have just as many calories as their regular counterparts. Sometimes the low-fat or fat-free version of the food may be the best choice, but not always.

Myth: I should eat more fish but avoid salmon because it is relatively high in fat.

Fact: Americans should eat more fish, especially fatty fish. Salmon is high in heart-healthy omega-3 fatty acids. Based on much research, the American Heart Association recommends two or more servings of fish (preferably oily fish such as salmon) twice a week.

Myth: Eggs have too much cholesterol to be a healthy food.

Fact: Eggs are a great inexpensive source of protein. The yolk is high in cholesterol but the fat in egg is mostly healthy unsaturated fat. Consuming eggs in moderation (up to one a day) is a healthy choice.

Myth: I can use all of the olive oil I want because it is a healthy monounsaturated fat.

Fact: Although olive oil is a healthy choice for cooking and in salads, it still has 120 calories per tablespoon. Moderation is the key, even with healthy oils and fats.

Back to the Story

Jane has a family history of heart disease. There is nothing she can do about who her relatives are, but she can do something about other risk factors for heart disease that are in her control. Jane needs to eat smart and move more to get her weight within normal range. Eating a healthy diet will also help reduce her cholesterol. Specifically, Jane needs to decrease the amount of fat in her diet and increase her consumption of fruits, vegetables, whole grains, and lean sources of protein. Although she may not be able to avoid the family legacy of heart disease, she will have a better chance of lifelong good health by addressing the risk factors that are within her control. What other suggestions do you have for Jane?

References

1. Institute of Medicine, Food and Nutrition Board. *Dietary Reference Intakes for Energy, Carbohydrate, Fiber, Fat, Fatty Acids, Cholesterol, Protein, and Amino Acids*. Washington, DC: National Academies Press, 2005.
2. US Department of Health and Human Services and US Department of Agriculture. *Dietary Guidelines for Americans, 2010*, 7th ed. Washington, DC: US Government Printing Office, December 2010.
3. Hu, FB, Willett WC. Optimal diets for prevention of coronary heart disease. *JAMA*. 2002;288(20):2569–2578.
4. Lichtenstein AH, Appel LJ, Brands M, et al. Diet and lifestyle recommendations revision 2006: a scientific statement from the American Heart Association Nutrition Committee. *Circulation*. 2006;114:82–96.
5. Grundy SM, Denke MA. Dietary influences on serum lipids and lipoproteins. *J Lipid Res*. 1990;31:1149–1172.
6. Kris-Etherton PM, Yu S. Individual fatty acid effects on plasma lipids and lipoproteins: human studies. *Am J Clin Nutr*. 1997;65(suppl 5):1628S–1644S.
7. Mensink RP, Katan MB. Effects of dietary fatty acids on serum lipids and lipoproteins: a meta-analysis of 27 trials. *Arterioscler Thromb*. 1992;12:911–919.
8. Ginsberg HN, Kris-Etherton P, Dennis B, et al., for the Delta Research Group. Effects of reducing dietary saturated fatty acids on plasma lipids and lipoproteins in healthy subjects: the Delta Study, Protocol 1. *Arterioscler Thromb Vasc Biol*. 1998;18:441–449.
9. Walden CE, Retzlaff BM, Buck BL, Wallick S, McCann BS, Knopp RH. Differential effect of National Cholesterol Education Program (NCEP) Step II diet on HDL cholesterol, its subfractions, and apoprotein A-I in hypercholesterolemic women and men after 1 year: the beFIT study. *Arterioscler Thromb Vasc Biol*. 2000;20:1580–1587.
10. Walden CE, Retzlaff BM, Buck BL, McCann BS, Knopp RH. Lipoprotein lipid response to the National Cholesterol Education Program Step II diet by hypercholesterolemic and combined hyperlipidemic women and men. *Arterioscler Thromb Vasc Biol*. 1997;17:375–382.
11. National Cholesterol Education Program. *Third Report of the Expert Panel on Detection, Evaluation, and Treatment of High Blood Cholesterol in Adults (Adult Treatment Panel III), Final Report*. NIH publication 02-5215. Washington, DC: US Department of Health and Human Services, 2002.
12. Briefel RR, Johnson CL. Secular trends in dietary intake in the United States. *Ann Rev Nutr*. 2004;24:401–431.
13. Wright JD, Wang CY, Kennedy-Stephenson J, Ervin RB. Dietary intake of ten key nutrients for public health, United States: 1999–2000. *Advance data from Vital and Health Statistics*, no. 334. Hyattsville, MD: National Center for Health Statistics, 2003.
14. Cotton PA, Subar AF, Friday JE, Cook S. Dietary sources of nutrients among US adults, 1994–1996. *J Am Diet Assoc*. 2004;104:921–930.
15. Chanmuga, P, Guthrie JF, Cecilio S, Morton J, Basiotis PP, Anand R. Did fat intake in the United States really decline between 1989–1991 and 1994–1996? *J Am Diet Assoc*. 2003;103:867–872.
16. Wright JD, Hirsch R, Wang C. One-third of US adults embraced most heart healthy behaviors 1999–2002. *National Center for Health Statistics*. Data Brief No. 17. May 2009.
17. Centers for Disease Control and Prevention. National Center for Health Statistics. NHANES 1999–2000 data file documentation. http://www.nhlbi.nih.gov/guidelines/cvd_adult/background.htm. Accessed June 25, 2009.
18. Campbell TC, Parpia B, Chen J. Diet, lifestyle, and the etiology of coronary artery disease: The Cornell China Study. *Am J Cardiol*. 1998;82:18T–21T.
19. Singh RB, Ghosh S, Niaz AM, et al. Epidemiologic study of diet and coronary risk factors in relation to central obesity and insulin levels in rural and urban populations of north India. *Int J Cardiol*. 1995;47:245–255.
20. Tao SC, Huang ZD, Wu XG, et al. CHD and its risk factors in the People's Republic of China. *Int J Epidemiol*. 1989;18:S159–S163.

21. Walker AR, Walker BF. High high-density-lipoprotein cholesterol in African children and adults in a population free of coronary heart disease. *Br Med J*. 1978;2:1336–1337.
22. The Keystone Center. *The Keystone Forum on Away-From-Home Foods: Opportunities for Preventing Weight Gain and Obesity Final Report, May 2006*. http://www.keystone.org/spp/health-and-social-policy/chronic-disease-healthy-lifestyles. Accessed June 24, 2009.
23. Kant AK, Graubard BI. Eating out in America, 1987–2000: trends and nutritional correlates. *Prev Med*. 2004;38:243–249.
24. McLaughlin C, Tarasuk V, Kreiger N. An examination of at-home food preparation activity among low-income, food-insecure women. *J Am Diet Assoc*. 2003;103:1506–1512.
25. Gillman M, Rifas-Shiman SL, Frazier L, et al. Family dinner and diet quality among older children and adolescents. *Arch Fam Med*. 2000;9:235–240.
26. Thompson OM, Ballew C, Resnicow K, et al. Food purchased away from home as a predictor of change in BMI z-score among girls. *Inter J Obes*. 2004;28:282–289.
27. Guthrie JF, Lin BH, Frazao E. Role of food prepared away from home in the American diet, 1977–78 versus 1994–96: changes and consequences. *J Nutr Ed Behav*. 2002;34:140–150.
28. Bowman SA, Gortmaker SL, Ebbeling CB, Pereira MA, Ludwig DS. Effects of fast-food consumption on energy intake and diet quality among children in a national household survey. *Pediatrics*. 2004;113(1):112–118.
29. Bowman SA, Vinyard BT. Fast food consumption of US adults: impact on energy and nutrient intakes and overweight status. *J Am Coll Nutr*. 2004;23(2):163–168.
30. Neuhouser ML, Rock CL, Dristal AR, et al. Olestra is associated with slight reductions in serum carotenoids but does not markedly influence serum fat-soluble vitamin concentrations. *Am J Clin Nutr*. 2006;83(3):624–631.
31. American Dietetic Association. Position of the American Dietetic Association: fat replacers. *J Am Diet Assoc*. 2005;105:266–275.
32. Rosett J. Fat substitutes and health. An advisory from the nutrition committee of the American Heart Association. *Circulation*. 2002;105:2800–2804.
33. American Diabetes Association. Evidence-based nutrition principles and recommendations for the treatment and prevention of diabetes and related complication. *Diabetes Care*. 2004;27(suppl 1):S36–S46.
34. Bray GA, Lovejoy JC, Most-Windhauser M, et al. A nine-month randomized clinical trial comparing a fat substituted and fat-reduced diet in healthy obese men: The Ole Study. *Am J Clin Nutr*. 2002;76:928–934.
35. Roy HJ, Most MM, Sparti A, et al. Effect on body weight of replacing dietary fat with Olestra for two or ten weeks in healthy men and women. *J Am Coll Nutr*. 2002;21(3):259–267.
36. Hu FB, Stampfer MJ, Rimm EB, et al. A prospective study of egg consumption and risk of cardiovascular disease in men and women. *JAMA*. 1999;281:1387–1394.
37. Fernandez ML. Dietary cholesterol provided by eggs and plasma lipoproteins in healthy populations. *Curr Opin Clin Nutr Metab Care*. 2006;9:8–12.
38. Djousse L, Gaziano JM. Egg consumption and risk of heart failure in the Physicians' Health Study. *Circulation*. 2008; 117:512–516.
39. Mozaffarin D, Katan MB, Acherio A, Stampfer MJ, Willitt WC. Trans fatty acids and cardiovascular disease. *N Engl J Med*. 2006;345(15):1601–1613.
40. Ascherio A, Katan MB, Zock PL, Stampfer MJ, Willett WC. Trans fatty acids and coronary heart disease. *N Engl J Med*. 1999;340:1994–1998.
41. Pietinen P, Ascherio A, Korhonen P, et al. Intake of fatty acids and risk of coronary heart disease in a cohort of Finnish men: the Alpha-Tocopherol, Beta-Carotene Cancer Prevention Study. *Am J Epidemiol*. 1997;145:876–887.
42. Oomen CM, Ocke MC, Feskens EJ, van Erp-Baart MA, Kok FJ, Kromhout D. Association between trans fatty acid intake and 10-year risk of coronary heart disease in the Zutphen Elderly Study: a prospective population-based study. *Lancet*. 2001; 357:746–751.
43. Oh K, Hu FB, Manson JE, Stampfer MJ, Willett WC. Dietary fat intake and risk of coronary heart disease in women: 20 years of follow-up of the Nurses' Health Study. *Am J Epidemiol*. 2005;161:672–679.
44. Ascherio A, Rimm EB, Giovannucci EL, Spiegelman D, Stampfer M, Willett WC. Dietary fat and risk of coronary heart disease in men: cohort follow up study in the United States. *BMJ*. 1996;313:84–90.
45. DerSimonian R, Laird N. Meta-analysis in clinical trials. *Control Clin Trials*. 1986;7:177–188.
46. Aro A, Kardinaal AF, Salminen I, et al. Adipose tissue isomeric trans fatty acids and risk of myocardial infarction in nine countries: the EURAMIC study. *Lancet*. 1995;345:273–278.
47. Baylin A, Kabagambe EK, Ascherio A, Spiegelman D, Campos H. High 18:2 trans-fatty acids in adipose tissue are associated with increased risk of nonfatal acute myocardial infarction in Costa Rican adults. *J Nutr*. 2003;133:1186–1191.
48. Clifton PM, Keogh JB, Noakes M. Trans fatty acids in adipose tissue and the food supply are associated with myocardial infarction. *J Nutr*. 2004;134:874–879.

49. Bang HO, Dyerberg J, Nielsen AB. Plasma lipid and lipoprotein pattern in Greenlandic west-coast Eskimos. *Lancet*. 1971;1:1143–1146.
50. Bang HO, Dyerberg J. Plasma lipids and lipoproteins in Greenlandic west-coast Eskimos. *Acta Med Scand*. 1972;192:85–94.
51. Dyerberg J, Bang HO, Hjorne N. Fatty acid composition of the plasma lipids in Greenland Eskimos. *Am J Clin Nutr*. 1975;28:958–966.
52. Psota TL, Gebauer SK, Kris-Etherton P. Dietary omega-3 fatty acid intake and cardiovascular risk. *Am J Cardiol*. 2006;98[suppl]:3i–18i.
53. Kris-Etherton PM, Harris WS, Lawrence J. Fish consumption, fish oil, omega-3 fatty acids, and cardiovascular disease. *Circulation*. 2002;106:2747–2757.
54. Emken EA, Adlof RO, Gulle RM. Dietary linoleic acid influences desaturation and acylation of deuterium-labeled linoleic and linolenic acids in young adult males. *Biochim Biophus Acta*. 1994;1213:277–288.
55. Pawlosky RJ, Hibbeln JR, Novotny JA, Salem N. Physiological compartmental analysis of alpha-linolenic acid metabolism in adult humans. *J Lipid Res*. 2001;42:1257–1265.
56. Foran JA, Good DH, Carpenter DO, Hamilton MC, Kuth BA, Schwager SJ. Quantitative analysis of the benefits and risks of consuming farmed and wild salmon. *J Nutr*. 2005;135:2639–2643.
57. Mozffarian D, Rimm EB. Fish intake, contaminants, and human health, evaluating the risks and benefits. *JAMA*. 2006;296:1885–1899.
58. Foran JA, Good DH, Carpenter DO, Hamilton MC, Knuth BA, Schwager SJ. Quantitative analysis of the benefits and risks of consuming farmed and wild salmon. *J Nutr*. 2005;135:2639–2643.
59. Food and Drug Administration. Mercury levels in commercial fish and shellfish. http://www.fda.gov/Food/FoodSafety/Product-SpecificInformation/Seafood/FoodbornePathogensContaminants/Methylmercury/ucm115644.htm. Accessed: June 25, 2009.
60. Hamilton MC, Hites RA, Schwager SJ, Foran JA, Knuth BA, Carpenter DO. Lipid composition and contaminants in farmed and wild salmon. *Environ Sci Technol*. 2005;39(22):8622–8629.
61. Blanchet C, Lucas M, Julien P, Morin R, Gingras S, Dewailly E. Fatty acid composition of wild and farmed Atlantic salmon (Salmo salar) and rainbow trout (Oncorhynchus mykiss). *Lipids*. 2005;40(5):529–531.
62. Borresen T. Understanding the consumer's perception of aquaculture. *J Aquatic Food Product Tech*. 2009;181:191–192.
63. Centers for Disease Control and Prevention. Deaths: Final data for 2006. *National Vital Statistics Reports*. DHHS Publication No. (PHS) 2009-1120. 2009;57(1).
64. Statistics Canada. Leading causes of death in Canada, 2005. http://www.statcan.gc.ca/pub/84-215-x/84-215-x2009000-eng.htm. Accessed June 15, 2009.
65. Knoops KT, de Groot LC, Kromhout D, et al. Mediterranean diet, lifestyle factors, and 10-year mortality in elderly European men and women: the HALE project. *JAMA*. 2004;292:1433–1439.
66. Appel LJ, Moore TJ, Obarzanek E, et al. A clinical trial of the effects of dietary patterns on blood pressure. DASH Collaborative Research Group. *N Engl J Med*. 1997;336:1117–1124.
67. Appel LJ, Sacks FM, Carey VJ, et al. The effects of protein, monounsaturated fat, and carbohydrate intake on blood pressure and serum lipids: results of the OmniHeart randomized trial. *JAMA*. 2005;294:2455–2464.
68. VanHorn L, McCoin M, Kris-Etherton PM, et al. The evidence for dietary prevention and treatment of cardiovascular disease. *J Am Diet Assoc*. 2008;108:287–331.
69. Rashid MN, Fuentes F, Touchon RC, Wehner PS. Obesity and the risk for cardiovascular disease. *Prev Cardiol*. 2003;6:42–47.
70. US Department of Health and Human Services, National Institutes of Health, National Heart, Lung, and Blood Institute. Guidelines on Overweight and Obesity: Electronic Textbook. http://www.nhlbi.nih.gov/guidelines/obesity/e_txtbk/ratnl/23.htm. Accessed June 17, 2009.
71. Hill JO, Thompson H, Wyatt H. Weight maintenance: what's missing? *J Am Diet Assoc*. 2005;105(suppl 1):S63–S66.
72. Wing RR, Phelan S. Long-term weight loss maintenance. *Am J Clin Nutr*. 2005;82:222S–225S.
73. Expert Panel on Detection, Evaluation, and Treatment of High Blood Cholesterol in Adults. Executive summary of the third report of the National Cholesterol Education Program (NCEP) Expert Panel on Detection, Evaluation, and Treatment of High Blood Cholesterol in Adults (Adult Treatment Panel III). *JAMA*. 2001;285:2486–2497.
74. Kodama S, Tanaka S, Saito K, et al. Effect of aerobic exercise training on serum levels of high-density lipoprotein cholesterol. *Arch Intern Med*. 2007;167:999–1008.
75. Lewington S, Clarke R, Qizilbash N, Peto R, Collins R; Prospective Studies Collaboration. Age-specific relevance of usual blood pressure to vascular mortality: a meta-analysis of individual data for one million adults in 61 prospective studies. *Lancet*. 2002;360:1903–1913.
76. Appel LJ, Brands MW, Daniels SR, Karanja N, Elmer PJ, Sacks FM; American Heart Association. Dietary approaches to prevent and treat hypertension. A scientific statement from the American Heart Association. *Hypertension*. 2006;47:969–980.
77. Smith SC, Allne J, Blair SN, et al. AHA/ACC guidelines for secondary prevention for patients with coronary and other atherosclerotic vascular disease: 2006 update. *J Am Coll Cardiol*. 2006;47;2130–2139.
78. Chobanian AV, Bakris GL, Black HR, et al. Joint National Committee on Prevention, Detection, Evaluation, and Treatment of High Blood Pressure. National Heart,

Lung, and Blood Institute; National High Blood Pressure Education Program Coordinating Committee. Seventh report of the Joint National Committee on Prevention, Detection, Evaluation, and Treatment of High Blood Pressure. *Hypertension*. 2003;42:1206–1252.

79. Knowler WC, Barrett-Connor E, Fowler SE, et al. Reduction in the incidence of type 2 diabetes with lifestyle intervention or metformin. *N Engl J Med*. 2002;346:393–403.
80. Lindstrom J, Louheranta A, Mannelin M, et al. The Finnish Diabetes Prevention Study (DPS): lifestyle intervention and 3-year results on diet and physical activity. *Diabetes Care*. 2003;26:3230–3236.
81. Fogelholm M, Kukkonen-Harjula K. Does physical activity prevent weight gain—a systematic review. *Obes Rev*. 2000;1:95–111.
82. Maron BJ, Chaitman BR, Ackerman MJ, et al. Recommendations for physical activity and recreational sports participation for young patients with genetic cardiovascular diseases. *Circulation*. 2004; 109:2807–2816.
83. Centers for Disease Control. How much physical activity do adults need? http://www.cdc.gov/physicalactivity/everyone/guidelines/adults.html. Accessed July 13, 2009.
84. Ockene IS, Miller NH. Cigarette smoking, cardiovascular disease, and stroke: a statement for healthcare professionals from the American Heart Association, American Heart Association Task Force on Risk Reduction. *Circulation*. 1997;96:3243–3247.
85. Barnoya J, Glantz SA. Cardiovascular effects of secondhand smoke: nearly as large as smoking. *Circulation*. 2005;111:2684–2698.
86. Khuder SA, Milz S, Jordan T, Price J, Silvestri K, Butler P. The impact of a smoking ban on hospital admissions for coronary heart disease. *Prev Med*. 2007;45(1):3–8.
87. Kawachi I, Colditz GA, Speizer FE, et al. A prospective study of passive smoking and coronary heart disease. *Circulation*. 1997;95:2374–2379.

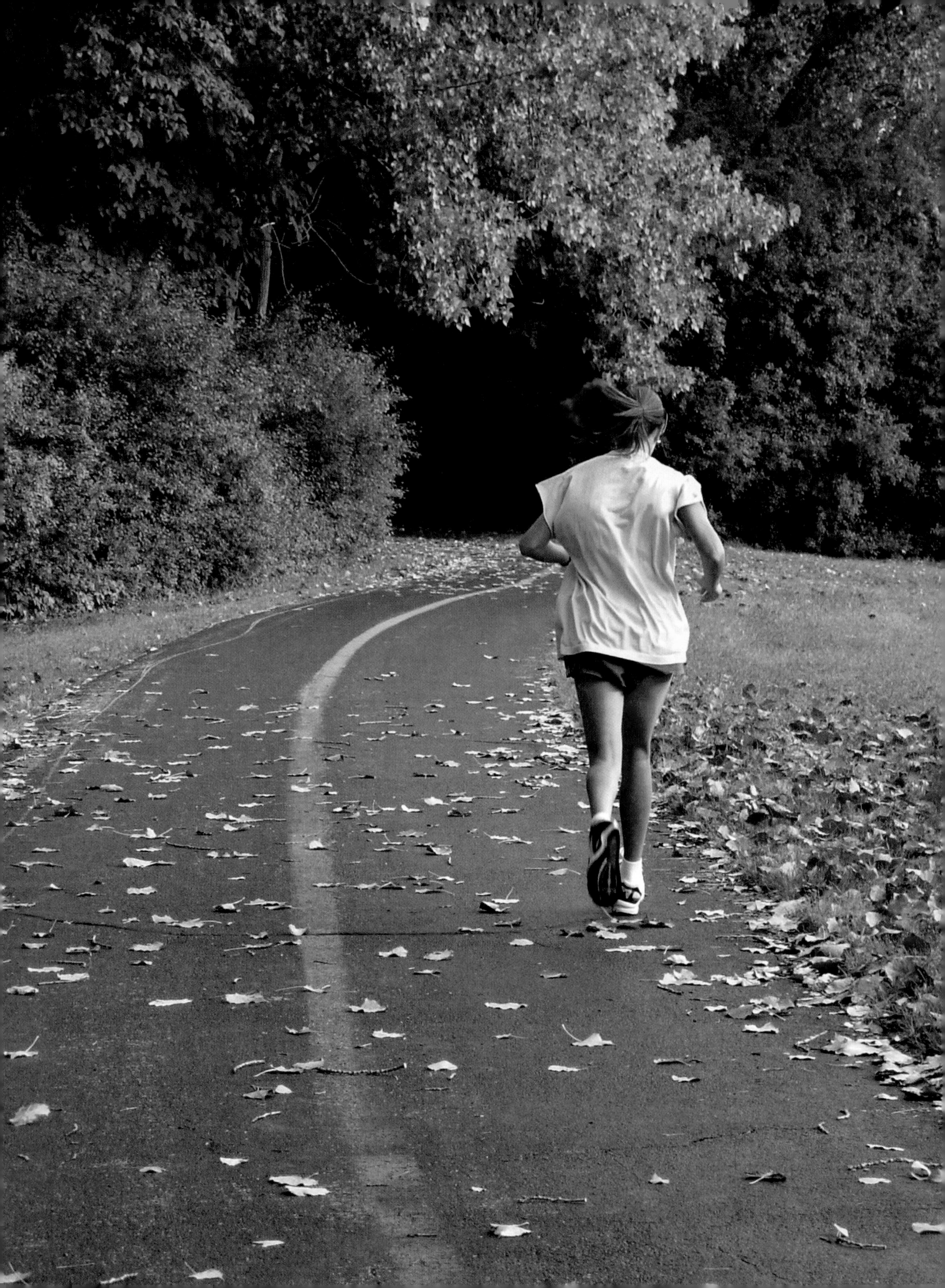

Chapter 11

Physical Activity and Exercise: Move More Every Day

Key Messages

- Physical activity is one of the most important components of a healthy lifestyle.
- Physical activity can reduce the risk of many chronic diseases and help you achieve and maintain a healthy weight.
- Cardiorespiratory endurance, muscular endurance, muscular strength, and flexibility are the components of physical fitness.
- Your personal physical activity plan should include aerobic activity, strength building, and stretching to achieve physical fitness.
- Your community has a role to play in helping you to be active for life.

Regular physical activity throughout the life span can produce many long-term health benefits. Ample evidence supports the recommendation that all people, regardless of age, gender, or ability, should engage in regular physical activity. There are cable television channels devoted to physical activity and fitness; fitness facilities are all over the landscape; bookstores are filled with fitness books; workout videos are available to help you walk, run, or lift or practice yoga or a martial art. Fitness gurus have websites to inspire you to move. With all of this, you would think that Americans would be active and fit; however, it is quite the opposite. Despite the known benefits of exercise, most people do not get the activity they need for good health.

This chapter will discuss physical activity: how much you need to be healthy, how much and what kind you need to be fit, how you can create a fitness plan to fit your lifestyle, and how the community plays a role in creating environments that support an active lifestyle.

Story

Katie and Roger are engaged to be married. They just finished their first two years of college and are ready to start a life together. They both plan on working while they finish their degrees. They are into all types of technology and live in front of their computer, smartphone, and iPad screens. Both are active on Facebook and Twitter and spend a lot of time on social networking websites. Katie and Roger have never been active. They were not athletic in high school and have never been into sports. They try to eat healthy foods but still carry a few extra pounds—maybe more than a few. Katie is overweight and would like to get into a smaller wedding dress or at least tone up a little. Roger is in the obese category and hopes his tuxedo will hide the pounds that have been creeping on since he started college. They know they should exercise, but because they have never been active, they don't know where to start. They don't remember much from gym class in high school; only one semester was required. What they do remember is that whatever sports they were playing were not much fun, and they were not good at any of them. They live about 2 miles from campus but drive in every day because they are usually running late for class. How can Katie and Roger incorporate physical activity into their busy lives? What advice do you have for these two nonathletes to get fit and healthy?

Physical Activity and Exercise

The terms *physical activity* and *exercise* are often used interchangeably. However, they do not mean exactly the same thing. **Physical activity** is any bodily movement that uses your muscles and increases the number of calories you burn. Physical activity can be divided into two categories: baseline activity and health-enhancing physical activity. **Baseline activity** is light-intensity activities that you do every day, such as standing, walking slowly, or lifting lightweight objects. Your job or lifestyle will dictate how much baseline activity you get each day. If you do only baseline activity, you are considered to be inactive. Even if you do bursts of moderate activity, such as climbing the stairs, it is not long enough to count toward meeting physical activity recommendations.

Another type of physical activity is **health-enhancing physical activity**. This is physical activity beyond baseline physical activity that produces health benefits. Brisk walking, climbing on playground equipment, and dancing are examples of health-enhancing physical activity. If you have a job that requires a lot of physical activity, such as construction work, you may get enough physical activity on your job to meet physical activity recommendations.

Exercise is a type of physical activity that is planned, structured, repetitive, and done for the purpose of improving physical fitness, physical performance, or health. Jogging, running, using cardio equipment, lifting weights, taking a yoga class, and swimming laps are all examples of exercise. In this chapter, the terms *exercise* and *physical activity* will both be used to describe activities done to meet physical activity recommendations.

How Physically Active Are Americans?

Many people do not get the physical activity they need each day. Only half of adults 18 and older get the minimum recommended amount of physical activity. This number is even lower (39%) in adults over age 65. One-quarter of people do not do any leisure time physical activity, such as walking, gardening, playing golf, or tennis.[1]

Children are also not as physically active as they should be. Less than 20% of middle and high school students participate in the recommended amount of physical activity. Boys do better than girls (25% versus 11%), but both genders could benefit from more physical activity.[2]

TERMS

physical activity Any movement that works the muscles and uses more energy than when the body is at rest.

baseline activity Light-intensity activities performed in everyday life, such as standing, walking slowly, or lifting lightweight objects.

health-enhancing physical activity Physical activity beyond baseline physical activity that produces health benefits.

exercise A type of physical activity that is planned, structured, repetitive, and done for the purpose of improving physical fitness, physical performance, or health.

How is it that so many people are not active at a level that would provide health benefits? What has changed in our culture and society to support inactivity? Many changes in the world point to why so many people are inactive. Many of the jobs today do not require any physical activity. Even jobs that once required physical activity now are performed by machines or are automated. We have labor-saving devices for virtually every aspect of our daily lives, from electric toothbrushes, electric sidewalks, elevators, and riding lawnmowers, to automatic dishwashers. Even children who once rode wheeled toys powered by their own energy now ride toys powered by electricity. Our cities and neighborhoods are built so that we have to drive everywhere instead of walking or biking. Sitting in front of some screen—computer, TV, iPod, phone, or video game—often comprises most of the day.

Your life is certainly not going to go back to manual labor, and the computer and other technologies are here to stay. Getting the amount of physical activity by completing daily tasks is not possible for most people. To be physically active at the recommended level, you must be mindful to add physical activity and exercise each day.

Benefits of Physical Activity

Being physically active is one of the most important steps you can take to improve your health. Being physically active at the minimum recommended levels brings a number of health benefits (**Table 11.1**). Strong evidence supports that physical activity reduces the risk of premature death from all causes.[3]

The number one killer in North America is cardiovascular disease (CVD; heart disease and stroke). Major risk factors for CVD are inactivity and poor cardiorespiratory fitness. Physical activity decreases the incidence of CVD as well as some of the risk factors for the disease.[4–11] Physical activity can help lower blood cholesterol and blood pressure.[12] Being physically active can also decrease the risk of type 2 diabetes and obesity.[13] Regular physical activity can decrease these risk factors in both men and women, regardless of age or weight status. Even moderate physical activity can greatly reduce the risk of CVD.

Physical activity decreases the risk of several forms of cancer. The evidence suggests that physical activity is protective against breast and colon cancer.[14,15] Some evidence suggests that it can also protect against endometrial and lung cancer.[15]

Physical activity has a profound effect on **musculoskeletal** health. Physical activity can decrease the risk of bone fractures and protect against the onset of osteoporosis.[16,17] It can also increase muscle mass and help maintain muscle mass as you age, which promotes healthy ageing.[17] Some evidence indicates that physical activity has a protective effect against the onset of arthritis. Ample evidence suggests that physical activity can help those with arthritis manage pain and maintain mobility.[18,19] Being physically active can also prevent or delay the onset of functional limitations as you age.[20] It can also reduce the risk of falls in older adults by helping maintain strength and balance.

Table 11.1

Health Benefits Associated with Regular Physical Activity

Children and Adolescents
Strong evidence
• Improved cardiorespiratory and muscular fitness
• Improved bone health
• Improved cardiovascular and metabolic health biomarkers
• Favorable body composition
Moderate evidence
• Reduced symptoms of depression
Adults and Older Adults
Strong evidence
• Lower risk of early death
• Lower risk of coronary heart disease
• Lower risk of stroke
• Lower risk of high blood pressure
• Lower risk of adverse blood lipid profile
• Lower risk of type 2 diabetes
• Lower risk of metabolic syndrome
• Lower risk of colon cancer
• Lower risk of breast cancer
• Prevention of weight gain
• Weight loss, particularly when combined with reduced calorie intake
• Improved cardiorespiratory and muscular fitness
• Prevention of falls
• Reduced depression
• Better cognitive function (for older adults)
Moderate to strong evidence
• Better functional health (for older adults)
• Reduced abdominal obesity
Moderate evidence
• Lower risk of hip fracture
• Lower risk of lung cancer
• Lower risk of endometrial cancer
• Weight maintenance after weight loss
• Increased bone density
• Improved sleep quality

Source: US Department of Health and Human Services. *2008 Physical Activity Guidelines for Americans*. Washington, DC: USDHHS, 2008. http://www.health.gov/paguidelines/default/aspx. Accessed May 26, 2010.

TERMS

musculoskeletal All of the muscles, bones, joints, and related structures that function in the movement of the body.

As part of the energy balance equation, physical activity can help you achieve and maintain a healthy weight. Being physically active is one of the factors associated with a healthy weight. It is very difficult to achieve and maintain a healthy weight without physical activity.[21]

Finally, physical activity plays a role in mental health. Regular physical activity has a protective effect against several negative aspects of mental health and can decrease the risk of depression and cognitive decline.[22] It can also decrease symptoms of anxiety, feelings of distress, and fatigue. Physical activity lowers the odds of disruptive and insufficient sleep. Most important, physical activity can enhance your overall sense of well-being.

Components of Physical Activity

There are different types of physical activity, and each type provides a unique benefit to your body. Aerobic activity works the large muscles and challenges your heart and lungs. Muscle-strengthening activities build and strengthen muscles. Bone-building activities help you maintain strong bone mass throughout your life. Flexibility activities help your joints to move in a full range of motion. Physical fitness requires all of these forms of physical activity.

Aerobic Activity

Aerobic activity is sometimes called *endurance activity* or *cardio*. The rows of treadmills, stair climbers, bicycles, and elliptical trainers in most gyms are there to help you to engage in aerobic activity. Aerobic activity uses the large muscles of the body for a sustained period of time. Brisk walking, running, jogging, bicycling, jumping rope, and swimming are all aerobic activities. Aerobic activity causes your heart rate to increase to meet the demands of increased body movement. Over time, aerobic activity will make your heart and lungs stronger. Aerobic activity requires more energy than most other activities because you are working the large muscles of your body. In other words, you burn more calories when doing aerobic activity than other activities. Aerobic activity has three components: intensity, frequency, and duration.

Intensity is how hard you are working (**Table 11.2**). You may hear intensity referred to as light, moderate, or vigorous. The talk test is a simple way for you to monitor exercise intensity. At a light intensity level, you should be able to sing while doing the activity. For most people, light daily activities such as shopping, cooking, and doing the laundry do not count toward the recommended amounts of physical activity. Your body is not working hard enough to get your heart rate up. At a moderate intensity level, you should be able to carry on a conversation comfortably while engaging in the activity, but not be able to sing. At a vigorous intensity level, you cannot say more than a few words without pausing for a breath. The higher the intensity, the more your heart rate and breathing will increase.

Perceived exertion is another simple way to monitor intensity (**Figure 11.1**). This is a scale from 0–10 that estimates your perceived intensity. When determining perceived exertion, think about your entire body, not just your legs or your breathing. Think about your overall effort and rate it on a scale from 0–10, with 0 being nothing at all and 10 being the absolute maximum you can do. Don't compare how hard you feel like you are working to anyone else; it is *your* rating of exertion. A 0 is sitting, a level of 5–6 is moderate, and a level of 7–8 is vigorous. Depending on your fitness level, a brisk walk is usually moderate intensity and running or jogging is vigorous intensity.

TERMS

aerobic activity Physical activity that requires the heart and lungs to work harder to meet the body's oxygen demands; includes brisk walking, jogging, running, swimming, and other activities that use the large muscle groups.

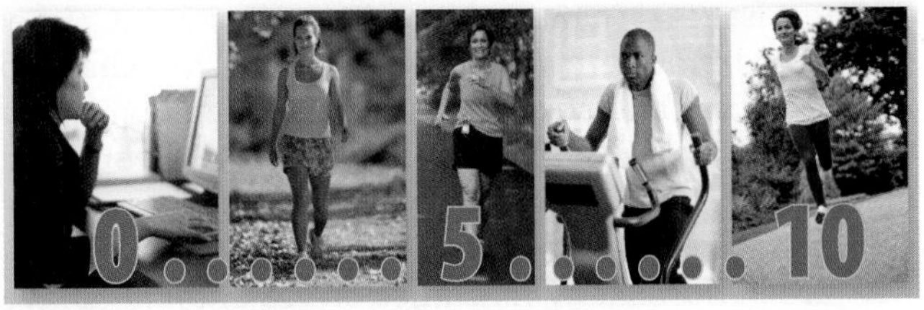

Figure 11.1

Perceived Exertion Is a Good Way to Estimate the Intensity of Your Aerobic Activity

Table 11.2

Examples of Aerobic Activities and Estimated Intensity Level

Moderate Intensity	Vigorous Intensity
Walking briskly (3 miles per hour or faster)	Fast walking (race walking) Jogging
Water aerobics	Running Swimming laps
Bicycling (slower than 10 miles per hour)	Tennis (singles) Aerobic dance (or other similar group exercise)
Tennis (doubles)	Bicycling (10 miles per hour or faster)
Ballroom dancing	Jumping rope
Gardening	Heavy gardening (continuous digging or hoeing, with heart rate increases)
Elliptical trainer at a moderate pace	Elliptical trainer at a vigorous pace

The *frequency* of aerobic activity is how often you do the activity, that is, daily, weekly, etc. The *duration* of aerobic activity is how long you do the activity. Together, intensity, frequency, and duration add up to the amount of benefit you will receive from the aerobic activity. Because aerobic activity uses the large muscle groups of your body, one benefit is the calories burned (**Table 11.3**). The actual calories that you burn will depend on your body size, the intensity of the activity, and the duration of the activity.

Muscle-Strengthening Activity

With **muscle-strengthening activity**, the muscles work against a force or weight. Muscle-strengthening activities can incorporate weights, elastic bands or tubes, or your own body weight. Muscle-strengthening activities make the muscles do more work than they are used to doing. The muscles respond by growing stronger over time. Muscle-strengthening activities provide benefits that cannot be achieved with aerobic activities alone. Muscle-strengthening activities help to maintain or increase muscle mass, increase muscular strength, and increase bone strength.

Table 11.3

Calories Burned per Minute per Pound for Common Activities

Activity	Calories Burned per Minute per Pound
Walking (3.5 miles per hour, approximately 17 minutes per mile)	.030
Walking (4.5 miles per hour, approximately 13 minutes per mile)	.050
Running (5 miles per hour, approximately 12 minutes per mile)	.064
Running (7.5 miles per hour, approximately 8 minutes per mile)	.095
Biking (< 10 miles per hour)	.031
Biking (> 10 miles per hour)	.064
Swimming (slow freestyle)	.058
Swimming (fast freestyle)	.071
Yard work (light gardening)	.036
Yard work (heavy digging, chopping wood)	.048
Ballroom dancing	.036
Aerobics	.052
Elliptical trainer (moderate pace)	.068
Elliptical trainer (vigorous pace)	.076
Weight lifting (light workout)	.024
Weight lifting (vigorous, heavy lifting)	.048

Use the following formula to get an estimate of the number of calories burned during exercise:

weight in pounds × minutes of activity × calories per minute per pound for given exercise = estimate of calories burned

For example, a 150-pound person who ran at a rate of 5 miles per hour for 30 minutes would burn:

150 × 30 × .064 = 288 calories

Inactive adults lose around 0.5 pounds of muscle per year, which adds up to 5 pounds per decade. You need to try to keep or even increase the amount of muscle tissue you have. Muscle tissue is active and burns calories even when at rest. Regular strength training can boost your basal metabolic rate as the amount of muscle you have increases. Strength training is effective in increasing lean body mass as you age; even older adults can benefit from strength training.[23]

Muscle-strengthening activities are especially important for someone who is trying to lose weight. When calories are reduced, lean tissue and muscle mass can be lost. Adding muscle-strengthening activities can help maintain lean body mass even while losing weight.

There are some common misconceptions about muscle-strengthening activities. If you are a woman, you may be worried that lifting weights will make you big and bulky. Most women lack the hormones and body structure to develop bulky muscles. Men, although they do have hormones that allow for building more muscle tissue, still have to work very hard to create large muscles. Resistance exercises can positively shape your body, creating a "fit" look. Another misconception is that that muscle will turn into fat. Fat cells and muscle cells are different; one cannot change into the other. If you stop exercising, you may gain weight due to consuming more calories than you need, but muscle cannot turn into fat.

Muscle-strengthening activities have three components: intensity, frequency, and repetition. In muscle-strengthening activities, *intensity* refers to the amount of weight or force that is used relative to the amount you can lift. *Frequency* is how often you do muscle-strengthening activities. *Repetition* is how many times you lift a weight or do a sit-up or pull-up. The effects of muscle-strengthening activities are limited to the muscle you are working. You need to work all the major muscle groups of the body: legs, hips, back, abdomen, chest, shoulders, and arms.

Bone-Strengthening Activity

Bone-strengthening activities are sometime called weight-bearing activities. These types of activities put force on the bones and cause them to grow stronger. Bone-strengthening activities can be aerobic activities, such as walking or running, or muscle-strengthening activities, such as lifting weights. Participating in bone-strengthening activities can decrease your risk of osteoporosis.

TERMS

muscle-strengthening activity Sometimes called *resistance training*; a type of physical activity that engages the muscles to do more work than they are used to doing, such as when lifting weights or using stretch bands.

Flexibility Activity

Flexibility activities are those that require reaching, bending, and stretching. Flexibility exercises increase the ability of a joint to move through a range of motion. A lack of flexibility may make it harder to be physically active or even to do regular day-to-day activities. Adding flexibility exercises to your routine offers a number of benefits. You will have greater freedom of movement, improved posture, increased physical and mental relaxation, and reduced muscle tension and soreness. Simple stretches are good flexibility activities to do before or after aerobic or muscle-building activities. Yoga and Pilates and some martial arts also increase flexibility.

Physical Fitness

Physical fitness is related to your ability to perform physical activity. Overall fitness includes cardiorespiratory endurance, muscular endurance, muscular strength, and flexibility. In order to be fit, you must address all of these components in your physical activity routine. A physical activity routine that only includes running addresses cardiorespiratory and muscular endurance but does little to increase muscle strength or flexibility. Similarly, only lifting weights addresses muscular strength but does not improve cardiorespiratory endurance or flexibility. Your physical activity choices should include a balance of activities that address all aspects of fitness.

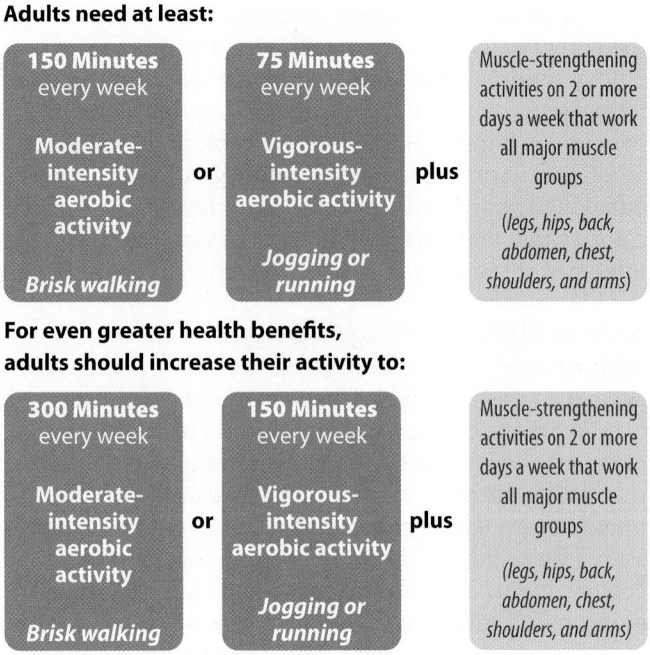

■ **Figure 11.2**

Physical Activity Guidelines for Adults

All adults should avoid inactivity. Some physical activity is better than none. Adults who participate in any amount of physical activity gain some health benefits.

Source: US Department of Health and Human Services. *2008 Physical Activity Guidelines for Americans*. Washington, DC: USDHHS, 2008. http://www.health.gov/paguidelines/default/aspx. Accessed May 26, 2010.

Physical Activity Recommendations

Physical activity recommendations are set by a group of experts assembled by the Centers for Disease Control and Prevention (CDC) and are based on all of the available research on the health benefits of exercise. Physical activity recommendations are set for children, adolescents, adults, older adults, and people with disabilities.

Adults

For substantial health benefits, you need at least 2 hours and 30 minutes (150 minutes) of moderate-intensity aerobic activity (e.g., brisk walking, water aerobics, riding a bike on level ground or with few hills, or playing doubles tennis) every week (**Figure 11.2**). Or, participate in 1 hour and 15 minutes (75 minutes) of vigorous-intensity aerobic activity (e.g., jogging or running, swimming laps, riding a bike fast or on hills, playing singles tennis, or playing basketball) every week.

For even greater health benefits (i.e., to manage body weight and/or to prevent gradual unhealthy weight gain), you should increase your activity to 5 hours (300 minutes) of moderate-intensity aerobic activity every week or participate in 2 hours and 30 minutes (150 minutes) of vigorous-intensity aerobic activity every week.[24]

This may sound like a lot, especially if you are not currently active, but you don't have to do it all at once, and keep in mind that this is the amount you need for the whole week. You can fit the activity into your schedule throughout the week. As long as you are doing your activity at a moderate or vigorous effort for at least 10 minutes at a time, it counts toward your weekly total. You don't have to choose between moderate or vigorous; an equivalent mix of moderate-intensity and vigorous-intensity aerobic activity is acceptable. A rule of thumb is that one minute of vigorous activity is about the same as two minutes of moderate activity.

All adults should avoid being inactive. Some physical activity is better than none, even if you don't reach the minimum recommended level. Even small amounts of physical activity can have some health benefits (see **Table 11.4**).

Muscle-strengthening activities should also be part of your physical activity routine. There is no specific recom-

TERMS

flexibility activities Physical activity done to increase the ability of a joint to move through a range of motion, such as bending, reaching, or stretching.

physical fitness A state of well-being with low risk of premature health problems and energy to participate in a variety of physical activities; includes cardiorespiratory endurance, muscular endurance, muscular strength, and flexibility.

Table 11.4

Classification of Total Weekly Amounts of Aerobic Physical Activity

Levels of Physical Activity	Range of Moderate-Intensity Minutes a Week	Summary of Overall Health Benefits	Comment
Inactive	No activity beyond baseline	None	Being inactive is unhealthy.
Low	Activity beyond baseline but fewer than 150 minutes a week	Some	Low levels of activity are clearly preferable to an inactive lifestyle.
Medium	150 minutes to 300 minutes a week	Substantial	Activity at the high end of this range has additional and more extensive health benefits than activity at the low end.
High	More than 300 minutes a week	Additional	Current science does not allow researchers to identify an upper limit of activity above which there are no additional health benefits.

Source: US Department of Health and Human Services. *2008 Physical Activity Guidelines for Americans*. Washington, DC: USDHHS, 2008. http://www.health.gov/paguidelines /default/aspx. Accessed May 26, 2010.

mendation for the amount of time you should spend on muscle strengthening. However, there are some guidelines as to how much you should do to see benefits. *Repetition* and *set* are terms used to describe the amount of resistance exercise. A repetition is how many times in a row an exercise is performed before resting. A set is a group of repetitions. For example, eight push-ups (repetitions), rest for one minute, eight push-ups (repetitions) would equal two sets of eight repetitions of push-ups. A minimum of one set of 8–12 repetitions of exercises for each major muscle group of the body—legs, hips, back, abdomen, chest, shoulders, and arms—at least twice a week on nonconsecutive days is recommended. Skipping at least a day in between training a muscle group will allow for that muscle to recover.

Choose a weight that is heavy enough to cause fatigue by the last repetition. Even with fatigue, you should still be using proper form. For example, if you are going to do one set of eight repetitions of bicep curls, choose a weight heavy enough that by the eighth repetition you can still use good form but feel like you need to rest before doing another. In order for muscle-strengthening activities to be effective, they should consistently and sufficiently fatigue the muscles without causing pain or discomfort. Whether you are using stretch bands, hand weights, or your own body weight, the muscle must be challenged for you to see gains in strength. Increase the amount of weight or resistance you use as you get stronger. You may want to build up from one set of exercises per muscle group to two to three sets per muscle group. Increase the number of sets from each muscle group or number of days you do muscle-strengthening exercises for even more benefit.

There are no recommendations for the amount of flexibility activities you should do. But there are some guidelines you can follow to make sure you maintain flexibility. Warm your muscles up before stretching by doing 5–10 minutes of low-intensity physical activity, such as walking or marching in place. Stretch to a point of tightness, without causing discomfort. Hold each stretch for 15 to 30 seconds without bouncing.

Older Adults

Regular physical activity is important for healthy aging.[25] Adults aged 65 and older can benefit, both mentally and physically, from regular physical activity. Older adults who are in generally good health can follow the guidelines for adults for physical activity. Older adults with chronic diseases or other health conditions that could limit activity should discuss appropriate physical activity with their healthcare provider (**Figure 11.3**).

- When older adults cannot do 150 minutes of moderate-intensity aerobic activity a week because of chronic conditions, they should be as physically active as their abilities and conditions allow.
- Older adults should do exercises that maintain or improve balance if they are at risk of falling.
- Older adults should determine their level of effort for physical activity relative to their level of fitness.
- Older adults with chronic conditions should understand whether and how their conditions affect their ability to do regular physical activity safety.

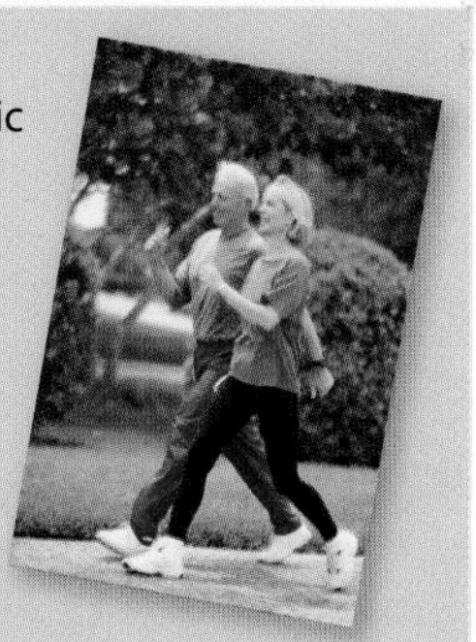

Figure 11.3

Physical Activity Guidelines for Older Adults

The guidelines for adults also apply to older adults. In addition, these guidelines are just for older adults.

Source: US Department of Health and Human Services. *2008 Physical Activity Guidelines for Americans*. Washington, DC: USDHHS, 2008. http://www.health.gov/paguidelines/default/aspx. Accessed May 26, 2010.

As with all adults, older adults should participate in both aerobic and strength-building exercise. Aging is associated with a loss of lean body mass; strength-building exercises can help slow this process.[23] Research suggests that regular physical activity can reduce the risk of falls.[26] Reduction of falls is seen when older adults participate in physical activities that promote balance, such as backward walking, sideways walking, or standing from a seated position.

Children and Adolescents

Children and adolescents should be physically active on a regular basis for physical and mental health and well-being. Children who are physically active are more likely to be active as adults. Children and adolescents ages 6–17 years old should participate in 60 minutes or more of moderate to vigorous age-appropriate activity each day.[25] The activities should include muscle- and bone-strengthening activities as well as aerobic activities (**Table 11.5**).

Children and adolescents should engage in a combination of moderate and vigorous or all vigorous activity for at least 60 minutes per day (**Figure 11.4**). Engaging only in moderate-intensity activity is not recommended, because it will not substantially improve cardiorespiratory fitness. Intensity can be estimated using techniques similar to those used by adults. Adults supervising children can observe the intensity of activity in children. For example, a child walking to school is moderate intensity, while running in a game of tag is vigorous intensity. Sed-

Table 11.5

Examples of Moderate- and Vigorous-Intensity Aerobic Physical Activities and Muscle- and Bone-Strengthening Activities for Children and Adolescents

	Age Group	
Type of Physical Activity	Children	Adolescents
Moderate–intensity aerobic	• Active recreation, such as hiking, skateboarding, rollerblading • Bicycle riding • Brisk walking	• Active recreation, such as canoeing, hiking, skateboarding, rollerblading • Brisk walking • Bicycle riding (stationary or road bike) • Housework and yard work, such as sweeping or pushing a lawn mower • Games that require catching and throwing, such as baseball and softball
Vigorous–intensity aerobic	• Active games involving running and chasing, such as tag • Bicycle riding • Jumping rope • Martial arts, such as karate • Running • Sports such as soccer, ice or field hockey, basketball, swimming, tennis • Cross-country skiing	• Active games involving running and chasing, such as flag football • Bicycle riding • Jumping rope • Martial arts, such as karate • Running • Sports such as soccer, ice or field hockey, basketball, swimming, tennis • Vigorous dancing • Cross-country skiing
Muscle-strengthening	• Games such as tug-of-war • Modified push-ups (with knees on the floor) • Resistance exercises using body weight or resistance bands • Rope or tree climbing • Sit-ups (curl-ups or crunches) • Swinging on playground equipment/bars	• Games such as tug-of-war • Push-ups and pull-ups • Resistance exercises with exercise bands, weight machines, hand-held weights • Climbing wall • Sit-ups (curl-ups or crunches)
Bone-strengthening	• Games such as hopscotch • Hopping, skipping, jumping • Jumping rope • Running • Sports such as gymnastics, basketball, volleyball, tennis	• Hopping, skipping, jumping • Jumping rope • Running • Sports such as gymnastics, basketball, volleyball, tennis

Source: US Department of Health and Human Services. *2008 Physical Activity Guidelines for Americans*. Washington, DC: USDHHS, 2008. http://www.health.gov/paguidelines/default/aspx. Accessed May 26, 2010.

Which Side Are You On?

Making the Case for Physical Activity in Schools

Physical activity is an important component of good health for all persons, regardless of age or ability. It is critical that children and adolescents engage in physical activity on a regular basis to improve their health. It is widely recognized that lack of adequate physical activity, along with poor eating habits, are the primary contributors to the childhood obesity epidemic. It is recommended that children and adolescents participate in 60 minutes and up to several hours of age-appropriate physical activity each day.[24] Ensuring that children and adolescents are physically active each day is one way to improve children's physical and mental health, as well as their ability to learn. Healthy, active children are likely to become healthy, active adults. Teaching children and adolescents the benefits of an active lifestyle and giving them the skills to remain active for life should be a common goal of preschools, schools, families, and communities.

Children and adolescents spend a large part of their day at school. Schools are places of extraordinary influence on the development of lifelong behavior patters. This influence stems not only from what children learn in the classroom, but also from environmental cues, role modeling, and peer influence.

Schools cannot be expected to solve all the problems associated with physical inactivity, but they do play a significant role. Many people feel that schools should be places where physical activity opportunities, consistent messages, and supportive environments are priorities.

Schools are under pressure for students to perform well in reading, writing, and math. This sometimes means more time in the classroom and less time for recess or physical education. Time at play is seen as taking time away from more important aspects of learning. Certainly, it is a challenge to meet students' academic and health needs. However, both are important, and many feel both should receive time and resources.

Taking time away from the classroom for physical activity can, in fact, help with students' academic performance. Physical activity, both recess and physical education class, have positive effects not only on physical health, but on mental health as well. Regular physical activity causes changes in the brain and brain chemistry that improve mood and cognitive function. Cognitive function includes brain-related abilities such as attention, concentration, memory, language, abstract reasoning, and calculation. Evidence suggests that students in elementary through high school perform better academically when they are physically active.[28–31] Physical activity is linked to many positive academic outcomes, including higher grade point averages, higher scores on standardized tests, increased concentration, better memory, improved classroom behaviors, reduced school dropout rate, and greater odds of attending college full time. Increased physical activity, even when it reduces academic instruction time, has been shown to have a favorable effect on students' academic achievement.[28–30]

It is important that physical activity in the form of recess and physical education be included in the school day. Although schools should provide opportunities for children to accumulate some of the physical activity they need each day, parents and communities also have a role in children's physical activity. Communities should provide safe places for children and families to play and be active. Parents should provide opportunities for daily movement and limit the amount of time children spend with inactive activities, such as playing video games or watching television.

entary activities, such as television or video games, should be replaced with activity whenever possible.

Less is known about the specific physical activity needs of children aged 0 to 5. However, the National Association of Sport and Physical Education states that all children from birth to age 5 should engage daily in physical activity the promotes movement skillfulness and establishes a foundation for health-related fitness.[27] Infants should interact with caregivers in daily physical activities that are dedicated to exploring movement and the environment. Caregivers should place infants in environments that encourage movement and promote skill development. Toddlers should engage in a total of at least 30 minutes of structured physical activity each day and at least 60 minutes of unstructured physically active play. Preschoolers should get at least 60 minutes of structured physical activity and at least 60 minute and up to several hours of unstructured physical activity each day. Except when sleeping, toddlers and preschoolers should not be inactive for more than 60 minutes at a time.

People with Disabilities

People with disabilities can gain health benefits from regular physical activity (see **Figure 11.5**). A healthcare provider should be consulted to discuss how a person's disability affects his or her ability to do certain physical activities. Some people with disabilities may be able to follow guidelines for adults. Others may need to adapt the guidelines to match their abilities.

How You Can Become More Physically Active

You have many options to become physically active and create an active lifestyle for the rest of your life. The first place to start is to assess how active you are. Use Table 11.4 to compare your current activity level with what is recommended. If you are inactive, work gradually toward the goal of 150 minutes of physical activity per week. Walking is a great place to start (**Table 11.6** and **Figure 11.6**). You can walk indoors on a treadmill or outside.

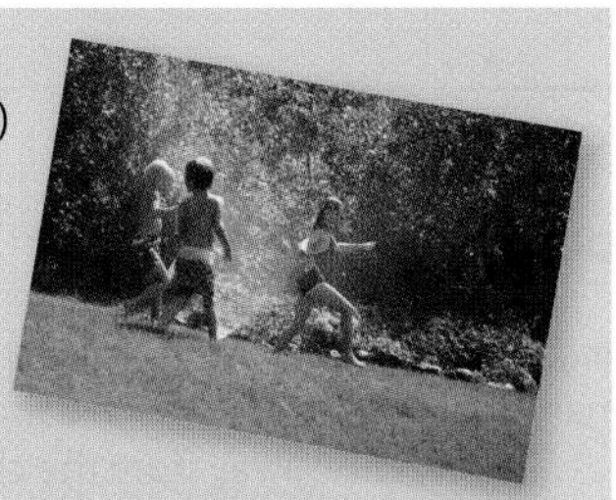

- Children and adolescents should do 60 minutes (1 hour) or more of physical activity daily.

  Aerobic: Most of the 60 or more minutes a day should be either moderate- or vigorous-intensity aerobic physical activity and should include vigorous-intensity physical activity at least 3 days per week.

  Muscle-strengthening: As part of their 60 or more minutes of daily physical activity, children and adolescents should include muscle-strengthening physical activity on at least 3 days of the week.

  Bone-strengthening: As part of their 60 or more minutes of daily physical activity, children and adolescents should include bone-strengthening physical activity on at least 3 days of the week.

- It is important to encourage young people to participate in physical activities that are appropriate for their age, that are enjoyable, and that offer variety.

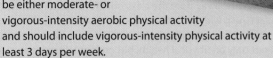

■ **Figure 11.4**

Physical Activity Guidelines for Children and Adolescents

Source: US Department of Health and Human Services. *2008 Physical Activity Guidelines for Americans*. Washington, DC: USDHHS, 2008. http://www.health.gov/paguidelines/default/aspx. Accessed May 26, 2010.

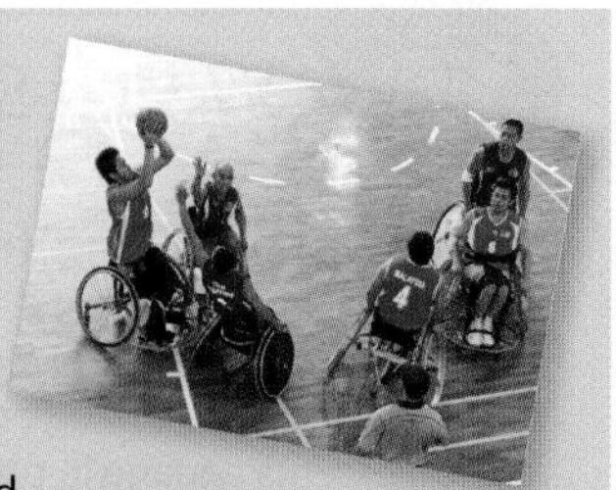

- Adults with disabilities, who are able to, should get at least 150 minutes a week of moderate-intensity, or 75 minutes a week of vigorous-intensity, aerobic activity, or an equivalent combination of moderate- and vigorous-intensity aerobic activity. Aerobic activity should be performed in episodes of at least 10 minutes, and preferably, it should be spread throughout the week.
- Adults with disabilities, who are able to, should also do muscle-strengthening activities of moderate or high intensity that involve all major muscle groups on 2 or more days a week, as these activities provide additional health benefits.
- When adults with disabilities are not able to meet the Guidelines, they should engage in regular physical activity according to their abilities and should avoid inactivity.
- Adults with disabilities should consult their healthcare provider about the amounts and types of physical activity that are appropriate for their abilities.

■ **Figure 11.5**

Physical Activity Guidelines for Adults with Disabilities

Source: US Department of Health and Human Services. *2008 Physical Activity Guidelines for Americans*. Washington, DC: USDHHS, 2008. http://www.health.gov/paguidelines/default/aspx. Accessed May 26, 2010.

Table 11.6

Sample Walking Program

	Warm up	Exercise	Cool down	Total time
Week 1				
Session A	Walk 5 min.	Walk briskly 5 min.	Walk more slowly 5 min.	15 min.
Session B	Repeat above pattern.			
Session C	Repeat above pattern.			
Continue with at least three exercise sessions during each week of the program.				
WEEK 2	Walk 5 min.	Walk briskly 7 min.	Walk 5 min.	17 min.
WEEK 3	Walk 5 min.	Walk briskly 9 min.	Walk 5 min.	19 min.
WEEK 4	Walk 5 min.	Walk briskly 11 min.	Walk 5 min.	21 min.
WEEK 5	Walk 5 min.	Walk briskly 13 min.	Walk 5 min.	23 min.
WEEK 6	Walk 5 min.	Walk briskly 15 min.	Walk 5 min.	25 min.
WEEK 7	Walk 5 min.	Walk briskly 18 min.	Walk 5 min.	28 min.
WEEK 8	Walk 5 min.	Walk briskly 20 min.	Walk 5 min.	30 min.
WEEK 9	Walk 5 min.	Walk briskly 23 min.	Walk 5 min.	33 min.
WEEK 10	Walk 5 min.	Walk briskly 26 min.	Walk 5 min.	36 min.
WEEK 11	Walk 5 min.	Walk briskly 28 min.	Walk 5 min.	38 min.
WEEK 12	Walk 5 min.	Walk briskly 30 min.	Walk 5 min.	40 min.

WEEK 13 ON: Gradually increase your brisk walking time to 30 to 60 minutes, three or four times a week. Remember that your goal is to get the benefits you are seeking and enjoy your activity.

Source: National Institutes of Health, National Heart, Lung, and Blood Institute. *The Practical Guide: Identification, Evaluation and Treatment of Overweight and Obesity in Adults.* 2000. http://www.nhlbi.nih.gov/guidelines/obesity/prctgd_c.pdf. Accessed April 10, 2011.

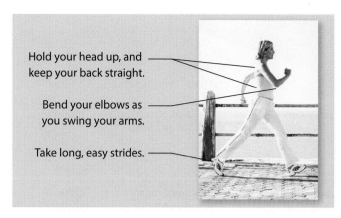

Hold your head up, and keep your back straight.
Bend your elbows as you swing your arms.
Take long, easy strides.

■ **Figure 11.6**
Use Good Form When Walking

You should also add muscle-strengthening actives and increase them gradually over time (**Table 11.7**). To start, you may want to do these active only one day a week and at a light or moderate level. Over time, increase the muscle-strengthening activities to two or more times each week. Increase the intensity (amount of weight or effort) each week as well. If you are new to muscle-strengthening activities, you may want to get the help of a personal trainer to develop a program that is appropriate for your fitness level and goals.

If you are already active and get the recommended minimum amount of physical activity and muscle-strengthening activities, you can gain even more health and fitness benefits by increasing your physical activity. You can do this by increasing the duration and/or the intensity. If time is a challenge, the best way to achieve more benefits is to increase the intensity of your physical activity. If you usually walk for 30 minutes for your cardio, step it up to a jog (**Table 11.8**). If you do the elliptical or bike for 30 minutes at a moderate pace, up the intensity so that you are working at a vigorous level. Generally, it is a 2 to 1 rule—two minutes of moderate intensity is equal to one minute of vigorous intensity. You can get twice the benefit in the same amount of time by increasing intensity.

Table 11.7

Strengthening Tips for Weights or Stretch Bands

- Perform exercises for each of the major muscle groups: legs, back, chest, shoulders, arms, and abdomen.
- Perform one set of each exercise to the point where you feel your muscles are fatigued, while maintaining proper form.
- Exercise each muscle group two to three nonconsecutive days per week if possible.
- Use good form. Using good form is as important as the amount of weight you use!
- Allow enough time between exercises to perform the next exercise in proper form.
- Perform both the lifting and lowering portion of the resistance exercises in a controlled manner.
- Maintain a normal breathing pattern; breath-holding can cause excessive increase in blood pressure. Breathe out during the lifting phase; breathe in during the lowering phase.
- If possible, exercise with a training partner who can provide feedback, assistance, and motivation.

Getting and Staying Motivated

You know you should be active. You may even make it to the gym or out the door for a walk on occasion. How can you get motivated to make physical activity a priority, and stay motivated to achieve your fitness goals? Here are some ideas that can help get you motivated and help you stay that way to create your physically active lifestyle:

Find a workout buddy. A workout partner can be valuable to keep you motivated. Find a friend or family member to be your workout buddy and to keep you on track with your activity goals. You may not make it to the gym or out the door for a walk if it is just you, but if you have someone counting on you to be there, you are more likely to show up. If you are a member of a gym, check into working out with a certified personal trainer for some of your workouts.

Focus on progress. If you want to increase your physical activity, it is important to start slowly and progress

Green and Healthy

Green Transportation

Making streets conducive to both pedestrian and bicycle travel is not only good for the health of residents, but it can also help to minimize the environmental impact of streets. Many aspects of street design can work in favor of both complete streets for all travelers and green streets for environmental sustainability.[40] Nearly half of the trips you take are 3 miles or less, and 28% are less than a mile, yet most are taken by car.[46] In fact, 65% of trips less than 1 mile are made by automobile.[46] Automobiles are the fastest growing carbon dioxide source in the United States. Even with improvements in vehicle and fuel economy, greenhouse gas emissions from transportation continue to climb.[47] One way to decrease carbon emissions is to take more trips on foot or by bicycle.

Complete streets are needed to reduce the need to drive everywhere. Cities and towns that provide residents with transportation options are seeing decreases in their carbon emissions. Changing existing streets to complete streets helps reduce pollution and can play a vital role in the fight against climate change.[40] One of the best ways you can make a contribution to a greener world is to bike or walk whenever you can instead of getting in the car. You will not only be helping the environment, but you will improve your health as well.

Table 11.8

Sample Jogging Program

	Warm up	Exercise	Cool down	Total time
WEEK 1				
Session A	Walk 5 min., then stretch and limber up.	Then walk 10 min. Try not to stop.	Then walk more slowly 3 min. Stretch 2 min.	20 min.
Session B	Repeat above pattern.			
Session C	Repeat above pattern.			
Continue with at least three exercise sessions during each week of the program.				
WEEK 2	Walk 5 min., then stretch and limber up.	Walk 5 min., jog 1 min., walk 5 min., jog 1 min.	Walk 3 min., stretch 2 min.	22 min.
WEEK 3	Walk 5 min., then stretch and limber up.	Walk 5 min., jog 3 min., walk 5 min., jog 3 min.	Walk 3 min., stretch 2 min.	26 min.
WEEK 4	Walk 5 min., then stretch and limber up.	Walk 4 min., jog 5 min., walk 4 min., jog 5 min.	Walk 3 min., stretch 2 min.	28 min.
WEEK 5	Walk 5 min., then stretch and limber up.	Walk 4 min., jog 5 min., walk 4 min., jog 5 min.	Walk 3 min., stretch 2 min.	28 min.
WEEK 6	Walk 5 min., then stretch and limber up.	Walk 4 min., jog 6 min., walk 4 min., jog 6 min.	Walk 3 min., stretch 2 min.	30 min.
WEEK 7	Walk 5 min., then stretch and limber up.	Walk 4 min., jog 7 min., walk 4 min., jog 7 min.	Walk 3 min., stretch 2 min.	32 min.
WEEK 8	Walk 5 min., then stretch and limber up.	Walk 4 min., jog 8 min., walk 4 min., jog 8 min.	Walk 3 min., stretch 2 min.	34 min.
WEEK 9	Walk 5 min., then stretch and limber up.	Walk 4 min., jog 9 min., walk 4 min., jog 9 min.	Walk 3 min., stretch 2 min.	36 min.
WEEK 10	Walk 5 min., then stretch and limber up.	Walk 4 min., jog 13 min.	Walk 3 min., stretch 2 min.	27 min.
WEEK 11	Walk 5 min., then stretch and limber up.	Walk 4 min., jog 15 min.	Walk 3 min., stretch 2 min.	29 min.
WEEK 12	Walk 5 min., then stretch and limber up.	Walk 4 min., jog 17 min.	Walk 3 min., stretch 2 min.	31 min.
WEEK 13	Walk 5 min., then stretch and limber up.	Walk 2 min., jog slowly 2 min., jog 17 min.	Walk 3 min., stretch 2 min.	31 min.
WEEK 14	Walk 5 min., then stretch and limber up.	Walk 1 min., jog slowly 3 min., jog 17 min.	Walk 3 min., stretch 2 min.	31 min.
WEEK 15	Walk 5 min., then stretch and limber up.	Jog slowly 3 min., jog 17 min.	Walk 3 min., stretch 2 min.	30 min.
WEEK 16 ON: Gradually increase your jogging time from 20 to 30 minutes (or more, up to 60 minutes), three or four times a week. Remember that your goal is to get the benefits you are seeking and enjoy your activity.				

Source: National Institutes of Health, National Heart, Lung, and Blood Institute. *The Practical Guide: Identification, Evaluation and Treatment of Overweight and Obesity in Adults.* 2000. www.nhlbi.nih.gov/guidelines/obesity/prctgd_c.pdf. Accessed April 10, 2011.

gradually. Remember to focus on progress, not perfection. You will progress at your own rate depending on your age, fitness level, health status, and goals. Gradually work toward reaching the recommended amounts of aerobic, muscle-strengthening, and flexibility exercises. If you miss some workouts or even have a week where you don't get any physical activity, don't criticize yourself. Pledge to get back on track with your physical activity.

Set physical activity and fitness goals. Setting defined goals can help you stay on track with your physical activity routine. Maybe you want to run in a 10K race or complete a triathlon. Your goal may be as simple as running for 30 minutes without stopping. Whatever your goal, write it down and look at it regularly. Chart your progress so you can see how you are doing. Once you reach your goal, set another one. Physical activity is for a lifetime.

Plan. Plan time every day for exercise (**Figure 11.7**). This means more than just making active choices. It means planning a block of time in your day when you will be physically active. Your time for physical activity is as important as other meetings and commitments in your life. Even if you have a busy work or school schedule, find time for physical activity each week. You will be better able to handle the stress of a busy life if you are at least moderately active. Your best time to work out may be first thing in the morning or after school. Figure out what schedule works best for you.

Listen to your body. Especially when you are first starting a physical activity routine, exercise can cause soreness. Being sore is a sign that your muscles have worked more than normal and are getting stronger. Pay attention to your body. If you feel pain, stop. Pain is a sign that you have done too much. The most important thing is to be good to yourself and to listen to your body. You are doing this to improve your health and to feel great. You want to push yourself to do more, without trying to do too much all at once. Being physically active is a lifelong journey. You want to stay healthy, not risk an injury. You also need to listen to your body to tell you that you can do more. You want to push yourself to get the most benefit without overdoing it and risking injury.

Find activities that you enjoy. Exercise means "planned and structured," not "boring and hard." Many different types of physical activity are possible, from team

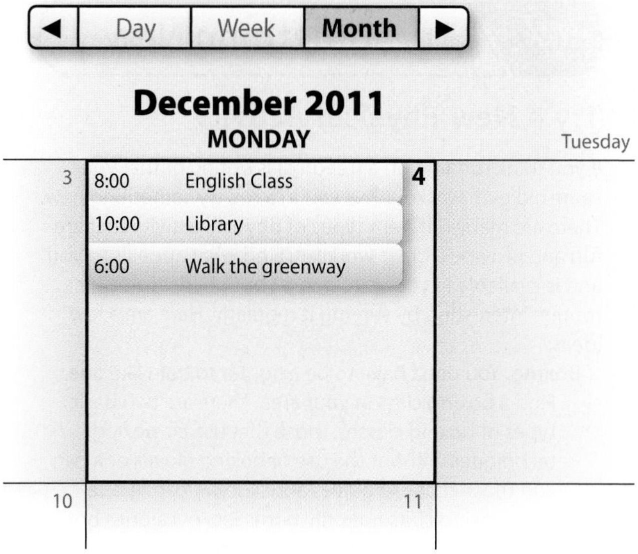

■ **Figure 11.7**

Plan Time for Exercise

Try a Pedometer

You are on the go all day running from home to school and work. You don't need to work out; you get plenty of exercise just living your life. You may think you are active when, in reality—thanks to cars and automation—you are not really moving very much. Using a pedometer can help you assess just how many steps you take during the day. A pedometer is a small device that is worn on your waistband or belt that counts the number of steps you take. Basic pedometers just count steps. More elaborate models can estimate miles, calories burned, or keep daily step totals over a week. Pedometers have been shown to be a great motivational tool. On average, those who wear pedometers walk 2,000 more steps than those who do not; 2,000 steps for most people is about a mile.[32] Using a pedometer has been shown to increase physical activity by as much as 27% per day.[32] Knowing how active you are (or are not) is a motivator to do a little bit more each day.

It is important for you to set a goal as to how many steps you will take each day. A good goal is 10,000 steps per day, or the equivalent of 5 miles of walking. Wear a pedometer for a few days and get your average steps per day. If you are under the 10,000-step goal, try to add 500 steps per day until you average 10,000 steps per day.

Pedometers are relatively inexpensive (less than $25) and can be found in sporting goods stores and department stores. Less expensive models use a spring-suspended system to count your steps and must be worn perpendicular on the body. More expensive models use a mechanism that senses acceleration and can be worn at any angle, even in your pocket.

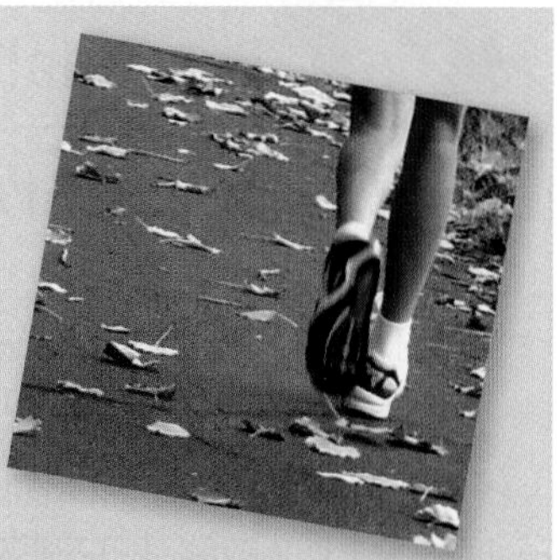

Face the traffic: If your walking routes do not have bike paths or sidewalks and you are forced to walk on the road, always walk facing oncoming traffic.

Use the buddy system: If at all possible, walk with someone. If you don't have someone to walk with, tell someone which route you will be walking and what time you expect to return.

Keep right: If you're walking on a pedestrian path, walk on the right side so that faster walkers, runners, and cyclists can pass.

Walk defensively: Don't assume that all road-users know about the "pedestrian has right-of-way" rule, especially at intersections.

Vary your routes: Don't establish regular patterns by walking the same route at the same time every day. Randomly vary your routes and the time you walk.

Self-defense: If you choose to use a hand-held spray device that contains mace or something similar, read the directions and make sure you know how to use it.

Carry ID: Always carry some form of ID in case of an accident or emergency.

Stay alert: Avoid listening to a Walkman™ or iPod™ at times when you need to be alert to your surroundings (traffic, people, pets, etc.).

Stay hydrated: Drink plenty of water before, during, and after activity.

Wear reflective clothing: If you are walking when it is dark, wear reflective clothing. Reflective belts are available at most retail stores.

■ **Figure 11.8**

Walking Safety Tips

sports to martial arts, dance, group fitness classes, and more. If your thing is working out in a gym, great; if not, find something else. You are more likely to stay with something you find enjoyable. Mix it up for added motivation. If you have been running for a while, try substituting a dance video one day a week. If you take aerobic dance three times a week, try a spin class.

Stay Safe

Engaging in physical activity does bring a risk of injury. However, strong scientific evidence indicates that physical activity is safe (**Figure 11.8**) for almost everyone and

Personal Health Check

Take the President's Challenge Adult Fitness Test

Knowing where you are with your level of fitness will help you set your physical activity goals. The President's Challenge Adult Fitness Test will help you estimate your level of aerobic fitness, muscular strength and endurance, flexibility, and body composition. To assess your aerobic fitness, you will participate in either a 1-mile walk or a 1.5-mile run. The number of push-ups and sits-ups you can perform in one minute will give you an estimate of your muscular strength and endurance. Flexibility is tested by measuring your reach in a sit-and-reach position. Finally, your BMI and waist circumference are used to estimate your body composition. Specifics on how to do the tests properly for an accurate measure can be found at www.adultfitnesstest.org (see page 217). You should only complete these tests if you are in good health. Once you have completed the tests, record your results. Enter your data online for an instant estimate of your fitness level. How did you do? Use the information to set fitness goals for the next month, year, or longer.

that the health benefits far outweigh the risks.[24] You can take a number of steps to avoid injury. First and foremost, you should not be active at a level that is not appropriate for your fitness level. You should start slow and build up gradually for both aerobic and strength-building activities. Wear appropriate protective gear, such as a bicycle helmet or other sport-specific equipment. You should make sensible choices about how, when, and where to be active. Consider weather, traffic, and air quality when exercising outside.

Try Something New

Try a New Physical Activity

If you think running on a treadmill is boring or that your same old gym workout has you in a rut, try something new. There are many different types of physical activity that are fun and provide a great workout. Find what appeals to you and is available in your area. Keep your physical activity routine interesting by varying it regularly. Here are a few ideas:

Boxing. You don't have to be a fighter to train like one. Find a boxing class in your area. There are two basic types of boxing classes: those that use air-boxing techniques without the use of boxing gloves or a bag and those that use gloves and a heavy bag. A one-hour boxing class not only burns lots of calories but is also a fun way to get both muscle-building and aerobic physical activity.

Pilates. A physical fitness system developed by Josef Pilates that promotes the use of core muscles to keep the body balanced. Pilates teaches awareness of breath and alignment of the back to develop strong muscles in the abdomen. Classes can be taught using only your body and a mat or through the use of specialized apparatus.

Martial arts. You can learn self-defense and get a good workout at the same time. There are many different forms of martial arts from which to choose. Check with your college physical education department or local parks and recreation to see if they offer classes.

Group fitness classes. Most gyms and many colleges offer group fitness classes. Group fitness can be aerobic, as with step aerobics or spin, or a combination of muscle-building and aerobic classes that use weights in addition to a cardio workout.

Physical Activity in the Community

The growing evidence as to the importance of physical activity has prompted researchers to investigate what can be done at the community level to encourage activity. How can we better build our communities, roads, and neighborhoods to make them places where being active is possible? What policies need to be in place so that we move from an inactive society to one that presents opportunities to move the body throughout the day? Simply telling someone to be more physically active without providing opportunity for physical activity will not create change. Addressing multiple levels of influence, including the individual, interpersonal, institution, and community, to increase physical activity can be effective.[33,34] This will take the efforts of all of us, including schools, policymakers, city planners, and businesses. A number of strategies have shown promise in increasing the physical activity of adults and children.[35–37]

Community-Wide Campaigns

Community-wide campaigns are large-scale, multicomponent efforts to engage a community to increase physical activity. They involve media efforts, such as TV, radio, and print, as well as on-the-ground efforts. Community events, support groups, and physical activity counseling can be part of a community-wide campaign. Successful programs have a recognizable brand associated with the campaign. Most successful campaigns also coincide with policy change. An example of policy change that could support a community-wide campaign would be schools that make their facilities available to the community after hours or on weekends. Successful community-wide campaigns must be sustained over a longer period of time as opposed to one-shot, short-lived efforts. Community-wide campaigns require substantial resources for media and personnel to handle community outreach, but they have been proven to increase physical activity in community members.

THE PRESIDENT'S CHALLENGE

ADULT FITNESS TEST

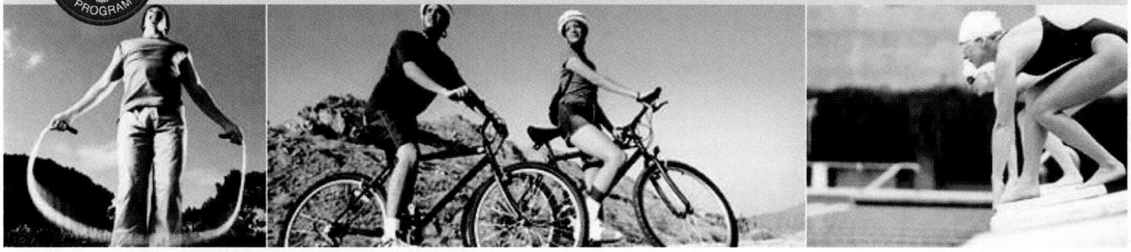

Get Your Adult Fitness Test Score!
As you complete each of the testing events, enter your data into the fields below. When all testing events are completed, transfer the data to the online data entry form and submit your data.

Please complete the form below. Mandatory fields are marked *

PERSONAL INFORMATION

State*

Gender * ❑ Male ❑ Female

Age * ____ yrs

AEROBIC FITNESS

Must enter either a 1-mile walk time and heart rate or enter a 1.5-mile run time.

Mile Walk Time ____ minutes ____ seconds

Heart Rate (after walk) ____ beats per minute

Weight ____ lbs required for result calculation

OR

1.5-Mile Run Time ____ minutes ____ seconds

MUSCULAR STRENGTH

Half Sit-Ups ____ (in one minute)

Push-Ups ____

FLEXIBILITY

Sit and Reach ____ inches

BODY COMPOSITION

BMI/BODY MASS INDEX

Enter height in feet AND inches.

Height ____ feet ____ inches

Weight ____ lbs

Waist Measurement ____ inches

The President's Challenge Adult Fitness Test

Take the President's Challenge adult fitness test and enter your results online at www.adultfitnesstest.org to see your fitness level.

Source: © The President's Council on Fitness, Sports & Nutrition. The President's Challenge Adult Fitness Test. www.adultfitnesstest.org. Accessed April 10, 2011.

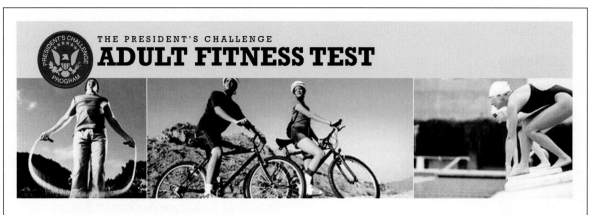

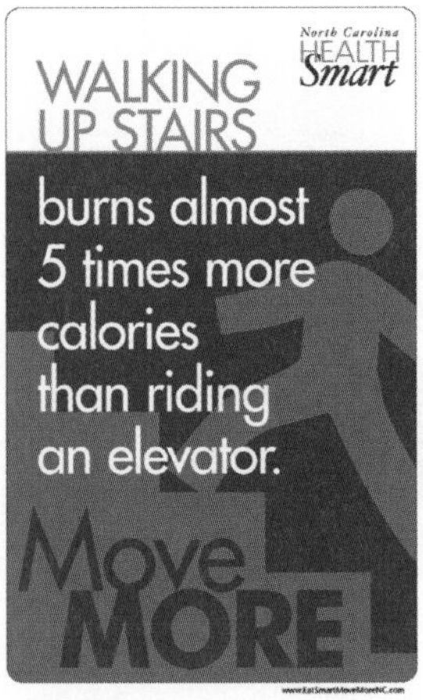
North Carolina
HEALTH
Smart
WALKING UP STAIRS
burns almost 5 times more calories than riding an elevator.
Move MORE

■ **Figure 11.9**

Point-of-Decision Prompts

Point-of-decision prompts encourage the use of the stairs instead of the elevator or escalator.

Source: © Eat Smart, Move More, North Carolina. www.eatsmartmovemorenc.com. Accessed April 10, 2011.

Point-of-Decision Prompts

Point-of-decision prompts (PODP) are signs posted by elevators and escalators to encourage people to choose to use the stairs (**Figure 11.9**). Because stairs are required in any multilevel building, PODP can be used by many organizations. The type of signs used as PODP vary, but they usually have a motivational message about the health or weight-loss benefits of physical activity. PODP have been proven to be effective at increasing physical activity. PODP require few resources; signs are available for free on the Internet. They can be used in multiple settings, including airports, malls, universities, and worksites. Enhancements to stairwells, such as paint, artwork, or carpet, can also be added to make taking the stairs a more pleasurable experience (**Figure 11.10**).

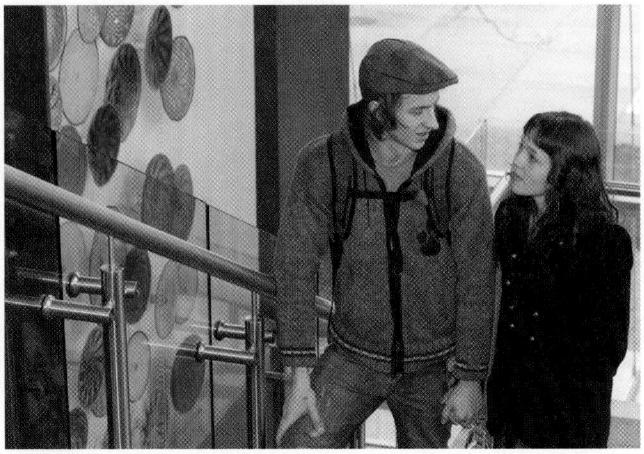

■ **Figure 11.10**

Enhancements to Stairways Encourage Their Use

Social Support Interventions in Community Settings

Most people are more likely to be physically active if they have social support. Social support interventions build and maintain social networks that provide supportive relationship for physical activity. New networks can be formed or existing networks, such as those in the workplace or in schools, can be strengthened. Components of a successful intervention may include setting up buddy systems, contracts between coworkers, or walking groups in the community.

Create or Enhance Access to Places for Physical Activity Combined with Informational Outreach

Individuals may have the knowledge, skills, and even the motivation to be active but they also need a place to be active that is safe and convenient. Opportunities for physical activity such as walking trails, bike paths, or exercise facilities can be created or enhanced to improve access. If there are physical activity opportunities in a city but some residents live far away, is there public transportation to get them there? Are walking trails perceived by residents as safe to use? If not, can more frequent patrol from law enforcement or better lighting enhance safety? Safe, accessible places to be active can help citizens be more physically active.[38] Building or enhancing places for physical activity is the first step. Then, residents need to be informed about where they can be active. Outreach to the community about what opportunities there are for physical activity

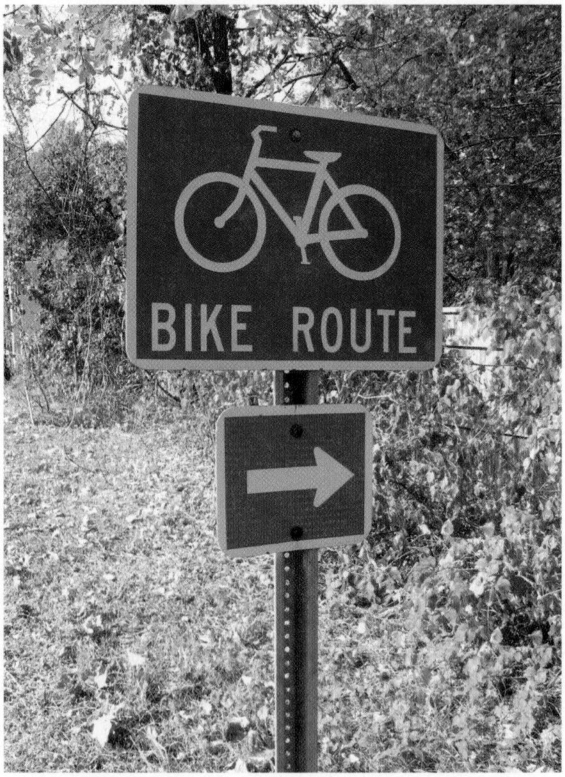
BIKE ROUTE

■ **Figure 11.11**

Way-Finding Signs Promote the Use of Walking and Biking Trails

How Policy and Environment Affect My Choices

Complete Streets

The layouts of most cities and towns tend to favor automobile travel over walking and biking. Neighborhoods are built so they do not connect to shopping or services for residents. Speeding traffic, large intersections, and a lack of sidewalks and bike lanes discourage any type of transportation other than by automobile. Even short trips may be unsafe or impossible without the use of a car. The health implications of relying more and more on cars for transportation are clear. Each additional hour spent in the car is associated with a 6% increase in the likelihood of obesity.[39]

Complete streets are designed not just for cars, as most streets are, but for all users. Pedestrians, bicyclists, transit riders, and motorists of all ages and abilities must be able to use a street for it to be complete. Streets designed only for cars make biking and walking more difficult, or sometimes impossible.

Each community and street is unique, so the components needed for a street to be transformed into a complete street vary. Some elements of a complete street may be sidewalks, bike lanes (or wide paved shoulders), special bus lanes, comfortable and accessible transit stops, frequent crossing opportunities, median islands, accessible pedestrian signals, and curb extensions.[40] Urban complete streets will look different from those in rural areas. Regardless of venue, complete streets are designed to balance safety and convenience for everyone using the street, whether they are on foot, on a bicycle, or in a car.

Complete streets make active living possible. The most effective policy for encouraging bicycling and walking is incorporating sidewalks and bike lanes into community design.[41,42] People with safe places to walk are more likely to meet recommended activity levels.[43] People who live in walkable neighborhoods are more active and less likely to be overweight or obese than similar people living in neighborhoods where walking is difficult or not possible.[44,45]

Many states and cities have adopted pedestrian and bicycling plans to support complete streets. Some have gone as far as to pass complete streets policies that allocate funding to improve streets for walkers and bikers. In March 2010, the U.S. Department of Transportation (DOT) announced a policy statement on bicycle and pedestrian accommodations that supports fully integrated active transportation networks and recognizes the importance of well-connected walking and bicycling networks for livable communities. The DOT policy is to incorporate safe and convenient walking and bicycling facilities into transportation projects. DOT will also encourage states, local governments, professional associations, community organizations, public transportation agencies, and other government agencies to adopt a similar position on making biking and walking safe, attractive, sustainable, accessible, and convenient.

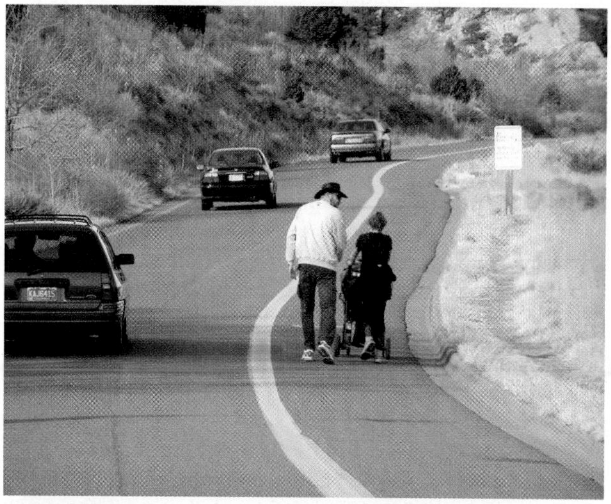

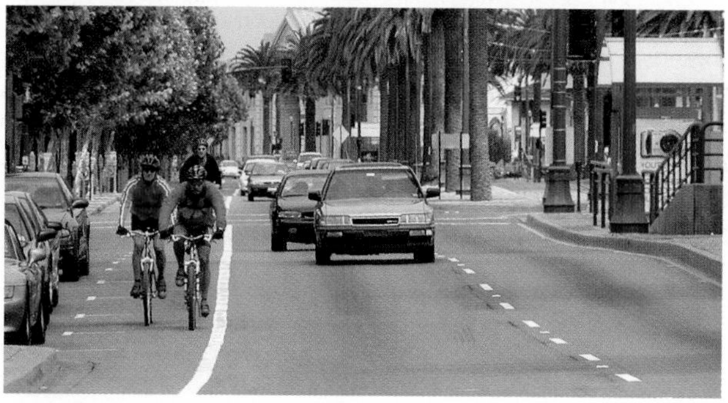

Complete Streets
Complete streets may include different elements but all are designed to allow for safe walking and biking. (a) In rural areas, a wide shoulder helps pedestrians, bicyclists, and families with strollers travel from one place to another without needing a car. (b) Cyclists on an off-road bike trail can easily cross pedestrian and automobile areas thanks to good striping, curb cuts, and signals.

and how they can access it will increase use. Way-finding signs should be posted to let people know where walking or biking trails are located (**Figure 11.11**). Maps of all physical activity opportunities in a community will inform residents of their options for physical activity. The combination of increased availability of places to be active and communicating this to residents will increase physical activity.

TERMS

complete streets Streets designed and operated to accommodate all users, including bicyclists, public transportation vehicles and riders, and pedestrians of all ages and abilities.

Special Report

Nutrition for Optimal Athletic Performance

Whether you frequent the gym for regular workouts, are training for a 10K run, or are a competitive athlete, proper nutrition is important for optimal performance and recovery.[48] A poor diet will negatively affect performance in the gym or during competition. The good news is that a diet for optimal athletic performance does not differ from that suggested for nonathletes. In general, athletes should consume a balanced diet with adequate calories to maintain body weight. Following the *Dietary Guidelines for America* and MyPlate will ensure that adequate carbohydrates, proteins, and fats are consumed. Vitamin and mineral supplements are usually not needed, provided that adequate energy to maintain body weight is consumed from a variety of foods.[48] Adequate food and fluid should be consumed before, during, and after exercise to help maintain blood glucose concentration during exercise, provide for optimal performance, and improve recovery time.[48] Special attention should be given to proper hydration (see Chapter 7 for more information on hydration, water, and sports drinks).

Before Exercise or an Athletic Event

Michael Jordan always ate steak and French fries before a game. Did this meal make him the greatest basketball player ever? No, hard work and genetics did that, but a pre-event or pre-workout meal help you perform your best.

Timing is important; exercising on a full stomach is not recommended. You have to learn what your body can tolerate and how long you must wait from eating a meal to having a good workout. Depending on the size and composition of the meal, this may be three to four hours prior to the event or workout. Choose foods that you know you can digest and tolerate well. Meals that are higher in fat will take longer to digest than high-carbohydrate meals.

It is also not recommended to work out on a totally empty stomach, because you might not have the energy needed to have a good workout or to perform well in an event. Try eating a few nuts, a piece of fruit, or a granola bar 30 minutes prior to your workout so you have the fuel your body needs to perform. If you have an early morning event or workout, you may want to get up early enough to have at least a snack so that you don't have a totally empty stomach.

What you eat, when you eat, and how much you eat just prior to exercise is something that you will have to work out for yourself by trial and error. You will need to find out what best fuels your workouts and athletic events so you have the energy you need for peak performance.

During Exercise or an Athletic Event

What you should consume during exercise is related to the intensity and duration of the activity and the weather conditions. Proper hydration is critical. If you are exercising for less than 90 minutes, drink plain water during exercise. Try to drink 8–10 ounces of water for every 15 minutes of exercise. If you are exercising in hot weather or for more than 90 minutes, you may want to consume a beverage with some carbohydrates, such as a sports drink.

Following Exercise or an Athletic Event

After you work out or participate in an athletic event, you need to replace the fluid you lost. One way to determine whether you are properly hydrated is to check the color of your urine. Dark, concentrated urine may indicate that you have not replaced the fluid you lost. Your urine should be pale yellow. You also need to replace carbohydrates after exercise. After an intense workout, game, or event, eat a healthy meal within one to two hours to replace the glycogen you used during the activity.

Supplements and the Athlete

An overwhelming number of supplements are on the market that claim to enhance athletic performance. Although they are highly prevalent and readily available, few have been proven to improve performance.[49] As long as a supplement has a label that lists all the ingredients and indicates the active ingredient, it can claim that it provides enhanced performance, even if that claim is not valid. In other words, a supplement can claim that you will increase muscle mass even if this may not be true, as long as it lists the ingredients that are in the product. Several supplements do perform as they claim, but many others do not, and some are even dangerous.

Creatine is widely used among athletes who want to build muscle.[50] It has been shown to have some benefits with high-intensity weight lifting and may help the muscle recover faster.[50,51] The safety of creatine is heavily debated, and long-term effects are still unknown. Common side effects are cramping, nausea, diarrhea, and fluid retention.

Caffeine is used by some athletes to boost their energy level during a workout. Caffeine's effect as a stimulant may decrease perception of effort. Athletes may not feel they are working as hard as they actually are and may be able to sustain a higher level of activity for a short period of time. High levels of caffeine have adverse effects such as rapid heartbeat and gastrointestinal distress.[48]

Protein is the most widely used supplement among athletes. Although such supplements do perform as they suggest on the label—they provide protein to the body—they are no more or less effective than consuming foods that contain protein.[48,49]

The majority of supplements on the market do not perform as they claim. Amino acids, branched-chain amino acids, carnitine, chromium picolinate, coenzyme Q10, conjugated linoleic acid, ginseng, medium-chain tryiglycerides, and oxygenated water are all substances that you can find at your local supplement store that make claims that have no proven benefit to body composition or athletic performance. Literally hundreds of others could be added to this list. Many of these supplements can have adverse effects. Although scientific evidence may someday prove that some of these are beneficial to athletes, to date none has surfaced.

Several supplements are dangerous or are illegal. Anabolic steroids are extremely dangerous and should not be taken without a physician's supervision. The temptation for rapid muscle growth and fast recovery makes the use of steroids too common in athletics. However, the risk of serious side effects and even death should make these off limits to even the most competitive of athletes. Some claim that *Tribulus terrestris* will increase testosterone production and thus aid in muscle development. These claims are unfounded, and the substance has been shown to be harmful. Ephedra-containing supplements were once touted as increasing athletic performance and facilitating weight loss. The dangerous side effects and deaths attributed to ephedra caused them to be removed from the market.

Ready to Make a Change

Are you ready to make a change, small or large, in your physical activity? Make the commitment to take the first step. Whether it is a small, medium, or large change, it is a step in the right direction toward healthier behaviors.

I commit to a small first step. If you are not physically active, commit to adding physical activity into your daily life. Take the stairs instead of the elevator, park further away when you shop, use the drive-through less often. Although these small bouts of physical activity don't count towards the minimum recommendations, it is a step in the right direction to a more active lifestyle. Try this for a while, and then you may be ready to add more physical activity to meet the minimum levels needed to improve health.

I am ready to take the next step and make a medium change. Commit to getting the recommended amount of physical activity each week. If you are not active, start slow and build up to the recommended minutes. If you already do some physical activity but don't meet the minimum recommendations or are not consistent with your activity, commit to making it part of your life each week. Cardio is important, but don't forget to add the strength training to help you build and maintain lean body mass. Find a friend to be your workout buddy to keep you motivated.

I have been making changes for some time and am ready to make a large change in physical activity. Commit to increase the amount of physical activity or increase the intensity of your physical activity. Aim for 300 minutes of moderate or 150 minutes of vigorous activity each week plus strength training at least twice a week. To keep it interesting, try some new types of physical activity, such as boxing, group fitness classes, or martial arts. To stay motivated, sign up for an upcoming event such as a 10K run or triathlon.

Myth Versus Fact

Myth: Lifting weights will make you bulky. You should only lift weights if you want to gain muscle mass.

Fact: Lifting weights or doing other types of muscle-strengthening activities can help you gain and maintain lean body mass. Most women lack the hormones and body structure to develop bulky muscles. Men, although having the hormones that allow for building more muscle tissue, still have to work very hard to create large muscles. Resistance exercise can shape your body and help you create a body that is fit and strong.

Myth: Because I am on the go all day, I don't need to exercise.

Fact: Even if you are very busy, it is not likely that you get the amount of physical activity that you need. You may be physically tired at the end of the day, but this does not mean that you have done activities that count toward the minimum amount needed to be healthy.

Myth: Working out at the gym for one hour, three times a week is plenty to stay fit.

Fact: That would depend on what you do in that hour. Fitness includes aerobic or cardiorespiratory fitness, muscle strength, and flexibility. If that hour is spent only lifting, you would be missing cardiorespiratory fitness; if you do cardio only, you would not gain muscle strength. You need to spend that hour doing some cardio, some weights, and some stretching to be fit.

Myth: I am not an athlete; physical activity is not for me.

Fact: Physical activity and sports are two different things. You don't have to be an athlete to get the health benefits from being physically active. Even the most nonathletic person can find some form of physical activity to enjoy.

Myth: I hate to run and going to a gym is too intimidating; there is no way I can be physically active.

Fact: Running is only one of many options for being physically active, and you don't have to go to a gym. Find something you enjoy to meet your physical activity goals. There are many options to choose from: fitness DVDs, Wii Fit, dance classes, television shows that get you moving, and martial arts, just to name a few.

Myth: Children are naturally active. You don't have to worry about them getting enough activity.

Fact: Many children are not active at recommended levels. Thanks to television, video games, and hours in front of a screen, many children need to be more active. Activity for children means active play, both structured and unstructured. If you have children, you can benefit from being active with them.

Myth: I don't have time to be physically active.

Fact: Everyone has the same 24 hours in the day. What you do with them is up to you. It is not easy to carve out time to be active; however, with a little planning and commitment to make physical activity a priority, you can do it. Find the time of day that is best for you—early morning, lunch break, after school or work—just schedule your physical activity like you would a class or meeting and keep your appointment with yourself.

Back to the Story

Katie and Roger are not unlike many nonathletes who are not active. However, they don't have to be athletes or into sports to add physical activity into their lives. They have a big event coming up—their wedding. They can use that as motivation to start (and stick with) a physical activity routine. They have the advantage of having a built-in workout buddy and can provide one another with social support. One way to get moving would be for them to plan their day so that they can walk to school if there is a safe route. This would be a total of 4 miles a day; depending on their pace, this would be about an hour of moderate activity. If there are no safe routes to school, they could start a walking program after they get home. They could use the time together to make wedding plans or to catch up on each other's day. Once they have worked up to the recommended amount of aerobic activity, they can add some strength training. They may even want to check out whether they can take a class at school on strength training or fitness to get them started. Because they are into technology, they may want to try some of the applications that are available for their smartphones (or other similar devices) to monitor their physical activity and food intake. Finding the time and motivation to get and stay active will get them on the way to a smaller wedding dress, a smaller tuxedo, and a healthy start to their life together.

References

1. National Center for Chronic Disease Prevention and Health Promotion, Centers for Disease Control and Prevention. Behavioral Risk Factor Surveillance System, Prevalence and Trends data, Physical Activity—2009. http://apps.nccd.cdc.gov/brfss/list.asp?cat=PA&yr=2009&qkey=4418&state=All. Accessed June 2, 2010.
2. Eaton DK, Kann L, Kinchen S, et al. Youth risk behavior surveillance—United States, 2009. *MMWR Surveillance Summaries*. 2010;59:1–142.
3. Lee IM, Skerrett PJ. Physical activity and all-cause mortality: what is the dose-response relation? *Med Sci Sports Exerc*. 2001;33(6 suppl):S459–S471.
4. Manson JE, Hu FB, Rich-Edwards JW, et al. A prospective study of walking as compared with vigorous exercise in the prevention of coronary heart disease in women. *N Eng J Med*. 1999;341(9):650–658.
5. Lee IM, Rexrode KM, Cook NR, Manson JE, Buring JE. Physical activity and coronary heart disease in women: is "no pain, no gain" passe? *JAMA*. 2001;285(11):1447–1454.
6. Tanasescu M, Leitzmann MF, Rimm EB, Willett WC, Stampfer MJ, Hu FB. Exercise type and intensity in relation to coronary heart disease in men. *JAMA*. 2002;288(16):1994–2000.
7. Oguma Y, Shinoda-Tagawa T. Physical activity decreases cardiovascular disease risk in women: review and meta-analysis. *Am J Prev Med*. 2004;26(5):407–418.
8. Kohl HW, III. Physical activity and cardiovascular disease: evidence for a dose response. *Med Sci Sports Exer*. 2001;33(6 Suppl):S472–S483.
9. Williams PT. Physical fitness and activity as separate heart disease risk factors: a meta-analysis. *Med Sci Sports Exerc*. 2001;33(5):754–761.
10. Sundquist K, Qvist J, Johansson SE, Sundquist J. The long-term effect of physical activity on incidence of coronary heart disease: a 12-year follow-up study. *Prev Med*. 2005;41(1):219–225.
11. Church TS, Earnest CP, Skinner JS, Blair SN. Effects of different doses of physical activity on cardiorespiratory fitness among sedentary, overweight or obese postmenopausal women with elevated blood pressure: a randomized controlled trial. *JAMA*. 2007;297(19):2081–2091.
12. Cornelissen VA, Fagard RH. Effects of endurance training on blood pressure, blood pressure-regulating mechanisms, and cardiovascular risk factors. *Hypertension*. 2005;46(4):667–675.
13. Knowler WC, Barrett-Connor E, Fowler SE, et al. Reduction in the incidence of type 2 diabetes with lifestyle intervention or metformin. *N Engl J Med*. 2002;346(6):393–403.
14. Monninkhof EM, Elias SG, Vlems FA, et al. Physical activity and breast cancer: a systematic review. *Epidemiology*. 2007;8(1):137–57.
15. Lee IM, Oguma Y. Physical activity. In: Schottenfeld D, Fraumeni JF, eds. *Cancer Epidemiology and Prevention*, 3rd ed. New York: Oxford University Press, 2006:449–467.
16. Feskanich D, Willett W, Colditz G. Walking and leisure-time activity and risk of hip fracture in postmenopausal women. *JAMA*. 2002;288(18):2300–2306.

17. Sinaki M, Itoi E, Wahner HW, et al. Stronger back muscles reduce the incidence of vertebral fractures: a prospective 10-year follow-up of postmenopausal women. *Bone*. 2002;30(6):836–841.
18. Wilcox S, Der AC, Abbott J, et al. Perceived exercise barriers, enablers, and benefits among exercising and nonexercising adults with arthritis: results from a qualitative study. *Arthritis Rheum*. 2006;55(4):616–627.
19. Fransen M, Nairn L, Winstanley J, Lam P, Edmonds J. Physical activity for osteoarthritis management: a randomized controlled clinical trial evaluating hydrotherapy or Tai Chi classes. *Arthritis Rheum*. 2007;57(3):407–414.
20. Singh MA. Exercise to prevent and treat functional disability. *Clin Geriatric Med*. 2002;18(3):431–462.
21. Centers for Disease Control and Prevention. *Overweight and Obesity: Contributing Factors, 2006*. www.cdc.gov/nccdphp/dnpa/obesity/contributing_factors.htm. Updated December 7, 2009. Accessed April 19, 2011.
22. Harris AH, Cronkite R, Moos R. Physical activity, exercise coping, and depression in a 10-year cohort study of depressed patients. *J Affect Disord*. 2006;93(1–3):79–85.
23. Peterson MD, Sen A, Gordon PM. Influence of resistance exercise on lean body mass in aging adults: a meta-analysis. *Med Sci in Sports and Exercise*. 2011; 42(2):249–258.
24. US Department of Health and Human Services. 2008 *Physical Activity Guidelines for Americans*. Washington, DC: USDHHS, 2008. http://www.health.gov/PAGUIDELINES. Updated November 4, 2009. Accessed April 19, 2011.
25. Nelson ME, Rejeski J, Blair SN, et al. Physical activity and public health in older adults. Recommendation from the American College of Sports Medicine and the American Heart Association. *Circulation*. 2007;116:1194–1105.
26. Warburton DER, Nicol CW, Bredin SSD. Health benefits of physical activity: the evidence. *CMAJ*. 2006;174(6):801–809.
27. National Association for Sport and Physical Activity. *Active Start: A Statement of Physical Activity Guidelines for Children from Birth to Age 5*, 2nd ed. Reston, VA: NAESPA, 2009.
28. Sallis JF, McKenzie T L, Kolody B, Lewis M, Marshall S, Rosengard P. Effects of health-related physical education on academic achievement: Project SPARK. *Res Quart Exerc Sport*. 1999;70(2):127–134.
29. Shephard R. Curricular physical activity and academic performance. *Ped Exerci Sci*. 1997;9:113–126.
30. Tremblay M, Inman W, Willms JD. The relationship between physical activity, self-esteem, and academic achievement in twelve-year old children. *Ped Exerci Sci*. 1998;12:312–324.
31. Centers for Disease Control and Prevention. *The Association Between School-Based Physical Activity, Including Physical Education, and Academic Performance*. Atlanta, GA: US Department of Health and Human Services, 2010.
32. Bravata DM, Smith-Spangler C, Sundaram V, et al. Using pedometers to increase physical activity and improve health, a systematic review. *JAMA*. 2007;298(19):2296–2304.
33. Brownson RC, Haire-Joshu D, Luke DA. Shaping the context of health: a review of environmental and policy approaches in the prevention of chronic diseases. *Annu Rev Public Health*. 2006;27:341–370.
34. Sallis JF, Cervero R, Ascher W, Henderson KA, Kraft MK, Kerr J. An ecological approach to creating active living communities. *Annu Rev Public Health*. 2006;27:297–322.
35. Centers for Disease Control and Prevention. Increasing physical activity: a report on recommendations of the Task Force on Community Preventive Services. *MMWR*. 2001;50(No. RR 18).
36. The Community Guide. Guide to community preventive services. http://www.thecommunityguide.org/pa/index.html. Updated January 20, 2011. Accessed April 19, 2011.
37. Kahn EB, Ramsey LT, Brownson RC, et al. Task Force on Community Preventive Services. The effectiveness of interventions to increase physical activity: a systematic review. *Am J Prev Med*. 2002;22(4S):73–96.
38. Addy CL, Wilson DK, Kirtland KA, Ainsworth BE, Sharpe P, Kimsey D. Associations of perceived social and physical environmental supports with physical activity and walking behavior. *Am J Public Health*. 2004;94(3):440–443.
39. Frank LD, Andersen MA, Schmid TL. Obesity relationships with community design, physical activity, and time spent in cars. *Am J Prev Med*. 2004;27(2):87–96.
40. National Complete Streets Coalition. http://www.completestreets.org. Accessed April 29, 2010.
41. Robbins LT, Morandi L. Promoting biking and walking: the legislative role. National Conference of State Legislatures, December 2002.
42. Brennan Ramirez LK, Hoehner CM, Brownson RC, et al. Indicators of activity-friendly communities, an evidence-based consensus process. *Am J Prev Med*. 2006;31(6):515–524.
43. Powell KE, Martin L, Chowdhury PP. Places to walk: convenience and regular physical activity. *Am J Public Health*. 2003;93:1519–1521.
44. Giles-Corti B, Donovan RJ. The relative influence of individual, social, and physical environment determinants of physical activity. *Soc Sci Med*. 2001;54:1793–1812.
45. Sallis JF, Saelens BE, Frank LD, et al. Neighborhood built environment and income: examining multiple health outcomes. *Soc Sci Med*. 2009;68:1285–1293.
46. US Department of Transportation. National Household Transportation Survey. 2001.
47. US Department of Transportation. Transportation's role in climate change, transportation and climate

change clearing hours. http://climate.dot.gov/about/transportations-role/overview.html. Accessed April 19, 2011.

48. American College of Sports Medicine, American Dietetic Association, Dietitians of Canada, Joint Position Statement. Nutrition and athletic performance. *Med Sci Sports. Exerc.* 2009;47(3):709–731.
49. Dunford M, Smith M. Dietary supplements and ergogenic aids. In: Dunford M, ed. *Sports Nutrition: A Practice Manual for Professionals.* Chicago: American Dietetic Association, 2006:116–141.
50. Bemben MG, Lamont HS. Creatine supplementation and exercise performance: recent findings. *Sports Med.* 2005;35:107–125.
51. Candow DG, Little JP, Chilibeck PD, et al. Low-dose creatine combined with protein during resistance training in older men. *Med Sci in Sports and Exercise.* 2008;40(9):1645–1652.

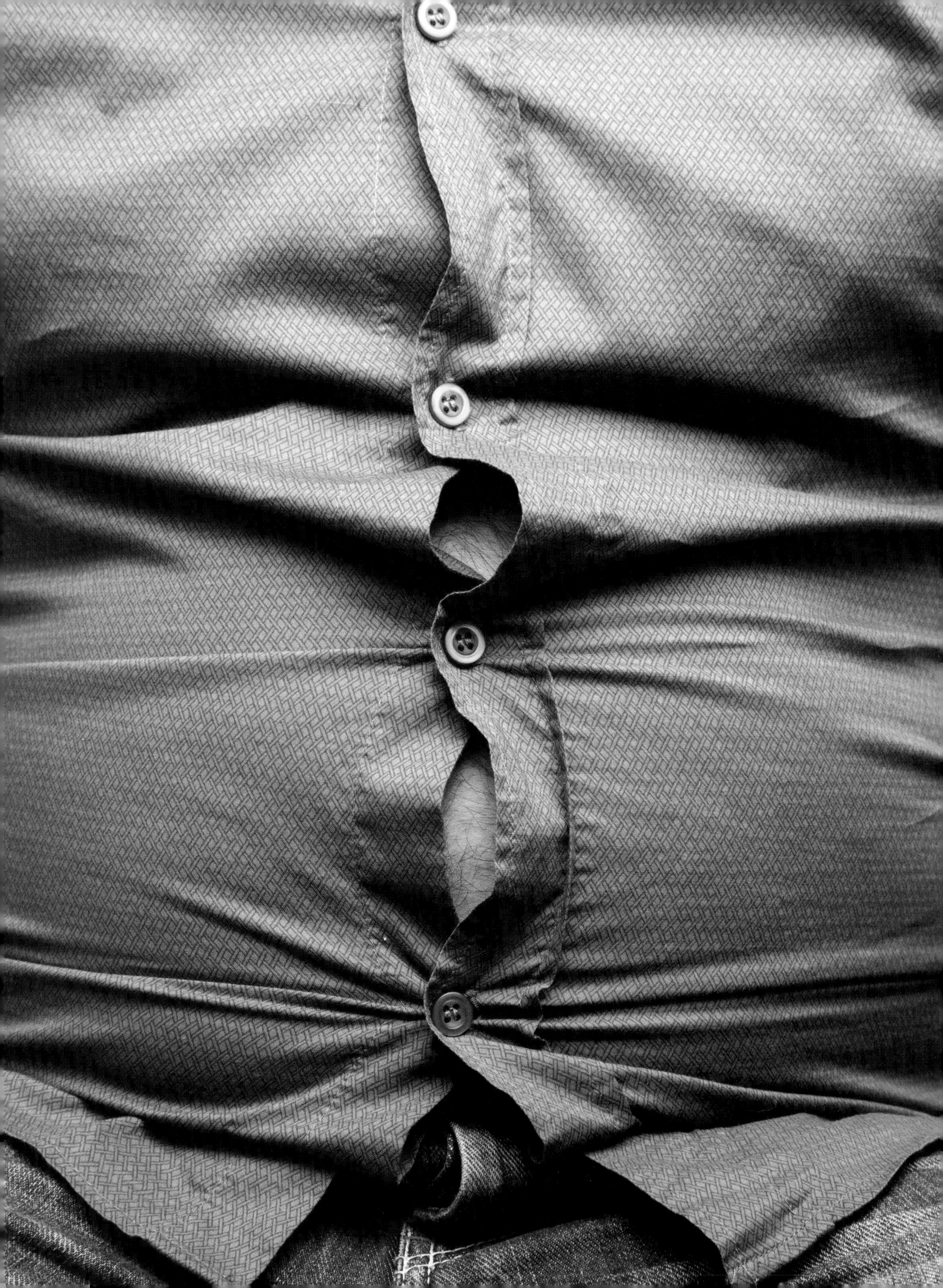

Chapter 12

Overweight and Obesity: The Public Health Crisis of Our Time

Key Messages

- Obesity is one of the biggest public health concerns of our time.
- Overweight and obesity increase the risk of heart disease, type 2 diabetes, and some forms of cancer.
- Healthy eating and physical activity are important behaviors to achieve and maintain a healthy weight.
- Many factors affect your decisions and abilities to practice positive behaviors with respect to healthy eating and physical activity.

You would have had to have been on an uninhabited island or in the middle of the desert for the past 10 years not to have heard about the crisis of overweight and obesity. It is a constant topic of conversation in the media. Reports run the gamut, from describing a condition that can increase risk of serious disease to explaining how to lose 10 pounds in 10 days. Overweight and obesity have become part of our culture. We have reality shows about losing weight, tens of thousands of books and websites on the subject, magazines devoted to weight loss, and an insatiable quest for a "cure." This chapter will explore the causes of overweight and obesity; the prevalence of overweight and obesity; what this means for the health of the U.S. population; how we can address the problem as a country; and how you, as an individual, can adopt healthy behaviors not only to achieve and maintain a healthy weight, but also to have lifelong good health and wellness.

Story

Sue is a 30-year-old wife, mother, and part-time college student. She also works part time as an administrative assistant at a local business. She has one daughter who is 3 and a son who is 9. Her husband, Tom, is 35 and works for the city as a police officer. A recent trip to the doctor was devastating for Sue. Her doctor told her she was obese. She knew she was overweight but would never have used the word *obese* to describe herself. Armed with new knowledge, she checked online to see if Tom or her children's weights were above normal. Tom was borderline between overweight and obese, and the children were both classified as overweight according to the growth charts. How did this happen? How could the whole family be overweight or obese?

Sue began to examine their lives and consider how she could make some changes to eat smart and move more. Her close examination revealed some interesting findings. The family either eats out or eats takeout food five nights a week, on average. Other dinners are usually foods that can be prepared quickly, such as frozen entrees or box dinners. Breakfast is always cereal for the children and nothing for Sue and Tom. Lunch for Sue is usually fast food or a sandwich from the deli near school. Tom's lunch is either from a diner near the police station or fast food. The family does not have many opportunities to be physically active. They enjoy television and watch it each night until bedtime. Sue and Tom get very little activity during the day. Sue is busy running between work, home, and school. She has very little time for herself, let alone time to exercise. How can Sue and Tom create a family environment that is more conducive to healthy eating and physical activity to move the family toward healthier weights?

TERMS

overweight For adults, a BMI between 25.0 and 29.9. For children under the age of 20, a BMI for age that is greater than the 85th percentile but less than the 95th percentile.

obese For adults, a BMI of 30 or higher. For children under the age of 20, a BMI for age at or greater than the 95th percentile.

Overweight and Obesity in America

The problem of overweight and obesity is arguably the number one public health crisis of our time. According to the Centers for Disease Control and Prevention, overweight and obesity are ranges of body weight that are greater than what is considered healthy for a given height (**Table 12.1** and **Figure 12.1**).[1–3] Over the past 30 years, the number of adults who are **overweight** or **obese** has increased dramatically. It is estimated that nearly 70% of adults in the United States are overweight or obese.[4–7] The rate has doubled since the early 1980s. Most of the increase in the rate of overweight and obesity is due to the increase in the number of Americans who are obese. **Figure 12.2** illustrates how obesity has increased dramatically in the United States.

Although some states have higher obesity rates than others, all states have seen sharp increases over time. There has been much speculation about whether the trend will continue. Recent data indicates that the rate of increase may have slowed, especially among women.[7] However, rates continue to rise in all segments of the population. If the upward trend continues, some researchers estimate that in less than 15 years 80% of all Americans will be overweight or obese.[8]

Table 12.1

Overweight and Obesity Defined for Adults, Children, and Teens

Weight Status Category	
Adults	**BMI**
Underweight	< 18.5
Healthy weight	18.5–24.9
Overweight	25.0–29.9
Obese	≥ 30
Children and Teens Ages 2–20	**Percentile Range**
Underweight	< 5th percentile
Healthy weight	5th to < 85th percentile
Overweight	85th to < 95th percentile
Obese	≥ 95th percentile

Source: Centers for Disease Control and Prevention. Defining overweight and obesity. http://www.cd.gov/obesity/defining.html. Accessed April 10, 2011. Centers for Disease Control and Prevention. About BMI for children and teens. http://www.cdc.gov/healthyweight/assessing/bmi/childrens_bmi/about_childrens_bmi.html. Accessed April 10, 2011.

Height \ Weight	100	110	120	130	140	150	160	170	180	190	200	210	220	230	240	250	260	270	280	290	300	310	320	330
5'0"	20	21	23	25	27	29	31	33	35	37	39	41	43	45	47	49	51	53	55	57	59	61	63	65
5'1"	19	21	23	25	27	28	30	32	34	36	38	40	42	44	45	47	49	51	53	55	57	59	61	62
5'2"	18	20	22	24	26	27	29	31	33	35	37	38	40	42	44	46	48	49	51	53	55	57	59	60
5'3"	18	19	21	23	25	27	28	30	32	34	36	37	39	41	43	44	46	48	50	51	53	55	57	59
5'4"	17	19	21	22	24	26	28	29	31	33	34	36	38	40	41	43	45	46	48	50	52	53	55	57
5'5"	17	18	20	22	23	25	27	28	30	32	33	35	37	38	40	42	43	45	47	48	50	52	53	55
5'6"	16	18	19	21	23	24	26	27	29	31	32	34	36	37	39	40	42	44	45	47	49	50	52	53
5'7"	16	17	19	20	22	24	25	27	28	30	31	33	35	36	38	39	41	42	44	46	47	49	50	52
5'8"	15	17	18	20	21	23	24	26	27	29	30	32	34	35	37	38	40	41	43	44	46	47	49	50
5'9"	15	16	18	19	21	22	24	25	27	28	30	31	33	34	36	37	38	40	41	43	44	46	47	49
5'10"	14	16	17	19	20	22	23	24	26	27	29	30	32	33	35	36	37	39	40	42	43	45	46	47
5'11"	14	15	17	18	20	21	22	24	25	27	28	29	31	32	34	35	36	38	39	41	42	43	45	46
6'0"	14	15	16	18	19	20	22	23	24	26	27	29	30	31	33	34	35	37	38	39	41	42	43	45
6'1"	13	15	16	17	19	20	21	22	24	25	26	28	29	30	32	33	34	36	37	38	40	41	42	44
6'2"	13	14	15	17	18	19	21	22	23	24	26	27	28	30	31	32	33	35	36	37	39	40	41	42
6'3"	13	14	15	16	18	19	20	21	23	24	25	26	28	29	30	31	33	34	35	36	38	39	40	41
6'4"	12	13	15	16	17	18	20	21	22	23	24	26	27	28	29	30	32	33	34	35	37	38	39	40

Underweight | Healthy Weight | Overweight | Obese | Severely Obese

■ **Figure 12.1**

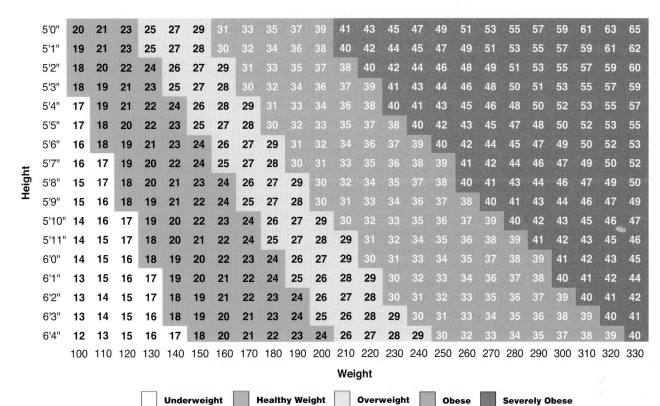

Are You at a Healthy Weight?

Find the column closest to your weight in pounds. Read the column until it crosses the row that most closely matches your height in feet and inches. That number is your body mass index. The healthiest BMI range for adults is 18 to 24.

Source: Data from Eat Smart, Move More North Carolina. http://www.eatsmartmovemorenc.com. Accessed April 10, 2011.

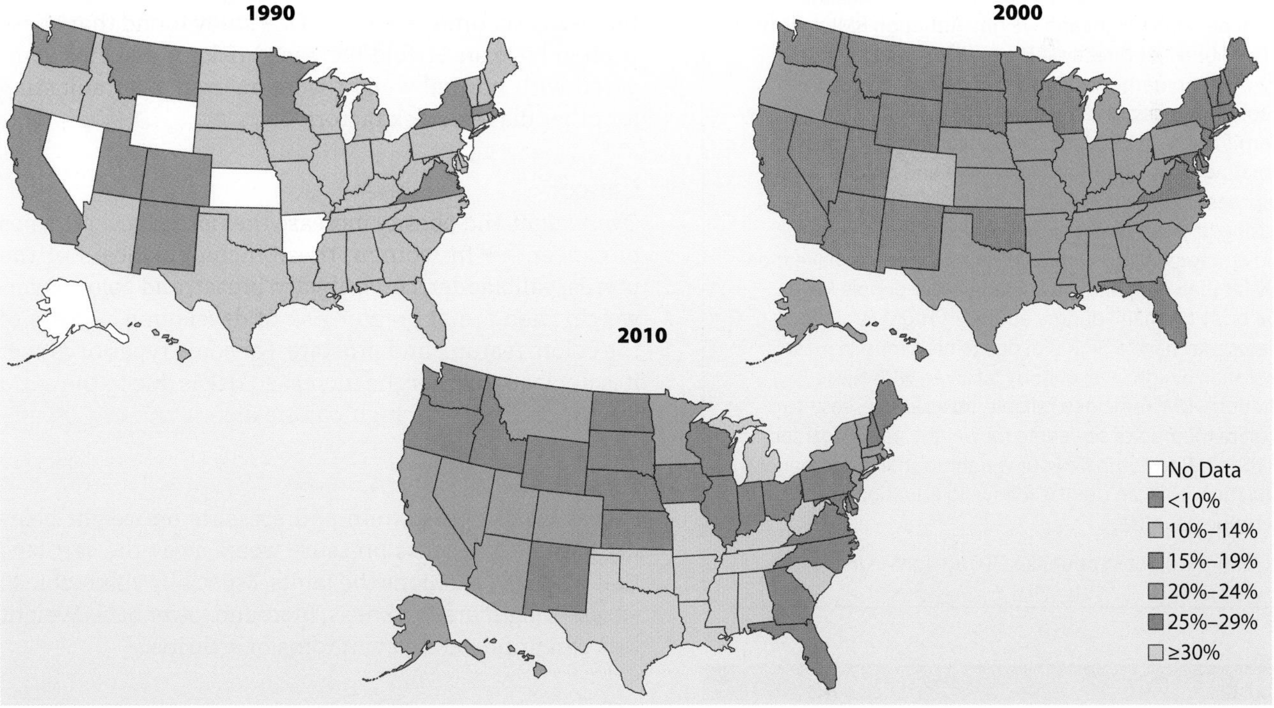

■ **Figure 12.2**

Obesity Trends in the United States, 1990, 2000, 2010

Source: Centers for Disease Control and Prevention. Obesity Trends Among U.S. Adults, BRFSS, 1990, 2000, 2010.

The rate of increase of all levels of overweight and obesity is a concern. Of grave concern is the increase in Americans who are extremely obese (BMI > 40). The rate of extreme obesity has increased from less than 1% in 1960 to 3% in the 1980s to 6% today.[6,7] Extreme obesity is highest among African American women, with 14% having a BMI over 40.[7]

Overweight and obesity affect all segments of society, regardless of race, gender, or socioeconomic status. Certain racial/ethnic populations, however, are affected disproportionally.[5,9–11] African Americans (74%) and Hispanics (78%) have higher rates of overweight and obesity than whites (67%). There are gender differences as well. Hispanic men (79%) have higher rates of overweight and obesity compared to white men (73%) and African American men (69%). The highest rates of overweight and obesity for are found in African American women (78%) compared to white women (61%) and Hispanic women (76%).[7] Overweight and obesity rates are higher in lower socioeconomic status populations, regardless of gender or race/ethnicity.

Children's levels of overweight and obesity have also risen sharply. Since 1980, the rate of overweight and obesity in children and adolescents has tripled.[11–13] Today, 32% of children ages 2–19 are overweight or obese; 17% fall into the obese category. Rates are slightly higher for African American and Hispanic children.[14]

What Is the Body Mass Index?

Body mass index (BMI) is a number that is calculated using a person's height and weight. Although BMI does not measure body fat directly, it is a good estimate of body fat.[13,14] Other methods of measuring body fat, such as skinfold thickness, underwater weight, or dual-energy x-ray absorpitometry (DEXA) are more accurate methods of estimating body fat but are expensive and require special equipment.

Using BMI to estimate body fat does have some disadvantages. At the same BMI, women tend to have more body fat than men and, on average, older people have more body fat than younger adults.[1,17] Highly trained athletes may have a high BMI due to high muscle mass rather than a high level of body fat. Even with these limitations, BMI remains a reliable, inexpensive, easy-to-calculate method of screening for weight status. You can use your BMI to compare your weight to that of the general population. You can use the following equation to determine your BMI:

$$\text{BMI} = \text{weight in pounds} \times 703/(\text{height in inches})^2$$

TERMS

body mass index (BMI) A measure of body fat based on height and weight.

Health Consequences of Overweight and Obesity

The primary concern related to overweight and obesity is the health risks they pose. The life expectancy of Americans has decreased for the first time in 100 years. One contributing factor to this trend is the rising rate of overweight and obesity.[18] An estimated 300,000 deaths per year may be attributable to obesity. Obese individuals have a 50–100% increased risk of premature death from all causes, compared to individuals of healthy weight.[19] The risk of premature death related to overweight is less clear; however, some studies suggest that overweight, especially in the upper ranges, is associated with premature death from some causes.[20] It is clear that overweight and obesity increase the risk of chronic disease and other health factors.

Heart Disease

Being overweight or obese increases the incidence of heart disease. People who are overweight or obese are more likely to have high blood pressure, elevated bad cholesterol (LDL), and low good cholesterol (HDL)—all risk factors for heart disease.[21,22]

Diabetes

Obesity is a well-established risk factor for type 2 diabetes.[23,24] Overweight individuals are more than twice as likely to develop diabetes as healthy weight individuals. Obese individuals have three times the risk. For someone who is 100 pounds or more overweight (morbidly obese), the risk is six times greater.[23] One study found that obese women have an 11-fold increased risk for diabetes compared with normal weight women, even after adjusting for other diabetes risk factors.[24]

Cancer

Overweight and obesity increase the risk for several types of cancer.[25,26] In women, these include cancers of the uterus, gallbladder, cervix, ovary, breast, and colon. Overweight men are at greater risk of developing cancers of the colon, rectum, and prostate. For some types of cancer it is unclear whether the increased risk is due to the extra weight or a high-fat, high-calorie diet.

Arthritis

Excess weight puts strain and pressure on weight-bearing joints. The excess pressure wears away the cartilage that normally cushions the joints. Especially vulnerable to excess weight are the knees, hips, and lower back. Weight loss can improve the symptoms of arthritis.[27]

Sleep Apnea

Sleep apnea is a condition that causes a person to stop breathing for short periods of time during sleep. Breathing can pause for just a few seconds to up to a minute or more. This can occur multiple times in an hour. When normal breathing starts again, there is sometimes a choking sound or a loud snore. Sleep apnea results in poor sleep quality and daytime drowsiness. Overweight and obesity are strong risk factors for sleep apnea.[28] The extra soft fat tissue can thicken the walls of the windpipe, causing the opening to narrow.

Gallbladder Disease

Obesity and overweight increase the risk of developing gallbladder disease or gallstones. Both men and women who are overweight or obese are more likely to develop gallstones than their healthy weight counterparts.[29]

Reproductive Complications

Overweight and obesity in women can cause reproductive problems. Excess weight is associated with menstrual irregularity and amenorrhea (absence of a menstrual cycle). Obese women are at a higher risk of infertility.[27]

Economic Consequences of Overweight and Obesity

As the health consequences of overweight and obesity continue to rise, so, too, do the healthcare costs related to excess weight. A clear relationship exists between rising rates of overweight and obesity and increases in medical spending.[30] The cost of overweight, obesity, and their associated health problems have a significant economic impact on the U.S. healthcare system, and thus the U.S. economy.[31] The costs associated with overweight and obesity involve both direct and indirect costs. Direct costs include diagnostic, preventive, and treatment services related to obesity. Indirect costs include income lost from decreased productivity, restricted activity, and absenteeism.[32,33]

It was estimated that in 1998 medical costs associated with overweight and obesity accounted for 9% of total U.S. medical expenditures, or more than $78 billion. Today, it is estimated that the bill for overweight and obesity has risen to over $140 billion per year. The increased cost of overweight and obesity puts an economic burden on both public and private healthcare payers. Per capita spending for an obese person is roughly 42% higher than for someone of normal weight.[30] Medicaid and Medicare pay approximately half of the medical costs associated with obesity.[31,34]

It is projected that the direct healthcare costs attributable to overweight and obesity will more than double every decade. By 2030, costs could be as high as $900 billion a year, or one in every six healthcare dollars.[30] As we search for ways to decrease healthcare costs, it is clear that reducing the rate of overweight and obesity should be a pillar of national healthcare reform.

How Did We Become an Overweight Nation?

How has it happened that today over two-thirds of adults and one-third of children are overweight or obese? The answer is simple. People are consuming more calories than they burn. But *why* is this happening? The answer to that question is more complex. To begin to understand the overweight crisis, we must look at our environment and government policies to see why it is so easy for any American—regardless of age, race, gender, or socioeconomic status—to be overweight. What has happened to our society and our culture over the past 20, 30, 40, or even 50 years? How has our environment contributed to being overweight being the norm for adults and so many children having an unhealthy weight?

Many factors in American culture have made it possible for so many people to be overweight. The number of fast-food outlets has increased dramatically over the past two decades. Twenty years ago, McDonald's had about 8,000 restaurants. Today, over 14,000 McDonald's outlets in the United States serve an estimated 25 million customers a day.[35] Every day, one in every four Americans eats a fast-food meal,[36] which is not surprising considering that the number of fast-food establishments in the country has increased from 70,000 in 1970 to almost 200,000 today.[37]

Not only are we choosing fast food more often, but what we eat when we go to fast-food restaurants has changed. The normal fast-food meal of 20 years ago is the Happy Meal of today; fries, hamburgers, and drinks have all gotten larger and larger. Americans are eating more meals away from home in general. Eating away from home often means meals that are high in calories and fat.[38] In schools, high-fat, high-sugar foods are sold to children in competition with the healthy school lunch.

Americans' consumption of soft drinks continues to rise. What was in years past an occasional treat, served in small quantities, is now an everyday, with every meal norm, often with free refills. Each year enough soft drink is produced in the United States to supply every person with 14 ounces of soft drink per day.[39]

The physical activity patterns of Americans have also changed. In an attempt to make our lives easier, we have removed many of the opportunities to move our bodies. Physical activity for all ages has decreased, especially in young children.

In 1980, there were just over 161 million cars on the road in the United States; today there are well over 225 million.[40] We build our neighborhoods and communities so that walking and biking are not safe alternatives to riding in a car. Physical activity for all ages has decreased, but especially among children. Children's bikes are often motorized and require little or no effort to ride. Physical activity opportunities during the school day have decreased or have been eliminated.

No one could have predicted the impact that television has had on our society. Today, virtually all U.S. households have at least one TV, with close to 80% having multiple sets.[41] The viewing options for TV have increased from three network channels to endless options on cable, pay per view, on demand, and DVD.

The 1980s marked the first time in history when people of all segments of society used television as their number one leisure time activity. Today, Americans spend an average of four hours each day inactive sitting in front of the television.[42] That means hours of inactivity as well as hours of exposure to the marketing of high-fat, high-calorie foods. Many of these ads are aimed directly at children.

Similarly, the 1970s were the beginning of the video game era. The video game industry has grown from the introduction of Pong in the 1970s to a $6.3 billion industry. Today, 90% of households with children own or rent video and computer games.[43]

Empowering individuals, families, and communities with knowledge and skills to change their eating and physical activity patterns is imperative. However, knowledge only addresses part of the problem. People must have the opportunity to eat healthy and be active. People must live in an environment that supports healthy eating and physical activity.

Other Contributors to Obesity

There is certainly ample support for the premise that lack of physical activity and unhealthy eating are the causes of the rise in obesity rates. However, a growing body of evidence indicates that there may be more factors in play, factors that, until now, we didn't see as being related to obesity.[44] The first of these "other" factors is sleep. For children and adults, hours of sleep each night are inversely related to weight status.[45,46] The average amount of sleep each night has been steadily decreasing in both adults and children.[47,48]

The reduction in variability of inside temperature is another factor that may be related to overweight and obesity.[49,50] We have moved to a society where the temperature inside our houses and workplaces remains constant year round thanks to air conditioning and better heating systems. This requires very little work to maintain body temperature. In the past, the body had to burn calories to stay warm in the winter and cool in the summer.

In addition, certain drugs induce weight gain. Many drugs in common use today, such as antidepressants, mood stabilizers, antidiabetics, antihypertensives, contraceptives, and antihistamines, can induce weight gain. Prescriptions for many of these medications have increased dramatically over the past 20 to 30 years.[51–53]

Researchers are exploring other factors that may contribute to obesity, such as exposure to smoke in utero, maternal obesity during pregnancy, increasing age of pregnancy, and chemical contamination in the water, soil, and food supply.[44] When the book is closed on the obesity crisis, we are likely to see a long list of contributors. Nevertheless, the two at the top remain eating and physical activity patterns.

The Socioecological Approach to Addressing Overweight and Obesity

Many factors affect individuals' decisions and abilities to practice positive behaviors with respect to healthy eating and physical activity. People must have opportunities to eat healthy and be physically active. Factors that affect whether people will eat healthy and be active include the physical and social environments of their families, communities, and organizations; the policies, practices, and norms within their social and work settings; and their access to reliable information. Certainly, personal responsibility has a role to play in eating smart and moving more. However, the responsibility is shared with local, state, and federal governments to create possibilities and help remove barriers to good health behaviors.

The multilevel model, also called the *socioecological model*, provides a framework that includes multiple factors that influence individuals' ability to change their health behaviors (**Figure 12.3**). Lasting change in health behaviors requires physical environments and social systems that support positive lifestyle habits.[54] At the base of the model is the two-sided equation of energy in (calories eaten) and energy out (calories expended). Although this is certainly what ultimately dictates body weight, the model explains the complex system that influences both sides of this important equation.

To reverse the rising tide of overweight and obesity, changes need to be made in organizational, community, social, and physical environments. Without such changes, successful health behavior change will be difficult to achieve and sustain. Confidence to adopt and maintain a behavior may be strengthened when the physical and social environments support the new behavior.

Policy changes and environmental intervention can improve the health of all people, not just small groups of motivated or high-risk individuals. They can impact a broad audience and produce long-term changes in health behaviors. These interventions are supported by enhanced public awareness of the need for healthy eating and increased opportunities for physical activity. By collectively focusing on policy and environmental changes, individuals can reduce or eliminate barriers to healthy eating and physical activity.

All levels of the socioecological model must be addressed to affect change. Individuals must be informed and motivated to eat healthy and be active. Behavioral settings—where people live, work, or go to school—must support these behaviors and provide opportunities for healthy eating and physical activity. For example, school and workplace cafeterias should serve healthy foods, cities should provide sidewalks and bike lanes, and employers

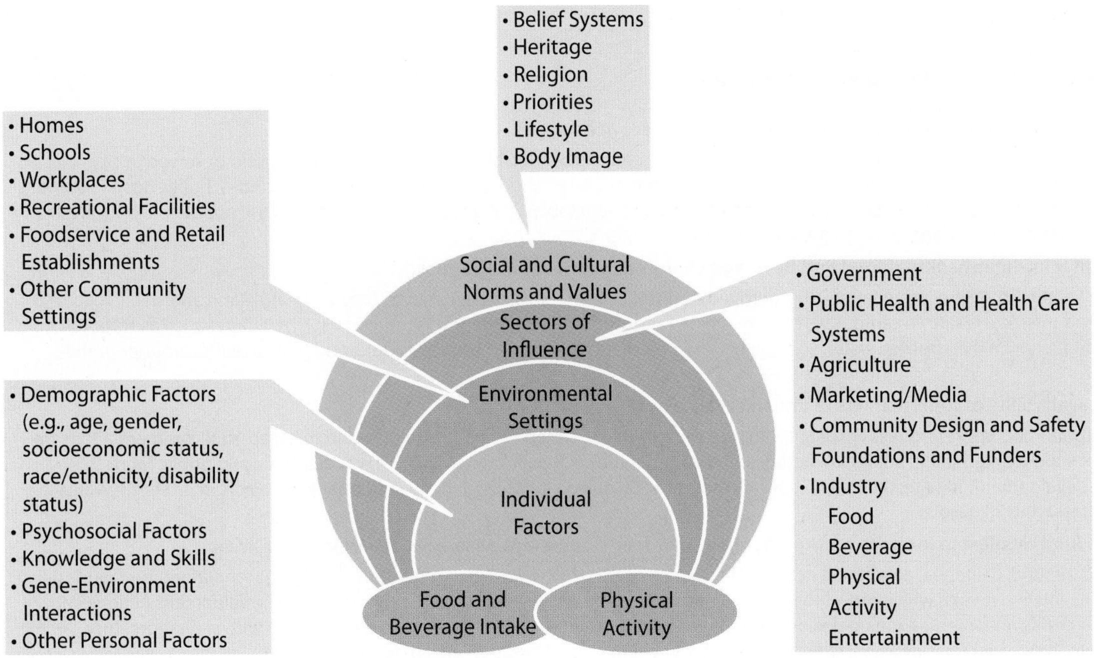

Figure 12.3

A Framework to Prevent and Control Overweight and Obesity

Sources: Adapted from Centers for Disease Control and Prevention. Division of Nutrition, Physical Activity, and Obesity. State Nutrition, Physical Activity and Obesity (NPAO) Program: Technical Assistance Manual. January 2008, page 36. Accessed April 21, 2010. http://www.cdc.gov/obesity/ downloads/TA_Manual_1_31_08.pdf. Institute of Medicine. *Preventing Childhood Obesity: Health in the Balance*. Washington, DC: National Academies Press, 2005; 85. M Story, KM Kaphingst, R Robinson-O'Brien, K Glanz. Creating healthy food and eating environments: Policy and environmental approaches. *Annu Rev Public Health*. 2008;29:253–272.

should offer flex time so their employees can be active. The various sectors of influence must support healthy behaviors. For example, the food and beverage industry can offer healthier options; the media can use its power to inform the public about healthy eating and physical activity; and local governments can pass zoning laws to limit the number of fast-food establishments.

Often, such actions are driven by policy changes. Policy change can be a federal law, such as requiring menu labeling on all restaurant foods. It can be a state law, such as not allowing the sale of sugar-sweetened beverages in schools. It can also be a local ordinance, such as requiring developers to have sidewalks in new housing developments. Policy change, however, is not limited to a law or statute. It can be a policy in a workplace, such as providing worksite wellness classes for all employees, or at a place of worship, such as not serving sugar-sweetened beverages at communal meals. Change can even occur at the family level. Families can change or adopt new standards of practice, such as no TV on school nights, weekly family outings that include physical activity, or planning meals together for the week. All of the levels of the socioecological model work together to create a shift in social norms and values so that eating healthy and being physically active are possible for all people.

Recommended Community Strategies to Prevent Obesity

The Centers for Disease Control and Prevention has suggested strategies that can be implemented at the local level to address overweight and obesity (**Figure 12.4**).[55] The 24 recommendations are designed to offer guidelines to change the physical and food environments to provide more opportunities for people to eat healthy foods and to be physically activity on a daily basis (**Table 12.2**). These recommendations suggest that healthy policies lead to healthy environments, which influence health behaviors, ultimately resulting in healthy people.[56] Most, if not all, of these recommended strategies require support by local, state, or federal policy changes.

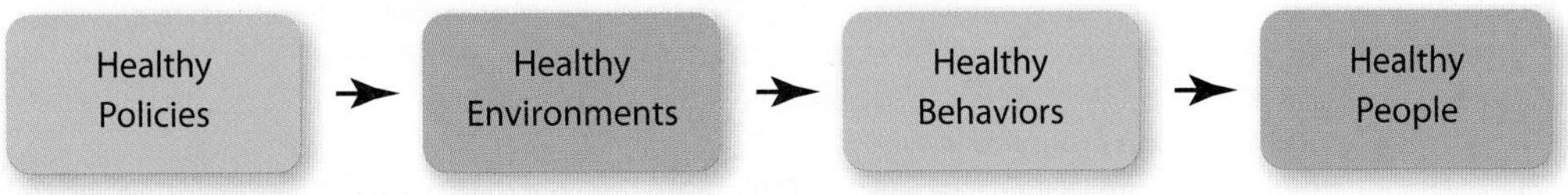

Figure 12.4

Policies That Promote Healthy Behaviors Ultimately Lead to Healthy People

Table 12.2

Recommended Community Strategies for Obesity Prevention

1. **Increase availability of healthier food and beverage choices in public service venues.**

   Example: In 2008, New York City became the first major city in the United States to set nutrition standards for all foods sold or served in city agencies, including schools, senior centers, homeless shelters, child care centers, afterschool programs, correctional facilities, public hospitals, and parks. The standards require city agencies to include two serving of fruits and vegetables in every lunch and dinner, phase out deep frying, lower salt content, serve healthier beverages, and increase the amount of fiber in meals.

2. **Improve availability of affordable healthier food and beverage choices in public service venues.**

   Example: In 2004, the Seattle School Board unanimously approved nutrition-related policies designed to provide healthy and affordable food and beverage options to students. As a result, all campus vending machines and student stores are now required to sell beverages such as soda, juice, and sports drinks at a higher price than bottled water. The policy was implemented in all elementary, middle, and high schools throughout the Seattle School District.

3. **Improve geographic availability of supermarkets in underserved areas.**

   Example: The Philadelphia Food Marketing Task Force investigated the lack of supermarkets in Philadelphia and released 10 recommendations to increase the number of supermarkets in Philadelphia's underserved communities. A new funding initiative was created using public funds to leverage supermarket development. To date, the initiative has committed $67 million in funding for 69 supermarket projects in 27 Pennsylvania counties, creating or preserving 3,900 jobs.

4. **Provide incentives to food retailers to locate in and/or offer healthier food and beverage choices in underserved areas.**

   Example: The city of Richmond, California, attracted a national discount grocery store to an urban retail center with adjacent affordable housing by offering an attractive incentive package, which included land sold at a reduced cost to the developer; a Federal Urban Development Action Grant of $3.5 million for commercial development; a zoning designation that provided tax incentives; assistance in negotiations with state regulatory agencies; improvements to surrounding sidewalks, streetscape, and traffic signals; and concessions on design standards.

5. **Improve availability of mechanisms for purchasing foods from farms.**

   Example: The Food Trust's Farmers' Market Program operates a network of 30 farmers' markets serving more than 125,000 customers in the Philadelphia region of Pennsylvania. Many of the farmers' markets are located in neighborhoods underserved by supermarkets, grocery stores, and other fresh food outlets. All of the farmers' markets accept food stamps (EBT/Access cards) and Farmers' Market Nutrition Program vouchers.

6. **Provide incentives for the production, distribution, and procurement of foods from local farms.**

   Example: The New North Florida Cooperative (NNFC) serves as a regional lead agency for the National Farm to School Network and is the hub for farm-to-school activities in the southern region of the United States. The mission of NNFC is to facilitate the sale of locally grown produce to local school districts for school lunch and breakfast programs by acting as an intermediary between local farmers and school districts. The cooperative markets, handles, processes, and delivers fresh produce on behalf of participating local farmers at competitive prices so schools are not paying more to buy local. To date, the cooperative has served fresh fruits and vegetables to over one million students in 72 school districts.

7. **Restrict availability of less healthy foods and beverages in public service venues.**

   Example: In 2003, Arkansas passed comprehensive legislation to combat childhood obesity. One component of Act 1220 prohibits student access to food and beverage vending machines in all Arkansas elementary schools. The fourth annual evaluation of the law found a significant increase in policies to prohibit the sale of "junk foods" in schools and less availability of high-fat, high-sugar items and more availability of healthy food and beverage options in school vending machines.

8. **Institute smaller portion size options in public service venues.**

   Example: The Texas Department of State Health Services developed the *Tex Plate* program to assist Texas restaurants in serving healthier portion sizes to consumers. Participating restaurants receive specialized 9-inch plates that indicate proper portions of key food groups, such as vegetables, proteins, and whole grains. The program is designed to encourage participating restaurants to increase the vegetable portion of the meal and decrease the entrée and starch portions of the meal.

9. **Limit advertisements of less healthy foods and beverages.**

   Example: The Mercedes Independent School District in Mercedes, Texas, adopted a comprehensive Student Nutrition/Wellness Plan in 2005 that includes a marketing component. The policy states that schools will promote healthy food choices and will not allow advertising that promotes less nutritious food choices. The plan also defines and prohibits possession of foods of minimal nutritional value at school.

10. **Discourage consumption of sugar-sweetened beverages.**

    Example: In 2006, the New York City Board of Health adopted regulations that provide nutrition standards and limit the serving size for beverages served to children in licensed day care centers. Specifically, the New York City Health Code prohibits serving beverages with added sweeteners and limits the serving size of 100% fruit juice to 6 ounces per day for children 8 months of age and older. When milk is served, children 2 years of age and older must receive low-fat 1% or nonfat milk, and water must be made easily available to children throughout the day.

11. **Increase support for breastfeeding.**

    Example: In 2008, Navajo Nation lawmakers passed a bill that requires employers on the reservation to provide a place for working mothers to breastfeed. The Navajo Nation Healthy Start Act allows mothers unpaid time during work hours to breastfeed their children or to use a breast pump.

12. **Require physical education in schools.**

    Example: In 2007, the State of Mississippi passed the Mississippi Healthy Students Act, which includes a requirement for public schools to provide 150 minutes per week of physical activity-based instruction and 45 minutes per week of health education in grades K–8. The act also requires 60 hours per year of physical education and 60 hours per year of health education in grades 9–12 to meet graduation requirements.

13. **Increase the amount of physical activity in physical education programs in schools.**

    Example: Equestrian Trails Elementary School, located in Wellington, Florida, received a STARS award from the National Association for Sport and Physical Education in recognition of its outstanding PE program. The PE staff at Equestrian Trails Elementary designed a yearly plan of instruction using physical activity and fitness components as the primary foundation for its curriculum. The curriculum teaches students the basic skills of several movement forms, including team, dual, and individual sports, and dance.

Table 12.2

Recommended Community Strategies for Obesity Prevention *(Continued)*

14. Increase opportunities for extracurricular physical activity.

Example: Pitt County, North Carolina, formed the Community Schools and Recreation Program (CSR) in 1978 to provide recreation and physical activity opportunities for all citizens. As a result of ongoing collaboration between the CSR and the Pitt County School District, all school facilities are available for free or a small service charge to community organizations, civic groups, private nonprofit agencies, commercial businesses, faith organizations, private and commercial sport leagues, and individuals.

15. Reduce screen time in public service venues.

Example: In 2007, Delaware's Office of Child Care Licensing promulgated regulations that set limits on the amount of screen time allowed in child care facilities. Specifically, child care facilities must limit screen time to one hour per day, while screen time for children younger than 2 years of age is prohibited. In addition, Delaware and Colorado are the only two states that require parental permission to use television during child care hours.

16. Improve access to outdoor recreational facilities.

Example: The Healthy Choice Program in Duarte, California, undertook a project that rehabilitated and revitalized local hiking trails and increased access for local residents. The Fish Canyon Trail Crew, which primarily consisted of youth and adolescents, gathered to clear, widen, and repair a mile of hiking trails that led to the local park's waterfall. In addition, the program initiated the development of nine walking/jogging routes in the city and distributed maps of the routes in the community's fitness center, the Chamber of Commerce, and along the Duarte multipurpose trail. As a result of these efforts, a Teen Trekkers program was created and Bike Ride-Alongs were promoted for residents in lower-income neighborhoods.

17. Enhance infrastructure supporting bicycling.

Example: In May 2005, Boulder, Colorado, was awarded Gold status as a Bicycle-Friendly Community by the League of American Bicyclists. The city committed 15% of its annual transportation budget, $3.1 million, toward bicycle enhancement and maintenance activities. More than 95% of Boulder's arterial streets have bicycle facilities and all local and regional buses are equipped with bike racks. In addition, Boulder has created an online bike routing system that provides cyclists a direct and safe bike route to travel within city limits.

18. Enhance infrastructure supporting walking.

Example: In an effort to increase physical activity for residents, four towns in northern Maine created walking and biking trails from preexisting winter ski trails. The towns of Van Buren, Caribou, Stockholm, and New Sweden all had limited sidewalks or paved shoulders for community members to use. The ski trails consisted of rough brush and mud in spring, summer, and fall but are now refurbished with packed dirt and can be enjoyed by residents year-round.

19. Support locating schools within easy walking distance of residential areas.

Example: In 2005, the City of Milwaukee began its Neighborhood Schools initiative. As a result of this initiative, the city decided to build six new schools from the ground up and spent millions of dollars revamping and expanding dilapidated schools that were located in and around community neighborhoods. The goals of the initiative were to reduce the number of students being bused to schools around the city and to increase the number of students walking or biking to schools that were centrally located and close to their neighborhoods.

20. Improve access to public transportation.

Example: Local business owners and residents of the South Park neighborhood of Tucson, Arizona, received funding from the local government and the Federal Transit Administration (FTA) to implement a series of improvements to the existing public transit system. Funds were used to install six new artistic bus shelters, new traffic signals, and additional sidewalk and curb access ramps for public transit users, bicyclers, and pedestrians. As a result of the efforts to revitalize its public transit infrastructure, South Park has experienced renewed pride in its community and helped to rebuild its local economy.

21. Zone for mixed-use development.

Example: King County, Washington, developed a comprehensive land use plan that encourages zoning for mixed-use development as a way to support active living among residents. The land use plan outlines specific design components for mixed-use developments, such as integrating retail establishments and business offices into the same buildings as residential units, ensuring the availability of parking lots or parking garages either within or close to buildings, and having safe pedestrian connections and bicycle facilities throughout the area.

22. Enhance personal safety in areas where persons are or could be physically active.

Example: Detroit, Michigan, has one of the highest home foreclosure rates in the country, resulting in a dramatic increase in the number of abandoned buildings and boarded-up homes, which attract vandals and petty crime. In response, Urban Farming, an international nonprofit organization, joined forces with the local county government to transform 20 abandoned properties into active fruit and vegetable garden plots that feed the homeless and improve the aesthetic appeal of city neighborhoods. Since establishing the gardens, residents report less vandalism and blight in their community and the local county government donates water to maintain the city gardens on an ongoing basis.

23. Enhance traffic safety in areas where persons are or could be physically active.

Example: After noting an increase in motor vehicle crashes resulting in pedestrian injuries and fatalities, a public official in Montgomery County, Maryland, appointed a 40-member Blue Ribbon Panel on Pedestrian and Traffic Safety. The panel developed an action-oriented set of recommendations to reduce pedestrian deaths and injuries and their associated economic costs by addressing ways to create pedestrian-friendly, walkable communities. The panel also developed a pedestrian safety toolbox for community planners.

24. Participate in community coalitions or partnerships to address obesity.

Example: A Food Policy Council (FPC) is a type of coalition that brings together stakeholders from diverse food-related areas to examine how the food system is working. In Knoxville, Tennessee, an FPC monitors and evaluates the performance of the city's food system and recommends actions to improve it. A major accomplishment of the FPC was improving access to competitively priced nutritious foods by changing the city bus routes so that poorer inner city residents could reach outlying supermarkets.

Source: D Keener, K Goodman, A Lowry, S Zaro, L Kettel Khan. *Recommended Community Strategies and Measurements to Prevent Obesity in the United States: Implementation and Measurement Guide*. Atlanta, GA: U.S. Department of Health and Human Services, Centers for Disease Control and Prevention, 2009.

Which Side Are You On?

The Soda Tax: Passing the Blame or a Tool to Curb Obesity?

The increased burden of obesity has prompted policymakers to explore many different approaches to addressing the problem. Taxing sugar-sweetened beverages is one policy that is under consideration by the federal government, as well as many state and city governments. Several states and cities already have a tax on sugar-sweetened beverages.

Would a tax on sugar-sweetened beverages eliminate obesity? Certainly not. As you have learned, obesity is a multifaceted problem. Taxes on tobacco have not totally eliminated smoking or diseases related to tobacco consumption, and seatbelt laws have not eliminated deaths from car accidents; however, they are sound policies nonetheless. Sharp reductions in the obesity rate are unlikely to result from any one intervention or policy. A tax on sugar-sweetened beverages will not eliminate obesity, but could it help? Let's examine that question.

Government agencies and professional organizations, including the Centers for Disease Control and Prevention, the U.S. Department of Agriculture, the Institute of Medicine, the American Academy of Pediatrics, the American Medical Association, the American Heart Association, and the World Health Organization, have all called for consumers to decrease consumption of sugar-sweetened beverages. It is estimated by some researchers that consumption of sugar-sweetened beverages may be the single largest driver of the obesity epidemic.[57] A clear association exists between sugar-sweetened beverages and increased consumption of calories, increased body weight, poor nutritional status, and incidence of diabetes.[58,59] Calories from sugar-sweetened beverages make up a significant percentage of daily calories for most Americans and is as high as 13% in adolescents.[58] Critics of the tax on sugar-sweetened beverages cite reports that run counter to the majority of research in the area of obesity and sugar-sweetened beverages, noting that some researchers have found that consumption of sugar-sweetened beverages has little or no effect on weight. These studies have been criticized because they were funded by the soft drink industry.[60] Most everyone can agree, however, that sugar-sweetened beverages are not a necessary food. Plus, there is a low- or no-cost alternative—water.

What effect would a soft drink tax have on consumption? Manipulating what consumers buy by altering prices is certainly possible. One of the best examples is that of tobacco. The increase in tobacco taxes has been identified as a major contributor to decreased smoking rates.[61,62] Policies that have decreased the prices of healthy foods simultaneous to increasing the prices of unhealthy foods have seen a shift in consumption toward healthier foods.[63–66] Soft drinks have been identified as one of the foods most responsive to price changes; that is, as price goes up, consumption goes down.[67] It is estimated that for every 10% increase in the price of sugar-sweetened beverages, consumption will decrease 8–10%.

The ultimate effect of a tax on sugar-sweetened beverages on obesity rates is unknown. Will consumers choose other foods and beverages that are not taxed but that are just as high in calories? This has yet to be answered, as some states and cities have just begun to implement this strategy.

In addition to possibly decreasing consumption of soft drinks, a sugar-sweetened beverage tax could raise considerable funds. A tax of 1 cent per ounce on sugar-sweetened beverages would raise an estimated $14.88 billion a year.[68] Revenue from a sugar-sweetened beverage tax could be used to address childhood obesity or other health concerns. Public sentiment for a sugar-sweetened beverage tax is more positive if the funds are earmarked for a specific health cause.[69,70] Revenue from a sugar-sweetened beverage tax could be used to decrease the cost of healthier foods, something that is under consideration at the federal level.

Several arguments against a tax on sugar-sweetened beverages have been raised, and, as you might imagine, there has been vigorous opposition by the beverage industry. Some argue that the tax is regressive and will hurt poor people more. Although this is true, what is also true is that sugar-sweetened beverages are not a necessary part of anyone's diet. People, regardless of income, do not have to consume sugar-sweetened beverages. Others indicate that it is wrong to blame soft drinks for obesity. True, sugar-sweetened beverages are not solely responsible for the rise in obesity; a single cause does not exist. However, sugar-sweetened beverages do represent one of the contributors to overweight and obesity. Finally, one of the arguments against a tax on sugar-sweetened beverages is that the government should not try to regulate what people eat or drink. The fact is, however, that the government already has considerable influence on what you consume. It subsidizes some commodities, including corn that makes high-fructose corn sweetener; sets standards for school meals; and requires labels on foods.

Now that you know more about a tax on sugar-sweetened beverages, where do you stand? Do you think this is a good strategy to address overweight and obesity, or is it an unnecessary government mandate?

How You Can Achieve and Maintain a Healthy Weight

By now, you understand what it will take to make the nation a place where people have the opportunity to eat smart and move more. Changing policies and environments is key in helping all people achieve and maintain a healthy weight, but what can you do as an individual in your day-to-day life to live healthy, make good choices, and be a healthy weight? For some of you, it will mean not gaining any weight over time. For others of you, it may mean losing weight to get your weight in line with

Personal Health Check

Your BMI and Daily Calorie Needs

What Is Your BMI?

To assess your personal BMI you need two pieces of information: your height without shoes and your weight in pounds. Use the equation presented in the sidebar earlier in this chapter to calculate your BMI. Then use the color-coded BMI chart in Figure 12.1 to see into what category your BMI falls. You can also find several BMI calculators online. If you are in the overweight or obese category, how many pounds would you need to lose to be in the healthy weight category?

How Many Calories Do You Need Each Day?

Your **basal metabolic rate (BMR)** and physical activity level dictate the number of calories you need each day. Your BMR is the number of calories that you need at rest to keep your body alive. These are the calories needed to keep you breathing, your heart beating, your temperature normal, and all body systems functioning. Your BMR is affected by several factors.[71] Genetics dictates some of what your BMR will be. Some people simply have a faster metabolism than others. Gender also affects BMR, with males having a higher BMR than females. Body fatness greatly effects BMR; the more muscle you have, the higher your BMR. Age effects BMR as well. As you get older, your BMR will decrease; however, some of this depends on how much lean body mass you lose as you age. Finally, diet can affect BMR. If you are on a low-calorie diet, your BMR will decrease. The body is able to sense when calories are at a deficit and slows everything down to conserve energy. This safety mechanism helped keep us alive thousands of years ago when we had to hunt for food. In times of low food intake, our bodies held on to every calorie they could in order to survive until food would be available again. Today, even though food is readily available, perhaps even too available, our bodies still have this mechanism. This is one reason why ultra-low-calorie diets are not recommended.

The other factor that dictates the number of calories you need each day is your physical activity level. Your daily physical activity level includes all the times you move your body in a given day. On one end of the spectrum would be someone who sits at a desk all day and moves very little to someone who is training for an athletic event or does manual labor most of the day. The *Dietary Guidelines for Americans* has ranges of calories based on gender, age, and activity level.[72]

Estimate of Daily Calorie Needs

This table estimates the number of calories that you need each day. It is only an estimate; individual calorie needs vary based on body size, gender, and activity level.

		Activity Level		
Gender	Age	Sedentary	Moderately Active	Active
Female	19–30	1,800–2,000	2,000–2,200	2,400
	31–50	1,800	2,000	2,200
	51+	1,600	1,800	2,000–2,200
Male	19–30	2,400–2,600	2,000–2,200	3,000
	31–50	2,200–2,400	2,400–2,600	2,800–3,000
	51+	2,000–2,200	2,200–2,400	2,400–2,800

Source: P Britten, K Marcoe, S Yamini, C Davis. Development of food intake patterns for the MyPyramid Food Guidance System. *J Nutr Educ Behav*. 2006;38(6 Suppl):S78–S92.

what is healthy for you. The first step is to assess where you are. See the Personal Health Check to assess your current BMI.

Once you know your BMI and have determined what your weight status is, you can set realistic goals. For those of you who are underweight, ask your physician or healthcare provider if you need to gain weight to be a healthy weight. Those of you in the normal weight category, congratulations! Your goal is to avoid gaining weight over time. Those of you in the overweight or obese categories may want to take steps to lose weight. No matter what your weight status, the behaviors discussed in this chapter are ones that you all should adopt for a lifetime of good health, including achieving and maintaining a healthy weight.

Setting your goal should be about good health, not achieving an unrealistic goal. You may never look like

TERMS

basal metabolic rate (BMR) The amount of energy the body expends at rest to maintain bodily functions, such as breathing.

Personal Health Check

Calculate Your Total Daily Energy Expenditure

Use the following equation and steps provided to calculate your daily energy expenditure.

total daily energy expenditure = BMR × physical activity multiplier

1. **Calculate your BMR.**
   Female BMR: −161 + 10(weight in pounds ÷ 2.2) + 6.25(height in inches × 2.54) − 5(age)
   Male BMR: 5 + 10(weight in pounds ÷ 2.2) + 6.25(height in inches × 2.54) − 5(age)
2. **Assess your physical activity level and calculate physical activity multiplier.**
   Sedentary (little or no exercise, desk job) = BMR × 1.2
   Light activity (light exercise/sports one to three days/week) = BMR × 1.375
   Moderate activity (moderate exercise/sports three to five days/week) = BMR × 1.55
   Very active (hard exercise/sports six to seven days/week) = BMR × 1.75
   Extremely active (hard daily exercise/sports and physical job OR twice daily athletic training) = BMR × 1.9
3. **Calculate total daily energy expenditure by multiplying BMR by the appropriate physical activity multiplier.**
   EXAMPLE:
   Female
   Age: 35
   Weight: 206 pounds
   Height: 5 foot, 7 inches
   Light activity level
   BMR = −161 + 10(206 ÷ 2.2) + 6.25(67 × 2.54) − 5(35)
   BMR = −161 + 936 + 1064 − 175
   BMR = 1,664
   2,143(1.375) = 2,288

Based on these calculations, this woman's daily calorie needs are 2,288. This is an estimate of the number of calories she needs to consume each day to maintain her weight at 206. If she consumes less and maintains her activity level, she will lose weight. If she eats more than 2,288 calories and maintains her activity level, she will gain weight.

Source: MD Mifflin, ST St Jeor, LA Hill, BJ Scott, SA Daugherty, YO Koh. A new predictive equation for resting energy expenditure in healthy individuals. *Am J Clin Nutr.* 1990;51:241–247.

the images you see in magazines or in the movies, few do. Some basic tenants of size acceptance are presented in **Table 12.3**.

Accepting yourself will improve your self-esteem. Improved self-esteem can help you in all aspects of your life. However, along with self-acceptance, you need to make a commitment to eating healthy and being physically active for a lifetime of good health.

Table 12.3

Basic Tenets of Size Acceptance

- Human beings come in a variety of sizes and shapes. We celebrate this diversity as a positive characteristic of the human race.
- There is no ideal body size, shape, or weight that every individual should strive to achieve.
- Every body is a good body, whatever its size or shape.
- Self-esteem and body image are strongly linked. Helping people feel good about their bodies and about who they are can help motivate and maintain healthy behaviors.
- Appearance stereotyping is inherently unfair to the individual because it is based on superficial factors which the individual has little or no control over.
- We respect the bodies of others even though they might be quite different from our own.
- Each person is responsible for taking care of his/her own body.
- Good health is not defined by body size; it is a state of physical, mental, and social well-being.
- People of all sizes and shapes can reduce their risk of poor health by adopting a healthy lifestyle.

Source: Fact sheet developed by dietitians and nutritionists who are advocates of size acceptance. Their efforts are coordinated by Joanne P. Ikeda, MA, RD, Nutrition Education Specialist, Department of Nutritional Sciences, University of California, Berkeley, CA.

If your goal is to lose weight, set a SMART goal. A SMART goal is specific, measurable, attainable, realistic, and timely. Healthy weight loss should be at a rate of between 0.5 to 2.0 pounds per week. To set a SMART goal, first think of the number of pounds you want to lose. Be specific: "I want to lose 10 pounds," as opposed to "I want to lose weight." Make sure your goal is measurable; weight is pretty easy to measure provided that you have access to a scale. To be attainable and realistic, your weight loss goal should be 0.5 to 2.0 pounds a week. Setting a goal to lose 50 pounds in a month is not attainable by most people, is not realistic, and could be dangerous. Finally, your goal should be timely, when are you going to do this. An example of a SMART weight loss goal is: *I will lose 10 pounds between July 1 and September 1.*

You know your BMI and your weight status and have set your goals; now comes the strategies that will help you achieve your goals. Although there are many pills, potions, powders, and so-called quick fixes on the market, none are a substitute for healthy eating and physical activity. Adopting the behaviors outlined here is the safe and healthy way to a lifestyle that can decrease your risk of disease and promote lifelong health. Most of these concepts are discussed in greater detail elsewhere in this text. However, when examined together you can see how these behaviors collectively are the foundation for a healthy lifestyle. Something else that can help you stay the course of healthy eating and physical activity is to find others who can support you. This may be your family or friends, but it often is another group that you may join that can provide the social support you need.

Healthy Weight Behaviors

There are a number of research-based strategies that have been proven to be effective in helping you achieve and maintain a healthy weight. Planning and tracking will help you be more mindful about your eating and physical activity patterns. Other behaviors you can choose to achieve and maintain a healthy weight include balancing calories, eating more fruits and vegetables, eating more whole grains, eating breakfast, consuming the right-sized portions, eating more meals at home, drinking fewer calorie-containing beverages, moving more, and watching less television.

Plan Planning is an important part of a healthy lifestyle. You should plan what you are going to eat, which means planning trips to the grocery store or farmers' market for healthy foods. You can't eat what you don't have on hand. When you are hungry and ready for a meal or snack, you will most likely grab the most convenient choice. Make that choice a healthy one by planning for healthy foods. Fast food is just a phone call or drive-through away, so keep that choice off the radar with good choices that are just as quick. See Chapter 3 for more information about preparing healthy meals at home.

Planning is also important when it comes to physical activity. Set aside time during your day when you can be active. Use your calendar to plan out your week of physical activity. Make every effort to keep the dates and times you set for yourself to be active, just as you would a scheduled meeting or class.

Track Keeping track of eating, physical activity, and body weight is one of the most successful techniques to promote weight loss and weight maintenance.[73–75] Keep a food journal and write down everything you eat and drink. You will be amazed how more mindful it will make you about the choices you make. Find a convenient way to track your eating and physical activity. It can be as simple as a mark you make on your calendar or as sophisticated as a smartphone or iPad application. Use whatever works for you. Be sure to track the type of food, the amount, and the way it is prepared. Don't forget extras like salad dressings, sauces, and condiments. You may do this for only a few days, or it may become something you do on a daily basis to help you stay on track with healthy eating. Do the same with tracking your weight. Even if you are normal weight, periodically keeping track of where you are will help you maintain a healthy weight throughout your life.[75]

One way to track your eating and physical activity is to use the food tracker at www.choosemyplate.gov.[76] This online dietary and physical activity assessment tool can help you assess your diet quality and physical activity status (**Figure 12.5**). It also provides nutrition facts and links to nutrition and physical activity information. The Food Calories/Energy Balance feature automatically calculates your energy balance by subtracting the energy you expend from physical activity from your food calories/energy intake. Use of this tool helps you better understand your energy balance status and enhances the link between good nutrition and regular physical activity. You can keep track of your energy balance history and view it for up to one year.

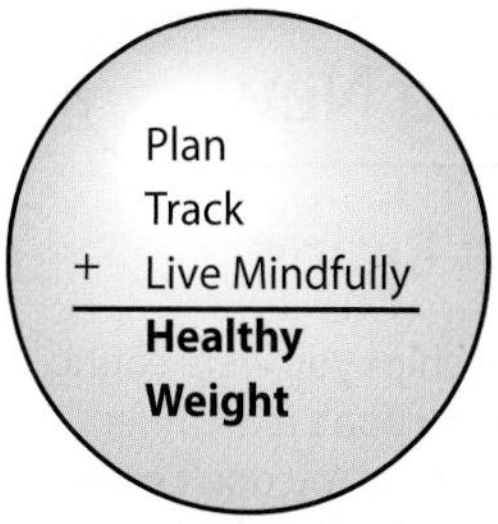

Figure 12.5

Plan, Track, and Live Mindfully to Achieve and Maintain a Healthy Weight

> ### Healthy Weight Behaviors
>
> Follow healthy weight behaviors to achieve and maintain a healthy weight and to decrease your risk of many chronic diseases:
>
> - Plan.
> - Track.
> - Live mindfully.
> - Balance calories.
> - Eat more fruits and vegetables.
> - Eat more whole grains.
> - Eat breakfast.
> - Right-size portions.
> - Eat more meals at home.
> - Drink fewer calorie-containing beverages.
> - Move more.
> - Watch less television.

Balance Calories Numerous fad diets promise success if you just eat low carb or high protein or low fat. The bottom line is that there must be a calorie deficit in order to lose weight or a calorie balance to maintain weight. So, it may not be very catchy, but balancing the calories you consume with physical activity is the strategy for weight management that is supported by research.[87,88]

Many studies have found that people do achieve short-term weight loss on low-carb diets. The reason for the weight loss, however, is most often due to a lower calorie intake, not just a low carbohydrate intake.[88] If you think about a low-carbohydrate diet in the context of all we know about health and nutrition, it does not make

Try Something New

Mindful Versus Mindless Eating

Have you ever looked down at a bag of chips you were eating and wondered where the chips went? You don't remember eating that many chips, yet they are all gone. You don't even remember if the chips tasted good or not. This is called *mindless eating* or *distracted eating*. Eating breakfast while watching the morning news, having a snack while surfing the web, and gobbling down a burger at a stoplight are all examples of mindless eating. You may not even be aware of the number of food decisions you make in a day. Research indicates that we overlook as many as 200 food decisions each day.[77] These overlooked food decisions are made without you even being aware that you are making them. Your decision of what to eat, whether to eat, and how much to eat is based on what you usually do; external cues, such as seeing or smelling food; or simply eating what is there. Moving from mindless eating to mindful eating can make a big difference in how you relate to food and ultimately impact your weight. A growing body of evidence suggests that mindful eating can enhance weight loss efforts.[78–85]

The concept of mindfulness comes from Buddhism. You may wonder what we might learn from the round-bellied Buddha about healthy eating. When it comes to mindfulness, there is plenty to be learned. Buddha said that right mindfulness is a step on the path to nirvana. **Mindfulness** is living with greater awareness of moment-to-moment thoughts, feelings, and actions.

Mindful eating can be a step towards healthy eating. Mindful eating means paying close attention to every detail of the eating experience. Being mindful can increase your awareness of the internal and external cues that guide your eating behavior. These cues may be physical, emotional, or cognitive. Often, we eat almost automatically, giving little thought to what or how much we are eating. The candy jar is there, so you grab some. You are served a large plate of food, and you eat it all. You order the number one combo because that is what you usually eat. Mindfulness can lead to making intentional choices when eating instead of responding to external cues, emotions, or your environment.

The theory of mindfulness is based on several assumptions. Many people operate on autopilot. This means that you may be unaware of your moment-to-moment experiences. The mind processes experiences and reacts to them with a specific action or behavior. However, you may not be fully engaged in the progression of the action. It is possible to learn to become more aware of moment-to-moment experiences and cues and to actively identify the experiences and cues of daily living. Learning to do this will take time and practice. By becoming more mindful, you can make your life better and more purposeful. By no longer acting on autopilot, you will become more engaged in your daily life. Being mindful can help you gain awareness so you can identify specific cues that influence your eating behavior. Practicing mindfulness can change your actions so that you have greater control over your eating. It allows you to make deliberate decisions about eating instead of acting without thinking.

According to the Center for Mindful Eating, mindful eating is based on several principles.[86] Allow yourself to become aware of the positive and nurturing opportunities that are available through food preparation and consumption by respecting your own inner wisdom. Choose to eat food that is both pleasing to you and nourishing to your body by using all your senses to explore, savor, and taste. Acknowledge responses to food likes and dislikes without judgment. Learn to be aware of physical hunger and satiety cues to guide your decision to begin eating and to stop eating.

You can take some simple steps to apply mindful eating:

- Eat without distractions—no cell phone, TV, work, computer, or newspaper.
- Don't eat while driving or working at your desk.
- Eat sitting down.
- Eat slowly and enjoy every bite.
- Make each meal last at least 20 minutes.

A good way to get started is to try this simple exercise with a raisin. Put the raisin in your mouth and close your eyes. Do not begin chewing yet. Try not to pay attention to the ideas running through your mind; just focus on the raisin. Notice the texture, temperature, and taste. Begin chewing slowly. Notice what it feels like. If you find your mind wandering away from the raisin and on to other things, gently bring your thoughts back to the raisin. Notice how your jaw moves each time you chew. Swallow slowly and sense the movement of muscles in your throat and tongue. Take a deep breath and open your eyes. You may find it helpful to do a similar exercise with the first bite of every meal.

good sense to recommend a diet high in animal fat and low in fruits and vegetables. Without exception, a diet that is high in complex carbohydrates and vegetable proteins is associated with low body mass. But before you head to the nearest pasta restaurant, remember that the majority of the carbohydrates you consume should be whole grains, fruits, and vegetables.

TERMS

mindfulness A state of active attention to the present, having greater awareness of moment-to-moment thoughts, feelings, and actions. Mindfulness means living in the moment and being aware of everything that makes up your day.

According to the latest analysis of the diet of the U.S. population, Americans are consuming more calories than they did 30 years ago, and the rate of increase is three times greater in women than men.[89] U.S. women have increased their daily calorie consumption by 22% over the past 30 years, from 1,542 to 1,877 calories per day. During the same period, calorie intake for men has increased

7%, from 2,450 to 2,618 calories per day. The increase in calories is mainly due to an increase in carbohydrate consumption. Men increased the percentage of their daily calorie intake from carbohydrates from 42.4% to 49%. Women increased their carbohydrate consumption from 45.4% of daily calorie intake to 51.6%.

To lose weight, you need to eat fewer calories and/or increase physical activity. To lose 1 pound, you have to consume 3,500 fewer calories than you need. For example, if you consume 500 fewer calories per day than you need, you would lose 1 pound per week. You have to bal-

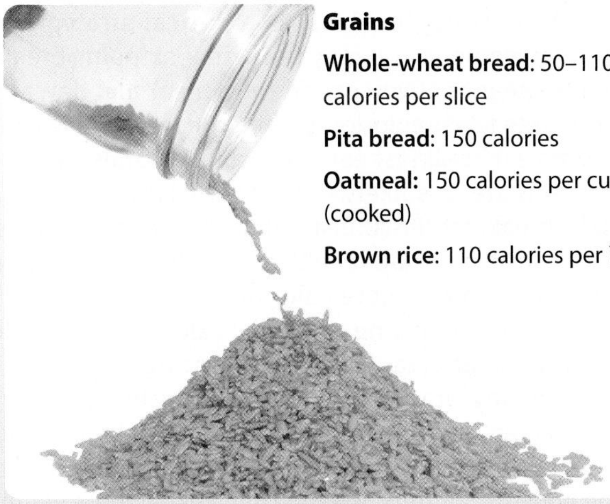

Grains

Whole-wheat bread: 50–110 calories per slice

Pita bread: 150 calories

Oatmeal: 150 calories per cup (cooked)

Brown rice: 110 calories per ½ cup

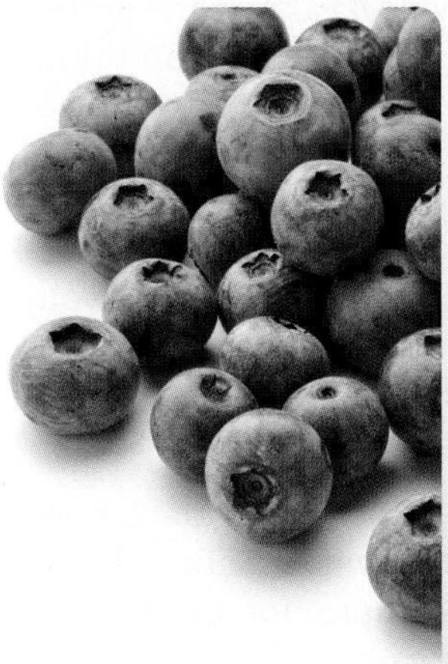

Dairy

Skim milk: 90 calories per cup

Non-fat, sugar-free yogurt: 90 calories per cup

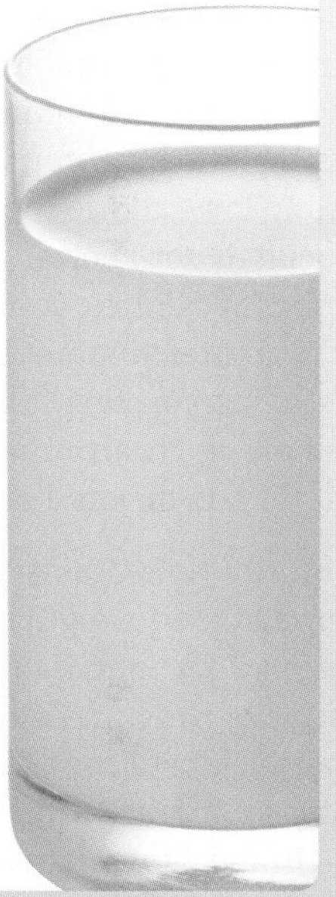

Vegetables

Most vegetables have between 15–25 calories per ½ cup.

Starchy vegetables such as peas, potatoes, and corn have between 60–90 calories per ½ cup.

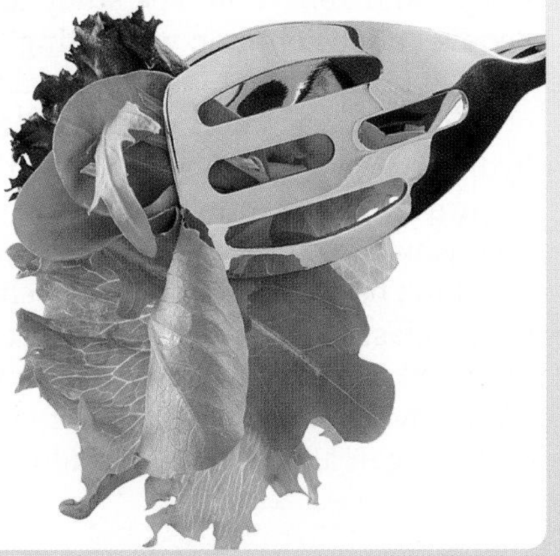

Fruit

Medium apple or pear: 80 calories

½ grapefruit: 40 calories

Medium orange: 60 calories

1 cup berries or melon: 50 calories

1 cup canned fruit: 60–100 calories

Meat and beans

- Choose lean beef and pork
- Choose light meat chicken
- Choose fish often

Lean cuts of beef

Several cuts of beef are low in calories and fat. These cuts have between 150–160 calories for 3 ounces.

- Eye of round
- Bottom round
- Round tip
- Chuck shoulder
- Flank steak
- Sirloin steak

- Remove visible fat from meat
- Remove skin from chicken
- Choose beans often

Lean cuts of pork

Several cuts of pork are low in calories and fat. These cuts have between 140–170 calories for 3 ounces.

- Pork tenderloin
- Pork boneless loin roast
- Pork loin chop

Cook low-calorie

- Grill
- Steam
- Stir fry
- Roast
- Bake

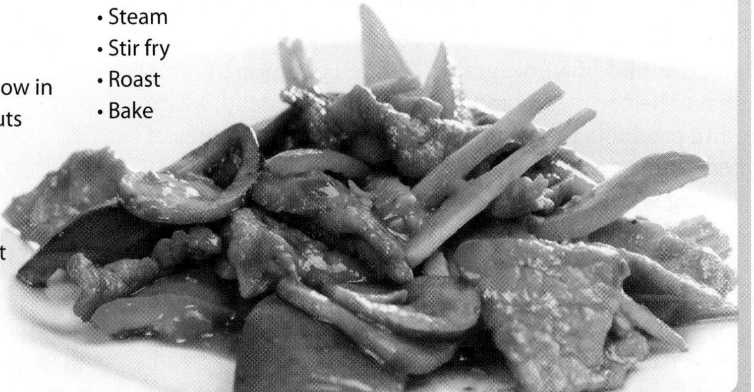

Figure 12.6

Lower-Calorie Options in Each Food Group

ance calories with physical activity to maintain your current weight.

We get calories from three major energy sources in foods: fat, carbohydrates (starches, sugars, and fiber), and proteins. Alcohol is another source of calories; it has 7 calories per gram. Fats provide 9 calories per gram. That is twice the number of calories supplied by carbohydrates and proteins. Carbohydrates provide 4 calories per gram. Protein also provides 4 calories per gram. You can think about it this way: Every tablespoon of olive oil you use in salad dressing or in cooking adds 120 calories. Every time you sprinkle a tablespoon of sugar in your coffee or on your cereal, you add 45 calories. When you choose a quarter-pound hamburger instead of the regular size, you double the calories from protein from 50 to 100 and from fat from 90 to 180 calories. The bottom line is to choose lower-calorie options from each food group (**Figure 12.6**).

Eat More Fruits and Vegetables Fruits and vegetables, in their natural state, are low in calories and fat. Eating plenty of fruits and vegetables is a good choice for weight loss and weight maintenance.[90–94] They are low in calories, but their high fiber content provides a feeling of fullness. Consuming low-calorie foods such as fruits and vegetables is associated with better weight management. For the same number of calories, you can eat foods with low energy density in greater volume than foods with high energy density. This helps you feel full and yet consume fewer calories. They are such an important part of a healthy diet that Chapter 6 is devoted entirely to fruits and vegetables.

Eat More Whole Grains Eating whole grains that are rich in fiber is a good weight management strategy. The *Dietary Guidelines for Americans* suggest that at least half of the grains we consume should be whole grains. More would be better. Most Americans need about six servings of grain a day, so at least three should be whole grain. Adults in the United States consume an average of almost seven servings of grain products per day—more than what many of us need. However, on average, only about one in seven of these servings is whole grain, well below what is recommended.[95]

Whole grains are grains that have the bran, endosperm, and germ intact. Whole wheat, oatmeal, and brown rice are all examples of whole grains. Refined grains are grains that have the germ and bran removed. White bread, white rice, and products made with white flour are examples of refined grains or foods made with refined grains.

Eating whole grains should be a part of your weight loss/weight maintenance plan. People who eat more whole grains have a lower body weight than people who eat primarily refined grains.[96–98] Often when people go on a weight-loss diet, their nutrition suffers because they may not be getting all the vitamins and minerals they need. Eating whole grains not only helps with weight loss, but it also helps improve the overall quality of the diet during weight loss.

Eating whole grains instead of refined grains has many nutritional advantages. One big benefit of consuming whole grains when you are trying to lose or maintain weight is that the dietary fiber content of whole grains helps you feel full longer. See Chapter 5 on carbohydrates for more information on whole grains and how you can incorporate them into your daily diet.

Eat Breakfast Eating breakfast is a critical strategy for weight management. You may think that skipping breakfast would mean that you eat one less meal that day, and thus consume fewer calories. In fact, the opposite is true. People who eat breakfast eat fewer total calories, eat less total fat, and are less likely to be overweight than those who skip breakfast. Breakfast-eaters weigh, on average, less than those who skip breakfast.[99,100] People who skip breakfast tend to eat more calorie-dense foods later in the day, more than making up for the calories they would have consumed at breakfast. Eating breakfast helps prevent binge eating later in the day by keeping hunger levels more stable; studies show that skipping breakfast slows the metabolic rate and causes blood sugar to drop, setting the body up for impulsive eating. Researchers examined hundreds of people across the country who had lost weight and kept it off. The study found that what these people had in common was eating breakfast.[101]

Get in the habit of eating breakfast to start your day off right. Choose a breakfast that has protein and carbohydrate to give you energy that will last all morning long (**Figure 12.7**). If you don't like eating when you first get up, take your breakfast with you and eat it mid-morning. If you don't have time for breakfast, choose a healthy cereal or breakfast bar for a quick breakfast on the go. If you don't like breakfast foods, choose something else. A peanut butter sandwich, a leftover piece of chicken, or cheese and crackers can also be breakfast foods.

Grain	Protein	Fruit
Whole-wheat toast	Low-fat milk	Banana
Oatmeal	Low-fat string cheese	Raisins
Whole-wheat toaster waffle	Low-fat cottage cheese	Apple
Whole-grain cereal	Low-fat yogurt	Grapes
	Hard-cooked egg	Orange slices
	Low-fat ham or turkey	Kiwi
		Tomato juice
		Other fruits in season

■ **Figure 12.7**

Breakfast Made Simple

Choose a grain, a protein, and a fruit for a healthy breakfast that will keep you going all morning.

Right-Size Portions How much we eat can be as important as what we eat. Controlling portions and making portions right-sized instead of super-sized is an important weight management strategy. Americans are eating larger portions than ever before. Portion sizes have increased significantly over the past ten years for people in all age groups.[102–104] The continuing trend of supersizing, huge portions, all-you-can-eat buffets, and extra-large single servings have all contributed to our expanding waistlines.

Portions, of course, impact the total number of calories consumed. That would not be a problem if you were able to recognize, both physically and psychologically, that you had eaten more calories than you need and compensated for it later in the day by eating less. However, that is not the way it works; generally, when you are served more food you eat more calories than you need over time.[105,106]

Most people are not adept at recognizing large portions and eating what they need. When served large portions, most people tend to eat more food and, therefore, more calories. Even if they don't eat the entire portion, most people eat more than they would have if they had been served a smaller portion.[103,105–108] Portion sizes are discussed in detail in Chapter 3.

Eat More Meals at Home As a country, we eat more of our meals away from home than ever before.[109] Over the past 30 years, the percentage of the total food budget spent on foods eaten away from home has risen from 17% to 49%.[110] Even if you are careful when you eat out, eating out generally means larger portions, more calories, more fat, fewer fruits and vegetables, fewer whole grains, fewer low-fat dairy products, and less fiber.[107,111–114] Although some restaurants now offer healthier options, eating simple foods prepared at home gives you more control over how your food is prepared and how much is served.

Of special concern for weight management is consumption of fast food. Every day, one in four Americans eats a fast-food meal. Fast food is usually high in fat and calories. So, it should be no surprise that consumption of fast food has been linked to an increased risk of overweight and obesity.[111,115] The more you eat fast food, the more likely you are to be overweight or obese.

It is clear that preparing and eating more meals at home is a good strategy for weight maintenance. The first step towards doing this is to plan. Planning meals is associated with a higher likelihood of preparing healthy meals at home.[116] Home-cooked meals don't have to be complicated, gourmet, or expensive. Plan simple meals, shop for the foods you need, and cook healthy foods for you and your family.

Drink Fewer Calorie-Containing Beverages Choosing healthy beverages is important for weight management both because of the calories that can be consumed and also because of how those calories are delivered—in liquid form.[117] According to the U.S. Department of Agriculture, per capita soft drink consumption has increased almost 500% over the past 50 years. Calories from soft drinks contribute an estimated 7% of total calorie intake. The most popular American beverage is the carbonated soft drink, which accounts for 28% of total beverage consumption. Enough regular soda is produced to supply every American with more than 14 ounces of soda every day.[118,119]

Soft drinks are available everywhere. They can be found in the workplace, schools, and convenience stores, and almost every public building has at least one soft drink machine. Soft drinks also come in larger sizes, which mean more calories.

People who drink sugar-sweetened beverages take in more calories than those who do not. A positive association exists between consumption of sugar-sweetened beverages and weight. Those who consume more sugar-sweetened beverages tend to weigh more.[120–123] Decreasing consumption of sugar-sweetened beverages is a good strategy to lower calorie intake and help manage weight.

Many types of beverages have calories. Any beverage that is sweetened with sugar or another calorie-containing sweetener (such as high-fructose corn sweetener) contains calories. This includes regular soda, lemonade, sweet tea, sports drinks, fruit drinks, and specialty coffee drinks. Milk, juice, and alcoholic beverages also contain calories. See Chapter 7 for a complete discussion of beverages, including the calories they contain.

Not only do sugar-sweetened beverages contain lots of calories, but your body does not respond to the calories in liquids the same way it does to calories in food. Your body has complex mechanisms in place to detect calorie needs and calorie consumption. These mechanisms allow the body to consume calories at a relatively stable rate over time. Liquid calories seem to go undetected by the body, or at least they are not as readily detected as those from food. The body's ability to detect calories in liquid form is not as accurate as it is in detecting calories in solid form. Your body may not register the calories you drink, so you could end up consuming calories you don't need on top of those you do. Another way of looking at this is that your body just doesn't "see or feel" the calories from beverages like it does from food. The calories in beverages are "stealth" calories and can cause you to consume more calories than you need.[124–127]

Liquid calories count towards the calories we need for the day. They may even cause us to consume more than we need because they don't trigger the body's mechanism for recognizing calories. Choosing low- or no-calorie beverages is a good strategy for weight management.[117]

Move More We have discussed many of the major dietary factors that are associated with achieving and maintaining a healthy weight. Let's look at the other side of the equation, energy expenditure. Physical activity is critical for lifelong weight management. Achieving and maintaining a healthy weight is about the balance between the calories you consume and the calories you use to function. Physical activity is important for achieving and maintaining a healthy weight because it burns calories. The evidence shows that we need a combination of healthy eating and physical activity to be successful with weight loss and weight maintenance. Physical activity is one of the best ways to keep off the pounds. Research shows that physical activity is one of the best predictors of maintaining weight loss.[128]

Most people do not get enough physical activity. Less than 30% of Americans are active at a vigorous level for 20 or more minutes on three or more days per week. More than half do not get even 30 minutes of moderate physical activity on most days.[129]

According to the conclusions of the comprehensive literature review conducted by the advisory committee in the development of the *2008 Physical Activity Guidelines for Americans*, there is clear evidence of a dose–response relationship between physical activity and weight loss.[130] This means that the more physical activity you engage in, the more likely you are to be a healthy weight and to maintain that weight over time. A dose of physical activity equivalent to walking at a 4 mile per hour pace for 150 minutes per week or jogging at a 6 mile per hour pace for 75 minutes per week results in modest weight loss of 1% to 3% of body weight. It is also clear that resistance training (e.g., weight lifting) results in weight loss; however, the amount of weight loss is modest (less than 2.2 pounds). The studies from which these conclusions were drawn were short term in nature, and the researchers recognize that many individuals gain fat-free mass (muscle), which impacts total weight lost. The research is quite clear that to achieve weight loss (i.e., more than 5% decrease in body weight) changes in both diet and exercise are necessary. If people simply maintain their current calorie intake, and/or reduce calorie intake, and incorporate regular physical activity, they will lose weight. The magnitude of change in weight due to physical activity adds to that associated with caloric restriction.

Most of the available literature indicates that "more is better" when it comes to the amount of physical activity needed to prevent weight regain following weight loss.

Special Report

Pills, Potions, and Surgery for Weight Loss

Lose all the weight you want without dieting, lose weight with no exercise, weight loss is as simple as this pill, lose 30 pounds in 30 days—sound familiar? If you have been in a drugstore in the weight-loss aisle or surfed the web for weight-loss aids, you have no doubt come across some of these slogans. Over-the-counter diet aids are a huge business. Consumers who are frustrated with conventional strategies for weight loss turn to what they hope is a quick fix. Unfortunately, there are no quick fixes; there are no short cut weight loss solutions.[136,137] Over-the-counter weight-loss aids may contain caffeine, benzocaine, or fiber. Caffeine is a stimulant and may act to blunt appetite. Benzocaine numbs the mouth and tongue and makes eating less pleasurable. Fiber pills can provide a feeling of fullness so, theoretically, you'll eat less. Most of the weight-loss aids sold over the counter have not been proven to be harmful—except for the harm they cause your wallet. Some, however, can be dangerous. You may remember back in 2004 when ephedra and ephedra-containing supplements were removed from drugstore shelves because of their association with strokes, seizures, and even death.

Although there are no quick fixes, pills, or potions that promote weight loss without diet and exercise, one of the newest diet aids on the market, Alli, has shown promise for modest help with weight loss. It must be used in conjunction with a low-fat, low-calorie diet and exercise to achieve weight loss goals. However, Alli has been linked to some serious side effects in some people, including severe kidney and liver problems.

What about prescription drugs? Are there any that can promote weight loss? Several prescription drugs can help to curb the appetite, such as siutramine (brand name Meridia), or block a percentage of fat absorption, such as orlistat (brand name Xenical). Literally hundreds of others are in the drug pipeline. Although these drugs may help some people, they are far from a quick fix. Nor do they allow for the patient to abandon traditional strategies of weight loss.

More drastic measures for weight loss include surgical procedures. Although these procedures are becoming more popular each year, surgery should be a last resort for weight loss and is only for patients who have a BMI greater than 40 or a BMI of 35 or greater with a serious medical problem. Weight-loss surgery, also called *bariatric surgery*, surgically alters the digestive system, limiting the amount of food that can be eaten. The most common bariatric surgery is the Roux-en-Y (roo-en-y). In this procedure, the stomach is stapled to create a small pouch about the size of an egg. In addition, part of the small intestine is bypassed to decrease absorption from food. Lap-band adjustable gastric banding is another procedure that works to reduce the size of the stomach. An inflatable band is used to divide the stomach into two parts. The band can be adjusted or removed, if needed. This procedure is much simpler than the Roux-en-Y, but weight loss results are much slower. Weight loss with either procedure can be dramatic. However, patients must monitor their intake of food the rest of their life. Patients can defeat the purpose of the surgery by consuming high-calorie foods or drinks. Over time, the pouch does stretch, but the hope is that healthy eating habits have been adopted and can continue. Most bariatric surgery patients require lifelong medical supervision.

However, the literature is limited in this area. Because of these limitations, the advisory committee recommends the equivalent of walking 54 minutes per day at a 4 mile per hour pace, walking 80 minutes per day at a 3 mile per hour pace, or jogging 26 minutes per day at a 6 mile per hour pace to maintain weight loss.[130] Chapter 11 contains detailed information on physical activity.

Watch Less Television One way to move more is to decrease the amount of time spent with sedentary activities, such as television, video games, computer use for fun—anything with a screen. On average, U.S. households have the TV on more than eight hours each day, and American adults watch more than four hours of TV, on average, per day. You have access to almost limitless channels on TV. Not home when the show you want to watch is on? No problem, you can record it on your DVR. Plus, you also have DVDs, pay-per-view, and streaming video on your TV or computer. Many homes have computers with high-speed Internet access, and kids and adults alike spend hours in front of screens. Overall, Americans spend 6.5 hours each day in front of some kind of screen.[127] Some of you spend more time with your computers at home than you do with your spouse or partner.

Adults and children who watch more than two hours of TV a day tend to weigh more than those who watch less than that.[132,133] This difference may be due to the hours of inactivity, exposure to food advertising, and mindless eating in front of the TV. Sitting in front of any kind of screen minimizes the amount of activity you get, and therefore limits the number of calories burned in any given day. Sitting for four to six hours in front of screens limits the amount of time you have to be active. Plus, sitting in front of a TV burns about the same number of calories as sleeping.

The second reason why screen time is correlated with higher body weight is exposure to food advertising.[134,135] A typical one-hour show on commercial television has about 20 minutes of commercials. Most of the advertisements are for foods and drinks that are high in sugar, fat, and calories. The food industry, particularly fast-food and beverage companies, spends billions of dollars advertising its food products on TV. Interestingly, the foods we overeat—sugary drinks, sweet and salty snacks, and fast food—are the very foods that are advertised heavily on TV. Exposure to advertising primes automatic eating behavior, thus contributing to the obesity epidemic.[136] We also know that eating in front of a screen of any kind is not mindful. Behavioral strategists have found that in order to eat less food, we must attend to the food we are eating, watching for feelings of fullness or satiety.

Ready to Make a Change

Are you ready to make a change, small or large, in your eating and physical activity to achieve and maintain a healthy weight? Make the commitment to take the first step. Whether it is a small, medium, or large change, it is a step in the right direction toward healthier behaviors.

I commit to a small first step. Choose one of the healthy weight behaviors to implement this week. If you are not a breakfast eater, maybe you are willing to commit to eating breakfast every day. If you currently eat lunch every day at a local fast-food restaurant, commit to bringing your lunch from home most days. Whatever behavior is the one that you feel you can make a lifelong commitment to—do it. It is a step in the right direction.

I am ready to take the next step and make a medium change. Plan all of your meals. You may think that this is a small change, but planning is a big step forward towards healthy eating. Planning all of your meals, including snacks, will help you be more mindful of what you are eating and where. You will be able to see at a glance how many meals you are going to eat out, what the meals will be that you will prepare at home, and the foods you need to buy to make it happen.

I have been making changes for some time and am ready to make a large change in physical activity and healthy eating to achieve and maintain a healthy weight. Adopt all of the healthy weight behaviors. Look at the complete list of healthy weight behaviors. Are there one or two that you need to address? You may be doing okay on the food side of the equation, but you may have slipped in the activity area. Or, you may be doing great with all the behaviors except that you need to work on eating more fruits and vegetables. Whatever your weak spot, commit to taking that step to eat smart and move more.

Myth Versus Fact

Myth: Skipping meals is a good way to cut calories and lose weight.

Fact: Skipping meals doesn't help you cut calories. In fact, it has the opposite effect. Eating regular meals, especially breakfast, helps you consume fewer calories than if you skip meal. Eat regular meals, at least three per day. You may even want to experiment with mini-meals, eating five to six times a day. This keeps your hunger low and your metabolism high.

Myth: If you work out regularly, you don't need to worry about your weight.

Fact: The equation for what you weigh has two sides, calories in and calories out. Although working out will certainly help keep you at a healthy weight, it is only one side of the equation. Plus, there are many reasons to eat healthy; what you weigh is only one. Even if you work out, you still need to eat healthy for overall health and well-being.

Myth: The obesity crisis is about personal responsibility. People know they should eat healthy and be active; they just need to do it.

Fact: Personal responsibility certainly has its role; you need to take responsibility for what you eat and how active you are. However, you also must have the opportunity to do this. If you go to the school cafeteria and there is only junk food and fast food, then it is hard to make a healthy choice. If your neighborhood has no place for you to be active, keeping your commitment to move more is difficult. The obesity crisis will not be solved by personal responsibility alone; it will take the work of many, including policymakers, to make it happen.

Myth: The government has no place in the obesity crisis. Don't tell me what to eat.

Fact: The government already plays a role in what you eat. The government provides subsidies for certain commodities, has rules about food labels, and offers guidelines for what can be served in schools. Just as the government has helped contribute to the obesity crisis, it has a role in helping correct it. The government can do many things to help that fall short of telling you what to eat. For example, the federal government could create price structures that make healthy foods more affordable, revise labeling laws to help consumers make better choices, or change guidelines as to what is served in schools.

Myth: Cutting carbs is the best way to lose weight.

Fact: It may not sound very exciting, but it is calories that ultimately matter in weight loss and weight maintenance. Cutting out carbohydrates can promote weight loss in the short run, but for sustained weight maintenance it is the balance of calories from carbohydrates, fats, and proteins that works.

Myth: If you eat healthy, you don't need to worry about exercise so much.

Fact: There are other health reasons to be active besides maintaining a healthy weight. If you are one of the lucky few who can maintain a healthy weight without being active, you still need physical activity for optimal health and to reduce your risk of chronic diseases such as heart disease, stroke, and some forms of cancer.

Myth: I don't have time to be mindful about what I eat. I have to eat on the go.

Fact: We all have the same 24 hours in the day. What you do with them is up to you. You have to make the time for healthy eating. Eating mindlessly while doing other things may seem to be a good idea from a time management point of view. From a health point of view, however, it is not a good idea. Make time, even 20 minutes, to sit and eat a healthy meal without other distractions.

Back to the Story

Sue is lucky. She found out her family was heading for possible medical problems before they happened. She now has an opportunity to change a few things in her life and her family's life to help them be healthier and to decrease their risk of serious health problems in the future. The first thing Sue and Tom can do is plan meals. They can take just 30 minutes each week and plan their evening meals. They need to rely less on convenience foods, such as frozen entrees, and eat more lean meats, fruits, vegetables, and whole grains. Planning the evening meals will also help them cut back on the number of meals they eat out. Eating at home as a family will allow for the children to learn good eating habits as well. If Sue and Tom don't know how to cook, they should see what is offered in their community to help them learn the skills they need to prepare simple, healthy meals.

Sue and Tom need to start their day off with breakfast. Cereal is a good choice as long as it is low in sugar, has moderate calories, and is topped with skim milk. This goes for the children as well. Some cereals marketed to children are more like candy than cereal due to the high sugar content. Sue and Tom need to plan for their meals away from home. Eating out every day for lunch makes it very difficult to eat healthy, not to mention the expense. They can each pack a small cooler with lunch and snacks for the day. That way they have control over what they are eating instead of mindlessly choosing what is most convenient.

Finally, the whole family should get moving. They can choose family activities once or twice a week that include some movement—a trip to a park for outside play, a walk around the block after dinner, dancing in the living room, whatever they choose, as long as they move. Tom and Sue should carve out at least 30 minutes on most days of the week to be active. It does not have to be in a gym, although that may be an option that they would enjoy. They should take just some of the TV time and turn it into time for Tom and Sue to move more. They should not try to do all of these suggestions at once. They should start slow and try to change one aspect of their lives each week. What other suggestions do you have for Sue, Tom, and their family?

References

1. Gallagher D, Visser M, Sepulveda D, Pierson RN, Harris T, Heymsfield SB. How useful is BMI for comparison of body fatness across age, sex and ethnic groups? *Am J Epidemiol*. 1996;143:228–239.
2. Centers for Disease Control and Prevention. Defining overweight and obesity. http://www.cdc.gov/obesity/defining.html. Accessed April 10, 2011.
3. Centers for Disease Control and Prevention. About BMI for children and teens. http://www.cdc.gov/healthyweight/assessing/bmi/childrens_bmi/about_childrens_bmi.html. Accessed April 10, 2011.
4. Flegal KM, Carroll MD, Ogden CL, Johnson CL. Prevalence and trends in obesity among US adults, 1999–2000. *JAMA*. 2002;288:1723–1727.
5. Ogden CL, Carroll MD, Curtin LR, McDowell MA, Tabak CJ, Flegal KM. Prevalence of overweight and obesity in the United States, 1999–2004. *JAMA*. 2006;295:1549–1555.
6. National Center for Health Statistics. Prevalence of overweight, obesity and extreme obesity among adults: United States, trends 1960–1962 through 2005–2006. http://www.cdc.gov/nchs/data/hestat/overweight/overweight_adult.htm. Accessed February 5, 2010.
7. Flegal KM, Carroll MD, Ogden CL, Curtin LR. Prevalence and trends in obesity among US adults, 1999–2008. *JAMA*. 2010;303(3):235–241.
8. Wang Y, Beydoun MA, Liang L, Caballero B, Kumanyika S K. Will all Americans become overweight or obese? Estimating the progression and cost of the US obesity epidemic. *Obesity*. 2008;16(10):2323–2330.
9. Wang Y, Beydoun MA. The obesity epidemic in the United States—gender, age, socioeconomic, racial/ethnic, and geographic characteristics: a systematic review and meta-regression analysis. *Epidemiol Rev*. 2007;29:6–28.
10. Centers for Disease Control and Prevention. Difference in prevalence of obesity among black, white, and Hispanic adults—United States, 2006–2008. *MMWR*. 2009;58(27)740–744.
11. Ogden CL, Carroll MD, Curtin LR, McDowell MA, Tabak CJ, Flegal KM. Prevalence of overweight and obesity in the United States, 1999–2004. *JAMA*. 2006;295:1549–1555.
12. Ogden CL, Flegal KM, Carroll MD, Johnson CL. Prevalence and trends in overweight among US children and adolescents, 1999–2000. *JAMA*. 2002;288(14):1728–1732.
13. Ogden CL, Carroll MD, Flegal KM. High body mass index for age among US children and adolescents, 2003–2006. *JAMA*. 2008;299(20):2401–2405.
14. Ogden CL, Carroll MD, Curtin LR, Lamb MM, Flegal KM. Prevalence of high body mass index in US children and adolescents, 2007–2008. *JAMA*. 2010;303(3):242–249.
15. Mei Z, Grummer-Strawn LM, Pietrobelli A, Goulding A, Goran MI, Dietz WH. Validity of body mass index compared with other body-composition

screening indexes for the assessment of body fatness in children and adolescents. *Am J Clin Nutr*. 2002;75(6):978–985.
16. Garrow JS, Webster J. Quetelet's index (W/H2) as a measure of fatness. *Inter J Obesity*. 1985;9:147–153.
17. Prentice AM, Jebb SA. Beyond Body Mass Index. *Obesity Rev*. 2001;2(3): 141–147.
18. Olshansky SJ, Passaro DJ, Hershow RC. A potential decline in life expectancy in the United States in the 21st century. *N Engl J Med*. 2005;352:1138–1145.
19. US Department of Health and Human Services. *The Surgeon General's Call to Action to Prevent and Decrease Overweight and Obesity*. Rockville, MD: U.S. Department of Health and Human Services, Public Health Service, Office of the Surgeon General, 2001.
20. Lewis CE, McTigue KM, Burke LE, et al. Mortality, health outcomes, and body mass index in the overweight range. *Circulation*. 2009;119:3263–3271.
21. Rashid MN, Fuentes F, Touchon RC, Wehner PS. Obesity and the risk for cardiovascular disease. *Prev Cardiol*. 2003;6:42– 47.
22. Lewington S, Clarke R, Qizilbash N, Peto R, Collins R; Prospective Studies Collaboration. Age-specific relevance of usual blood pressure to vascular mortality: a meta-analysis of individual data for one million adults in 61 prospective studies. *Lancet*. 2002;360:1903–1913.
23. Colditz GA, Willett WC, Stampfer MJ, et al. Weight as a risk factor for clinical diabetes in women. *Am J Epidemiol*. 1990;132:501–513.
24. Carey VJ, Walters EE, Colditz GA, et al. Body fat distribution and risk of non-insulin-dependent diabetes mellitus in women. The Nurses' Health Study. *Am J Epidemiol*. 1997;145:614–619.
25. Callee EE, Thun MJ. Obesity and cancer. *Oncogene*. 2004;23:6365–6378.
26. Renehan AG, Tyson M, Egger M, Heller RF, Zwahlen M. Body-mass index and incidence of cancer: a systematic review and meta-analysis of prospective observational studies. *Lancet*. 2008;371:569–578.
27. National Institutes for Health, Obesity Education Initiative. Clinical guidelines for the identification, evaluation and treatment of overweight and obesity in adults. 1998. NIH Publication No. 98-4083.
28. Schwartz AR, Patil SP, Laffan AM, Polotsky V, Schneider PL. Obesity and obstructive sleep apnea pathogenic mechanisms and therapeutic approaches. *Proc Am Thorac Soc*. 2007;5:185–192.
29. National Institutes of Health, National Institute of Diabetes and Digestive and Kidney Diseases. Do you know the health risks of being overweight? http://win.nidkk.nih.gov/publications/health_risks.htm#gallbladder. Accessed October 6, 2011.
30. Finkelstein EA, Trogdon JG, Cohen JW, Dietz W. Annual medical spending attributable to obesity: payer- and service-specific estimates. *Health Affairs*. 2009;28(5):w822–w831.
31. Finkelstein, EA, Fiebelkorn, IC, Wang, G. National medical spending attributable to overweight and obesity: How much, and who's paying? *Health Affairs*. 2003;W3;219–226.
32. Wolf AM, Colditz GA. Current estimates of the economic cost of obesity in the United States. *Obesity Res*.1998;6(2):97–106.
33. Wolf, A. What is the economic case for treating obesity? *Obesity Res*. 1998;6(suppl)2S–7S.
34. Finkelstein EA, Fiebelkorn, IC, Wang, G. State-level estimates of annual medical expenditures attributable to obesity. *Obesity Res*. 2004;12(1):18–24.
35. McDonald's Corporation. www.aboutmcdonalds.com. Accessed October 6, 2011.
36. Bowman SA, Vinyard BT. Fast food consumption of US adults: impact on nutrient and energy intakes and overweight status. *J Am Coll Nutr*. 2004;23(2):163–168.
37. US Census Bureau. US Department of Commerce. Food services and drinking places: 2002. October 2004. http://www.census.gov/. Accessed February 22, 2010.
38. The Keystone Center. The Keystone Forum on Away-From-Home Foods: Opportunities for Preventing Weight Gain and Obesity. Washington, DC: The Keystone Center, May 2006. http://www.keystone.org. Accessed February 20, 2010.
39. Nestle M. Soft drink "pouring rights": marketing empty calories. *Public Health Rep*. 2000;115:308–319.
40. US Department of Transportation, Federal Highway Administration, Office of Highway Policy Information. http://www.fhwa.dot.gov. Accessed February 10, 2010.
41. US Census Bureau. *Statistical Abstract of the United States, 2006*. Section 24: Communications and Information Technology. 737: Table 1117. http://www.census.gov/prod/2004pubs/04statab/infocomm.pdf. Accessed April 21, 2011.
42. US Census Bureau. *Statistical Abstract of the United States*, 2006. Section 24: Communications and Information Technology. 736: Table 1116. http://www.census.gov/prod/2005pubs/. Accessed February 5, 2010.
43. Song EH, Anderson JE. How violent video games may violate children's health. *Contemp Pediatr*. 2001;18(5):102–120.
44. Keith SW, Redden DT, Katzmarzyk PT, et al. Putative contributors to the secular increase in obesity: exploring the roads less traveled. *Int J Obesity*. 2006:30:1585–1594.
45. von Kries R, Toschke AM, Wurmser H, Sauerwald T, Koletzko B. Reduced risk for overweight and obesity in 5- and 6-year-old children by duration of sleep—a cross-sectional study. *Int J Obes Relat Metab Disord*. 2002;26:710–716.
46. Gangwisch JE, Malaspina D, Boden-Albala B, Heymsfield SB. Inadequate sleep as a risk factor for obesity: analysis of the NHANES I. *Sleep*. 2005;28:1289–1296.

47. Bonnet MH, Arand DL. We are chronically sleep deprived. *Sleep*.1995;18:908–911.
48. Iglowstein I, Jenni OG, Molinari L, Largo RH. Sleep duration from infancy to adolescence: reference values and generational trends. *Pediatrics*. 2003;111:302–307.
49. Westerterp-Plantenga MS, van Marken Lichtenbelt WD, Cilissen C, Top S. Energy metabolism in women during short exposure to the thermoneutral zone. *Physiol Behav*. 2002;75:227–235.
50. Saxton C. Effects of severe heat stress on respiration and metabolic rate in resting man. *Aviat Space Environ Med*. 1981;52:281–286.
51. Wysowski DK, Armstrong G, Governale L. Rapid increase in the use of oral antidiabetic drugs in the United States, 1990–2001. *Diabetes Care*. 2003;26:1852–1855.
52. Citrome L, Jaffe A, Levine J, Allingham B. Use of mood stabilizers among patients with schizophrenia, 1994–2001. *Psychiatr Serv*. 2002;53:1212.
53. Psaty BM, Manolio TA, Smith NL, et al. Time trends in high blood pressure control and use of antihypertensive medications in older adults. *Arch Intern Med*. 2002;162:2325–2332.
54. McLeroy KR, Bibleau D, Streckler A, Glanz K. An ecological perspective on health promotion programs. *Health Ed Quarterly*. 1988;15:351–378.
55. Keener D, Goodman K, Lowry A, Zaro S, Kellel Khan L. *Recommended Community Strategies and Measurements to Prevent Obesity in the United States: Implementation and Measurement Guide*. Atlanta, GA: US Department of Health and Human Services, Centers for Disease Control and Prevention, 2009.
56. Bell J, Rubin V. *Why Place Matters: Building a Movement for Healthy Communities*. Oakland, CA: PolicyLink, 2007.
57. Brownell KD, Frieden TR. Ounces of prevention—the public policy case for taxes on sugared beverages. *N Eng J Med*. 2009; 360(18):1805–1808.
58. Vartanian LR, Schwartz MB, Brownell KD. Effects of soft drink consumption on nutrition and health: a systematic review and meta-analysis. *Am J Public Health*. 2007;97(4):667–675.
59. Wang YC, Bleich SN, Gortmaker SL. Increasing caloric contribution from sugar-sweetened beverages and 100% fruit juices among US children and adolescents, 1988–2004. *Pediatrics*. 2008;121(6):e1604–e1614.
60. Forshee RA, Anderson PA, Storey ML. Sugar-sweetened beverages and body mass index in children and adolescents: a meta-analysis. *Am J Clin Nutr*. 2008;87:1662–1671.
61. Jha P, Chaloupka FJ, Corrao M, Jacob B. Reducing the burden of smoking worldwide: effectiveness of interventions and their coverage. *Drug Alcohol Rev*. 2006;25(6):597–609.
62. Chaloupka FJ, Wechsler H. Price, tobacco control policies and smoking among young adults. *J Health Econ*. 1997;16(3):359–373.
63. Epstein LH, Dearing KK, Paluch RA, Roemmich JN, Cho D. Price and maternal obesity influence purchasing of low- and high-energy dense foods. *Am J Clin Nutr*. 2001;86(4):914–922.
64. French SA. Pricing effects on food choices. *J Nutr*. 2003;133(3):841S–843S.
65. Herman DR, Harrison GG, Afifi AA, Jenks E. Effect of a targeted subsidy on intake of fruits and vegetables among low-income women in the Special Supplemental Nutrition Program for Women, Infants, and Children. *Am J Public Health*. 2008;98(1):98–105.
66. Horgen KB, Brownell KD. Comparison of price change and health message interventions in promoting healthy food choices. *Health Psychol*. 2002;2(5):505–512.
67. Andreyeva, Long MW, Brownell KD. The impact of food prices on consumption: a systematic review of research on the price elasticity of demand for food. *Am J Pub Health*. 2010;100(2):216–222.
68. Yale University Rudd Center for Food Policy and Obesity. Revenue calculator for soft drink taxes. http://yaleruddcenter.org/sodatax.aspx. Accessed February 24, 2010.
69. Cawley J. Contingent valuation analysis of willingness to pay to reduce childhood obesity. *Econ Hum Biol*. 2008;6(2):281–292.
70. Oliver JE, Lee T. Public opinion and the politics of obesity in America. *J Health Politics Policy Law*. 2005;30(5):923–954.
71. Mifflin MD, St Jeor ST, Hill LA, Scott BJ, Daugherty SA, Koh YO. A new predictive equation for resting energy expenditure in healthy individuals. *Am J Clin Nutr*. 1990;51:241–247.
72. Britten P, Marcoe K, Yamini S, Davis C. Development of food intake patterns for the MyPyramid Food Guidance System. *J Nutr Educ Behav*. 2006;38(6 Suppl):S78–S92.
73. Tinker LF, Rosal MC, Young AF, Perri MG, Paatterson RD, VanHorn L, Assaf AR, Bowen DJ, Ockene J, Hays J, Wu L. Predictors of dietary change and maintenance in the women's health initiative dietary modification trial. *J Am Diet Assoc*. 2007;107:1155–1165.
74. National Institute of Health, National Heart Lung and Blood Institute, North American Association for the Study of Obesity. The Practical Guide Identification, Evaluation, and Treatment of Overweight and Obesity in Adults. 2000. http://www.nhlbi.nih.gov/guidelines/obesity/practgde.htm. Accessed February 6, 2010.
75. O'Neil PM, Brown JD. Weigh the evidence: benefits of regular weight monitoring for weight control. *J Nutr Educ Behavior*. 2005;37:319–322.
76. US Department of Agriculture. MyPyramid Tracker. http://www.mypyramidtracker.gov. Accessed February 22, 2010.
77. Wansink B, Sobal J. Mindless eating: the 200 daily food decisions we overlook. *Environ Behav*. 2007;39(1):106–123.

78. Lillis J, Hayes SC, Bunting K, Masuda A. Teaching acceptance and mindfulness to improve the lives of the obese: a preliminary test of a theoretical model. *Ann Behav Med*. 2009;37:58–69.
79. Froman EM, Butryn ML, Hoffman KL, Herbert JD. An open trial of acceptance-based behavioral intervention for weight loss. *Cogn Behav Pract*. 2009;16(2):223–235.
80. Singh NN, Lancioni GE, Singh AN, et al. A mindfulness-based health wellness program for managing morbid obesity. *Clin Case Studies*. 2008;7(4):327–339.
81. Bly T, Hammond M, Thomson R, Bagdade P. Exploring the use of mindful eating training in the bariatric population. *Bariatric Times*. 2007. http://www.bariatrictimes.com. Accessed February 26, 2010.
82. Ludwig DS, Kabat-Zinn J. Mindfulness in medicine. *JAMA*. 2008;300(11):1350–1352.
83. Hammond M. Ways dietitians are incorporating mindfulness and mindful eating into nutrition counseling. *The Digest, Public Health/Community Nutrition Practice Group*. 2007; Fall:1–9.
84. Tapper K, Shaw C, Ilsley J, Hill AJ, Bond FW, Moore L. Exploratory randomized controlled trial of a mindfulness-based weight loss intervention for women. *Appetite*. 2009;52:396–404.
85. Willard K, Klatt M. Mindfulness based therapies for healthy long term weight loss. *J Am Diet Assoc*. 2009;109(9):A111.
86. The Center for Mindful Eating. The principles of mindful eating. http://www.tcme.org. Accessed February 1, 2009.
87. Sacks FM, Bray GA, Carey VJ, et al. Comparison of weight-loss diets with different compositions of fat, protein, and carbohydrates. *N Engl J Med*. 2009;360:859–873.
88. Merchant AT, Vatanparast H, Barlas S, et al. Carbohydrate intake and overweight and obesity among healthy adults. *J Am Diet Assoc*. 2009;109:1165–1172.
89. Centers for Disease Control and Prevention. Trends in intake of energy and macronutrients, United States, 1971–2000. *MMWR*. 2004;53(4):80–82.
90. Rolls BJ, Ello-Martin JA, Tohill BC. What can intervention studies tell us about the relationship between fruit and vegetable consumption and weight management? *Nutr Reviews*. 2004;62(1):1–17.
91. Yao M, Roberts SB. Dietary energy density and weight regulation. *Nutr Reviews*. 2001;59:247–258.
92. Gustafsson K, Asp N-G, Hagander B, Nyman M. Effects of different vegetables in mixed meals on glucose homeostasis and satiety. *Eur J Clin Nutr*. 1993;47:192–200.
93. Howarth NC, Saltzman E, Roberts SB. Dietary fiber and weight regulation. Energy density of foods affects energy intake across multiple levels of fat content in lean and obese women. *Am J Clin Nutr*. 2001;73:1010–1018.
94. Center for Disease Control and Prevention, National Center for Chronic Disease Prevention and Health Promotion, Division of Nutrition and Physical activity. Can eating fruits and vegetables help people to manage their weight? *Research to Practice Series*, no.1. http://www.cdc.gov/nutrition/professionals/researchtopractice/index.html. Updated March 11, 2011. Accessed April 21, 2011.
95. Cleveland LE, Moshfegh AJ, Albertson AM, Goldman JD. Dietary intake of whole grains. *J Am College of Nutr*. 2000;19(3):331S–338S.
96. Liu S, Willett WC, Manson JE, Hu FB, Rosner B, Cloditz. Relation between changes in intakes of dietary fiber and grain products and changes in weight and development of obesity among middle-aged women. *Am J Clin Nutr*. 2003;78:920–927.
97. McKeown NM, Meigs JB, Liu S, Wilson P, Jacques PF. Whole-grain intake is favorably associated with metabolic risk factors for type 2 diabetes and cardiovascular disease in the Framingham Offspring Study. *Am J Clin Nutr*. 2002;76(2): 390–398.
98. Melanson KJ, Angelopoulos TJ, Nguyen VT, et al. Consumption of whole-grain cereals during weight loss: effects on dietary quality dietary fiber, magnesium, vitamin B_6, and obesity. *J Am Diet Assoc*. 2006;106:1380–1388.
99. Ma Y, Bertone ER, Stanek EJ, et al. Association between eating patterns and obesity in a free-living US adult population. *Am J Epidemiology*. 2003;158(1):88–92.
100. Schlundt DG, Hill JO, Sbrocco T, Pope-Cordle J, Sharp T. The role of breakfast in the treatment of obesity: a randomized clinical trial. *Am J Clin Nutr*. 1992;55:645–651.
101. Wyatt HR, Grunwald GK, Mosca CL, Klem ML, Wing RR, Hill JO. Long-term weight loss and breakfast in subjects in the National Weight Control Registry. *Obesity Res*. 2002;10(2):78–82.
102. Smiciklas-Wright H, Mitchell DC, Mickle SJ, Goldman JD, Cook A. Foods commonly eaten in the United States, 1989–1991 and 1994–1996: are portion sizes changing? *J Am Diet Assoc*. 2003;103:41–47.
103. Young LR, Nestle M. The contribution of expanding portion sizes to the US obesity epidemic. *Am J Pub Health*. 2002;92:246–249.
104. Nielsen SJ, Popkin BM. Patterns and trends in food portion sizes, 1977–1998. *JAMA*. 2003;289(4):450–453.
105. Rolls BJ, Roe LS, Kral TVE, Meengs JS, Wall DE. Increasing the portion size of a packaged snack increases energy intake in men and women. *Appetite*. 2004;42(1):63–69.
106. Rolls BJ, Morris EL, Roe LS. Portion size of food affects energy intake in normal-weight and overweight men and women. *Am J Clin Nutr*. 2002;76:1207–1213.
107. Rolls BJ, Roe LS, Meengs JS, Wall DE. Increasing the portion size of a sandwich increases energy intake. *J Am Diet Assoc*. 2004;104:367–372.
108. Wansink B, Park SB. At the movies: how external cues and perceived taste impact consumption volume. *J Database Marketing*. 1996;60:1–14.

109. Kant AK, Graubard BI. Eating out in America, 1987–2000: trends and nutritional correlates. *Prev Med*. 2003:38(2):243–249.
110. USDA Economic Research Service. Food COI, prices and expenditure: food service as a share of food expenditures. http://www.ers.usda.gov/briefing/cpi foodandexpenditures/data/table12.htm. Accessed February 22, 2010.
111. Bowman SA, Vinyard BT. Fast food consumption of US adults: impact on energy and nutrient intakes and overweight status. *J Am Coll Nutr*. 2004;23(2):163–168.
112. Gutherie JF, Lin BH, Frazao E. Role of food prepared away from home in the American diet, 1977–78 versus 1994–96: changes and consequences. *J Nutr Educ Behav*. 2002;34:140–150.
113. Boutelle KN, Birnbaum AS, Lytle LA, Murray DM, Story M. Associations between perceived family meal environment and parent intake of fruit, vegetables, and fat. *J Nutr Ed Behavior*. 2003;35(1):24–29.
114. Gillman MW, Rifas-Shiman SL, Frazier AL, et al. Family dinner and diet quality among older children and adolescents. *Arch Fam Med*. 2000;9:235–240.
115. Bowman SA, Gortmaker SL, Ebbeling CB, Pereira MA, Ludwig DS. Effects of fast-food consumption on energy intake and diet quality among children in a national household survey. *Pediatrics*. 2004;113(1):112–118.
116. McLaughlin C, Tarasuk V, Kreiger N. An examination of at-home food preparation skills among low-income, food-insecure women. *J Am Diet Assoc*. 2003;103:1506–1512.
117. Centers for Disease Control and Prevention. Does drinking beverages with added sugars increase the risk of overweight? *Research to Practice Series*, no. 3, 2006. http://www.cdc.gov/nutrition/professionals /researchtopractice/index.html. Accessed April 8, 2009.
118. Block G. Foods contribute to energy intake in the US: data from NHANES III and NHANES 1999–2000. *J Food Composit Anal*. 2004;17:439–447.
119. Harnack L, Stang J, Story M. Soft drink consumption among US children and adolescents; nutritional consequences. *J Am Diet Assoc*. 1999;99(4):436–441.
120. Malik VS, Schulze MB, Hu FB. Intake of sugar-sweetened beverages and weight gain: a systematic review. *Am J Clin Nutr*. 2006;84:274–288.
121. Vartanian LR, Schwartz MB, Brownell KD. Effects of soft drink consumption on nutrition and health: A systematic review and meta analysis. *Am J Pub Health*. 2007;97:367–375.
122. Ebbeling CB, Feldman HA, Osganian SK, Chomitz VR, Ellenbogen SJ, Ludwig DS. Effects of decreasing sugar-sweetened beverages consumption on body weight in adolescents: a randomized, controlled pilot study. *Pediatrics*. 2006;117(3):673–680.
123. Schulze MB, Manson JE, Ludwig DS, et al. Sugar-sweetened beverages, weight gain, and incidence of type 2 diabetes in young and middle-aged women. *JAMA*. 2004;292:927–934.
124. Adriano J. In the drink—how beverages contribute to obesity. *Nutr Action Healthletter*. 2000;7–9.
125. Mouro DM, Bressan J, Campbell WW, Mattes RD. Effects of food form on appetite and energy intake in lean and obese young adults. *Inter J Obesity*. 2007;31:1688–1695.
126. Wellhoener P, Fruehwald-Schultes B, Kern W, Dantz D, Kerner W, Born J, Fehm HL, Peters A. Glucose metabolism rather than insulin is a main determinant of leptin secretion in humans. *J Clin Endo Metab*. 2000;85:1267–1271.
127. DiMeglio DP, Mattes RD. Liquid versus solid carbohydrate: effects on food intake and body weight. *Inter J Obesity*. 2000;24:794–800.
128. Centers for Disease Control and Prevention. *Overweight and Obesity: Contributing Factors, 2006*. http://www.cdc.gov/nccdphp/dnpa/obesity/contributing _factors.htm. Accessed April 2, 2009.
129. Centers for Disease Control and Prevention (CDC). *Behavioral Risk Factor Surveillance System Survey Data*. Atlanta, Georgia: U.S. Department of Health and Human Services, Centers for Disease Control and Prevention, 2007. http://www.cdc.gov/brfss/index .htm. Accessed February 22, 2010.
130. *Physical Activity Guidelines Advisory Committee Report*. Part G. Section 4: Energy balance.http://www.health .gov/paguidelines/Report/G4_energy.aspx#q2c. Accessed February 22, 2010.
131. Rideout, VJ, Vandewater, EA, Wartella, EA. Zero–six—electronic media in the lives of infants, toddlers and preschoolers. A Kaiser Family Foundation Report. 2003. http://www.kff.org. Accessed April 14, 2007.
132. Bowman SA. Television-viewing characteristics of adults: correlations to eating practices and overweight and health status. *Prev Chronic Dis*. 2006;3(2):1–11.
133. S. Gable, Y. Chang, J. Krull. Television watching and frequency of family meals are predictive of overweight onset and persistence in a national sample of school-aged children. *J Am Diet Assoc*. 2007;107(1):53–61.
134. French, SA, Story, M. Jeffery, RW. Environmental influences on eating and physical activity. *Ann Rev Publ Health*. 2001;2:309–335.
135. Harris JL, Bargh JA, Brownell KA. Priming effects of television food advertising on eating behavior. *Health Psychol*. 2009;28(4):404–413.
136. Dwyer, J, Allison DB, Coates PM, Dietary supplements in weight reduction. *J Am Diet Assoc*. 2005;105:580–586.
137. Pitter MH, Ernst E. Dietary supplements for body-weight reduction: a systematic review. *Am J Clin Nutr*. 2004; 79:529–536.

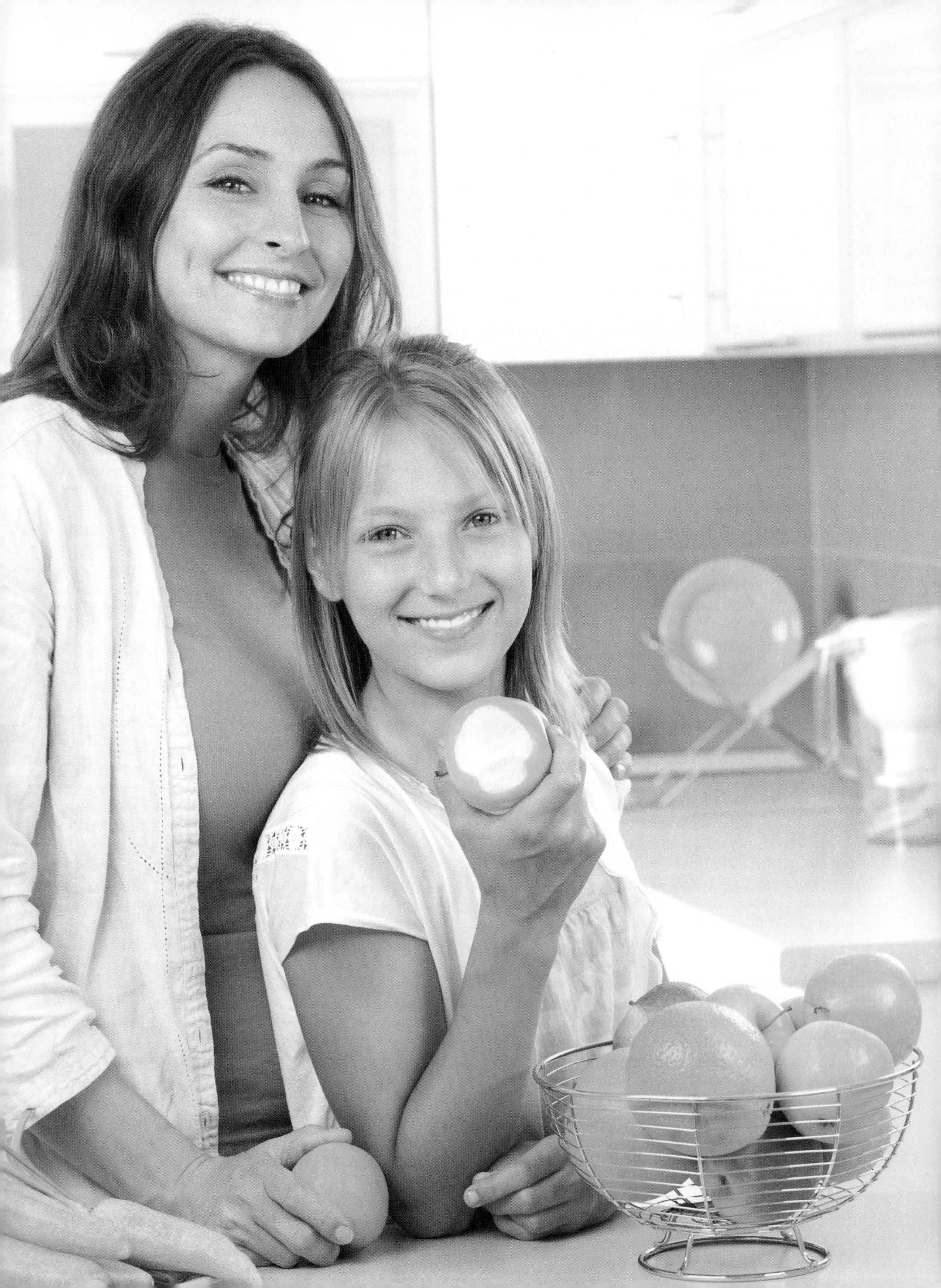

Chapter 13

Lifecycle Nutrition: Eating Smart Across the Life Span

Key Messages

- Eating healthy is important throughout the lifecycle.
- Pregnancy is an important time for good health habits, including healthy eating to support both mother and baby.
- Breast milk is the ideal food for infants.
- Children have special nutritional needs to support growth and development; healthy eating habits should be fostered to promote a lifetime of good health.
- Adolescents need optimal nutrition to support rapid growth and development.
- Nutrition in later years is critical for improved quality of life.

Story

Tasha and her husband Tim want to have a baby. They want to make sure that Tasha is healthy and eating right before she gets pregnant. Until now, Tasha and Tim's diet has not been great. They eat lots of fast food and often skip meals. They are also thinking about how they want to feed the baby once it is here. They have found online, from friends, and from Tasha's doctor that breastfeeding is best, but they are not sure if this will work for them.

Joan is the mother of two small children, one 5 and the other 7. As a single mom, she is busy with work, finishing her college degree, and taking care of her family. She relies on prepared foods from the deli at the grocery and too often orders pizza for the evening meal. It is quick, and the whole family enjoys it. The children only like a few foods, so she just serves them what they like so there are no hassles.

Anne is a typical 17-year-old girl. She is busy with school and a part-time job, and has lots of friends. Her busy schedule does not allow her to eat with her family very often. She skips breakfast, usually eats a protein bar for lunch, and dinner is whatever she can grab at the food court at the mall where she works. She is conscious about how many calories she eats, and if she feels like she has splurged the day before she may go without eating or not eat very much the next day.

Pam and Sean are in their late 60s. They are newly retired and ready to travel and enjoy life. Years of sedentary jobs have contributed to both of them being about 30 pounds overweight. Sean takes medicine for high blood pressure and Pam has been told that her blood cholesterol is too high.

All of these people are at different points in their life. However, all could benefit from some changes to their eating patterns. What changes can you suggest for Tasha and Tim, Joan and her family, Anne, and Pam and Sean to help them be healthy at their stage in life?

Nutrition During Pregnancy: Good Health for Mom and Baby

Pregnancy is the most important time in a woman's life for her to be conscious of what she eats. She is, after all, eating for two. Although this certainly does not mean eating twice as much, it does mean that all essential nutrients need to be consumed in the proper amounts. The only way that the fetus gets nutrients to grow and develop properly is from its mother. The mother's body is going through many physiological changes as well.

Before Conception

A women's nutrition and health status prior to conceiving is as important as eating healthy and adopting health habits during pregnancy. Potential parents need to think about the mother's health and nutrition prior to becoming pregnant. Preconception care can educate and encourage the prospective mother to get or stay healthy. It can also screen for and address risks such as smoking or alcohol.[1] Preconception care may also include stopping or changing prescription medications being taken by the mother that are known to cause problems in the fetus.

Everyone should be concerned with achieving and maintaining a healthy weight, especially a woman contemplating pregnancy. Overweight or underweight can complicate pregnancy.[2] Women who are underweight (BMI < 20) have an increased risk of delivering a low-birth-weight baby or delivering too early. Women who are overweight or obese also have an increased risk of preterm delivery. In addition, they are more likely to develop gestational diabetes and preeclampsia (these will be discussed later in this chapter).

Smoking and alcohol are widely known to put the unborn baby at risk of a multitude of problems or even fetal death. If a woman smokes, she should stop prior to becoming pregnant. Alcohol should be consumed in moderation, if at all, if a woman is considering pregnancy. Of course, once pregnant, alcohol should not be consumed at all.

An overall healthy diet prior to pregnancy is important for the optimal health of the mother. However, one nutrient may be needed in larger quantities than can be found in a normal diet. That nutrient is folic acid. Folic acid has been found to help prevent neural tube defects, major birth defects of the baby's brain and spine.[3–5] It is recommended that women get 400 micrograms of folic acid each day to protect against neural tube defects.[6] For folic acid to have this protective effect, a woman needs to take folic acid at least one month before she becomes pregnant and continue taking it through her pregnancy. Women can get the recommended amount of folic acid by taking a vitamin that has 400 micrograms of folic acid (most multivitamins contain folic acid) or by consuming foods that are fortified with folic acid. Many breakfast cereals contain the amount of folic acid that a woman needs each day. However, not every cereal has this amount; check the nutrition label on the side or back of the box to see if it has 400 micrograms of folic acid per serving.

Maternal Weight Gain

Once a woman becomes pregnant, how much weight she should gain is a common question. The answer to this question has varied over the years based on what has been shown to be the best outcomes for mothers and infants. Exactly how much weight a woman should gain during pregnancy depends on her prepregnancy weight (**Table 13.1**). For underweight women (BMI < 19), the recommended weight gain is 28–40 pounds; normal weight women (BMI 19–24.9) should gain between 25 and 35 pounds. Heavier women should gain less but still should gain at least 15 pounds.[7] Women who are pregnant with multiples need to gain more weight.

Table 13.1

Weight Gain During Pregnancy

Prepregnancy BMI	Recommended Pregnancy Weight Gain
< 19 (underweight)	28–40 pounds
19–24.9 (normal weight)	25–35 pounds
25–30 (overweight)	15–25
> 30 (obese)	≤ 15

Source: Data from Institute of Medicine, Food and Nutrition Board. *Nutrition During Pregnancy: Part I, Weight Gain: Part II, Nutrient Supplements*. Washington, DC: National Academies Press, 1990.

The pattern of weight gain is important. In the first trimester, weight gain should be relatively low, about 3–4 pounds. For the rest of the pregnancy, weight gain should be steady, usually just under a pound a week, depending on the woman's recommended overall weight gain.

What makes up the total weight gain is a combination of fetal and maternal tissue (**Figure 13.1**). Of course, there is the weight of the baby (7–9 pounds), but there is also the weight of the **placenta** (2 pounds), the **amniotic fluid** (2 pounds), the increased blood volume in the mother (4–5 pounds), the increased size of the uterus (2 pounds), increased breast size (1 pound), increased fluid in maternal tissue (3–4 pounds), and increased maternal fat stores (4–8 pounds).

Nutrient Needs During Pregnancy

The diet for a pregnant woman is not much different than that recommended for all adults. A variety of foods from each food group is the key for a well-balanced diet.

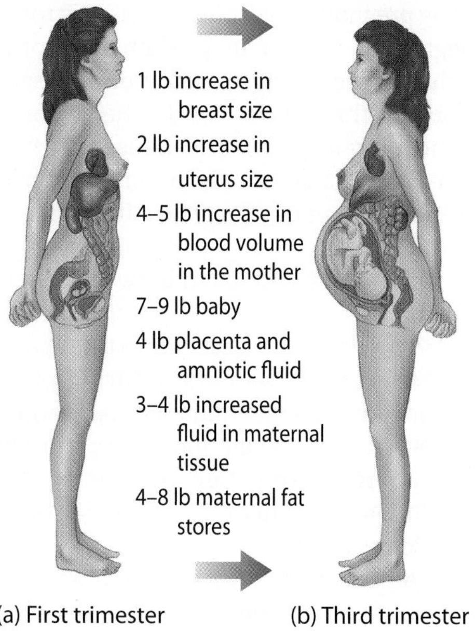

■ **Figure 13.1**
Components of Weight Gain During Pregnancy

The pregnant woman does have some additional calorie and nutrient needs to make sure that both she and the baby are healthy. Additional calories are needed to support fetal growth as well the increase in maternal tissues, including the placenta, uterus, and maternal fat stores. Approximately 340 calories more per day are needed in the second trimester and 450 calories more each day in the third trimester.[8] Because calorie needs can vary greatly from person to person, weight gain is the best indicator that calories are in line with what is needed. Protein needs are also increased. The pregnant woman needs about 25 grams of protein per day above that of a nonpregnant woman. Generally, this is easily met by a typical Western diet, because, more often than not, protein intake is above recommendations.

The pregnant woman has an increased need for many vitamins and minerals. The need for vitamins and minerals increases more than does energy needs. This means that pregnant women should choose foods that are nutrient dense and that provide lots of vitamins and minerals. Iron requirements increase dramatically during pregnancy. The amount needed during pregnancy (27 milligrams compared to 18 milligrams in the nonpregnant woman) is so high that it is almost impossible to get enough in food. Experts recommend taking an iron supplement during pregnancy.[7] A prenatal multivitamin is also commonly prescribed for women during pregnancy. See **Table 13.2** for some general guidelines of what women should eat during pregnancy.

Exercise During Pregnancy

Exercise is also important for the pregnant woman. Generally, whatever physical activity she engaged in prior to pregnancy can continue. Moderate physical activity, at least 30 minutes per day, is recommended on most days of the week.[7,9] Exercise can help prevent excessive weight gain and can help alleviate some of the discomforts of pregnancy, such as constipation and fatigue. Activities such as walking, jogging, swimming, or cycling are considered safe. Light to moderate activities may be acceptable even if the mother-to-be has not been active in the past. Contact sports should be avoided. All physical activity should be discussed with a physician to be sure it is safe for mother and baby.

Common Nutrition-Related Problems During Pregnancy

Several nutrition-related problems can arise during the nine months of pregnancy. Most are mild and can be tol-

TERMS

placenta The organ that develops during pregnancy that connects the fetus to the mother. It allows for nutrients and gases to pass to the fetus and for waste to be removed from the fetus.

amniotic fluid The fluid that surrounds the fetus.

Table 13.2

Nutrition During Pregnancy

Food Group	1st Trimester	2nd and 3rd Trimesters	What counts as 1 cup or 1 ounce?	Remember to . . .
	Eat this amount from each group daily.*			
Fruit Group	2 cups	2 cups	1 cup fruit or juice ½ cup dried fruit	*Focus on fruits*—Eat a variety of fruits.
Vegetable Group	2½ cups	3 cups	1 cup raw or cooked vegetables or juice 2 cups raw leafy vegetables	*Vary your veggies*—Eat more dark-green and orange vegetables and cooked dry beans.
Grains Group	6 ounces	8 ounces	1 slice bread 1 ounce ready-to-eat cereal ½ cup cooked pasta, rice, or cereal	*Make half your grains whole*—Choose whole instead of refined grains.
Protein Foods Group	5½ ounces	6½ ounces	1 ounce lean meat, poultry, or fish ¼ cup cooked dry beans ½ ounce nuts or 1 egg 1 tablespoon peanut butter	*Go lean with protein*—Choose low-fat or lean meats and poultry.
Dairy Group	3 cups	3 cups	1 cup milk 8 ounces yogurt 1½ ounces cheese 2 ounces processed cheese	*Get your calcium-rich foods*—Go low-fat or fat-free when you choose milk, yogurt, and cheese.

*These amounts are for an average pregnant woman. You may need more or less than the average. Check with your doctor to make sure you are gaining weight as you should. In each food group, choose foods that are low in "extras"—solid fats and added sugars.

Pregnant women and women who may become pregnant should not drink alcohol. Any amount of alcohol during pregnancy could cause problems for your baby.

Most doctors recommend that pregnant women take a prenatal vitamin and mineral supplement every day **in addition to** eating a healthy diet. This is so you and your baby get enough folic acid, iron, and other nutrients. But don't overdo it. Taking too much can be harmful.

Source: Data from US Department of Agriculture. http://www.choosemyplate.gov. Accessed October 9, 2011.

Women, Infants, and Children (WIC) Program

The Women, Infants, and Children (WIC) program targets low-income women, infants, and children up to age 5 who are at nutrition risk. The program supplies foods to supplement the diet of women, infants, and children and provides education on healthy eating to over 9 million participants each year.[10] This federally funded program is often administered by county health departments or community health centers. Participants must meet income requirements based on family income and location. They must also be determined to be at nutritional risk by a health professional. Participants receive supplemental foods designed to meet the special nutritional needs of low-income pregnant or breastfeeding women, infants, and children up to 5 years of age. The WIC food package has changed to address contemporary nutrition issues, including overweight and obesity, and now includes more fruits and vegetables. Participants can redeem food vouchers at most grocery stores and some farmers' markets. WIC foods include infant cereal, iron-fortified adult cereal, vitamin C–rich fruit or vegetable juice, eggs, milk, cheese, peanut butter, dried and canned beans/peas, canned fish, soy-based beverages, tofu, fruits and vegetables, baby foods, whole-wheat bread, and other whole-grain foods.[10]

erated with some dietary modifications, but others can be severe and pose a threat to mother and/or baby.

Gastrointestinal Issues Morning sickness and nausea are both common during pregnancy. Morning sickness is most common at the beginning of pregnancy, when the mother's body is adjusting to the change in hormones. Keeping food in the stomach throughout the day helps some women get over morning sickness and nausea. Eating crackers or dry cereal, especially first thing in the morning, also can help. Pregnant women may find it helpful to consume small frequent meals as opposed to three larger meals. It may also help to drink fluids in between meals instead of with meals.

The slower movement of the gastrointestinal tract often causes heartburn and constipation during pregnancy. To prevent heartburn, the pregnant woman should consume smaller, more frequent meals and remain upright for at least two hours after eating. Constipation can be helped by plenty of fluids and a diet that is high in fruits, vegetables, and whole grains.

Cravings are often associated with pregnancy. You have no doubt heard of pickles and ice cream or other strange food cravings in pregnant women. Also common are food aversions. Some pregnant women can't tolerate the smell or taste of meat or other specific foods. These cravings and aversions are most likely the result of alterations in taste caused by changes in the body during pregnancy. Unless the cravings or aversions are extreme, the pregnant woman can most likely work around them to consume a healthy diet.

Hypertension Hypertension during pregnancy (gestational hypertension) is defined as blood pressure greater than or equal to 140/90 mm Hg. A portion of women who develop gestational hypertension will also develop preeclampsia. **Preeclampsia** is gestational hypertension accompanied by increased protein in the urine.[11] Women who are over 35, under 19, first-time mothers, or who have a history of hypertension are more likely to develop preeclampsia. Mild cases of preeclampsia are usually treated by bed rest and careful monitoring. More severe cases may require hospitalization and drug therapy. Some women who have preeclampsia will develop eclampsia, which is life threatening for the mother and baby.

Diabetes Women with diabetes should work with their health care provider to get their diabetes under control prior to becoming pregnant. Once pregnant, their diabetes should be monitored and controlled closely. Uncontrolled diabetes places both the mother and baby at risk for severe complications.

Diabetes can develop during pregnancy, a condition called **gestational diabetes**. A woman with gestational diabetes has abnormal glucose tolerance during pregnancy that resolves when the baby is delivered. The hormones associated with pregnancy work against insulin in the body and interfere with normal glucose metabolism. Risk factors for gestational diabetes include obesity, a family history of diabetes, previous problems during pregnancy, or previously giving birth to a large infant. Gestational diabetes often can be controlled by diet or insulin therapy.[12]

Adolescent Pregnancy

Despite efforts to prevent unplanned teen pregnancy, the rates for teen pregnancy are considerably higher in the United States than in most other developed countries.[13] Teens are still growing and developing and often have diets that are low in essential nutrients. The demands of increased nutritional needs during pregnancy put the teen and the fetus at risk. Teen mothers have higher rates of preeclampsia, anemia, and preterm birth, and their infants have higher rates of low birth weight and infant death.[14] The children of teen mothers are more likely to have lower cognitive attainment at kindergarten entry, exhibit behavior problems, have chronic medical conditions, drop out of high school, and be unemployed as a young adult.[15] Pregnant adolescents should get prompt prenatal care so that a healthcare provider can assess the calorie needs of both the mother and child. Often, pregnant teens are encouraged to gain at the upper end of recommended levels to ensure that maternal growth is supported as well as growth and development of the fetus.

Personal Health Check

Are You Eating Right for Your Stage in Life?

Be mindful of your stage in life and how that may affect what you should be eating. Healthy eating is not something with which you are ever finished. It is something you do each day and can change from year to year. As you transition from one stage of life to another, changes that occur may require you to adjust your eating habits. Think about the stage of life you are in now; what are your specific nutrition needs? How will your needs change as you think about starting a family or get older? If you have children or plan to, how can you help them develop healthy eating habits?

Other Concerns During Pregnancy

Alcohol, Tobacco, and Drugs Alcohol should not be consumed by pregnant women and is associated with birth defects.[16] Even moderate drinking is not recommended and may have consequences for the development of the infant. Fetal alcohol syndrome (FAS) is caused when the mother consumes alcohol during pregnancy. Children affected by FAS have marked growth deficiencies, mental retardation, heart defects, and certain facial deformities. The greater the alcohol consumption in the mother, the more severe the outcomes of FAS seem to be. However, there is no safe level of alcohol consumption during pregnancy.

Smoking during pregnancy limits oxygen supplied to the fetus. Smoking during pregnancy is associated with a greater risk of many complications in the mother and child, including spontaneous abortion, fetal growth retardation, and sudden infant death syndrome.[16] Women should stop smoking prior to becoming pregnant. If the pregnancy is unplanned, women should stop smoking immediately upon learning they are pregnant.

Marijuana, cocaine, and other illicit drugs should not be consumed during pregnancy. Illicit drug use increases the risk of low birth weight, prematurity, and other developmental problems.[17]

TERMS

preeclampsia A condition in pregnancy that is characterized by high blood pressure, edema, and protein in the urine.

gestational diabetes A diabetic condition that results in high blood glucose levels during pregnancy.

Artificial Sweeteners Research has not indicated a link between artificial sweeteners and problems during pregnancy. Consumption of aspartame, saccharine, and sucralose within acceptable daily intakes is considered safe for pregnancy.[18]

Food Safety Everyone should use good food safety practices (see Chapter 14). Pregnancy is a particularly important time for proper food handling. Pregnant women are at a higher risk for foodborne illness. Pregnant women, due to their increased risk for foodborne illness, should not consume some foods that are fine for the general population. Pregnant women should avoid soft cheeses not made with pasteurized milk. They should only eat deli meats, luncheon meats, bologna, and hot dogs that have been heated to steaming hot. They should not consume unpasteurized milk or milk products, raw or partially cooked eggs, raw or undercooked meat, unpasteurized juice, raw sprouts, or raw or undercooked fish or shellfish. They should not consume fish that is known to have high levels of mercury, such as shark, swordfish, king mackerel, and tilefish, and should limit the consumption of albacore tuna to 6 ounces per week. Even fish with lower levels of mercury, such as shrimp, canned light tuna, salmon, catfish, and pollock, should be limited to 12 ounces or less per week.

Breastfeeding: The Ideal Choice for Mother and Child

Breastfeeding is widely accepted by health and scientific organizations as the best way to feed infants. Ideally, infants should be exclusively breastfed for six months, followed by continued breastfeeding while adding age-appropriate foods for at least the first year of life. Despite the virtually undisputed advantage of breastfeeding, many women still do not breastfeed. The rate of breastfeeding initiation in the United States is around 75%. However, only 50% of women are still breastfeeding at 6 months and 25% are still breastfeeding at 12 months. The rate of exclusive breastfeeding is low.[22] Breastfeeding offers many benefits for both mother and child.

Benefits of Breastfeeding

Breast milk is the best food for a growing infant. It contains antibodies that can help protect infants from infections and even sudden infant death syndrome (SIDS). Breastfeeding is linked with lower risk for ear infections, stomach viruses, diarrhea, respiratory infections, asthma, and diabetes in infants.[23–30] Breast milk changes over time to meet the baby's needs. The first breast milk (colostrum) is thick and yellow in color. It is rich in nutrients and antibodies. After a few days, the milk changes to contain just the right amount and type of fats and nutrients needed by the baby.

Breastfeeding has benefits for the mother as well. Breastfeeding doesn't require the mother to sterilize bottles and nipples. With no formula to purchase, breastfeeding can save money as well. The energy needed to make breast milk can help the mother lose the weight gained during pregnancy, helping her to quickly get back to her prepregnancy weight. Breastfeeding is also associated with a lower risk of type 2 diabetes, breast cancer, ovarian cancer, and postpartum depression.[31–35]

Breastfeeding and Childhood Overweight

Research suggests that initiation of breastfeeding is associated with a reduction in overall risk of overweight.[36,37] The longer the duration of breastfeeding, the lower the risk for overweight. For each month of breastfeeding, up to nine months, the risk of overweight is decreased by 4%, which translates to a 30% decrease in risk of overweight for a child who was breasted for nine months compared to a child who was never breastfed.[38] Exclusive breastfeeding appears to have a stronger protective effect than combining breastfeeding with formula.[37]

Several theories have been proposed as to why breastfeeding is associated with lower rates of overweight and obesity. One theory is that formula-fed infants have higher plasma insulin concentrations. Formula may stimulate the secretion of insulin that, in turn, stimulates more fat to be deposited.[39,40] Another possible explanation for the protective effect of breastfeeding on obesity is self-regulation of energy intake. Breastfed infants may be better able to respond to internal cues of hunger and satiety and stop eating when they are full. Bottle-fed infants may be encouraged to eat until the bottle is empty, regardless of hunger level.[41]

Barriers to Breastfeeding

Several barriers may keep a woman from successfully breastfeeding. One common barrier is lack of knowledge about the importance of breastfeeding and inaccurate information about how to breastfeed. Mothers may become discouraged if they do not have support as to how to initiate and continue breastfeeding. They may discontinue breastfeeding due to pain, lack of support, or fear that they may not have adequate milk. Hospital practices may include separating mother and infant in a manner that does not support early and positive initiation of breastfeeding. Infant formulas are heavily marketed and easily accessible. Clever marketing campaigns may leave mothers with the false impression that these products are better for their infants than their own milk. As mothers return to work or school and the infant is placed in child care or with a family member, breastfeeding may become more difficult.

Eliminating barriers to allow more women to exclusively breastfeed is an important health issue. Women must be informed and supported to make good decisions about how to feed their infants. More employers need to provide appropriate space for women to pump milk while at work. Child care facilities need to provide moth-

Early Life Indicators of Obesity

To prevent obesity, you need to start early to establish good eating and physical activity habits. How early is early enough? New research indicates that events very early in a child's life, before birth, can mean the difference between healthy weight and obesity. Smoking is a known risk factor for low birth weight and preterm births. However, even though babies are generally smaller when the mother smokes, they are at an increased risk of becoming overweight as a child.[19] Similarly, a fetus that is exposed to diabetes in the womb is more likely to become overweight or obese as a child.[20,21] Babies born to mothers who gained either too much or too little weight during pregnancy are also more likely to be overweight or obese as children.[19] The research into the effects of events prior to birth on overweight and obesity are relatively recent. However, it points to the importance of early prevention efforts.

ers with ways to continue to provide breast milk to their child, including training for staff in handling and storing breast milk.

Almost all women who want to breastfeed can do so successfully. In some instances, breastfeeding is not possible because of disease or infection in the mother or baby. Some medications can pass into the breast milk that may not allow the mother to breastfeed.

Alternatives to Breastfeeding

Women who decide not to breastfeed, cannot breastfeed, or who breastfeed for only a short time can use infant formula. Infant formula is designed to provide adequate nutrition for the infant. Most infant formula is cow's milk with added nutrients. Specialized formulas are available that contain soy or different proteins or nutrients for infants with special nutritional needs. Infant formula attempts to mimic human milk. Although formula is close to human milk, it is not an exact copy, thus the mother's milk remains the preferred feeding method.

Infant formula comes in three varieties: ready-to-feed, concentrate, and powdered. When mixing concentrate or powdered formula, good food safety practices need to be followed. Once mixed, formula needs to be refrigerated immediately and should be used within 48 hours. For the first two months of life, bottles should be sterilized. Formula should not be overdiluted; doing so deprives the infant of needed calories and nutrients.

Introduction to Solids

Once an infant is able to sit up, foods other than breast milk or infant formula can be introduced. This usually happens around 6 months of age. By this age, infants have the digestive enzymes to handle other foods and are able to maintain hydration. Introduction of foods prior to 6 months of age is not recommended and can have adverse health effects in the infant, such as dehydration. When solid foods are introduced, they should be complementary and not replace breast milk or formula altogether (**Figure 13.2**). The first food for a baby is usually iron-fortified cereal mixed with breast milk or formula. Foods should be introduced slowly, one at a time at one- to two-week intervals. This will allow caregivers to see how a given food is tolerated.

The order in which foods are introduced varies widely and is often dictated by culture. Foods should be soft in texture to avoid choking. Foods that are common allergens in children, such as cow's milk, egg whites, and wheat, should not be consumed in the first year.

Nutrition for Breastfeeding Women

The best diet for breastfeeding women is to continue the healthy, varied diet followed during pregnancy. Energy needs are as high or higher than they were during pregnancy. Some of the energy needed to produce breast milk comes from fat that was stored during pregnancy. Protein, vitamin, and mineral needs are all elevated. However, the increased need can easily be met by a well-selected diet. A breastfeeding woman will need to make sure that she gets plenty of fluids, especially water. Beverages that contain caffeine should be limited to one to two per day, because caffeine is passed into the breast milk. Supplements are generally not needed but may be prescribed by a healthcare provider as a precaution.

Nutrition During Childhood: Building Lifelong Habits for Good Health

Childhood is a time of rapid growth and development. It is also a time for the development of positive eating habits for a lifetime of good health. Developing good eating habits during childhood is critical, not just for health and proper growth, but because eating habits follow children into adolescence and eventually into adulthood.[42,43] Over the past three decades, great improvements have been made in some areas of child health. Nutrient-deficiency diseases are all but a thing of the past.[43] Although children should still be monitored, iron deficiency anemia has decreased thanks to fortification of common foods and early detection.[44]

Issues of deficiency, undernutrition, and poor growth have been overshadowed by issues of excess and overconsumption. The number one nutrition issue facing children today is overweight and obesity. In the past 30 years, the number of children who are overweight or obese has increased dramatically. Almost one-quarter of children

Development Stage	Newborn	Head Up	Supported Sitter	Independent Sitter	Crawler	Beginning to Walk	Independent Toddler
	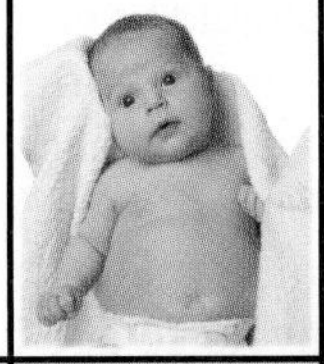	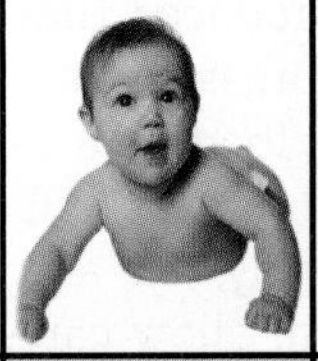	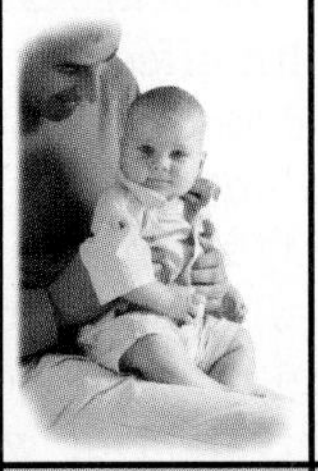	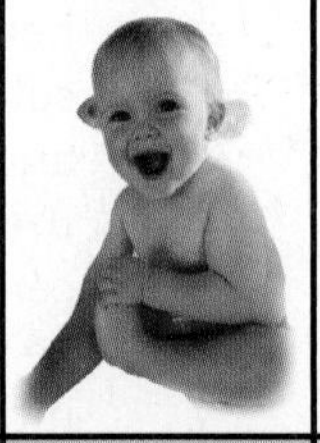	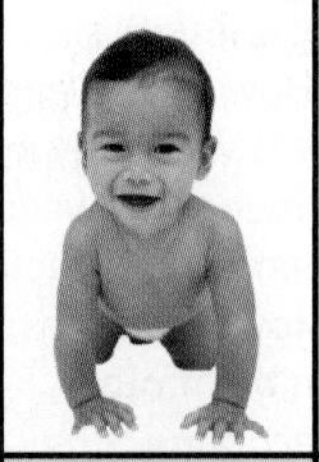	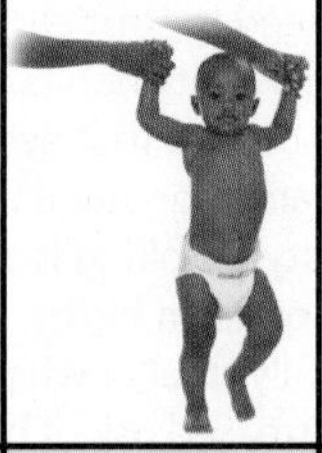	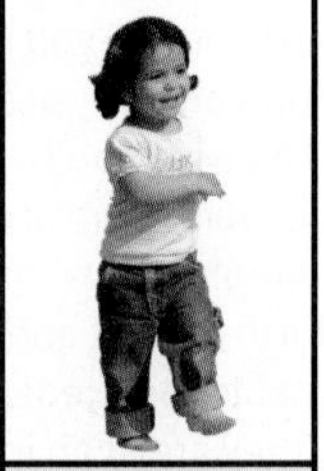
Physical Skills	• Needs head support	• More skillful head control with support emerging	• Sits with help or support • On tummy, pushes up on arms with straight elbows	• Sits independently • Can pick up and hold small object in hand • Leans toward food or spoon	• Learns to crawl • May pull self to stand	• Pulls self to stand • Stands alone • Takes early steps	• Walks well alone • Runs
Eating Skills	• Baby establishes a suck-swallow-breathe pattern during breast or bottle feeding	• Breastfeeds or bottle feeds • Tongue moves forward and back to suck	• May push food out of mouth with tongue, which gradually decreases with age • Moves pureed food forward and backward in mouth with tongue to swallow • Recognizes spoon and holds mouth open as spoon approaches	• Learns to keep thick purees in mouth • Pulls head downward and presses upper lip to draw food from spoon • Tries to rake foods toward self into fist • Can transfer food from one hand to the other • Can drink from a cup held by feeder	• Learns to move tongue from side to side to transfer food around mouth and push food to the side of the mouth so food can be mashed • Begins to use jaw and tongue to mash food • Plays with spoon at mealtime, may bring it to mouth, but does not use it for self-feeding yet • Can feed self finger foods • Holds cup independently • Holds small foods between thumb and first finger	• Feeds self easily with fingers • Can drink from a straw • Can hold cup with two hands and take swallows • More skillful at chewing • Dips spoon in food rather than scooping • Demands to spoon-feed self • Bites through a variety of textures	• Chews and swallows firmer foods skillfully • Learns to use a fork for spearing • Uses spoon with less spilling • Can hold cup in one hand and set it down skillfully
Baby's Hunger & Fullness Cues	• Cries or fusses to show hunger • Gazes at caregiver, opens mouth during feeding indicating desire to continue • Spits out nipple or falls asleep when full • Stops sucking when full	• Cries or fusses to show hunger • Smiles, gazes at caregiver, or coos during feeding to indicate desire to continue • Spits out nipple or falls asleep when full • Stops sucking when full	• Moves head forward to reach spoon when hungry • May swipe the food toward the mouth when hungry • Turns head away from spoon when full • May be distracted or notice surroundings more when full	• Reaches for spoon or food when hungry • Points to food when hungry • Slows down in eating when full • Clenches mouth shut or pushes food away when full	• Reaches for food when hungry • Points to food when hungry • Shows excitement when food is presented when hungry • Pushes food away when full • Slows down in eating when full	• Expresses desire for specific foods with words or sounds • Shakes head to say "no more" when full	• Combines phrases with gestures, such as "want that" and pointing • Can lead parent to refrigerator and point to a desired food or drink • Uses words like "all done" and "get down" • Plays with food or throws food when full
Appropriate Foods & Textures	• Breastmilk or infant formula	• Breastmilk or infant formula	• Breastmilk or infant formula • Infant cereals • Thin pureed foods	• Breastmilk or infant formula • Infant cereals • Thin pureed baby foods • Thicker pureed baby foods • Soft mashed foods without lumps • 100% Juice	• Breastmilk or infant formula • 100% Juice • Infant cereals • Pureed foods • Ground or soft mashed foods with tiny soft noticeable lumps • Foods with soft texture • Crunchy foods that dissolve (such as baby biscuits or crackers) • Increase variety of flavors offered	• Breastmilk or infant formula or whole milk • 100% Juice • Coarsely chopped foods, including foods with noticeable pieces • Foods with soft to moderate texture • Toddler foods • Bite sized pieces of food • Bites through a variety of texures	• Whole milk • 100% Juice • Coarsely chopped foods • Toddler foods • Bite-sized pieces of food • Becomes efficient at eating foods of varying textures and taking controlled bites of soft solids, hard solids, or crunchy foods by 2 years

Figure 13.2

The Start Healthy Feeding Guidelines

Summary of physical and eating skills, hunger and fullness cues, and appropriate food textures for children 0–24 months of age.

Source: N Butte, K Cobb, J Dwyer, L Graney, W Heird, K Rickard. The start healthy feeding guidelines for infants and toddlers. *J Am Diet Assoc.* 2004;104(3):442–454.

Green and Healthy

Community Gardens

No matter where you are in the life cycle, community gardens offer a great opportunity for young and old to come together for good health. Grandparents can get some activity while teaching the younger generation how to garden. Young children can learn where foods come from before they get to the grocery store. Teens can help revitalize their community while growing healthy food. A community garden is any piece of land that is gardened by a group of people. Community gardens can be located in schools, parks, housing projects, places of worship, vacant lots, private property, or anywhere there is open land and sunlight. Community gardens can be as large as a 2- or 3-acre garden or just a few pots or raised beds in an urban setting. Community gardens can grow a range of fruits, vegetables, flowers, herbs, and other plants.

Community gardens have a variety of purposes. They offer an opportunity to improve a community's appearance by turning vacant lots into green and vibrant spaces.[114] They provide the opportunity for community members to be physically active as they plant and care for the garden.[114] They are a way to build a sense of community, bringing people together with a common goal and enhancing personal satisfaction in a neighborhood.[115–119] They offer opportunities for intergenerational interactions as elders in the community teach children and visa versa. Community gardens even have the potential to increase neighborhood property values.[120]

One of the positive benefits of community gardens on nutrition is that they can increase the availability of fruits and vegetables to those who participate. Community gardens can remove one of the barriers to fruit and vegetable intake, that of access.[121] Community gardens can offer affordable and convenient access to fresh produce, specifically in urban areas that may have limited access to stores that offer fresh produce for sale or where prices are high.[121–123] Household participation in a community garden may improve fruit and vegetable intake in adults who live in urban areas.[121]

Other barriers to fruit and vegetable consumption, such as preference, quality, selection, and cost, also can be addressed by community gardens. Participation in school gardens has been shown to increase children's preference for vegetables.[124,125] Involving children in the planting, growing, harvesting, and cooking of fruits and vegetables is a great way to encourage consumption. Another barrier to fruit and vegetable consumption that is addressed by community gardens is preference. Community gardens often provide fruits and vegetables of higher quality than may be available in many neighborhoods. Furthermore, the selection and cost can be better with participation in community gardens.

Many resources are available that can help you start a community garden in your neighborhood, at your child's school, at your faith community, or on campus. The American Community Gardening Association is a good place to start (www.communitygarden.org). Resources are also available at www.eatsmartmovemorenc.com. Check with your local Cooperative Extension Service to see if they have resources on starting a community garden.

Benefits of Community Gardens

Participating in a community garden offers a wide range of benefits:

Builds community. Thriving community gardens are a great way to bring people together and create healthy and strong communities. Gardens can increase community involvement and development and enhance personal satisfaction in a neighborhood.

Strengthens bonds. Gardening brings families and neighbors closer to nature and helps children and adults learn how to care for the environment.

Saves money. Gardeners can lower their grocery store bills and earn extra income by growing their own food.

Creates opportunities to connect. Gardens help us meet people who live nearby. People can share their interests and desire to garden. From potluck dinners to community service, opportunities to build relationships are abundant at gardens.

Increases fruit and vegetable consumption. Adults who participate in community gardening may increase fruit and vegetable consumption. Children who participate in school gardens are more likely to eat fruits and vegetables.

Improves skills in food preparation. Fruits and vegetables are a quick, easy, and nutritious snack. They can be prepared in a number of ways in salads, soups, sauces, sandwiches, and desserts. Community gardens are a good place to teach people how to prepare nutritious and delicious foods. At community potlucks, gardeners can share recipes and enjoy the fruits of their labor with one another.

Increases physical activity. Gardening not only burns calories, it tones muscles and increases flexibility.

Teaches life and business skills. Participating in community gardening helps teach valuable life skills such as discipline, timeliness, pride, patience, leadership, and responsibility. In gardens that function as businesses, gardeners can learn skills such as marketing, packaging, customer service, troubleshooting, and leadership.

Source: Data from K Baldwin, D Beth, L Bradley, N Cave, S Jakes, M Nelson. Eat Smart, Move More North Carolina: growing communities through gardens. NC Department of Health and Human Services, Division of Public Health, Raleigh, NC; 2009.

ages 2 through 5 are overweight or obese. More than one-third of children ages 6 to 11 are overweight or obese.[45] Overweight and obese children face health issues both as children and as adults. Obesity has been shown to track from childhood to adolescence and ultimately to adulthood. Children who are overweight or obese are more likely to be overweight or obese adults.[46–48] See Chapter 12 for more information on overweight and obesity.

What Children Eat

Many children's eating patterns are not consistent with current recommendations for a healthy diet.[49] Children consume too much fat and too many sugar-sweetened beverages. They also consume many meals away from home, which too often means large portions of high-fat fast food. In turn, their diets are too low in fruits and vegetables.[50–52] Over the past 20 years, total energy intake has increased in children.[53] For many children, this means that they are consuming more calories than they need each day. Although the percentage of fat in the diet of children has decreased, the actual intake of fat has not.[54] The increase in total calories has caused the lowering of the percentage of calories from fat. Thanks to the availability of a wide variety of foods, some of which are fortified, most children get the vitamins and minerals they need each day. However, overall, children's diets in the United States need improvement.[55]

Nutrition Recommendations for Children

A healthy diet for children that supports growth and development as well as optimal health is not very different than what you, as an adult, should be eating. Children should consume a diet that is moderate in fat, low in saturated fat, and high in complex carbohydrates (**Table 13.3**).

Nutritionists were once concerned that if children were fed a moderate-fat diet, the overall nutrient composition of the diet would be compromised. However, studies have consistently shown that children can follow a moderate-fat diet and still have adequate energy, vitamins, and minerals. Strategies should be used to moderate the fat in children's diets by selecting nonfat or low-fat milk after the age of 2 and choosing lower-fat dairy options, such as cheese and yogurt, and lower-fat meat options.

MyPlate offers guidance as to specifically what and how much children should be eating. Once calorie requirements have been determined (**Table 13.4**), MyPlate can be

Table 13.3

Nutrition Needs During Childhood

Nutrient	Recommendation
Carbohydrates	45–65% of total calories
Fats	
1–3 years	30–40% of total calories
4–18 years	25–35% of total calories
Protein	
Young children	5–20% of total calories
Older children	10–30% of total calories
Added sugar	Should not exceed 25% of total calories
Saturated fat, trans fatty acids, and cholesterol	As low as possible while maintaining a nutritionally adequate diet
Total fiber	
1–3 years	19 grams per day
4–8 years	25 grams per day
Boys 9–13 years	31 grams per day
Girls 9–13 years	26 grams per day

Source: Data from Institute of Medicine, Food and Nutrition Board. *Dietary Reference Intakes for Energy, Carbohydrate, Fiber, Fat, Fatty Acids, Cholesterol, Protein, and Amino Acids*. Washington, DC: National Academies Press, 2005.

Table 13.4

Estimated Calorie Needs for Children by Age, Gender, and Physical Activity Level[a]

Estimated amounts of calories needed to maintain calorie balance for various gender and age groups at three different levels of physical activity. The estimates are rounded to the nearest 200 calories. An individual's calorie needs may be higher or lower than these average estimates.

			Physical Activity Level[b]	
Gender	Age (years)	Sedentary	Moderately Active	Active
Child (female and male)	2–3	1,000–1,200[c]	1,000–1,400[c]	1,000–1,400[c]
Female	4–8	1,200–1,400	1,400–1,600	1,400–1,800
	9–13	1,400–1,600	1,600–2,000	1,800–2,200
	14–18	1,800	2,000	2,400
Male	4–8	1,200–1,400	1,400–1,600	1,600–2,000
	9–13	1,600–2,000	1,800–2,200	2,000–2,600
	14–18	2,000–2.400	2,400–2,800	2,800–3,200

a. Based on Estimated Energy Requirements (EER) equations, using reference heights (average) and reference weights (healthy) for each age/gender group. For children and adolescents, reference height and weight vary. For adults, the reference man is 5 feet 10 inches tall and weighs 154 pounds. The reference woman is 5 feet 4 inches tall and weighs 126 pounds. EER equations are from the Institute of Medicine. *Dietary Reference Intakes for Energy, Carbohydrate, Fiber, Fat, Fatty Acids, Cholesterol, Protein, and Amino Acids*. Washington (DC): The National Academies Press; 2002.

b. Sedentary means a lifestyle that includes only the light physical activity associated with typical day-to-day life. Moderately active means a lifestyle that includes physical activity equivalent to walking about 1.5 to 3 miles per day at 3 to 4 miles per hour, in addition to the light physical activity associated with typical day-to-day life. Active means a lifestyle that includes physical activity equivalent to walking more than 3 miles per day at 3 to 4 miles per hour, in addition to the light physical activity associated with typical day-to-day life.

c. The calorie ranges shown are to accommodate needs of different ages within the group. For children and adolescents, more calories are needed at older ages. For adults, fewer calories are needed at older ages.

Source: Institute of Medicine. *Dietary Reference Intakes for Energy, Carbohydrate, Fiber, Fat, Fatty Acids, Cholesterol, Protein, and Amino Acids*. Washington, DC: National Academies Press, 2005.

used to determine the amount that should be eaten from each food group (**Table 13.5**).

The American Heart Association also provides guidance as to what children older than age 2 should eat (**Table 13.6**). The recommendations emphasize a dietary pattern that meets nutrition requirements for growth and development while minimizing the development of cardiovascular risk factors, primarily high blood cholesterol, blood pressure, and glucose levels and overweight and obesity.[56]

Guide for Parents The family is the most influential aspect of a child's life and provides the cornerstone for the development of healthy eating patterns.[57–62] Few issues get parents' attention like that of how to feed their children. Helping children develop lifelong habits for good health is important. However, for many families mealtime is a battle to get their children to eat what they should eat. Parents and children have clear roles in the feeding environment. Parents decide what the children will eat and when. Children decide whether to eat and how much to eat.[63] It is important for parents to stay in their role as food provider and not force food or try to dictate how much is eaten. Parents should encourage healthy food choices. The 5-3-2-1-Almost None Campaign provides parents with simple messages about how children can eat healthy and be physically active (**Figure 13.3**; also see Chapter 11 on physical activity). In addition, parents can follow some simple steps to help their children develop lifelong healthy habits:

Table 13.6

American Heart Association Dietary Strategies for Children Over 2 Years of Age

- Balance dietary calories with physical activity to maintain normal growth.
- Engage in 60 minutes of moderate to vigorous play or physical activity daily.
- Eat vegetables and fruits daily and limit juice intake.
- Use vegetable oils and soft margarines low in saturated fat and trans fatty acids instead of butter or most other animal fats in the diet.
- Eat whole-grain breads and cereals rather than refined-grain products.
- Reduce the intake of sugar-sweetened beverages and foods.
- Use nonfat (skim) or low-fat milk and dairy products daily.
- Eat more fish, especially oily fish, broiled or baked.
- Reduce salt intake, including salt from processed foods.

Source: Data from SS Gidding, AH Lihtenstein, MS Faith, et al. Implementing American Heart Association Pediatric and Adult Nutrition Guidelines. *Circulation* 2009;119:1161–1175.

Table 13.5

Plan for Preschool Children Based on Calorie Needs

The 1,200 Calorie Plan	Total Amount for the Day
Grains Group	4 ounces
Vegetable Group	1½ cups
Fruit Group	1 cup
Dairy Group	2 cups
Protein Foods Group	3 ounces
The 1,400 Calorie Plan	**Total Amount for the Day**
Grains Group	5 ounces
Vegetable Group	1½ cups
Fruit Group	1½ cups
Dairy Group	2 cups
Protein Foods Group	4 ounces
The 1,600 Calorie Plan	**Total Amount for the Day**
Grains Group	5 ounces
Vegetable Group	2 cups
Fruit Group	1½ cups
Dairy Group	2 cups
Protein Foods Group	5 ounces
The 1,000 Calorie Plan	**Total Amount for the Day**
Grains Group	3 ounces
Vegetable Group	1 cup
Fruit Group	1 cup
Dairy Group	2 cups
Protein Foods Group	2 ounces

Source: Data from US Department of Agriculture. http://www.choosemyplate.gov. Accessed October 9, 2011.

5-3-2-1-Almost None

5	5 or more servings of fruits and vegetables daily
3	3 structured meals daily— eat breakfast, less fast food, and more meals prepared at home
2	2 hours or less of TV or video games daily
1	1 hour or more of moderate to vigorous physical activity daily
Almost None	Limit sugar-sweetened drinks to "almost none"

■ **Figure 13.3**

5-3-2-1-Almost None

The 5-3-2-1-Almost None campaign provides simple messages for parents about healthy eating and physical activity for their children.

Source: Eat Smart, Move More, North Carolina. www.eatsmartmovemorenc.com. Accessed April 1, 2011. Adapted from National Initiative for Children's Healthcare Quality. Childhood obesity. http://www.nichq.org/areas_of_focus/childhood_obeisty_topic.html. Accessed April 11, 2011.

Try Something New

Getting Children to Eat Fruits and Vegetables

Children, like adults, do not eat enough fruits and vegetables. To make matters worse, the vegetables they eat the most are potatoes, fried. The number one vegetable consumed by children is french fries. The healthful benefits of fruits and vegetables, including protection against overweight and decreased risk of chronic disease, make increasing fruit and vegetable consumption in children an important public health issue. Why don't children consume more fruits and vegetables, and how are we going to get them to eat more?

This section is called "try something new," which is difficult for children, because they are generally neophobic.[64,65] This means they have a fear of trying new foods. **Neophobia** in children is linked to decreased fruit and vegetable consumption.[66,67] They simply don't want to try something they have not eaten before. Another barrier to vegetable consumption in children is taste. Children are born with the desire for sweet tastes, so consumption of fruit is not a problem.[68,69] They are also born, however, with a dislike of bitter tastes, which makes vegetable consumption more of a challenge. Over time, children's tastes change, but they generally continue to prefer sweet, fatty, starchy foods over vegetables.[67]

With neophobia and an inborn preference for sweet, starchy foods working against parents, how can children be encouraged to consume more fruits and vegetables? Exposure is very important. It may take multiple—ten or more—exposures to a fruit or vegetable for a child to try it, and even more exposures before they like it.[70–72] Although it may be discouraging, continued exposure may eventually lead to consumption. Positive reinforcement can also encourage children to try and ultimately like fruits and vegetables. Encouragement related to taste seems to be the most effective. Saying things such as "this tastes good" or "you will like the way this tastes" are more helpful than messages about how healthy a food is.[73] Rewards for eating a certain food, whether it is a nonfood reward or a food reward, seem to have the opposite effect on consumption. Children like the food less when they are rewarded for eating it.[74] Engaging children in food purchasing and food preparation can sometimes encourage consumption. Finally, changing the method of preparation may help with their willingness to eat a fruit or vegetables. If they don't like it cooked, try it raw; if raw is not working, try it lightly cooked or with a low-fat sauce.

Be patient. Young children may not be interested in trying new foods. Parents may need to offer a new food more than once. It will help for children to see that others in the family enjoy the food. The food may be accepted when it becomes more familiar to the child.

Be a planner. Most young children need a snack or two in addition to three regular daily meals. Parents should offer foods from three or more food groups for breakfast and lunch. Foods from four or more of the five major food groups should be offered for the main meal. Parents should plan snacks so they are not served too close to mealtime and offer foods from two or more of the five major food groups.

Be a good role model. Parents must practice and model what they say. Children learn from their parents about how and what to eat. Parents should eat meals with their children whenever possible. They should try new foods and new ways of preparing them. Both parent and child can be healthier by eating more dark-green leafy vegetables, deep-yellow vegetables, fruits, and whole-grain products.

Be adventurous. Allowing young children to choose a new vegetable or fruit is a good way to encourage consumption. At home children can help wash and prepare the food.

Be creative. Children should be encouraged to invent a new snack or sandwich from three or four healthy ingredients. They may want to try a new bread or whole-grain cracker. Parents should talk to their children about what food groups the new snack includes and why it tastes good.

Farm to School

One effort currently under way to improve the quality of school meals is farm-to-school programs. Farm-to-school programs work to integrate locally gown food into school meals as well as support educational activities such as field trips to farms, in-cafeteria education, and visits from local farmers.[79,80] Farm-to-school programs involve students, teachers, parents, and food service staff with the goal of providing fresh local fruits and vegetables in the school cafeteria. The farm-to-school movement has the potential to improve children's diets without breaking the food service budget.[81] Farm-to-school may also allow schools to purchase produce that is fresher than what they can buy from other vendors. It also allows the school to support the community by purchasing foods grown locally or at least in the proximity of the school. This allows for students to make a connection with where the food they eat comes from.

TERMS

neophobia Dislike of anything new or unfamiliar.

How Policy and Environment Affect My Choices

School Lunch: Is It Making the Grade for Children?

Schools can play a vital role in improving children's dietary habits and are in a unique position to promote healthy eating.[75,76] However, the words *school lunch* no doubt elicit visions of fish sticks, hot dogs, pizza, and sloppy joes. The stereotype of a school lunch is not one that is healthy and filled with fruits, vegetables, and the foods children should be eating on a regular basis.

Over 31 million children are served lunch at school each day. The school lunch has been in existence for over 60 years. President Harry Truman signed the National School Lunch Act into law in 1946. It was precipitated by boys not being strong enough to serve in the military due to poor nutrition. Today, the school lunch program continues; however, our children face very different issues. The issue today is one of excess and overweight as opposed to nutritional deficiencies. Has the school lunch program kept pace with contemporary nutrition concerns in children? If not, why not, and what can be done to change policies to help adapt the school lunch program to better serve children?

Since being signed into law in 1946, the school lunch program has undergone many changes. In 1966, the Child Nutrition Act was passed and now governs the National School Lunch Program (NSLP) and School Breakfast Program (SBP). In 1995, Nutrition Standards and Meal Requirements were put in place to ensure that the meals offered are of high nutritional quality. The Institute of Medicine has recommendations for school meals based on science and the nutrition issues children face today and has set targets for calories, fat, sodium, and other nutrients in school meals.[77] Although these guidelines have improved the quality of school meals, the overall school food environment is still lacking.[76,78]

The barrier to sweeping improvement is funding. School food service in the United States is funded primarily by federal subsidies based on the number of reimbursable meals served. Reimbursable meals are those that meet USDA guidelines for what is served. Schools need to serve as many reimbursable meals as possible to generate the revenue needed to stay in business. In most cases, school food service is responsible for paying for workers, equipment, and food and sometimes even the cafeteria itself. The need to remain in the black financially has caused most schools to offer à la carte items to generate revenue. The pizza, fries, flavored waters, ice cream, and cookies are sold to keep the cafeteria open. Selling these foods has turned school cafeterias into convenience stores as they struggle to have enough funding to remain open. The reimbursable meals that meet USDA guidelines may very well fall within a healthy range for many nutrients. However, it is all the other foods that are available in the cafeteria, sometimes in large portion sizes, that the children are drawn to and often consume.

What can be done to change the face of the school lunch? One possibility for change lies in the Child Nutrition Act. This act is reauthorized every five years and offers the opportunity for changing what is served in the school lunch. For example, in the most recent reauthorization the type of milk served was changed. Milk is the biggest single source of saturated fat on the lunch line. The Child Nutrition Act now only allows skim and 1% milk to be offered, banning whole and 2% milk. In addition, schools are required to ensure that children have water with their meals. The Child Nutrition Act also now allows the USDA to have some oversight in foods sold other places on campus besides the cafeteria, such as vending machines and school stores. Perhaps most important, the Child Nutrition Act has for the first time limited the number of calories in each reimbursable meal. Of course, these new changes are only one step. Many states have taken bolder steps towards funding healthier meals for students. Local schools have developed their own strategies for healthier meals. Changing the school food service environment for all children will take time, money, and the support of politicians and parents alike. We must create a system where decisions regarding foods and beverages can be made based on students' health and well-being, not profit.

High School lunch: **$2.00** (*chicken filet sandwich, lettuce and tomato, baked beans, raspberry applesauce, low-fat chocolate milk*) This menu provides 16% of calories from protein and 21% or calories from fat.

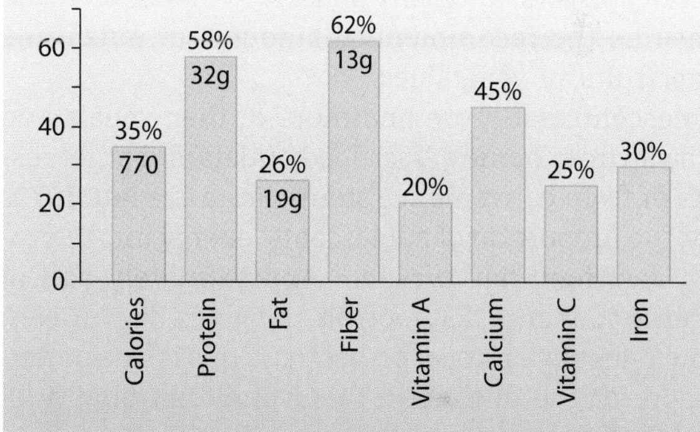

High School à la carte purchases: **$4.00** (*chicken filet sandwich, large french fries, 20-oz. sports drink*)
This menu provides 8% of calories from protein and 38% or calories from fat.

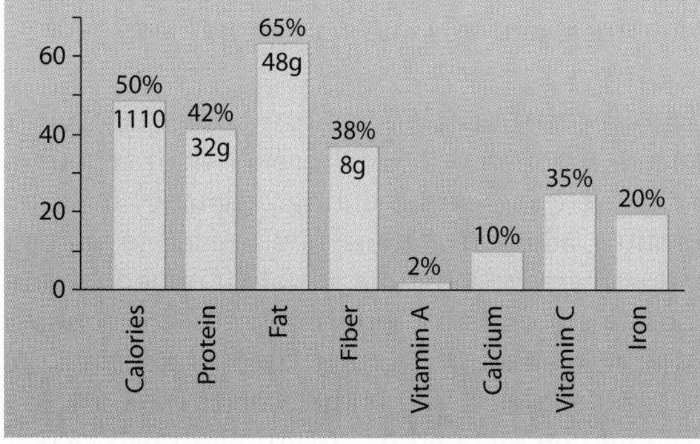

Comparison of a Reimbursable Meal and a Meal from à la Carte Purchases
Percentages are based on 2,200 calories per day.

Source: K Andersen, D Caldwell, C Dunn, L Hoggard, S Thaxton, C Thomas. Eat Smart: NC's Recommended Standard for All Foods Available in School. North Carolina SHHAS, NC Division for Public Health, Raleigh, NC. 2004.

Nutrition During Adolescence

Adolescence is defined as the period between the onset of puberty and adulthood, usually the ages of 9–18. Adolescence is a critical time for the development of dietary behaviors that continue into adulthood.[82–84] You have no doubt heard of (and have most likely experienced) the adolescent growth spurt, a time of rapid growth and development. Growth during adolescence includes increases in height and weight and changes in body composition. Until puberty, body composition in girls and boys is similar. During puberty, however, boys develop more lean body mass and girls develop hips and breast tissue that is mostly made up of fat. Not only are adolescents' bodies changing, but there are many emotional changes going on as well. Adolescence is also a time of increased peer influence, social changes, and independence.

What Adolescents Eat

Over the past few decades, the quality of adolescents' diets has declined. Consumption of calories has increased along with the consumption of sugar-sweetened beverages, pizza, burgers, and salty snacks.[85–87] Most teens do not consume the recommended amounts of milk, milk products, fruits, or vegetables.[85,87,88]

Adolescents eat more and more of their meals and snacks away from home at fast-food outlets and other restaurants or from convenience stores. From the late 1970s to today, the proportion of adolescents' energy intake provided by fast food has tripled.[85] Approximately half of adolescents consume fast food on any given day.[85] Given the known negative impact of fast food, this is one potential reason for the decline in the overall diet quality of adolescents.[89–92]

The replacement of the family dinner table with the fast-food drive-through puts adolescents at nutritional risk not only during their teens but also into adulthood. Eating meals prepared at home with family during adolescence may have a lasting, positive influence on dietary quality and meal patterns into young adulthood.[84]

Nutrition Recommendations for Adolescents

Energy needs are greater in adolescence than any other time in the life cycle except during pregnancy or lactation. Certainly, adequate calories are needed to support growth. However, a much more prevalent issue for teens than undernutrition is too many calories; the number of overweight teens in the United States has tripled in the past two decades.[93] The number of calories that are needed should be dictated by growth and may need to be adjusted to support growth without contributing to overweight, obesity, or increased risk of chronic diseases such as diabetes.[94]

Protein needs are greater during adolescence to support growth and development. A typical North American diet is generally more than adequate in protein, so special attention to protein intake during adolescence is usually not necessary.

Most nutrient needs increase as calorie needs increase. Nutrients of special concern are vitamin A, calcium, and iron. Vitamin A is essential for proper growth and development. Teens can increase their vitamin A intake by including fruits and vegetables in their diet daily. Especially high in vitamin A are deep-green, orange, and yellow fruits and vegetables.

Calcium is critical to the development of strong bones. It is also important so that maximum bone density can be achieved, helping to protect bones later in life. It is very difficult to achieve the needed daily intake of calcium without consuming three to four servings of dairy products each day. Skim milk, yogurt, and cheese need to be part of adolescents' diets for proper bone growth.

Iron is needed in higher amounts during adolescence. Boys need extra iron to help in the development of muscle mass. Girls need extra iron to make up for the blood lost during menstruation. Both boys and girls should be able to achieve needed iron intake if they consume a varied diet with adequate calories.

Adolescents and Body Image

Adolescence is a time of rapid change in the size and shape of both boys' and girls' bodies. It is also a time of intense peer pressure to look a certain way. Magazines, television programs, and movies show perfect bodies that are unattainable by most people. Teens are pressured to attain a certain social and cultural ideal of beauty, which can lead to poor **body image**. A person with a negative body image has a distorted perception of his or her shape and size or general unhappiness with his or her appearance. Poor body image can lead to emotional stress, low self-esteem, unhealthy dieting habits, anxiety, depression, and eating disorders. Developing a healthy body image is crucial to overall wellness. Adolescents (and adults) should work to develop a body image that is based on what is realistic, not what is on the cover of fashion magazines. Teens need to recognize that their body is unique and does not have to look a certain way. Adults should help teens develop a positive body image by being supportive and helping them see the positive aspects of their body and being careful to not be overly critical.

TERMS

body image A person's perception of his or her physical appearance.

anorexia nervosa An eating disorder that involves an inability to stay at the minimum body weight considered to be healthy. Persons with this disorder may have an intense fear of weight gain, even when they are underweight. They may use extreme dieting, excessive exercise, or other methods to lose weight.

Special Report

Eating Disorders

Severely distorted body image can lead to an eating disorder. Eating too little, binging and purging, extreme distress about body weight, all of these are disturbances in the relationship between food and eating. Eating disorders are characterized by the extremes of eating too little or too much. Someone with an eating disorder may have started out with just a small change in eating patterns, but for some reason the urge to eat to extremes, either too little or too much, spirals out of control.

Although eating disorders manifest themselves in food behaviors, they are complex mental illnesses. Eating disorders are complicated and not fully understood. Even though they have been studied for decades, the reason why someone would develop an eating disorder remains unclear. Although treatment is successful for some, for others effective treatment remains somewhat elusive.

The three main types of eating disorders are anorexia nervosa, bulimia nervosa, and binge-eating disorder. The prevalence of these disorders is very low. Anorexia nervosa affects approximately 0.9% of women and 0.3% of men; bulimia nervosa affects 1.5% of women and 0.5% of men. Binge-eating disorder affects 3.5% of women and 2% of men.[95] Although these disorders are relatively uncommon, they do represent a public health concern because they coexist with other mental and physical health issues and are frequently undertreated.[95]

Some people may be concerned that increased messages about healthy eating and prevention of overweight will cause an increase in eating disorders. Eating disorders are mental health issues whose cause is not entirely understood. However, the increased attention to healthy eating and preventing overweight and obesity has not been associated with an increased incidence of eating disorders. It should be noted that the prevalence of eating disorders has remained relatively unchanged over the past few decades.

Anorexia Nervosa

Anorexia nervosa is a visible eating disorder; it is characterized by emaciation and relentless pursuit of thinness. People with anorexia nervosa have an unwillingness to maintain a healthy weight and have a distorted body image.[96] They may believe themselves to be overweight even when they are clearly underweight. Some people with anorexia nervosa lose weight by extreme dieting and exercise; others lose weight through self-induced vomiting or abuse of laxatives, diuretics, or enemas.

Those with anorexia nervosa have extremely disturbed eating behaviors. They may portion out food or even weigh their food. They may have "safe" foods and limit consumption to only four or five foods that they deem to be acceptable for them to eat. They may weigh themselves frequently and/or have rituals about eating, exercise, and tracking their behavior. *Anorexia nervosa* literally means "nervous loss of appetite." This is somewhat misleading, because the person with anorexia nervosa has an appetite, but he or she just chooses not to eat or to eat very little. The peak age for onset of anorexia nervosa is between 15 and 19 years old.[97] However, growing numbers of cases are occurring in mid- and late life.[98,99]

Anorexia Nervosa

Weight	Refusal to maintain body weight at or above minimally normal weight for age and height (less than 85% of expected weight). OR Failure to make expected weight gain during growth period, leading to weight < 85% of expected normal body weight.
Phobia/associated disorders	Intense fear of gaining weight or becoming fat even though underweight.
Body perception	Disturbance in the way in which one's body weight and shape are experienced; undue influence of body weight or shape on self-evaluation. OR Denial of the seriousness of the current low body weight.
Amenorrhea/ fluctuations	Loss of menstrual period in women for at least three hormonal consecutive cycles.

Source: Data from American Psychiatric Association. *Diagnostic and Statistical Manual of Mental Disorders*, 4th ed (DSM-IV). Washington, DC: American Psychiatric Association, 1994.

Many people with anorexia nervosa have coexisting mental and physical problems. Depression, anxiety, obsessive behavior, substance abuse, cardiovascular complications, and impaired physical development are common in those with anorexia nervosa.[100] As the body deals with a constant lack of calories, persons with anorexia may develop other chronic health issues over time, including osteoporosis, brittle hair and nails, yellow or dry skin, growth of fine hair over their entire body, anemia, muscle weakness, severe constipation, low blood pressure, slowed breathing, fatigue, and a drop in internal body temperature, which causes them to feel cold all the time. Anorexia nervosa can cause severe health issues and even death. The most common complications that lead to death are cardiac arrest, electrolyte and fluid imbalance, and suicide.

Treating anorexia nervosa is difficult and must address three underlying issues. A specific, successful treatment strategy continues to elude medical professionals. However, any potentially successful treatment program must address the following: First, weight must be restored to a healthy level. Second, the psychological issues related to the disorder must be treated. Third, the behaviors and thoughts that lead to

(continues)

disordered eating must be reduced or eliminated.[101] The use of medications in treating anorexia nervosa has shown mixed results. Some studies have found antidepressants or mood stabilizers to be helpful, but others have not.[102] Overall, it is unclear what role medication may play in treating anorexia nervosa. Different forms of therapy, including individual, group, or family, can help address psychological reasons for the illness. No one therapy has been found to be consistently effective for treating anorexia nervosa. Over time, many people with anorexia nervosa no longer have the disorder. However, many continue to suffer for a long period of time from a lesser form of the disease.[103]

Bulimia Nervosa

Although a person with anorexia nervosa will be emaciated, one with **bulimia nervosa** will be normal weight or even slightly overweight. Bulimia nervosa is characterized by frequent episodes of binging and purging. Persons with bulimia nervosa will have episodes of eating unusually large amounts of food and feel that they lack control over their eating. Purging, either by self-induced vomiting, abuse of laxatives, fasting, or excessive exercise, follows the binge. The binge–purge cycle is usually done several times per week. This behavior is almost always done in secret. Bulimics often feel intensely ashamed of their behavior. Like those with anorexia nervosa, bulimics fear weight gain and want to lose weight. They, too, are very unhappy with their body size and shape.

Like those with anorexia nervosa, those with bulimia nervosa often have coexisting mental illnesses, such as depression, anxiety, or substance abuse. A number of physical conditions result from purging on a regular basis. Those with bulimia nervosa can have electrolyte imbalances, gastrointestinal problems, tooth decay from regurgitated stomach acid, a chronically inflamed throat, intestinal distress and irritation from laxative abuse, kidney problems from diuretic abuse, or severe dehydration.[104]

Bulimics require nutritional counseling and psychotherapy to address the binge–purge behavior. The most successful type of therapy for bulimia nervosa is cognitive behavioral therapy.[102] Many bulimics are prescribed antidepressants, which may help those who also have depression and/or anxiety. Antidepressants also may help reduce the binge–purge behavior and improve attitudes about eating.

Bulimia Nervosa

Weight	Normal or overweight
Phobia/associated behaviors	Recurrent episodes of binge eating, characterized by eating a substantially larger amount of food in a discrete period of time than would be eaten by most people and sense of lack of control over eating during the binge. Recurrent inappropriate compensatory behavior to prevent weight gain (i.e., self-induced vomiting, use of laxatives, diuretics, fasting, or excessive exercise). Binges or inappropriate compensatory behaviors occurring, on average, at least twice weekly for at least three months.
Body perception	Disturbance in the way in which one's body weight and shape are experienced. Undue influence of body weight or shape on self-evaluation.

Source: Data from American Psychiatric Association. *Diagnostic and Statistical Manual of Mental Disorders*, 4th ed (DSM-IV). Washington, DC: American Psychiatric Association, 1994.

Binge-Eating Disorder

Binge-eating disorder is characterized by a loss of control over eating and recurring binge-eating episodes. It differs from bulimia nervosa in that the binge is not followed by a purge. People with binge-eating disorder are often overweight or obese and may experience guilt or shame when they binge. This can lead to even more binge-eating episodes.

As with other eating disorders, binge-eating disorders can coexist with other mental illnesses, such as anxiety or depression. Treatment of the disorder is similar to that of bulimia and often includes prescription antidepressants and psychotherapy.[103]

What to Do If You Suspect Someone Has an Eating Disorder

Before you approach a friend or family member you suspect has an eating disorder, educate yourself. Eating disorders are complex and not easily solved without the help of trained medical professionals. Remember that eating disorders are mental illnesses and are not just about food and weight. Talk with your friend or family member in a private, nonthreatening setting. Avoid talking about the person's weight or appearance; this may only make matters worse. Let the person know you are concerned and that you are there to provide help and support. Listen to the person and don't be too quick with your own opinions. Encourage the person to get help and be ready to suggest resources in your community. If you are not a trained therapist, don't take on that role. Help your friend or family member get the professional help he or she needs.

Nutrition Later in Life: Eating Well and Staying Well

Diet and nutrition play an important role in maintaining health and preventing disease. This is especially important for older adults. Many of the chronic conditions in older adults, such as obesity, hypertension, heart disease, and diabetes, are diet related. The prevalence of obesity is increasing in all age groups, including older adults. Obesity can exacerbate the age-related decline in physical function and lead to frailty.[104] Older adults may be vulnerable to poor nutrition due to physical limitations, limited income, drug interactions, or living situation. Proper nutrition in older adults is critical to maintain health and function to help not only add years of life, but to make those added years filled with health and vitality.

Which Side Are You On?

Calorie Restriction: A Great Anti-Aging Strategy, or Does It Just Feel Like a Longer Life?

Benjamin Franklin once provided his advice for living a long life: if you eat only nutritious foods, don't consume alcohol, and stay away from the opposite sex, you will live to be 100, but it will feel like 200. This may be your sentiment about one anti-aging theory called calorie restriction, or CR.

CR is the practice of limiting daily calorie intake to improve health and slow down the aging process. Depending on a person's gender, body size, and activity level, calories are restricted to 1,700–1,900 calories, or even lower in some cases. It was first introduced as a possible anti-aging process by researchers in the 1930s who observed that laboratory rats who were fed a severely reduced calorie diet with optimal nutrients had life spans up to twice as long as expected.[111] Research that followed found that CR improved life expectancy in other species. CR is the only known dietary measure that can extend the maximum, and not the average, life span.

Why CR works is a topic of some debate. Many theories as to why CR works have been disproven. A theory that has some plausibility is the Hormesis Hypothesis. This theory states that CR places a person in a defensive state so that the body can survive adversity, which results in improved health and longer life.[112] Whatever the theory, the fact remains that most research points to the fact that CR in adult men and women causes beneficial metabolic, hormonal, and functional changes, including a longer life. CR in humans is also associated with reduction of multiple chronic disease risk factors, even when restriction is not started until midlife.[113]

There are some problems with CR, however. Precisely the amount of restriction of calories that is needed to optimize longevity in humans is not known. Compliance is an issue as well; consumption of calories below what your body needs for an extended period of time is difficult, if not impossible, for most people. It is difficult to reduce calories while still getting the needed nutrients to support life. In addition, it could be harmful to some people who are very lean already.[113]

TERMS

bulimia nervosa An eating disorder in which a person binges on food or has regular episodes of significant overeating and feels a loss of control. The affected person then uses various methods, such as vomiting or laxative abuse, to prevent weight gain.

binge-eating disorder An eating disorder characterized by a loss of control over eating and recurring binge-eating episodes.

What Older Adults Eat

Not unlike younger adults' diets, older adults' diets are not always consistent with what is recommended. Using the Healthy Eating Index, a tool developed by U.S. Department of Agriculture to assess overall diet quality, 68% of Americans over age 60 have diets that "need improvement," with 14% rated as poor.[105] Only 17% of older adults have diets considered to be "good." Many older adults consume too much sodium and saturated fat. They also have diets that are low in fiber, fruits, vegetables, and whole grains.[106]

Nutrition Recommendations for Older Adults

Nutrition recommendations for older adults are similar to those for adults of any age. However, some changes that occur as we age can make eating a healthy diet more of a challenge. The National Institute for Health recommends four simple steps for older adults to eat healthy: know how much to eat, choose nutrient-dense foods, limit some foods, and enjoy meals.[107]

One of the biggest changes with respect to nutrition as we get older is the number of calories needed. Aging is associated with considerable changes in body composition. After 20 to 30 years of age, muscle mass decreases and fat mass increases. Some of this decline in muscle mass may be halted or at least slowed by increased resistance training (see Chapter 11 on physical activity). This change in body composition has a direct impact on the number of calories needed to maintain weight. The resting metabolic rate (RMR), the calories needed while at rest, declines by 2–3% per decade after age 20.[105] About 75% of this decline is due to the change in body composition.[107] Simply put, as muscle mass declines so does the number of calories needed to maintain weight. If calories are consumed at the same rate, weight gain will occur without an increase in physical activity.

Choosing nutrient-dense foods is especially important for older adults. Although calorie needs decrease with increasing age, most nutrients needed for good health do not. This makes it even more important to choose lower-calorie foods that have lots of nutrients. Older adults should choose fruits, vegetables, whole grains, skim milk and dairy products, and lean meats to ensure that they consume adequate nutrients but not too many calories.

It is also important for older adults to limit certain foods. Foods high in saturated fat and cholesterol should be consumed only occasionally. Foods with high sodium or added sugars should also be avoided. This means limiting the consumption of processed foods and foods prepared outside the home.

Older adults should try to maintain their interest in eating so that they enjoy their meals. Eating is one of life's greatest pleasures. Many older adults, however, find that they have lost interest in food and cooking. They may not enjoy meals because they have to eat alone. Eating with others is a way to return some of the joy of eating. Older adults should be encouraged to find ways to eat with friends or family members as often as possible. They may

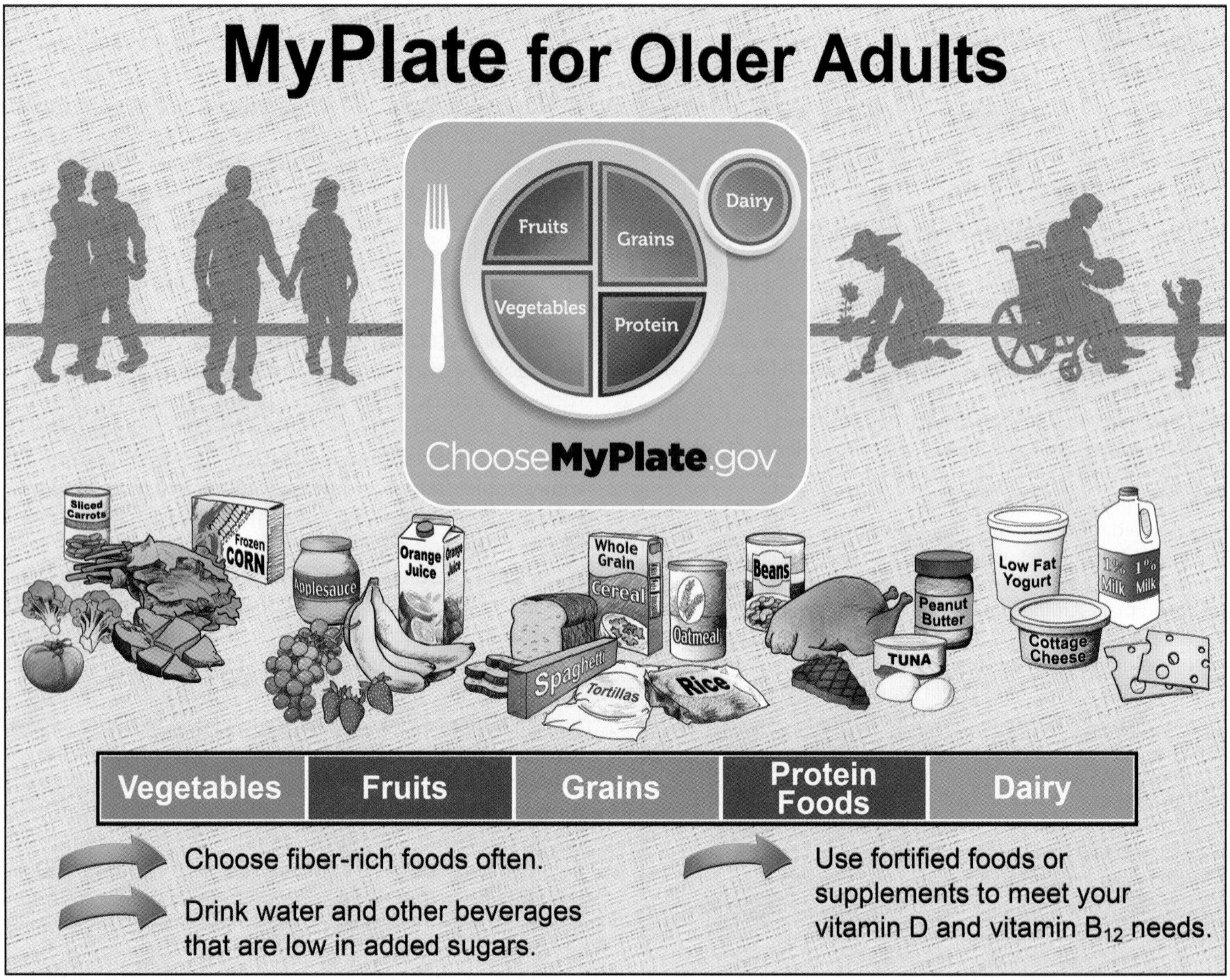

■ **Figure 13.4**
MyPlate for Older Adults
Source: © University of Florida, Elder Nutrition and Food Safety.

want to join or start a dinner club or find neighbors to share meals with on a regular basis.

Older adults may not enjoy eating due to trouble chewing. A doctor or dentist should be consulted to ensure that everything is being done to make eating as pleasurable as possible. Chewing problems can sometimes be resolved by changing the foods that are eaten. Raw vegetables can be replaced with cooked vegetables. Canned or frozen fruit without added sugar can replace fresh fruits. Choosing ground meat or meat that can be shredded will help older adults with trouble chewing. Beans, eggs, or tuna can be high-protein easy-to-chew substitutes to meat.

Another reason some older adults lose interest in foods is because they have a decreased sense of taste and/or smell. Adding additional or different herbs or spices can enhance food flavors. Older adults, and those who care for them, may want to experiment with bold flavors so that food regains its appeal.

To help older adults understand their unique nutrition needs, nutrition professionals have created the MyPlate for older adults (**Figure 13.4**).[108] It uses graphics that are consistent with an older adult population. It also highlights the need for decreased calories while maintaining high nutrient intake. Specifically, it highlights the need for consumption of fruits, vegetables, and other high-fiber foods, as well as the need for consumption of foods fortified with vitamins D and B_{12}, two vitamins often lacking in the diet of older adults.[109,110]

VEGETABLES Vary your veggies	FRUITS Focus on fruits	GRAINS Make half your grains whole	PROTEIN FOODS Go lean with protein	DAIRY Get your calcium-rich foods
Eat more dark-green veggies, like broccoli, salad greens, and cooked greens. Eat more orange vegetables, such as carrots and sweet potatoes. Eat more dried beans and peas, like pinto, black, or kidney beans, and lentils.	Eat a variety of fruits, like bananas, berries, grapes, and oranges. Choose fresh, frozen, canned, or dried fruit. Eat fruit rather than drinking juice for most of your fruit choices.	Eat at least 3 oz. of whole-grain cereals, breads, rice, crackers, or pasta every day. 1 oz. is about 1 slice of bread, 1 cup of cold breakfast cereal, or ½ cup of cooked cereal, rice, or pasta. Eat cereals fortified with vitamin B_{12}.	Choose low-fat or lean meats and poultry. Bake, broil, or grill. Vary your protein sources. Include eggs, dried beans, tofu, fish, nuts, and seeds.	Choose low-fat or fat-free milk, yogurt, and other milk products. If you don't or can't consume milk, choose lactose-free products or other calcium sources, such as fortified foods and beverages.

For an 1,800-calorie diet, you need the amounts below from each food group. To find the amounts that are right for you, go to ChooseMyPlate.gov.

Vegetables	Fruits	Grains	Protein Foods	Dairy
Eat 2½ cups every day	Eat 1½ cups every day	Eat 6 oz. every day	Eat 5 oz. every day	Eat 3 cups every day

Eat Right

- **Choose foods rich in fiber to help keep you regular.**
- **Drink plenty of fluids to stay hydrated.**
- **Limit sweets to decrease empty calories.**
- **Get your oils from fish, nuts, and liquid oils such as canola, olive, corn or soybean oils.**
- **Choose and prepare foods with less salt or sodium.**
- **Talk to your doctor or pharmacist about supplements you are taking.**

Be Active

- **Go for a walk.**
- **Play with your grandchildren and/or a pet.**
- **Work in your yard or garden.**
- **Take an exercise or dance class at a community center or gym.**
- **Share a fun activity with a friend or family member.**
- **Remember: all activity adds up! You don't have to do it all at once.**

Enjoy Life: **Spend time with caring people doing things you enjoy.**

UF UNIVERSITY of FLORIDA
IFAS Extension

MyPlate for Older Adults was adapted from USDA's MyPlate by nutrition faculty in the Department of Family, Youth and Community Sciences, IFAS, University of Florida, Gainesville, Florida 32611.
2011

ENAFS Elder Nutrition and Food Safety

■ **Figure 13.4**
MyPlate for Older Adults *(Continued)*
Source: © University of Florida, Elder Nutrition and Food Safety.

Myth Versus Fact

Myth: It is impossible to get kids to eat vegetables.

Fact: Although it may seem impossible to many parents, with repeated offerings and creativity in preparation, children can be encouraged to eat more vegetables.

Myth: If someone has an eating disorder, they will always have one, because eating disorders are almost impossible to treat.

Fact: Eating disorders are very difficult to treat. However, with proper care from a mental health professional and the support of family and friends, those with eating disorders can get better and lead normal lives.

Myth: Most teens have terrible diets; as long as they start eating better as an adult they will be fine.

Fact: The first part is true; most teens have terrible diets high in fast food, sugar-sweetened beverages, burgers, and pizza. It is never too late to develop good eating habits, but developing them early is certainly advised. Eating habits developed in the teen years tend to track into adulthood. That means that those bad habits will follow teens as they get older. It is best to start early in developing positive eating habits for a lifetime of good health.

Myth: The school lunch is unhealthy; students should bring their lunch from home.

Fact: The school lunch can offer a healthy meal to students. It is the à la carte items of large servings of pizza, fries, cookies, and chips that push the limits of good nutrition. These items are sold to help keep the cafeteria operating within budget. Students should select the regular school meal as opposed to other foods for a healthier choice.

Myth: When a woman is pregnant, she needs to eat for two.

Fact: Calorie needs are increased during pregnancy, but eating for two is not entirely accurate. The desired weight gain during pregnancy is a good guide for the number of calories that are needed.

Myth: A pregnant woman needs to eat really healthy during the last three months of pregnancy, because that is when the baby gains the most weight.

Fact: The entire pregnancy is a time of increased nutritional needs for a healthy mom and baby. However, the most critical time for healthy eating is the first few weeks of pregnancy, or even the period prior to conception. This makes eating healthy during all periods of life critical for mom and baby.

Myth: Formula is just as healthy for the baby as breast milk.

Fact: Formula companies can get close to breast milk, but they have yet to replicate all of the advantages of breast milk. Breastfeeding is best for mother and child.

Back to the Story

Tasha and Tim are to be commended for thinking about their baby's health even before Tasha becomes pregnant. Tasha should make sure she is eating healthy now as well as when she gets pregnant. This is a great time to make some lifetime changes for the whole family. She may want to talk to her doctor about taking a folic acid supplement to help decrease the risk of neural tube defects in the baby. They should also talk with Tasha's doctor about how they want to feed the baby. Experts agree that breastfeeding is best for both mother and baby.

Joan is not unlike many moms struggling with work, school, and a family. No matter how hectic the schedule, good nutrition needs to be on the to-do list. Joan should try to prepare simple meals at home instead of relying on highly processed foods and takeout pizza. She should get the children involved whenever possible in selecting and preparing meals. Now is the time for her to try (and try again) to expand the food choices her children enjoy. They are developing eating patterns that will be with them for many years to come.

Anne can make some simple changes to improve her diet. First, she needs to get into the breakfast habit. If she is not hungry when she wakes up, she can take a breakfast bar or peanut butter sandwich with her on her way out the door. She needs to plan more for her lunch and dinner meals. Eating fast food too often is not a good way for Anne to maintain her weight, nor is skipping meals. Planning meals and taking foods with her will help. She should try to schedule dinner with her family on at least one or two nights a week.

Pam and Sean are ready to relax and enjoy all of their hard work as they prepare to retire. However, high blood pressure and high cholesterol threaten to make their retirement years less than healthy. It is never too late to begin to adopt healthy eating habits. Pam and Sean would benefit greatly from a slight reduction in body weight. Most likely, losing a few pounds by making small changes in diet and exercise would get their blood pressure in check and may lower Pam's blood cholesterol.

All of these people are at different points in their life. However, they all can benefit from some changes to their eating patterns. What other changes can you suggest for Tasha and Tim, Joan and her family, Anne, and Pam and Sean to help them be healthy at their stage in life?

References

1. Johnson K, Posner SF, Biermann J, et al. Recommendations to improve preconception health and health care United States. *MMWR*. 2006;55(RRo6):1–23.
2. Cnattingius S, Bergstrom R, Lipworth L, Kramer MS. Prepregnancy weight and the risk of adverse pregnancy outcomes. *N Engl J Med*. 1998;338:147–152.
3. Shaw GM, Schaffer D, Velie EM, Morland K, Harris JA. Periconceptional vitamin use, dietary folate, and the occurrence of neural tube defects. *Epidemiology*. 1995;6:219–26.
4. Mulinare J, Cordero JF, Erickson JD, Berry RJ. Periconceptional use of multivitamins and the occurrence of neural tube defects. *JAMA*. 1988;260:3141–3145.
5. Milunsky A, Jick H, Jick SS, Bruell CL, MacLaughlin DS, Rothman KJ, Willett W. Multivitamin/folic acid supplementation in early pregnancy reduces the prevalence of neural tube defects. *JAMA*. 1989;262:2847–52.
6. Institute of Medicine. Food and Nutrition Board. *Dietary Reference Intakes: Thiamin, Riboflavin, Niacin, Vitamin B_6, Folate, Vitamin B_{12}, Pantothenic Acid, Biotin, and Choline*. Washington, DC: National Academies Press, 1998.
7. Institute of Medicine, Food and Nutrition Board. *Nutrition During Pregnancy: Part I, Weight Gain: Part II, Nutrient Supplements*. Washington, DC: National Academies Press, 1990.
8. Institute of Medicine, Food and Nutrition Board. *Dietary Reference Intakes for Energy, Carbohydrate, Fiber, Fat, Fatty Acids, Cholesterol, Protein, and Amino Acids*. Washington, DC: National Academies Press, 2005.
9. American Dietetic Association. Position of the American Dietetic Association: nutrition and lifestyle for a healthy pregnancy outcome. *J Am Diet Assoc*. 2008;108(3):553–561.
10. US Department of Agriculture. Nutrition program facts. Food and Nutrition Service. 2009. http://www.fns.usda.gov/wic/wic-fact-sheet.pdf. Accessed April 21, 2011.
11. American College of Obstetricians and Gynecologists. Committee on Practice Bulletins—Obstetrics. ACOG practice bulletin. Diagnosis and management of preeclampsia and eclampsia. *Obstet Gynecol*. 2002;99(33):159–167.
12. American Diabetes Association. Nutrition recommendations and interventions for diabetes. *Diabetes Care*. 2007;30(suppl 1):S4–S40.
13. Singh S, Darroch JE. Adolescent pregnancy and childbearing: levels and trends in developed countries. *Fam Plan Perspect*. 2000;32(1):14–23.
14. Ventura SJ, Mathews TJ, Hamilton BE. Births to teenagers in the United States, 1940–2000. *Nat Vital Stats Rept*. 2001;49(10).
15. Hoffman SD. *Kids having kids: economic costs and social consequences of teen pregnancy*. Washington, DC: The Urban Institute Press, 2008.
16. Greenfield SF, Manwani SG, Nargiso JE. Epidemiology of substance use disorders in women. *Obstet Gynecol Clin North Am*. 2003;30:413–446.
17. Bolnick JM, Rayburn WK. Substance use during pregnancy. *Obstet Gynecol Clin North Am*. 2003;30:545–558.
18. Duffy VB, Sigman-Grant M. Position of the American Dietetic Association: use of nutritive and nonnutritive sweeteners. *J Am Diet Assoc*. 2004;104:255–275.
19. Gillman MW, Rifas-Shiman SL, Kleinman K, Oken E, Rich-Edwards JW, Taveras EM. Developmental origins of childhood overweight: potential public health impact. *Obesity*. 2001;16(7):1651–1656.
20. Lamb MM, Dabelea D, Yin X, et al. Early-life predictors of higher body mass index in healthy children. *Ann Nutr Metab*. 2010;56(1):16–22.
21. Dabelea K, Hanson RL, Lindsay RS, et al. Intrauterine exposure to diabetes conveys risks for type 2 diabetes and obesity: a study of discordant sibships. *Diabetes*. 2000;49(12):2208–2211.
22. Li R, Darling N, Maruie E, Barker L, Grummer-Strawn LM. Breastfeeding rates in the United States by characteristics of the child, mother, or family: the 2002 national immunization survey. *Pediatrics*. 2005;115:e31–e37.
23. Duncan B, Ey J, Holberg CJ, et al. Exclusive breast-feeding for at least 4 months protects against otitis media. [see comment]. *Pediatrics*. 1993;91(5):867–872.
24. Howie PW, Forsyth JS, Ogston SA, et al. Protective effect of breast feeding against infection. *BMJ*. 1990;300(6716):11–16.
25. Teele DW, Klein JO, Rosner B. Epidemiology of otitis media during the first seven years of life in children in greater Boston: a prospective, cohort study. *J Infect Dis*. 1989;160(1):83–94.
26. Bachrach VR, Schwarz E, Bachrach LR. Breastfeeding and the risk of hospitalization for respiratory disease in infancy: a meta-analysis. *Arch Pediatr Adolesc Med*. 2003;157(3):237–243
27. Chien PF, Howie PW. Breast milk and the risk of opportunistic infection in infancy in industrialized and non-industrialized settings. *Adv Nutr Res*. 2001;10:69–104.
28. Lucas A, Cole TJ. Breast milk and neonatal necrotising enterocolitis. *Lancet*. 1990;336:1519–1523.
29. Owen CG, Martin RM, Whincup PH, et al. Does breastfeeding influence risk of type 2 diabetes in later life? A quantitative analysis of published evidence. *Am J Clin Nutr*. 2006;84(5):1043–1054.

30. Mitchell EA, Tuohy PG, Brunt JM, et al. Risk factors for sudden infant death syndrome following the prevention campaign in New Zealand: a prospective study. *Pediatrics*. 1997;100(5):835–840.
31. Bernier MO, PluBureau G, Bossard N, et al. Breastfeeding and risk of breast cancer: a metaanalysis of published studies. *Hum Reprod Update*. 2000;6(4):374–386.
32. Collaborative Group on Hormonal Factors in Breast Cancer. Breast cancer and breastfeeding: collaborative reanalysis of individual data from 47 epidemiological studies in 30 countries, including 50,302 women with breast cancer and 96,973 women without the disease. *Lancet*. 2002;360:187–195.
33. Lipworth L, Bailey LR, Trichopoulos D. History of breast-feeding in relation to breast cancer risk: a review of the epidemiologic literature. *J Natl Cancer Inst*. 2000;92(4):302–312.
34. Whittemore AS, Harris R, Itnyre J. Characteristics relating to ovarian cancer risk: collaborative analysis of 12 U.S. case-control studies. II. Invasive ovarian cancers in white women. Collaborative Ovarian Cancer Group. *Am J Epidemiol*. 1992;136:1184–1203.
35. Stuebe AM, Rich-Edwards JW, Willett WC, et al. Duration of lactation and incidence of type 2 diabetes. *JAMA*. 2005;294(20):2601–2610.
36. Arenz S, Ruckerl R, Koletzko B, von Kries R. Breastfeeding and childhood obesity—a systematic review. *Int J Obes Relat Metab Disord*. 2004;28:1247–1256.
37. Owen CG, Martin RM, Whincup PH, et al. Effect of infant feeding on the risk of obesity across the life course: a quantitative review of published evidence. *Pediatrics*. 2005;115:1367–1377.
38. Harder T, Bergmann R, Kallischnigg G, Plagemann A. Duration of breastfeeding and risk of overweight: a meta-analysis. *Am J Epidemiol*. 2005; 162:397–403.
39. Lucas A, Boyes S, Bloom R, Aynsley-Green A. Metabolic and endocrine responses to a milk feed in six-day-old term infants: differences between breast and cow's milk formula feeding. *Acta Paediatr Scand*. 1981;70:195–200.
40. Odeleye OE, de Courten M, Pettitt DJ, Ravussin E. Fasting hyperinsulinemia is a predictor of increased body weight gain and obesity in Pima Indian children. *Diabetes*. 1997;46:1341–1345.
41. Fisher JO, Birch LL, Smiciklas-Wright H, Picciano MF. Breast-feeding through the first year predicts maternal control in feeding and subsequent toddler energy intakes. *J Am Diet Assoc*. 2000;100:641–646.
42. Singer MR, Moore LL, Garrahie EJ, Ellison RC. The tracking of nutrient intake in young children: The Framingham Children's Study. *Am J Pub Hlth*. 1995;85:1673–1677.
43. Public health Service, US Department of Health and Human Services. *Mid-Term Review of Nutrition Objectives 2000*. Washington, DC: Government Publishing Office, 1994.
44. Centers for Disease Control and Prevention. Iron deficiency—United States, 1999–2000. *MMWR*. 2002;51:897–920.
45. Ogden CL, Carroll MD, Curtin LR, Lamb MM, Flegal KM. Prevalence of high body mass index in US children and adolescents, 2007–2008. *JAMA*. 2010;303(3):242–249.
46. Guo SS, Chumlea W. Tracking of body mass in children in relation to overweight in adulthood. *Am J Clin Nutr*. 1999;70:145S–148S.
47. Must, A, Jacques PF, Dallal GE, Bajema CJ, Dietz WH. Long-term morbidity and mortality of overweight adolescents. A follow-up of the Harvard Growth Study of 1922 to 1935. *NEJM*. 1992;327:1350–1355.
48. Whitaker RC, Wright JA, Pepe MS, Seidel KD, Dietz WH. Predicting obesity in young adulthood from childhood and parental obesity. *NEJM*. 1997;337:869–873.
49. Munoz KA, Krebs-Smith SM, Ballard-Barbash R, Cleveland LE. Food intakes of US children and adolescents compares with recommendations. *Pediatrics*. 1997;100(3 pt 1):323–339.
50. Fox MK, Pac S, Devaney B, Jankowski L. Feeding Infants and Toddlers Study: what foods are infants and toddlers eating? *J Am Diet Assoc*. 2004;104:S22–S30.
51. Dennison BA, Rockwell HL, Baker SL. Fruit and vegetable intake in young children. *J Am Coll Nutr*. 1998;17:371–378.
52. Ludwig DS, Peterson KE, Gortmaker SL. Relationship between consumption of sugar-sweetened drinks and childhood obesity: a prospective, observational analysis. *Lancet*. 2001;357(9255):505–508.
53. Nielsen SJ, Siega-Riz AM, Popkin BM. Trends in energy intake in the US between 1977 and 1996: Similar shifts seen across age groups. *Obes Res*. 2002;10:370–378.
54. Morton JF, Guthrie JF. Changes in children's total fat intakes and their food group sources of fat, 1989–91 versus 1994–95: implications for diet quality. *Family Econ Nutr Rev*. 1998;11:45–57.
55. Carlson A, Lino M, Gerrior S, Basiotis P. Report card on the diet quality of children ages 2 to 9. *Nutrition Insights*, USDA Center for Policy and Promotion. September 2001.
56. Gidding SS, Lihtenstein AH, Faith MS, et al. Implementing American Heart Association Pediatric and Adult Nutrition Guidelines. *Circulation*. 2009;119:1161–1175.
57. Wardle J. Parental influences on children's diets. *Proc Nutr Soc*. 1995;54:747–758.
58. Hursti UKK. Factors influencing children's food choice. *Ann Med*. 1999;31(suppl 1):S26–S32.
59. Burt JV, Hertzler AA. Parental influences on the child's food preference. *J Nutr*. 1978;10:127–128.
60. Koivisto HUK. Factors influencing children's food choice. *Annu Med*. 1999;31(suppl 1):S26–S32.

61. Crockett JS, Sims LS. Environmental influences on children's eating. *J Nutr Ed*. 1995;27:235–249.
62. Nicklas TA, Baranowski T, Baranowski J, Cullen K, Rittenberry L, Olvera N. Family and child-care provider influences on preschool children's fruit, juice, and vegetable consumption. *Nutr Rev*. 2001; 59:224–235.
63. Satter E. *How to Get Your Kid to Eat But Not Too Much*. Boulder, CO: Bull Publishing, 1987.
64. Cashdan E. A sensitive period for learning about food. *Human Nature*. 1994;5:279–291.
65. Nicklaus S, Boggio V, Chabane C, Issanchou S. A prospective study of food variety seeking in childhood, adolescence and early adult life. *Appetite*. 2005;44:289–297.
66. Pelchat ML, Pliner P. Antecedents and correlates of feeding problems in young children. *J Nutr Ed*. 1986;18:23–29.
67. Cooke LJ, Wardle J. Age and gender differences in children's food preferences. *Bri J Nutr*. 2005;93:741–746.
68. Rosenstein D, Oster H. Differential facial responses to four basic tastes in newborns. *Child Dev*. 1988;59:1555–1568.
69. Kaijura H, Cowart BJ, Beauchamp GK. Early developmental change in bitter taste responses in human infants. *Dev Psychobiology*. 1992;25:375–386.
70. Birch LL, McPhee L, Shoba BC, Pirok E, Steinberg L. What kind of exposure reduces children's food neophobia? Looking vs. tasting. *Appetite*. 1987;9:171–178.
71. Zajonc RB. Mere exposure: a gateway to the subliminal. *Curr Dir Psychol Sci*. 2001;10:224–228.
72. Skinner JD, Carruth BR, Bounds W, Ziegler PJ. Children's food preferences: A longitudinal analysis. *J Am Diet Assoc*. 2002;102:1638–1647.
73. Pelchat ML, Pline P. "Try it. You'll like it." Effects of information on willingness to try novel foods. *Appetite*. 1995; 24:153–166.
74. Wardle J, Herrera ML, Cooke L, Gibson EL. Modifying children's food preferences: the effects of exposure and reward on acceptance of an unfamiliar vegetable. *Eur J Clin Nutr*. 2003;57:341–348.
75. Koplan JP, Liverman CT, Draak VI. *Preventing Childhood Obesity: Health in the Balance*. Washington, DC: National Academies Press, 2005.
76. Story M, Kaphingst KM, French S. the role of schools in obesity prevention. *Future Child*. 2006; 16:109–142.
77. Institute of Medicine Committee on Nutrition Standards for National School Lunch and Breakfast Programs. *School Meals: Building Blocks for Healthy Children*. Washington, DC: The National Academies Press, 2010.
78. O'Tools TP, Anderson S, Miller C, Guthrie J. Nutrition services and foods and beverages available at school: Results from the school health policies and programs study 2006. *J Sch Health*. 2007;77:500–521.
79. Allen P, Guthman J. From "old school" to "farm-to-school": neoliberalization from the ground up. *Agic Human Values*. 2006;23:401–415.
80. Urban Environmental Policy Institute. Farm to school. http://www.farmtoschool.org. Accessed April 13, 2010.
81. Izumi BT, Alaimo K, Hamm MW. Farm-to-school programs: perspectives of school food service professionals. *J Nutr Educ Behav*. 2010;42:83–91.
82. Diet, Nutrition, and the Prevention of Chronic Diseases: Report of a joint WHO/FAO expert consultation. WHO Technical Report Series 916. Geneva: World Health Organization, 2003. http://whqlibdoc.who.int/trs/WHO_TRS_916.pdf. Accessed April 21, 2010.
83. Kelder SH, Perry CL, Klepp KI, Lytle LL. Longitudinal tracking of adolescent smoking, physical activity, and food choice behaviors. *Am J Public Health*. 1994;84:1121–1126.
84. Larson NI, Neumark-Sztainer D, Hannan PJ, Story M. Family meals during adolescence are associated with higher diet quality and healthful meal patterns during young adulthood. *J Am Diet Assoc*. 2007;107:1502–1510.
85. Nielsen SJ, Siega-Riz AM, Popkin BM. Trends in food locations and sources among adolescents and young adults. *Prev Med*. 2002;35:107–113.
86. Nielsen SJ, Siega-Riz AM, Popkin BM. Trends in energy intake in US between 1977 and 1996: similar shifts seen across age groups. *Obes Res*. 2002;10:370–378.
87. Cavadini C, Siega-Riz AM, Popkin BM. US adolescent food intake trends from 1965 to 1996. *Arch Dis Child*. 2000;83:18–24.
88. Larson NI, Neumark-Sztainer D, Hannan PJ, Story M. Trends in adolescent fruit and vegetable consumption, 1999–2004: Project EAT. *Am J Prev Med*. 2007;32(2):147–150.
89. Bowman SA, Gortmaker SL, Ebbeling CB, Pereira MA, Ludwig DS. Effects of fast-food consumption on energy intake and diet quality among children in a national household survey. *Pediatrics*. 2004;113:112–118.
90. French SA, Story M, Neumark-Sztainer D, Fulkerson JA, Hannan P. Fast food restaurant use among adolescents: Associations with nutrient intake, food choices and behavioral and psychosocial variables. *Int J Obes*. 2001;25:1823–1833.
91. Paeratakul S, Ferdinand DP, Champagne CM, Ryan DH, Bray GA. Fast-food consumption among US adults and children: Dietary and nutrient intake profile. *J Am Diet Assoc*. 2003;103:1332–1338.
92. Schmidt M, Affenito SG, Striegel-Moore R, et al. Fast-food intake and diet quality in black and white girls: The National Heart, Lung, and Blood Institute Growth and Health Study. *Arch Pediatr Adolesc Med*. 2005;159:626–631.

93. Ogden CL, Carroll MD, Curtin LR, McDowell MA, Tabak CJ, Flegal KM. Prevalence of overweight and obesity in the United States, 1999–2004. *JAMA*. 2006;295:1549–1555.
94. Rodriguez BL, Fujimoto WY, Mayer-Davis EJ, et al. Prevalence of cardiovascular disease risk factors in US children and adolescents with diabetes: The SEARCH for diabetes in youth study. *Diabetes Care*. 2006;29:1891–1896.
95. Hudson JI, Hiripi E, Pope HG, Kessler RC. The prevalence and correlates of eating disorders in the national comorbidity survey replication. *Biol Psychiatry*. 2007;61(3):348–358.
96. American Psychiatric Association. *Diagnostic and Statistical Manual of Mental Disorders*, 4th ed (DSM-IV). Washington, DC: American Psychiatric Association, 1994.
97. Lucas AR, Beard CM, O'Fallon WM, et al. 50-year trends in the incidence of anorexia nervosa in Rochester, Minn.: a population-based study. *Am J Psychiatry*. 1991;148:917–922.
98. Inagaki T, Horiguchi J, Tsubouchi K, Miyaoka T, Uegaki J, Seno H. Late onset anorexia nervosa: two case reports. *Int J Psychiatry Med*. 2002;32(1):91–95.
99. Beck D, Casper R, Andersen A. Truly late onset of eating disorders: a study of 11 cases averaging 60 years of age at presentation. *Int J Eat Disord*. 1996;20(4):389–395.
100. Kaye WH, Bulik CM, Hornton L, Barbarich N, Masters K. Comorbidity of anxiety disorders with anorexia and bulimia nervosa. *Am J Psychiatry*. 2004;161(12):2215–2221.
101. Yager J, Devlin MJ, Halmi KA, et al. *Practice Guideline for the Treatment of Patients with Eating Disorders*, 3rd ed. Arlington, VA: American Psychiatric Association, 2006. http://www.psychiatryonline.com/pracGuide/PracticePDFs/EatingDisorders3ePG_04-28-06.pdf. Accessed April 19, 2011.
102. US Department of Health and Human Services, National Institutes of Health, National Institute for Mental Health. *Eating Disorders*. Publication No. 07-4901. 2007
103. Berkman ND, Lohr KN, Bulik CM. Outcomes of eating disorders: a systematic review of the literature. *Inter J Eating Dis*. 2007;40(4):293–308.
104. Villareal DT, Apovian CM, Kushner RF, Klein. Obesity in older adults: technical review and position statement of the American Society for Nutrition and NAASO, the obesity society. *Am J Clin Nutr*. 2005;82:923–934.
105. National Institutes of Health. NIH senior health. http://nihseniorhealth.gov/. Accessed April 20, 2011.
106. Ervin RB. Healthy eating index scores among adults, 60 years of age and over, by sociodemographic and health characteristics: United States, 1999–2002. *Adv Data*. 2008;20(395):1–16.
107. Tzankoff SP, Norris AH. Effect of muscle mass decrease on age-related BMR changes. *J Appl Physiol*. 1977;43:1001–1006.
108. Shelnutt KP, Bobroff LB, Diehl DC. MyPyramid for older adults. *J Nutr Ed Behav*. 2009;41(4):300–302.
109. Moore C, Murphy MM, Keast DR, Holick MF. Vitamin D intake in the United States. *J Am Diet Assoc*. 2004;104:980–983.
110. Lichtenstein AH, Rasmussen, Yu WW, Epstein SR, Russell RM. Modified MyPyramid for older adults. *J Nutr*. 2008;138:5–11.
111. McCay CM. Cellulose in the diet of mice and rats. *J Nutr*. 1935:435–447.
112. Sinclair DA. Toward a unified theory of caloric restriction and longevity regulation. *Mech Aging Dev*. 2005;126:987–1002.
113. Fontana L, Klein S. Aging, adiposity, and calorie restriction. *JAMA*. 2001;297:986–994.
114. Armstrong D. A survey of community gardens in upstate New York: implications for health promotion and community development. *Health Place*. 2000;6:319–327.
115. Saldivar-Tanaka L, Krasny M. Culturing community development, neighborhood open space, and civic agriculture: the case of Latino community gardens in New York City. *Agric Human Values*. 2004;21:399–412.
116. Schukoske JE. Community development through gardening: state and local policies transforming urban open space. *Leg Public Pol*. 2000;351:351–392.
117. Ferris J, Norman C, Sempik J. People, land, and sustainability: community gardens and the social dimension of sustainable development. *Soc Policy Admin*. 2001;35:559–568.
118. Twiss J, Dickinson J, Duma S, Kleinman T, Paulsen H, Riveria L. Community gardens: lessons learned from California Healthy Cities and Communities. *Am J Public Health*. 2003;93:1435–1438.
119. Glover TD. Social capital in the lived experiences of community gardeners. *Leisure Sci*. 2004;26:143–162.
120. Been V, Voicu I. The effect of community gardens on neighboring property values. New York: New York University School of Law, NYU Center for Law and Economics, 2006. Working Paper No. 06-09.
121. Alaimo k, Packnett E, Miles RA, Kruger DJ. Fruit and vegetable intake among urban community gardeners. *J Nutr Educ Behav*. 2008;40:94–101.
122. Zenk SN, Schulz AJ, Israel BA, James SA, Bao S, Wilson ML. Fruit and vegetable access differs by community racial composition and socioeconomic position in Detroit, Michigan. *Ethn Dis*. 2006;16:275–280.
123. Zenk SN, Schulz AJ, Hollis-Neely T, et al. Fruit and vegetable intake in African Americans: income and store characteristics. *Am J Prev Med*. 2005;29:1–9.

124. Baxter SD, Thompson WO. Fourth-grade children's consumption of fruit and vegetable items available as part of school lunches is closely related to preferences. *J Nutr Ed Behav*. 2002;34:166–171.

125. Cullen KW, Baranowski T, Owens E, Marsh T, Rittenberry L, de Moor C. Availability, accessibility, and preferences for fruit, 100% fruit juice, and vegetables influence children's dietary behavior. *Health Ed Behav*. 2003;30:615–626.

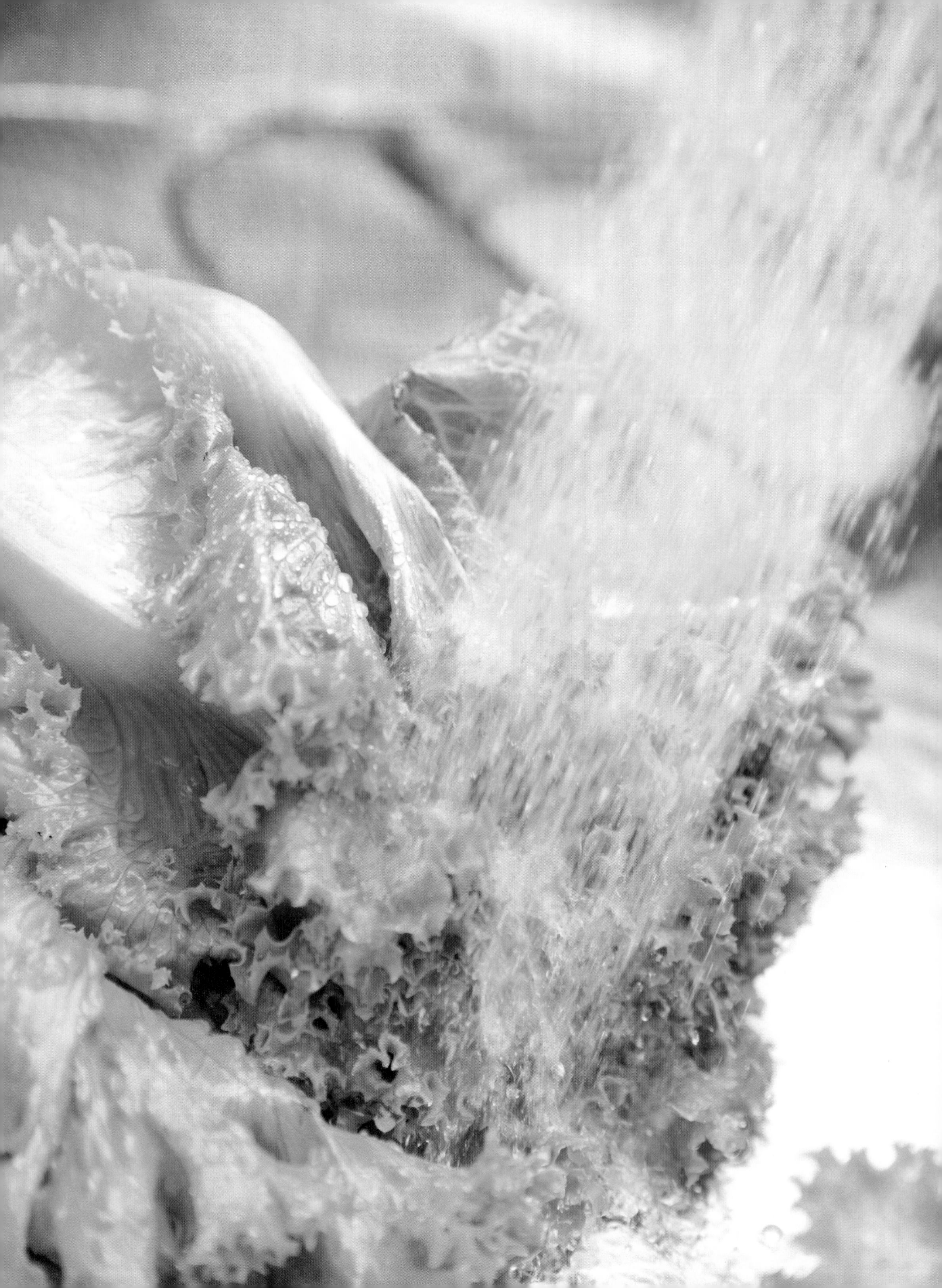

Chapter 14

Safety of the Food Supply: Keep Your Food Safe

Key Messages

- The three types of food risks are physical, chemical, and biological.
- The Food and Drug Association, the U.S. Department of Agriculture, and the Environmental Protection Agency work together to keep our food and water safe.
- The basic food safety rules of clean, separate, cook, and chill can help the home cook keep food safe.
- Certain populations are at increased risk of foodborne illness and should take special precautions.

What does it mean to have "safe" food? Food safety has many meanings. To some, it means food that is organic or produced with only natural pesticides. To others, it means food that is fresh and not spoiled. To others still, it means food that does not contain harmful bacteria and viruses that could cause serious illness. Literally, *food safety* means food that does not cause a health risk. How do you know which foods are safe? Simply looking at a food does not always work. Spoiled foods such as molded bread or cheese that look unsafe usually do not present a health risk, but some foods that may appear normal may not be safe to eat. What can you do when you shop, prepare, and store food to keep it safe? How can you make informed decisions about what foods to choose for the sake of food safety? What about all the foodborne-illness outbreaks you hear about on the news? Is there anything to learn from these, or is it just to scare us into not eating certain foods? In this chapter, you will explore all of these questions as well as learn kitchen skills to keep your food safe.

Story

George is learning to cook. He is tired of pizza and burgers and wants to try his hand at cooking some simple meals for himself and his girlfriend. He likes to grill outside when the weather is nice and is getting good at barbeque chicken. His usual routine is to come home from class, take the chicken out of the freezer, and put it on the counter to thaw while he goes to the gym. When he gets back, he marinates the chicken in barbeque sauce for about an hour on the counter while it finishes thawing. He takes the chicken to the grill on a cutting board. While the chicken cooks, he makes a salad to go with the meal. He turns the chicken once and cooks it until he thinks it is done. The meal is complete with the barbeque chicken, salad, and the rest of the marinade as a dipping sauce. George is to be commended for his foray into the culinary world. However, he has broken some cardinal rules of food safety. What tips can you give Geroge to help him keep him and his girlfriend from getting a foodborne illness?

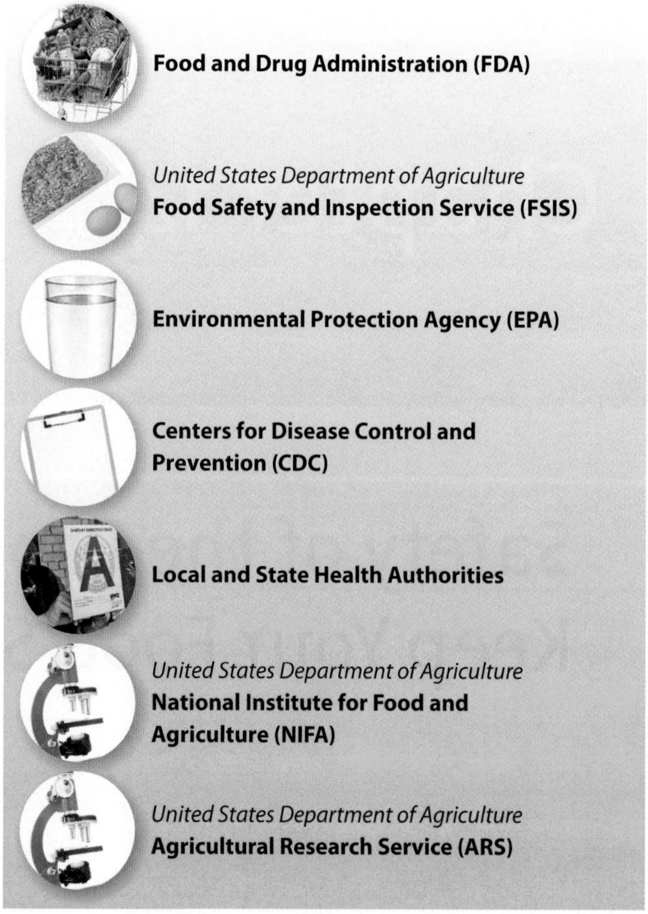

Figure 14.1

Government Agencies Work Together to Keep the Food Supply Safe

Oversight to Keep the Food Supply Safe

The coordination of keeping food safe requires several government agencies working together from farm to fork (**Figure 14.1**). Regulations and oversight are required at the farm, at the processing plant, during transportation, and at the point of sale. In the case of prepared foods, additional regulations are required for restaurants and other establishments that prepare food to ensure food safety. The following are the key federal agencies tasked with the safety of the U.S. food supply:

- **Food and Drug Administration (FDA).** The FDA is responsible for protecting the public health by ensuring the safety, efficacy, and security of the nation's food supply. The FDA is responsible for ensuring the safety of domestic and imported foods, except meat, poultry, and catfish, which are regulated by the USDA.
- **U.S. Department of Agriculture Food Safety and Inspection Service (FSIS).** The FSIS is the public health agency responsible for ensuring that the nation's commercial supply of meat, poultry, and egg products is safe, wholesome, and correctly labeled and packaged.
- **Environmental Protection Agency (EPA).** The EPA protects human health and the environment. The EPA regulates public drinking water supplies and approves pesticides and other chemicals that can be used in the environment.
- **Centers for Disease Control and Prevention (CDC).** The CDC monitors foodborne illnesses and investigates the causes of outbreaks. The CDC uses information gathered in its investigations to determine how outbreaks can be prevented in the future.

- **State and local health authorities.** In addition to these federal agencies, state and local health authorities oversee food safety in their area. They often work with federal agencies to make sure foods grown and produced in their area follow food safety standards. Restaurant inspection requirements vary from state to state, but often fall under local or state departments of health. Many states provide consumers with a grading system so that they can easily see how a restaurant did on inspection.

HACCP

The Hazard Analysis and Critical Control Point (HACCP) system was developed as a result of the need to have safe food for the space program. Although only a few men and women ever travel in space, HACCP has helped all of us have a safer food supply. HACCP is a food safety management tool used to control significant hazards. It functions by designing food safety into a product and controlling the process by which that product is produced. The HACCP method focuses on preventing hazards and relies on proven scientific principles of food safety. By law, the use of HACCP is required for seafood, juice, and meat. However, many other food manufacturers use the HACCP principles as their food safety program.

HACCP includes conducting a hazard analysis and identifying critical points in production. Plans are then put in place to control those critical points with specific limits of tolerance. A plan is put in place for correcting procedures if the tolerance limits are not met. HACCP also provides for record keeping so that data are available on the methods used.

Food Safety Research and Education

Food safety research is imperative to continue to inform everyone from farm to fork how to keep food safe. The National Institutes for Health, the USDA Agricultural Research Service (ARS), and other federal agencies fund research on food safety. The food industry also performs a great deal of research on food safety. The food industry has an interest in the best food safety practices to ensure that they are producing safe, high-quality products.

The USDA National Institute of Food and Agriculture (NIFA) supports research, education, and extension activities that address current priority issues in food safety. NIFA provides food safety education directly to consumers through the Cooperative Extension System. The Partnership for Food Safety Education (PFSE) informs consumers about the important steps they can take to reduce the risk of foodborne illness. Its Fight BAC campaign (**Figure 14.2**) is used by educators across the country to help consumers learn the basics of good food safety.

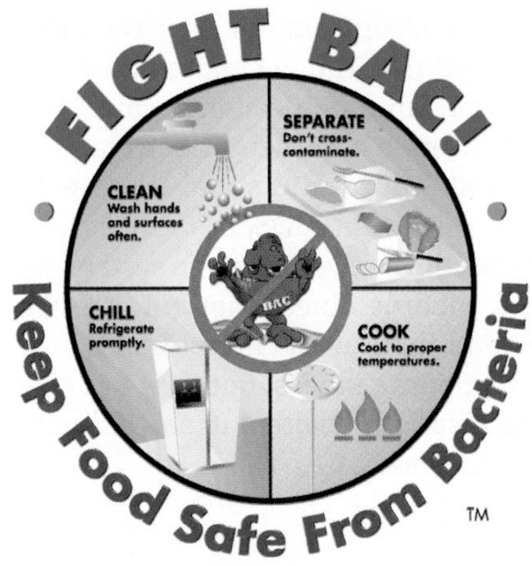

Clean: Wash hands and surfaces often
Separate: Don't cross-contaminate
Cook: Cook to safe temperature
Chill: Refrigerate properly

Figure 14.2

Fight BAC!

The Fight BAC! program encourages people to follow four basic food safety practices: clean, separate, cook, and chill.

Source: Illustration courtesy of Partnership for Food Safety Education. http://www.fightbac.org.

How Prevalent Is Foodborne Illness?

Foodborne illness is sickness caused by food that is contaminated with microorganisms, chemicals, or other substances harmful to human health. Foodborne illness affects more than 38 million people in the United States each year, resulting in more than 50,000 hospitalizations and 1,351 deaths.[1] This means that roughly four people die every day in the United States because of foodborne illness. The annual cost of foodborne illness is estimated at $152 billion.[2] The **World Health Organization** reports that up to 30% of individuals in developed countries acquire illness from food or water annually.[3]

In addition to the reported and documented cases of foodborne illness, many other cases go unreported. Often a foodborne illness is attributed to a stomach virus, because symptoms (vomiting, cramping, and diarrhea) are similar for both. Many foodborne illnesses take days to manifest, making it very difficult to isolate the offending food. Even if a case of foodborne illness is reported to public health authorities, there may be no clear link to the food that could have caused it, and thus it may not get counted as a foodborne illness.[4]

TERMS

foodborne illness Any illness that is caused by consuming food that is contaminated by a pathogen; commonly called *food poisoning*.

World Health Organization The public health arm of the United Nations; monitors disease outbreaks and assesses the performance of health systems around the world.

Everyone is at risk of foodborne illness. However, some groups are at an increased risk. Young children are at an increased risk because their immune systems may not be fully formed. Pregnant women and their unborn fetuses are also at increased risk. Older adults and those with chronic illnesses such as cancer, AIDS, or other health problems that may compromise their immune system are at increased risk for foodborne illness. Not only are the young, pregnant, old, and those with chronic conditions more susceptible to foodborne illness, but they are also at a much greater risk of serious health outcomes should they acquire a foodborne illness.

Substances in Food That Can Be Harmful

What causes foodborne illness? Foods can carry three types of substances that can cause harm to humans: biological, chemical, and physical. Biological contaminants include pathogens, which are bacteria, viruses, and parasites that cause illness. Chemical contaminants include pesticides, pollutants, and natural toxins. Finally, physical contaminants include nonfood substances such as glass, staples, or wood.

Pathogens

Pathogens are responsible for most foodborne illnesses in North America. Foodborne pathogenic microorganisms include bacteria, viruses, and parasites. Although most foodborne illnesses caused by **pathogens** result in a few days of misery of vomiting and diarrhea, others can be much more severe. A pathogen may be introduced into a food as it is produced or it may grow to harmful levels due to improper handling of a food. For example, a cooked hamburger may be fine to consume at 2 PM, but if left unrefrigerated until 7 PM it may contain bacteria in large enough numbers to cause foodborne illness. The warm environment allows bacteria to grow to numbers that can cause a foodborne illness. Foods can also become contaminated with human or animal feces that contain bacteria. Improper hand washing after using the toilet, improperly handled tomatoes fertilized with animal manure, vegetables cut on a cutting board that had raw meat, all have the possibility of causing contamination that can lead to foodborne illness.

The most common form of foodborne illness is caused by norovirus. Norovirus can be found in foods such as fresh produce and raw or undercooked shellfish. However, the usual transmission is from food handlers. Norovirus is highly contagious and can be easily passed from person to person with food as the vehicle. If a food worker is infected with norovirus and she comes to work, doesn't use good food safety practices, such as proper hand washing, and you eat a sandwich she made—you are likely to get norovirus. Luckily, unless you are **immunocompromised**, you will have a few days of illness but will recover.

Many different organisms can cause foodborne illness. Several other common pathogens that cause foodborne illness are *Campylobacter*, *Salmonella*, and *E. coli* O157:H7.[5] See **Table 14.1** for a summary of common pathogens found in food.

Chemical Contaminants

Chemical contamination includes pesticides, drugs, pollutants, and natural toxins. Most food safety experts agree that the threat to human health is far greater from pathogens in food than from chemical contaminants. Nonetheless, consumers continue to turn to foods produced using organic methods that limit the use of manmade chemicals. Organic produce cultivated with natural pesticides and fertilizer, milk produced without hormones or antibiotics, eggs from chickens fed organic diets, all are available and popular in the marketplace. All are being sold to consumers who want fewer manmade chemicals in their food. More specific details on organic fruits and vegetables, organic meat, and organic milk can be found in Chapters 6, 8, and 9.

Pesticides Pesticides are used to increase crop yields. They protect plants against disease and insects, as well as control weeds. The FDA sets standards for acceptable levels of pesticides on food. Since 1987, the FDA has collected and analyzed samples from domestic and imported fruits and vegetables. Results from these reports continue to demonstrate that levels of pesticide residues in the U.S. food supply are well below established safety standards.[10]

Children and infants are particularly vulnerable to hazards associated with pesticide residues. To address this, Congress passed the **Food Quality Protection Act** in 1996, the most comprehensive of the pesticide and food safety laws passed in recent decades. Some of the major requirements of the law are stricter safety standards, especially for infants and children, and a complete reassessment of all existing pesticide tolerances.[11]

Drugs Many drugs are used to keep food-producing animals healthy and disease free and to increase production. The FDA is responsible for monitoring what drugs can be used in animals that produce meat, milk, or eggs. It is also responsible for monitoring how much of any given drug ends up in a particular food and making sure the level

TERMS

pathogen An agent, such as a bacteria or virus, that causes disease or illness.

immunocompromised A person who is less capable of fighting infection due to an immune system that is impaired because of illness, life stage, or treatment for illness.

Food Quality Protection Act Federal law that mandates health-based standards for pesticides used in foods.

Table 14.1

Pathogens That Cause Foodborne Illness

Organism	Most Common Sources	Illness
Bacteria		
*Campylobacter**	Raw or undercooked poultry	Campylobacteriosis: fever, diarrhea, and abdominal cramps
Clostridium botulinum	Improperly canned food, garlic in oil, honey (acid in the stomach kills the small amount present; honey should not be given to infants for this reason)	Botulism (rare): progressive paralysis, can lead to death
Escherichia coli O157:H7 (*E. coli*)*	Raw or undercooked meat, vegetables contaminated with fecal matter	*E. coli* infection: bloody diarrhea, painful abdominal cramps, especially dangerous in young children and can cause kidney failure and death
Listeria	Soft cheese, unpasteurized milk, luncheon meats	Listeriosis: fever, nausea, vomiting; more common in pregnant women, infants, older adults, and people with compromised immune systems
*Salmonella**	Raw or undercooked meat, poultry, or eggs; raw sprouts; foods containing raw eggs	Salmonellosis: diarrhea, stomach cramps, fever, vomiting
Shigella	Water or food contaminated with feces	Shigellosis (bacillary dysentery): diarrhea, fever, stomach cramps, vomiting, blood in stools
Virus		
Hepatitis A	Food handled by infected person, raw shellfish from polluted water	Hepatitis A: nausea, vomiting, and fever; after 3–10 days, jaundice and darkened urine
Norwalk*	Foods handled by infected person	Gastroenteritis: vomiting, diarrhea
Parasites		
Cryptosporidia	Food or water contaminated with feces	Cryptosporidiosis: watery diarrhea, vomiting, fever
Giardia lamblia	Food or water contaminated with feces	Giardiasis: diarrhea, abdominal cramps, nausea

*Most common

is safe. If a producer uses antibiotics, regulations govern how they can be administered and how much can be used. Some are concerned that overuse of antibiotics in animals will result in antibiotic-resistant strains of bacteria. The FDA has urged producers to decrease the amount of antibiotics used on animals for this reason, stating that is poses a public health threat. It suggests that antibiotics should only be used on animals that are sick, not on all animals just to boost production.[12] These are just suggestions and are not yet regulations that must be used by food producers.

Hormones are another class of drugs used in animals. Of course, all animals have hormones naturally, so hormone-free products means free of added or synthetic hormones. Hormones are not allowed in pork or poultry production. Packages of chicken, turkey, other poultry, or pork cannot be labeled "hormone-free," because the use of hormones is not allowed. Hormones are allowed in beef and lamb production. It is not clear how these added hormones affect human health. Some evidence suggests that added hormones in beef may be one of the reasons that increased consumption of red meat increases the risk of breast and other cancers.[13,14] Hormone levels in milk from cows that have been given hormones are very low and similar to those of cows not given hormones.[15,16] Without definitive evidence as to harm to human health, hormones are allowed under USDA regulations for beef and lamb.

Pollutants and Natural Toxins Although industrial waste, runoff from farms that raise livestock, and human sewage can all contaminate places where food is grown, natural toxins can also be a danger. Fungi, under certain temperature and humidity conditions, produce **aflatoxins**. The most common foods to be contaminated are tree nuts, peanuts, and corn. Consumption of too much aflatoxin in developed countries is not a big concern. However, in countries where food and water are frequently contaminated with the fungus, aflatoxin consumption is associated with a higher risk of liver cancer.[17]

Methyl mercury is a common natural toxin. Mercury is found throughout the environment, from both natural sources and human activity. Mercury can dissolve in water and is found in rivers, streams, and oceans. Bacteria change mercury into the more toxic form of methyl mercury. Methyl mercury can be found in many fish species; however, it is most concentrated in large fish that consume fish that have eaten plankton contaminated with methyl mercury. Shark, swordfish, and some species of tuna have high methyl mercury levels. See Chapter 8 for more on mercury in fish.

TERMS

aflatoxin Toxin produced by food molds.

Special Report

Anatomy of an Outbreak

Outbreaks of foodborne illnesses make the news, especially those that involve large numbers of people or those that are potentially life threatening. The following is an analysis of three famous foodborne illness outbreaks that made national headlines and prompted heightened awareness of the importance of food safety from farm to fork.

Jack in the Box Wakes up the Food Service Industry

In 1993, *E. coli* O157:H7 was probably only known to food safety experts and scientists. After the foodborne illness outbreak at Jack in the Box in Washington State, however, it was on the minds of parents across North America. As many as 600 people fell ill, many were hospitalized, and 3 children died from eating improperly cooked hamburger.[6] When the outbreak occurred, state law in Washington required hamburgers be cooked to 155°F; federal law required hamburgers be cooked to 140°F. Investigation by local health officials traced the *E. coli* O157:H7 outbreak to the Jack in the Box chain. Further investigation revealed that the company did not follow Washington State law because, according to Jack in the Box officials, "if patties are cooked longer ... they tend to be tough." The company made a conscious decision to disregard Washington State law. When the court case ensued, Jack in the Box indicated that it was following federal guidelines for cooking ground meat. However, investigators found that its hamburgers were not even up to the federal standard of 140°F, let alone the state guideline of 155°F. It was also revealed that there had been consistent customer complaints about undercooked meat prior to the outbreak. Jack in the Box was held accountable for the illness of 600 and death of 3 for disregarding proper food safety guidelines. It sent shockwaves through the food service industry and forever changed the way ground beef is cooked in restaurants—no one wants to be the next Jack in the Box.

How can you, as a consumer, learn from this outbreak? Cook ground meat products thoroughly in your kitchen or backyard grill. When eating out, don't eat ground meat that is not cooked thoroughly to the recommended temperature of 155°F for three seconds or 160°F for one second. Ask to have your burger cooked to 160°F. Although the color of meat is not an exact indication of temperature, unless you have a meat thermometer with you, checking that there is no pink showing in ground meat may be the only indication you have when eating away from home.

Norovirus: Easy to Spread, Hard to Stop

A national chain restaurant was the site of a norovirus outbreak in 2006.[7] It is estimated that half of the known cases of norovirus infection are spread by food service workers.[8] As you examine the cause of this outbreak, you'll see why so many cases of norovirus can be traced to restaurants. In this Michigan case, several food service workers were ill between January 19 and February 3. One of these workers was a line cook who vomited in the kitchen at the restaurant on January 28. After the initial outbreak of norovirus in many patrons, the restaurant took action. It discarded all foods, required all ill employees to remain home until they were symptom free for at least 72 hours, and scrubbed the facility thoroughly. However, patrons continued to get sick. Health department officials discovered that the restaurant had used ammonia for the cleaning solution. Ammonia is ineffective against norovirus. The restaurant had to be recleaned with a chlorine bleach solution to effectively kill the remaining norovirus particles.

This outbreak highlights the importance of food service workers not working while ill. It also highlights the importance of proper hygiene by all food handlers. As a consumer, you can learn from this outbreak as well. You should not prepare food when ill, and you should wash your hands thoroughly with soap and water often, especially after visiting the toilet. If you use alcohol-based hand sanitizers, make sure that you also wash your hands with soap and water, because alcohol-based sanitizers are ineffective against norovirus.

When Spinach Turns Deadly

In 2006, 205 people in 26 states became ill from *E. coli* O157:H7. Half of the infected people required hospitalization, and three people died. The offending food was prewashed, bagged spinach. A massive nationwide recall began, and the FDA quickly issued warnings about consuming raw, bagged spinach. Although the recall included several brands, the outbreak was isolated to one brand of baby spinach from one set of farms. The investigation as to how *E. coli* O157:H7 got into the spinach was intense. Product codes from bags of contaminated spinach were used along with DNA fingerprinting. Investigators were able to isolate the specific field that yielded the spinach that was contaminated.[9] The exact reason why the spinach in this field became infected with *E. coli* O157:H7 is still unknown, but it is speculated that feces from wild pigs contaminated the crop. Even thought the spinach was washed, there was not enough chlorine in the wash water to kill the amount of *E. coli* that was present. People then became ill from eating the raw spinach.

Outbreaks of foodborne illness have also occurred with other fruits and vegetables. Should the threat of foodborne illness keep you from eating produce? Although there is a risk associated with all foods, the benefits of fruits and vegetables far outweigh the potential risk. In the case of the spinach and several other outbreaks, the only thing you, as a consumer, could have done to kill pathogens in the food would be to cook the food. Although this is possible, eliminating salads or raw fruits and vegetables is not a feasible answer. Following good food-handling practices, purchasing fruits and vegetables from reputable sources, and heeding food safety warnings from the FDA and other government agencies is your best defense as a consumer. Fresh fruit and vegetable safety is an issue that continues to be studied as to best farming and packaging practices to eliminate food safety issues.

How Policy and Environment Affect My Choices

Restaurant Service of Partially Cooked or Raw Foods

Many different policies affect the safety of the food supply. Government regulations and oversight work to keep the North American food supply as safe as possible. One aspect of this oversight is the FDA's Food Code. The **Food Code** provides scientifically sound technical information for the retail and food service industry. Many state agencies use the Food Code as a model to develop or update their own food safety rules to be consistent with national food regulatory policy.

One such regulation is the temperature at which ground meat must be cooked. Although each state sets its own standards, almost all restaurants in the United States must cook ground meat to 155°F for 15 seconds or 160°F for 1 second.[18] Cooking the meat to this temperature has been shown to kill bacteria that can cause severe foodborne illness, specifically *E. coli* O157:H7. The Food Code also suggests that if meat, poultry, seafood, shellfish, or eggs are not cooked to proper temperatures that the consumer be warned of the increased risk of foodborne illness.[18] Oysters on the half shell, steak tartar, eggs over easy, even rare hamburgers may still be on the menu in some states, but the consumer has to be informed of the increased risk of foodborne illness.

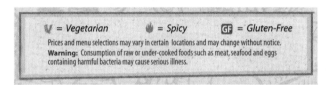

V = Vegetarian
= Spicy
GF = Gluten-Free
Prices and menu selections may vary in certain locations and may change without notice.
Warning: Consumption of raw or under-cooked foods such as meat, seafood and eggs containing harmful bacteria may cause serious illness.

Menu Warning for Raw or Undercooked Meat, Poultry, Seafood, Shellfish, or Eggs

Physical Contaminants

A physical contaminant in food is anything that can be visibly seen and is not part of the food originally. It is not clear how often physical contamination occurs, because problems are not usually reported unless major injuries occur. For example, you can probably recount finding a piece of plastic in your sandwich or a bug in your soup. Common physical contaminants include metal shards from kitchen equipment, staples from food containers, bugs (dead or alive), hair, and so on. You can take precautions in your home kitchen by keeping a watchful eye when preparing and storing food. When eating away from home, patronize establishments with a good sanitation rating.

Technology: Helping to Keep Food Safe

Technology has a large impact on the food we eat. Food science is used in the preservation, processing, packaging, and distribution of food. Technology has been an aspect of food production for more than a century. Without food technology, there would be no canned foods or packaged foods that were shelf-stable for more than a few days. Increasingly, technology is used to ensure that the foods available in the marketplace are safe. There is debate, however, about the risks and benefits associated with various technologies applied to food and whether the risks outweigh the benefits.

Food Preservatives

Preservatives are added to foods to prevent or delay spoilage, thus increasing the shelf life of food. Preservatives may inhibit the growth of bacteria or mold. Preservatives are regulated and monitored by the FDA. The FDA sets safety standards for the use of preservatives and determines whether a particular preservative is safe to use.

Examples of common preservatives are antioxidants, such as vitamin C and vitamin E, and sulfites. Two other common preservatives are butylated hydroxyanisole (BHA) and butylated hydroxytoluene (BHT). These preservatives are used to keep fats from going rancid. Some are concerned that BHA and BHT might increase the risk of cancer. However, the FDA states that there is no evidence that they are a health risk. The FDA continues to monitor the research on the impact of these and other preservatives on human health.

Food Irradiation

Food irradiation uses a source of ionizing energy that passes through food to destroy harmful bacteria and other organisms. Irradiation can destroy *E. coli* O157:H7, *Salmonella*, and *Campylobacter*. It can also destroy insects and parasites, prevent spoilage, and delay ripening of some fruits and vegetables. The FDA has approved the use of irradiation on spices and dry seasonings to control for insects and microorganisms, on fruits and vegetables to

TERMS

Food Code Guidelines released by the FDA every four years as a model for food safety for the retail and food service industry; used by local and state regulators to develop or update their own food safety rules to be consistent with national food regulatory policy.

food irradiation A food safety technology that eliminates pathogens from foods by treating food with ionizing radiation.

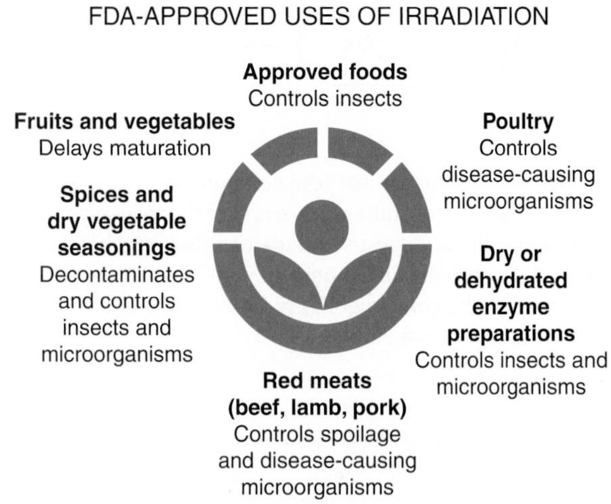

Figure 14.3

Irradiation Symbol

The international symbol for irradiation must be on all foods that have been irradiated.

delay ripening, on lettuce and spinach to control pathogens and extend shelf life, and on poultry and red meat to reduce pathogens. Irradiation is highly effective and can almost completely eliminate pathogens in poultry and meat. Although irradiation does not replace proper food handling and preparation, it can help deliver a safer product to the consumer. With the increase in foodborne illness, irradiation may become more prevalent and be demanded more frequently by consumers.[19]

The FDA requires that foods treated with irradiation be labeled with the international symbol for irradiation and indicate that the product was "treated with irradiation" or "treated by irradiation" (**Figure 14.3**).

Nanotechnology

Nanotechnology is the science of controlling substances at a very small scale, about 1 nanometer. One nanometer is about 1/80,000th the width of a human hair. Nanotechnology is being used in several aspects of food science, including how food is grown and how it is packaged. Nanotechnology can have an impact on a food's taste, safety, and health benefits. Examples of nanotechnology in food include storage bins with nanoparticles embedded in the plastic that will kill bacteria, nanoparticles that deliver vitamins or other nutrients in foods, and nanoparticles that can detect bacteria such as *Salmonella*. Research is ongoing to develop nanoparticles that protect food from bacteria that can cause illness or protect plants from pests.

How You Can Keep Your Food Safe

The food supply in the United States is among the safest in the world. However, if food is not handled properly pathogens can contaminate your food and cause illness, sometimes severe illness. The World Health Organization has identified five factors that contribute to foodborne illness:[23]

1. Cooking food to an improper temperature
2. Temperature abuse—not keeping foods cold or hot enough and not cooling them quickly enough
3. Improper hygiene by the food preparer
4. Cross-contamination between raw and fresh ready-to-eat foods
5. Purchasing food from unsafe sources

You can take steps when you purchase, store, cook, and serve food that will decrease your risk of foodborne illness. Good food safety practices should become standard in your kitchen. Make sure all food preparers in your home know and understand the importance of good food safety practices.

Shopping

The first rule of keeping your food safe is to buy foods from reputable sources. Grocery stores, whether chain or locally owned, have to pass sanitation standards in most states, and thus are reputable sources for your food purchases. Fruit and vegetable stands and farmers' markets that offer foods grown in your area are also a good choice for fresh local foods, but they may not be as regulated or inspected as strictly as retail stores. If you want to buy meat or eggs from local sources, make sure that they use good production and packaging practices. Talk to farmers about their practices to find out how their food was handled and processed prior to it coming to market. Use your instincts, shrimp from a market that has the fresh smell of the sea—good. Shrimp from a guy on the side of the road in a blue jeep—not so good.

When you are shopping, select nonperishable foods first. Next, choose perishable items such as meat, dairy, and eggs. The last thing to place in your basket should be frozen foods. When choosing meat, poultry, and seafood, make sure the package does not have tears, breaks, or leakage. Do not buy foods past the sell-by date (see the following section on checking the date). Place raw meat, poultry, and seafood away from other foods in your cart. Choose fruits and vegetables that are not bruised or damaged. Make sure that cut fruits and vegetables, such as packaged salad or precut melon, are refrigerated prior to purchase.

When bagging your food after purchase, there are a few rules to follow. Put meat, poultry, and seafood in separate bags. This will keep any juices that may leak from contaminating other food. If you are using your own reusable bags, put meat, poultry, and seafood in a plastic bag to keep your bag clean. Wash your reusable bags in the washing machine or by hand frequently. Go home immediately to refrigerate perishable items you have purchased. During hot weather or if you have a long distance to travel from the store to your refrigerator, use an insulated bag or cooler with ice or ice packs.

Check the Dates You may find several types of dates on food. Although there is no uniform system used for food

Which Side Are You On?

Genetically Engineered Foods

When you hear the term **genetically engineered food**, you may have a vision of some strange food that may be available in the distant future. In fact, genetically engineered foods have been in the food supply for decades. Over 80% of the soybeans and about one-third of the corn grown in the United States are genetically engineered.[20] So, chances are that you have eaten a genetically engineered food and have been doing so for many years. Many consumers are unaware of the widespread use of these foods.

A genetically engineered food is one where the DNA has been modified by technology; that is, the genetic makeup of the food has been modified. This can be done by rearranging the DNA in the food or by adding DNA from other foods. These changes result in a food that is different than the original food. Genetic engineering can be done to enhance the ability to store a food, to improve nutritional quality, or to make plants more resistant to diseases or insects. Examples of foods that have been genetically engineered are delayed-ripening tomatoes, pest-resistant vegetables, and many others.

Many professional organizations and regulatory bodies are in support of genetic engineering of food, including the American Medical Association[21] and the World Health Organization.[22] The World Health Organization indicates that genetically modified foods have the potential for increasing agricultural productivity and improving nutritional value. The FDA must approve genetically modified foods produced in the United States. Those available on the international market are governed by the country of origin but must pass safety assessments and, according to the World Health Organization, are not likely to present significant risks to human health.[22]

Despite the use of genetically engineered foods for decades and the high likelihood of safety, some consumers have concerns. The term *Frankenfood* has been used to characterize genetically engineered foods as not being natural. What are the threats to human health from genetic modification? One potential danger is food allergy. Proteins in milk, eggs, wheat, fish, tree nuts, peanuts, soybeans, and shellfish cause over 90% of food allergies. If a protein from one of these foods were to be used in the genetic modification of another food, people who are allergic to these proteins could unknowingly consume a protein that would cause an allergic reaction. To keep this from happening, the FDA requires producers of genetically engineered foods to present scientific evidence that they are not using any allergenic substances in their product. If this evidence cannot be provided, they are required to label the food to alert consumers. Another concern is that genes from genetically engineered foods could be transferred to the human body. If these genes were resistant to antibiotics, this would be of great concern for human health. The probability of gene transfer is small; however, the World Health Organization and others encourage producers not to use genes that are resistant to antibiotics. The debate about genetically engineered foods is likely to continue. How to balance costs, benefits, and safety issues will continue to be discussed.

dating in the United States, food dating is required in more than 20 states.[24] Dating is found primarily on perishable foods, such as meat, poultry, eggs, and dairy products. A **sell-by date** tells the store how long to display the food for sale. You should buy the product before the date expires (**Figure 14.4**).

How long you can keep a product after the sell-by date depends on the type of product, how it was handled prior to your purchase, and how you handle it once you buy it (**Table 14.2**). In the case of processed foods, such as lun-

TERMS

genetically engineered food A food that has been produced using plant or animal ingredients that have been modified using biotechnology.

sell-by date The date printed on a package of perishable food that indicates the date after which it should not be offered for sale.

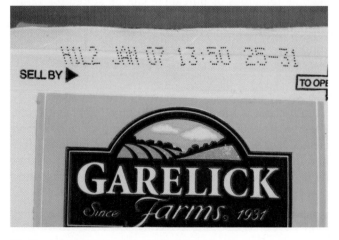

■ **Figure 14.4**

Sell-by Date

The sell-by date lets the store know how long to display to product for sale. Sell-by dates are most commonly found on perishable products, such as meat, milk, and eggs.

Table 14.2

Storage Time for Meat and Poultry Products

If a product has a sell-by date or no date, eat, cook, or freeze the product within the time frame noted in the table.

Product	Storage Time After Purchase
Poultry	1–2 days
Beef, veal, pork, and lamb	3–5 days
Ground meat and ground poultry	1–2 days
Eggs	3–5 weeks
Cooked poultry	3–4 days
Luncheon meat	2 weeks (3–5 days after opening)

Source: US Department of Agriculture, Food Safety and Inspection Service. Food product dating. http://www.fsis.usda.gov/factsheets/food_product_dating/index.asp. Accessed August 8, 2010.

cheon meat, it also depends on whether the product has been opened. For example, a package of turkey luncheon meat may have a date far into the future; however, once the package is opened, it should be used in three to five days. In addition, it is important that you get the food home and in the refrigerator quickly. Warm weather or an extra stop on your way home from the grocery store can make a big difference.

The **best if used by (or before) date** is a recommendation for best flavor or quality. It is not related to food safety. Usually the food will be safe to eat even after the date has passed, but it may not be at peak quality. These dates are usually found on nonperishable foods such as crackers, cookies, chips, and soft drinks.

Canned foods usually don't have a sell-by or best if used by date. They may have a code on the can that means something to the manufacturer but that is not meant for the consumer to interpret. In general, high-acid foods such as tomatoes or pineapple can be stored for 12–18 months. Low-acid foods, such as meat, fish, poultry, and vegetables, will keep indefinitely if the can is kept in good condition; however, quality is best if consumed within two to five years.

Clean

Keep it clean is the number one home food safety rule. Keep your hands, utensils, surfaces, and, of course, food clean. Wash your hands often: before handling food, after handling food, after using the bathroom, after changing a diaper, after tending to a sick person, after blowing your nose, after coughing or sneezing, and after handling pets. Wash your hands after handling raw meat, poultry, seafood, or eggs. Use warm water and soap for at least 20 seconds, and then dry using a clean cloth or paper towel. Keeping cooking tools clean is important as well. Wash cutting boards, dishes, utensils, and countertops with hot water and soap after preparing each food item before going on to the next food. Use paper towels to clean kitchen surfaces and then throw them away after one use. If you want to save paper and reduce your contribution to the landfill, use cloth towels. Just be sure to wash them often in the hot cycle of the washing machine. If you use sponges, replace them often and wash them in the dishwasher frequently.

TERMS

best if used by (or before) date A date usually found on nonperishable foods that indicates the date after which quality may be compromised; the date is not related to the safety of the food.

Can You Skip the Sink If You Use Hand Sanitizer?

Alcohol-based hand sanitizers are very popular. You see them at the gym, the doctor's office, and the school cafeteria. You may even have a bottle in your car, your backpack, or on your desk. Are these hand sanitizers a replacement for hand washing? The simple answer is absolutely not. Hand sanitizers can kill many types of bacteria and are great when soap and water are not available.[25] They are also a good supplement after hand washing to kill even more bacteria. Alone, however, hand sanitizers cannot kill the number one virus known to infect people through food—norovirus.[26] Norovirus and other viruses can be removed by proper hand washing with soap and water. Use hand sanitizers only when soap and water are not available, or in addition to proper hand washing with soap and water.

The best and least expensive cleaning solution for surface cleaning is a mixture of 3/4 teaspoon liquid chlorine bleach to 1 quart of water. The small amount of bleach adds extra protection against bacteria on countertops and cutting boards. Spray the solution on the surface and allow to stand for several minutes, then rinse with water and dry. Because bleach can lose its effectiveness over time, replace the bleach solution each week.

Clean your food as well as your hands, countertops, and utensils. Wash all fruits and vegetables under running water. Wash even those whose skin you don't intend to eat. Firm-skinned vegetables and fruits, such as potatoes, melons, or carrots, should be scrubbed with a vegetable brush. Fruits and vegetables that are packaged and labeled "ready-to-eat," "washed," or "triple washed" do not need to be washed. Washing fruits and vegetables with soap, detergent, or commercial produce wash is not recommended.[27]

Separate

Bacteria are often spread by cross-contamination. When raw foods that are to be cooked, such as meat, poultry, or

Hold the Sprouts

Ask most food safety specialists if there is any food that they do not consume due to food safety risks and you are likely to hear—raw sprouts. Bean sprouts are produced by sprouting seeds and beans. This requires warmth and moisture—the same environment that bacteria need to grow. Bean sprouts have been associated with at least 30 foodborne illness outbreaks over the past 15 years.[28,29] Growing your own sprouts is not necessarily safer than buying commercially produced sprouts, because the bacteria that cause the foodborne illness are usually already in the seed or bean. To reduce your risk of illness associated with sprouts, request that raw sprouts not be added to your food. If you do eat sprouts, make sue they are cooked thoroughly, because cooking will kill harmful bacteria.

seafood, come in contact with foods that are eaten raw, you have the potential to spread harmful bacteria. Use two cutting boards, one for raw meat, poultry, and seafood and the other for fruits and vegetables. If you only have one cutting board, make sure you carefully wash it with soapy water in between different types of foods. Remember to wash your knife well in between foods as well. If you put raw meat, poultry, or seafood on a plate, wash it before you put cooked foods on the same plate. Cross-contamination can also occur with marinades. Marinades used with raw meat, poultry, or seafood should not be used on cooked foods unless it is boiled first. When storing raw meat, poultry, or seafood make sure it is well wrapped or in a sealed container so that juices will not drip onto other foods. A common way that cross-contamination occurs is from your hands. You handle raw poultry, then touch the pantry door, then handle lettuce for a salad. Now you have potentially contaminated the pantry door handle and the lettuce. Remember to wash your hands well immediately after handling raw meat, poultry, seafood, or eggs.

Cook

Thawing foods properly is an important step to good home food safety. No matter how careful you are in the cooking process, if the foods have not been thawed properly bacteria may have a chance to grow to a level that can be harmful. There are three safe ways to defrost food. The safest is to thaw foods in the refrigerator. Depending on the size of the food, this can take 24 hours for small packages of meat or poultry to up to several days for a large turkey. If you are short on time, there are two other faster ways that are still safe. You can thaw meat or poultry in an airtight package in cold water. Change the water every 30 minutes so the water remains cool. Once the food is thawed, cook it immediately. You can also safely thaw food in the microwave. This method also requires that you cook the thawed food immediately. Never thaw food at room temperature or in warm or hot water. This can allow food to enter the danger temperature zone and allow bacteria to grow (**Figure 14.5**).

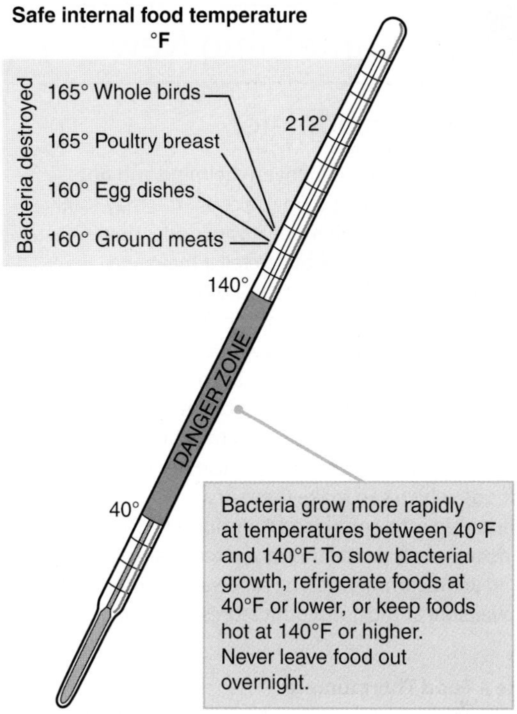

Figure 14.5

Keep Food out of the Danger Zone

To prevent bacterial growth, keep hot food hot and cold food cold. Bacteria grow rapidly between 40°F and 140°F.

Cooking foods to a proper internal temperature will kill harmful bacteria that cause foodborne illness (**Table 14.3**). Old methods of cooking chicken until the juices run clear or a hamburger until it is no longer pink are not

Table 14.3

USDA Recommended Safe Minimum Internal Temperatures

Food Item	Safe Minimum Internal Temperature
Steaks and roasts	145°F (higher for medium well or well done)
Ground Beef	160°F
Ground turkey or chicken	165°F
Chicken parts	165°F
Whole chicken or turkey	165°F
Pork	160°F
Fish	145°F
Egg dishes	165°F
Leftovers and casseroles	165°F

Source: US Department of Agriculture, Food Safety and Inspection Service. Food safety education: is it done yet? http://www.fsis.usda.gov/is_it_done_yet/brochure_text/index.asp. Accessed August 9, 2010.

Try Something New

Use a Food Thermometer

Using a thermometer may seem overwhelming and not something you need to do as a novice cook. You may think it is just easier to estimate when meats are done. However, it is very difficult, if not impossible, to tell if meat and poultry are cooked as well as they should be. Using the color of meat as a guide to doneness is not effective. Using a thermometer takes the guessing out of cooking and provides you with instant information as to the internal temperature of the food you are cooking.[30] Although it will make sure you cook foods long enough to achieve a safe temperature, using a thermometer will also help you not overcook foods, which can make them dry.

Your first step is to get a good thermometer. Tip-sensitive, instant-read, digital thermometers are the most accurate and are recommended by food safety experts. These are available at most discount stores or grocery stores.

How to Use a Food Thermometer

1. Use a digital, instant-read thermometer to check the internal temperature near the end of the cooking time, but before the food is expected to be done.
2. The food thermometer should be placed in multiple places in the thickest parts of the food and should not be touching bone, fat, or gristle. The thermometer should be inserted slowly to reveal if there are any cold spots.
3. Compare your thermometer reading to the temperatures in Table 14.3 to determine if your food has reached a safe temperature.
4. Make sure to clean you food thermometer with soapy water before and after each use.

There are many types of food thermometers. Follow the instructions for your specific food thermometer.

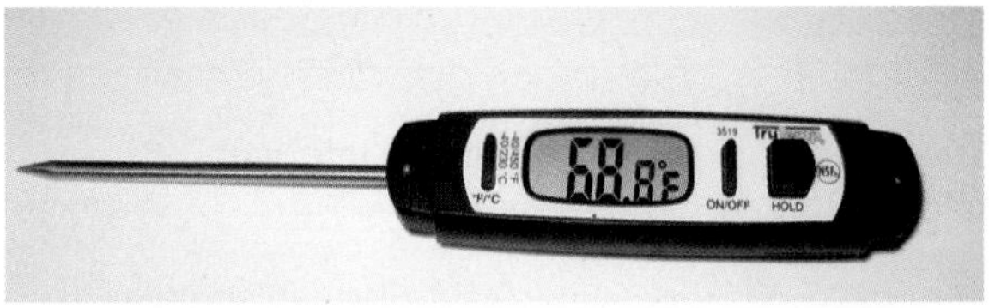

Food Thermometer
Use a tip-sensitive, digital thermometer to accurately gauge the internal temperature of meat, poultry, seafood, and leftovers.

Packing a Safe Lunch

One strategy for eating healthy is to plan your food away from home and take it with you. This will ensure that you have healthy options and are not tempted by fast food or pizza. But what about food safety? Keeping hot foods hot and cold foods cold is important for your to-go lunch. If you are packing hot soup or stew, use an insulated bottle. Cold foods are best kept cold by using a soft-sided insulated bag with an ice pack or frozen gel pack.

accurate and should not be used to judge internal temperature. The only way to accurately determine the internal temperature of meat, poultry, or seafood is to use a tip-sensitive thermometer. You can even use your thermometer to make sure that leftovers are properly heated.

Once you have properly prepared your food, you need to keep it at the proper temperature. Remember to keep cold foods cold and hot foods hot. Foods should not be kept at room temperature for longer than two hours. The two-hour time frame is a guide and not an absolute. Hot weather can greatly decrease the amount of time that foods can be held without being heated or cooled. Foods left out longer can enter the danger zone for temperature—the unsafe temperatures between 40°F and 140°F where bacteria can multiply rapidly.

Storage

Storing foods properly and promptly is one of the most effective ways to reduce the risk of foodborne illness. Refrigerate or freeze prepared foods and leftovers within two hours. Make sure your refrigerator is at 40°F or below and your freezer is at 0°F or below. Keeping your refrigerator and freezer at the correct temperature is critical in keeping microorganism growth down. Some refrigerators and freezers have built-in thermometers; if yours does not, you may want to get an appliance thermometer so you can monitor the temperature.

Hot foods can be placed directly in the refrigerator. You do not have to let them cool first. This practice of letting hot food get to room temperature prior to putting it

Green and Healthy

Don't Waste Food, But Keep It Safe

Being green is all about not wasting resources. Food, and the energy and water needed to produce that food, is among our most precious resources. Using the foods you buy and cook, as opposed to throwing them out, is a great green practice. However, you have to keep food safety in mind. Plan what you buy so that you don't purchase something just to have it spoil in the refrigerator. If plans change, some items, such as chicken or beef, can be frozen so you don't lose your investment. Plan your meals and food preparation so that when you have leftovers you eat them within three to five days. When reheating leftovers, use your thermometer to heat to make sure they are heated to a proper internal temperature (165°F).

Personal Health Check

Analyze Your Food Safety Practices

You can take many steps at home to keep food safe for you, your family, and your friends. Take the Home Food Safety Inspection Quiz and see how you do. Do you need to adjust some of your food safety practices?

Home Food Safety Inspection Quiz

Answer the questions below based on your usual practices in the kitchen. If you answer any of the questions NO, change your kitchen habits to keep food safe.

Yes	No	
□	□	I wash my hands before I begin to prepare food.
□	□	I wash my hands during food preparation if I handle raw meat or poultry.
□	□	I don't prepare food when I am sick.
□	□	I have hand soap in my kitchen.
□	□	I have soap for washing dishes in my kitchen.
□	□	Pets do not walk on countertops.
□	□	I wash dishes, pots, and pans as I use them and don't pile them in the sink.
□	□	My sink is clean and does not have bits of food.
□	□	I change the dishtowel and dishcloth often.
□	□	I wash the cutting board with soapy water in-between uses and after cutting raw meat or poultry.
□	□	I don't put cooked food onto a plate that held raw foods without washing it first.
□	□	The shelves and drawers in the refrigerator are clean and don't have spills, mold, or bits of food.
□	□	I refrigerate food quickly after a meal.
□	□	I thaw meat in the refrigerator or microwave and not on the counter.

in the refrigerator is a holdover from when we actually had ice in the refrigerator to keep it cool. Those days are long gone, as should be that practice. The refrigerator is designed to chill food rapidly and will not be overwhelmed by warm food.

If you have a large pot of soup or stew, you should put it in smaller or shallower containers so it can cool quickly. A large pot of food will take hours for the internal temperature to be below 40 °F. This can allow bacteria to begin to multiply.

Refrigerator drawers provide high-quality storage for fruits and vegetables. Vegetables need higher humidity, whereas fruits need lower humidity. Many refrigerators have controls that allow you to customize the drawers for their content.

Keep track of how long you have stored leftovers. Most cooked foods and mixed dishes should be eaten within three days. One of the best rules for home food safety is "when in doubt, throw it out." No food is worth risking a case of foodborne illness in yourself or your family.

Myth Versus Fact

Myth: When cooking chicken, you can tell that it is done when the juices run clear or the meat pulls away from the bone.

Fact: The only accurate way to tell if poultry or other meats are cooked properly is to use a thermometer. Using a thermometer will ensure that you cook poultry to a proper internal temperature.

Myth: Thawing meat on the counter is fine if you are going to use it right away.

Fact: Thawing meat on the counter is never a good practice. The outside of the meat gets warm faster than the inside, which can cause bacteria to grow. Thaw meat in the refrigerator, microwave, or in cold water that is changed every 30 minutes.

Myth: If you have leftover soup, let it cool to room temperature before you put it in the refrigerator.

Fact: Your refrigerator is well equipped to handle hot food and bring the temperature down quickly. Put large batches of food in smaller containers so they will cool quickly and make sure to refrigerate soon (within two hours) after you serve the meal.

Myth: Using hand sanitizer is just as good as hand washing.

Fact: There is no substitute for proper hand washing. Hand sanitizer is fine if there are no facilities to use soap and water. However, alcohol-based hand sanitizers do not kill all pathogens known to cause foodborne illness. Alcohol-based hand sanitizers do not kill norovirus, one of the most prevalent culprits in foodborne illness.

Myth: If it tastes fine, then it is safe to eat.

Fact: The taste or smell of a food is no guarantee that it is safe to eat. Most cases of foodborne illness are from foods that were handled improperly or that were contaminated with a pathogen. In most cases, these foods tasted fine. Follow proper food safety practices at home, and don't rely on your sense of smell and taste to keep you safe. When in doubt, throw it out.

Myth: Foodborne illness is no fun, but it is just a little vomiting and diarrhea.

Fact: Although most cases of foodborne illness result in some misery, vomiting, diarrhea, and mild dehydration, it can be more serious. Some cases of foodborne illness result in hospitalization and, in severe cases, can cause death.

Myth: If food is safe enough for one family member, it is safe for the entire family.

Fact: Several populations are at increased risk for foodborne illness. Infants, pregnant women, older adults, and those with chronic illness all have a greater risk of getting sick from pathogens in food. If you are preparing food for people in any of these groups, even greater care should be used to employ proper food handling practices. They should also be more careful about eating foods that are not cooked properly in restaurants.

Back to the Story

George is to be commended for preparing more meals at home. What he cooks will likely be healthier than pizza and burgers. However, he needs to follow good food safety practices to keep the food safe and decrease the risk of foodborne illness. His first mistake was to thaw the chicken on the counter. Food should be thawed in the refrigerator or microwave. A day or so prior to making his barbeque chicken meal, George should put the chicken in the refrigerator to thaw. It is a good idea to place it in a container on the bottom shelf to prevent juices from the raw meat from getting on other foods. If last-minute thawing is needed, the microwave is a quick way to thaw meat and poultry. Marinating the chicken is a great way to introduce lots of flavor. However, because the marinade has been in contact with raw poultry, it should not be used as a dipping sauce unless it is first boiled for several minutes. The cutting board that George uses to transport the raw chicken outside should be cleaned thoroughly with soapy water before he uses it with the cooked chicken. George should use another cutting board or a cleaned cutting board to prepare the salad or other foods that will be eaten raw. Finally, the only way to make sure that the chicken is cooked to the correct temperature is to use a thermometer. Looking at the chicken's color or texture or even timing cooking do not ensure that the proper temperature has been reached to kill harmful bacteria. Following these simple steps to good home food safety will make sure that George's meal is not only healthy, but also safe.

References

1. Scallan E, Griffin PM, Angulo FJ, Tauxe RV, Hoekstra RM. Foodborne illness acquired in the US—unspecified agents. *Emerg Infecti Dis*. 2011;17(1). http://www.cdc.gov/EID/content/17/1/16.htm. Accessed February 25, 2011.
2. Scharff RL. Health-related costs from foodborne illness in the United States. 2010. http://www.producesafetyproject.org/media?id=0009. Accessed October 4, 2010.
3. World Health Organization. Food safety and food-

borne illness. Fact sheet no. 237. 2007. http://www.who.int/mediacentre/factsheets/fs237/en/. Accessed August 17, 2010.

4. Mead PS, Slutsker L, Dietz V, et al. Food-related illness and death in the United States. *Emerg Infecti Dis.* 1999;5:607–625.
5. Centers for Disease Control and Prevention. Foodborne illness. 2005. http://www.cdc.gov/ncidod/dbmd/diseaseinfo/foodborneinfections_g.htm#mostcommon. Accessed August 16, 2010.
6. Porterfield E, Berliant A. Jack in the Box ignored safety rules. *The News Tribune*. Tacoma, WA. June 16, 1995.
7. Centers for Disease Control and Prevention. Norovirus outbreak association with ill food-service workers—Michigan, January–February 2006. *MMWR*. 2007;56(46):1212–1216.
8. Widdowson MA, Sulka A, Bulens S, et al. Norovirus and foodborne disease, United States, 1991–2000. *Emerg Infect Dis*. 2005;11:95–102.
9. Centers for Disease Control and Prevention. Ongoing multistate outbreak of *Escherichia coli* serotype O157:H7 infections associated with consumption of fresh spinach—United States, September 2006. *MMWR*. 2006;55:1–2.
10. US Food and Drug Administration. Residue Monitoring Reports, FDA Pesticide Program Residue Monitoring: 1993–2007. 2009. http://www.fda.gov/Food/FoodSafety/FoodContaminantsAdulteration/Pesticides/ResidueMonitoringReports/default.htm. Accessed August 16, 2010.
11. US Environmental Protection Agency. Pesticides: regulating pesticides—Food Quality Protection Act (FQPA) of 1996. http://www.epa.gov/opp00001/regulating/laws/fqpa/. Accessed August 16, 2010.
12. National Institutes of Health. FDA urges limiting antibiotics in meat. Medline Plus. June 28, 2010. http://www.nlm.nih.gov/medlinelus/news/fullstory_100474.html. Accessed August 16, 2010.
13. Andersson AM, Skakkebaek NE. Exposure to exogenous estrogens in food: possible impact on human development and health. *Eur J Endocrinol*. 1999;140:477–485.
14. Linos E, Willett WC, Cho E, Colditz G, Frizier LA. Red meat consumption during adolescence among premenopausal women and risk of breast cancer. *Cancer Epidemiol Biomarkers Prev*. 2008:17;2146–2151.
15. Vicini J, Etherton T, Kris-Etherton P, et al. Survey of retail milk composition as affected by label claims regarding farm-management practices. *J Am Diet Assoc*. 2008;108(7):1198–1203.
16. Pape-Zambito DA, Magliaro AL, Kensinger RS. Concentration of 17beta-estradiol in Holstein whole milk. *J Dairy Sci*. 2007;90:3308–3313.
17. Wild CP, Montesano R. A model of interaction: aflatoxins and hepatitis viruses in liver cancer etiology and prevention. *Cancer Letters*. 2009;286(1):22–28.
18. US Food and Drug Administration. FDA Food Code 2001: Chapter 3—Food. http://www.fda.gov/Food/FoodSafety/RetailFoodProtection/FoodCode/FoodCode2009/ucm186451.htm#part3-4. Accessed September 1, 2010.
19. Wood OB, Bruhn CM. Position of the American Dietetic Association: food irradiation. *J Am Diet Assoc*. 2000;100(2):246–253.
20. American Dietetic Association. Position of the American Dietetic Association: agricultural and food biotechnology. *J Am Diet Assoc*. 2006;106:285–293.
21. American Medical Association. Council on Scientific Affairs Report: genetically modified crops and foods. 2000. http://www.ama-assn.org/ama/no-index/about-ama/13595.shtml. Accessed September 1, 2010.
22. World Health Organization. Modern food biotechnology, human health and development: An evidence-based study. 2005. http://www.who.int/foodsafety/publications/biotech/biotech_en.pdf. Accessed September 1, 2010.
23. World Health Organization. Five keys to safer food manual. 2006. http://www.who.int/entity/foodsafety/publications/consumer/manual_keys.pdf. Accessed August 17, 2010.
24. United States Department of Agriculture, Food Safety and Inspection Service. Food product dating. http://www.fsis.usda.gov/factsheets/food_product_dating/index.asp. Accessed August 8, 2010.
25. Bloomfield SF, Aiello AE, Cookson B, O'Boyle C, Larson EL. The effectiveness of hand hygiene procedures in reducing the risks of infections in home and community settings including hand washing and alcohol-based hand sanitizers. *Am J Infect Contr*. 2007;35(10):S27–S64.
26. Liu P, Yuen Y, Hsio HM, Jaykus LA, Moe C. Effectiveness of liquid soap and hand sanitizer against Norwalk virus on contaminated hands. *App Environ Micro*. 2010;76(2):394–399.
27. US Department of Health and Human Services, Food and Drug Administration. Produce safety. http://www.fda.gov/Food/ResourcesForYou/Consumers/ucm114299. Accessed August 8, 2010.
28. US Department of Health and Human Services, Food and Drug Administration. Raw alfalfa sprouts linked to *Salmonella* contamination. http://www.fda.gov/NewsEvents/PublicHealthFocus/ucm150909.htm. Accessed August 8, 2010.
29. Centers for Disease Control and Prevention. Outbreak of *Salmonella* serotype saintpaul infections associated with eating alfalfa sprouts—United States, 2009. *MMWR*. 2009. http://www.cdc.gov/mmwr/pdf/wk/mm58e0507.pdf. Accessed August 9, 2010.
30. US Department of Agriculture, Food Safety and Inspection Service. Food safety education: is it done yet? http://www.fsis.usda.gov/is_it_done_yet/brochure_text/index.asp. Accessed August 9, 2010.

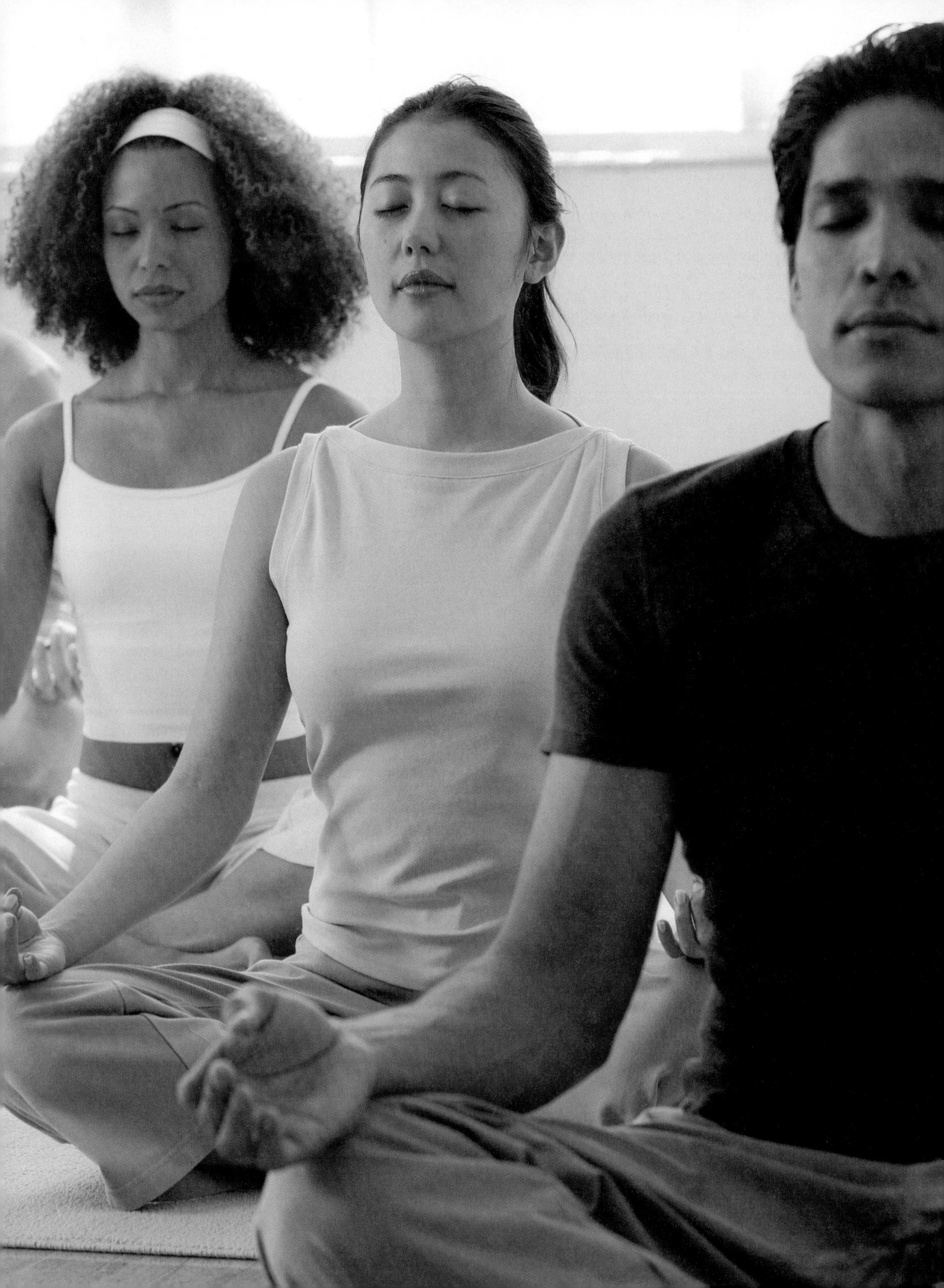

Chapter 15

Beyond Eating Smart and Moving More: Other Components of a Healthy Life

Key Messages

- Wellness has many components, including emotional, intellectual, spiritual, occupational, social, and physical.
- Stress has profound effects on overall health; managing stress is essential.
- Proper sleep habits are important for good health.
- Avoid unhealthy behaviors, such as unprotected sex, as well as tobacco and drug use.
- Be a good healthcare consumer, know important health numbers, and receive appropriate health screenings and immunizations.

Eating healthy, being physically active, and maintaining a healthy weight are cornerstones of good health. However, other aspects of health are important as well. To achieve optimal health, you must address not only physical health, but also all of the other components of wellness, including emotional, spiritual, intellectual, occupational, and social. Your overall health and wellness include not only healthy eating and physical activity, but also how well you manage stress and your sleep patterns and whether you engage in risky behaviors such as tobacco use. It also includes whether you get proper preventive medical care. This chapter will discuss how you can adopt healthy behaviors to achieve wellness and a high quality of life.

Story

Britney is a junior in college. She works 5 nights a week at a local restaurant to pay for tuition, books, and living expenses. She usually works from 4 PM until midnight or later on the weekends. Her job pays the bills, but it is not something she loves. Because of her job and school, she has very little time for friends or a social life. Her family lives in another state, so she only sees them a few times a year. Lately her schoolwork has been stressful, because she is taking several classes that have papers due around the same time. As a college student, she has health insurance through her parents, but she has not seen her doctor in a few years. She rarely gets sick, but if she does she usually goes to student health services on campus or to urgent care. Britney considers herself healthy. She eats healthy, exercises on most days, and is a normal weight. What do you think of Britney's overall health? Are there steps she can take to achieve a better quality of life?

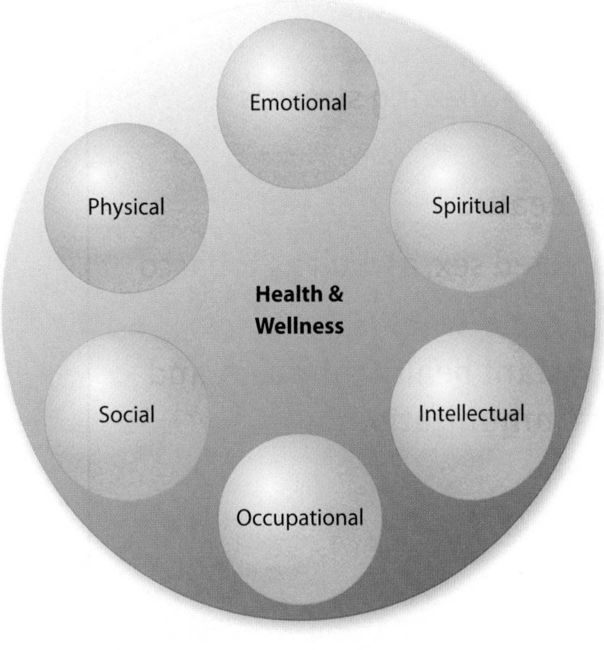

■ **Figure 15.1**
Components of Health and Wellness

What Are Health and Wellness?

Health and *wellness* are, no doubt, words that you have heard all of your life in many different contexts. But what do they really mean? *Health*, in the medical sense, means absence of disease. However, you probably want more out of life than just not being sick. The word *wellness* has no universally accepted definition, but most denote a state of well-being, positive health, or a high quality of life. Wellness is an active process of making choices that move you toward a successful, happy, healthy life. It includes all the choices you make throughout your life. It is not something you complete and mark off your to-do list. It is a lifelong process of being proactive about your health. Wellness includes making choices to keep you free from disease before you get sick and addressing health concerns early should they arise.

Components of Health and Wellness

The bulk of this text has addressed healthy eating and physical activity. Although these two behaviors are critical for wellness, wellness encompasses many behaviors beyond food and movement. Virtually every aspect of your life has a component of wellness and offers opportunities for you to make choices that can positively impact your health now and for the rest of your life. Emotional health, intellectual health, spiritual health, occupational health, social health, as well as physical health, are all components of wellness.

Emotional Health and Wellness

Emotional health and wellness include your enthusiasm for life, your ability to manage your feelings, and your ability to cope with stress. Daily, you go though a wide range of emotions. To be emotionally healthy, you must learn to cope with all those emotions and maintain an overall positive outlook on life. Accept your feelings and emotions instead of denying them. Approach life with optimism instead of pessimism. Looking at the glass as half full instead of half empty will help you have a more positive and hopeful outlook on your life. You can improve your emotional health by surrounding yourself with supportive family and friends. Positive social relationships are important to overall wellness. Be thankful for all the positive aspects of your life. Even if you are facing adversity, focus on what is good in your life instead of the negative.

Intellectual Health and Wellness

Continually challenging your mind is an important component of intellectual health and well-being. You must be a lifelong learner, not just in the classroom, but in everything you do. When a problem arises, use it as an opportunity to find a solution that is creative and uses all of your intellect. If you don't have the skills or knowledge to solve the problem, seek out what you need. Cultivate new interests and explore resources in your community to learn more about what interests you. Stretch your mind with books, magazines, newspapers, or websites on topics of interest.

Spiritual Health and Wellness

The components of spiritual health and wellness are different for each person. For some it means a faith-based practice. For others it means getting in touch with their purpose in life. Spiritual wellness includes asking hard questions such as, "Why am I here?" "How can I contribute to the common good?" "Am I the person I want to be?" On your own path to spiritual health and well-being you may explore how you can integrate your own beliefs into your daily actions or how you can best give your life purpose and direction. A good first step towards spiritual wellness is to explore your own values. Look for deeper meaning in the things you do. Spiritual health also includes recognizing that others' values may be different than your own and practicing acceptance. Everyone is on his or her own path to spiritual health and wellness.

Occupational Health and Wellness

Occupational health and wellness involve choosing a career path that is consistent with your values and beliefs. Choose work or volunteer activities that make you feel that you are making a contribution. This feeling of being a part something larger than yourself will contribute to your occupational wellness. It is much more important to choose work that gives your life meaning and that allows you to use your own unique skills than to choose work that is unrewarding.

Social Health and Wellness

Social health and wellness include the relationships you have with friends and family. It involves developing positive relationships with those around you, sharing your feelings, needs, wants, goals, and dreams. A strong social network is important for overall good health and well-being. People who have close friends and family to rely on are better equipped to handle stressful situations. Laughter, tears, hugging, and touching all make life richer and add to your overall well-being.

TERMS

stress Your body's reaction to a change that requires a physical, mental, or emotional adjustment or response. Stress can come from any situation or thought that makes you feel frustrated, angry, nervous, or anxious.

stressor An external stimulus that causes stress.

To be socially healthy, you must balance work and leisure and make time for the people who are important to you. If your social health is not what it should be, reach out to family and friends and make the time to create strong harmonious relationships that can enrich your life. Make an effort to stay in touch with the people who are supportive in your life.

Physical Health and Wellness

Most of this text has been about the physical aspects of health and wellness. Proper nutrition, regular physical activity, and moderate or no alcohol consumption all contribute to good physical health and wellness. Some other aspects of physical health and well-being include managing stress, not using tobacco, getting enough sleep, practicing safe sex, and wearing seat belts and bike helmets. We will discuss these aspects of health later in this chapter.

How Can You Be Well?

To be a healthy, happy, well person, consider taking a holistic approach that addresses both the mind and the body. To achieve wellness, you must eat healthy, stay active, mange stress, get adequate sleep, avoid unhealthy behaviors, and get proper medical care, including appropriate screenings and immunizations (**Figure 15.2**).

Manage Stress

Stress is the body's normal physical response to any stimulus that requires you to respond. A **stressor** is anything

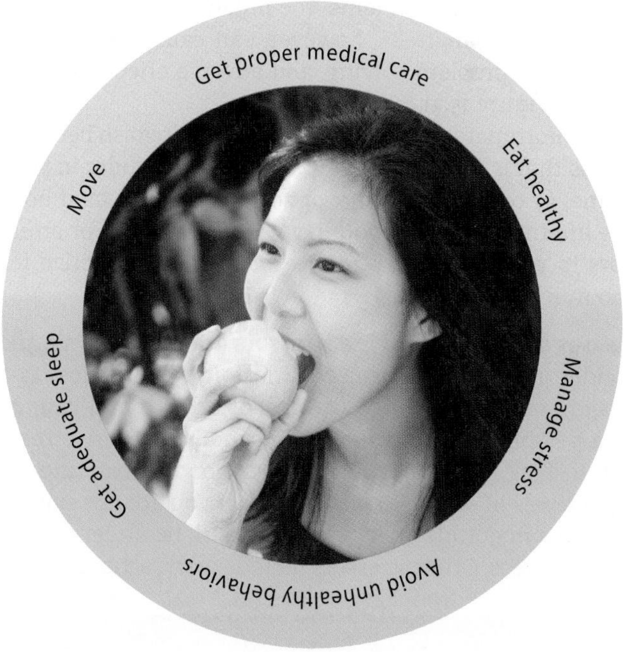

■ **Figure 15.2**

Components of a Healthy Life

What you eat and how you move are two components of a healthy life. For a healthy, happy life, you also must manage stress, get adequate sleep, avoid unhealthy behaviors, and seek proper medical care.

that is a source or cause of stress in your life. Stressors can be negative things in your life, such as too much work, an argument with your best friend, financial trouble, or the loss of a family member. Stressors can also be positive events in your life, such as the birth of a child, a new job, a vacation, graduation, or purchasing a new car.

Your body has an automatic response to stress. When you perceive a threat or get upset, your body moves into what is known as the fight-or-flight, or stress, response. For example, you walk into class and the professor announces a pop quiz and you know you have not done the reading for that class. Your nervous system responds by releasing the stress hormones adrenaline and cortisol. These hormones cause your heart to beat faster, muscles to tighten, blood pressure to rise, breathing to quicken, and senses to become sharper. Thanks to your body's response, you also have quicker reaction time and enhanced focus. Your body is now prepared to fight or flee from danger. In the case of the pop quiz, you more than likely take your seat and hope to be able to pull your grade up on other assignments. Your body's response may be a reminder of the importance of being prepared for class next time.

There is no such thing as being stress free. In fact, stress in small doses can help you perform better or motivate you to do your best. Too little stress can cause you to be bored, tired, or frustrated that your life is not as satisfying as it could be. The optimal amount of stress, or **eustress**, can increase your creativity, enhance your ability to problem solve, and help you finish a task on deadline. Stress is what keeps you focused to study for an exam or finish a paper. Stress is also what helps you find creative solutions to problems. Too much stress, sometimes referred to as **distress**, however, can cause exhaustion, ineffective problem solving, and adverse effects on your health (**Figure 15.3**).

Unfortunately, your body does not distinguish between stress that is life threatening, such as an intruder in your home, or overload at work or school. It reacts as if both are life threatening. If you have a lot of worries or stressors in your life, your stress response may be active for too much of the time.

Causes of Stress Major life stressors are relatively simple to identify. Losing a spouse or close family member is a major stressor. Marriage, divorce, or other major change to a person's relationship status can also be very stressful. In fact, any major life change, good or bad, means high levels of stress. However, even if you are not experiencing a major life change, you can still be under a great deal of stress. Other stressors include work, school, excessive obligations, financial problems, children, and family issues. All of these stressors are external; stressors can be internal as well. Having unrealistic expectations, being a perfectionist, engaging in negative self-talk, or an inability to accept change can also cause stress.

TERMS

eustress A level of stress that is healthy and gives you a feeling of fulfillment.

distress A level of stress that is too high and can cause emotional and physical problems.

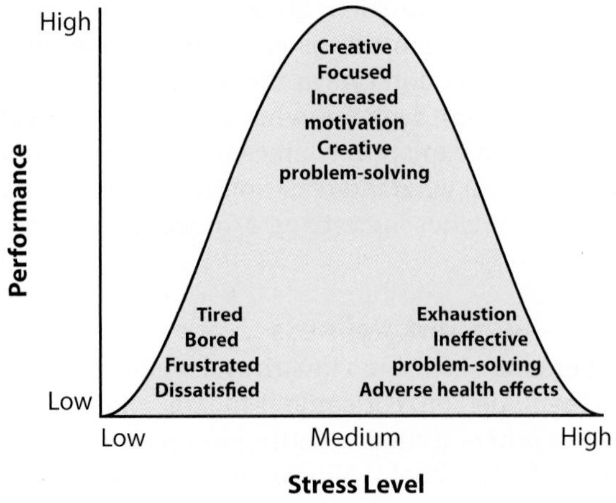

■ **Figure 15.3**

Stress Levels Can Affect Your Health and Performance
Stress can have positive effects in small amounts; however, high stress is associated with negative effects on health and well-being.

What is stressful for you may be not be stressful for someone else. You may be able to handle taking a full load at school, balancing family obligations, and working part time, whereas someone else may not be able to handle that much stress. Some people may find a change in responsibilities at work a welcome challenge; for others the added responsibilities may put them in stress overload. It is important for you to identify your stressors so that you can begin to address chronic stress in your life in a positive way.

How Much Is Too Much Stress? Because of the damage that stress can do to your health, it is important to know how much stress is too much for you. Your ability to handle stress will depend on your genetics, social support system, attitude, and ability to deal with your emotions and the strategies you have put in place to deal with stress. Only you can know how much is too much; however, there are some common signs you can look for to let you know that you may be under too much stress. If you are chronically exhausted or you are often impatient or short with those around you, these may be signs that stress is taking over your life. Other common signs of stress overload include sleep problems and a general lack of enjoyment in life. If you feel your life is just trying to hang on and get all of your obligations met, your stress level may be high enough to cause health problems.

Effect of Chronic Stress It would be difficult to overestimate the negative health effects that chronic stress can have on your body. It literally affects every body system.

It can cause health problems and make existing health issues worse. Chronic stress is considered to be the most damaging type of stress and the most likely to result in long-term health consequences.[1,2] One way that stress has an impact on health is through behavioral changes that occur as coping mechanisms to stress. Common responses to stress include increased use of tobacco or alcohol, decreased sleep and exercise, and not following medical advice. Another way stress impacts health is through the body's hormonal response to stress. Prolonged or repeated activation of stress hormones interferes with other body systems and results in increased risk for physical and mental health problems.

Chronic stress can cause you to have trouble sleeping. Constant tension in muscles due to chronic stress can lead to headaches and neck, shoulder, or back pain. Stress is also associated with a decrease in the immune system's ability to fight illness, so you may get sick more frequently if you are under a great deal of stress.[3,4] Chronic stress is also associated with high blood pressure, abnormal heartbeat, heart attacks, and an increase in coronary heart disease.[5–7] Chronic stress has also been linked to clinical depression.[8,9] Although is it not fully known if stress, in and of itself, can cause clinical depression, which is a chemical imbalance in the brain, stress can certainly make clinical depression worse and more difficult to manage. Chronic stress can make you more dissatisfied with your life, which can result in depressive symptoms, which should not to be confused with clinical depression.

Chronic stress can also make existing health problems worse. Skin problems, including acne and psoriasis, are worse and harder to manage in times of high stress.[10,11] High levels of stress exacerbate gastrointestinal problems, including ulcers, gastric reflux, and irritable bowel syndrome.[12] Asthma is also made worse by chronic stress.[13]

Strategies for Stress Management It is not possible to remove stress from your life. What you can do is learn to manage stress and recognize when you need to employ strategies to get your stress under control. Managing stress is often about taking charge of your life and your schedule. It also means taking charge of your thoughts and emotions. Find what works for you to manage your stress.

Take Care of Yourself When you are under stress you don't always do the best job of taking care of yourself. Make time to take care of yourself; include in your day time for the activities you enjoy, eat healthy, and stay active. All of these healthy behaviors will help you be better able to handle stress. Schedule time in the day for the things you love to do. You may not have time to do them every day, but cutting out your favorite activities is not a good way to handle stress. If you have a special TV show that you like to watch every week, make time for it in your schedule. If you love books, allow yourself a certain time each day to read. Set aside time for Facebook or emailing friends. The things that make your life interesting have a place on your to-do list.

Exercise is one of the best ways to care of yourself and at the same time take control of your stress. Any form of exercise, from walking around campus to lifting weights in the gym, is a great way to deal with stress. People who exercise report improved self-esteem, an improved sense of self-efficacy, improved information processing, decreased feelings of anxiety and depression, and an overall decrease in stress and tension.[14–17] During exercise, your brain produces endorphins. These are neurotransmitters that provide you with a sense of calm and well-being. You have probably heard of the "runner's high," a euphoric feeling that is achieved through running, usually long-distance running. You don't have to be a long-distance runner to experience the positive effects of exercise. An hour at the gym or a hike at a local park can produce endorphins as well. Exercise can also help you forget the stress you may be experiencing. It can also help you sleep better at night.

Relax Learning some relaxation techniques is important for stress management. You may find during times of high stress that you walk around like a ball of tension and nerves most of the day. There are many techniques you can try to help you relax. If you practice these techniques on a regular basis, you may find that you are better able to stay calm even during stressful situations.

Yoga Yoga originated in India more than 5,000 years ago. Today, yoga is practiced all over the world. Yoga is a combination of breathing, physical movements, and meditation. Yoga poses stretch the body in different ways in an effort to focus attention on the body and to become more aware of one's surroundings. The ultimate goal of yoga is to calm the mind in order to balance the mind, body, and spirit. In the western world, yoga is most often practiced in classes that are led by an instructor who guides students through a series of poses and breathing exercises. Yoga classes are offered at most gyms; you can even find yoga classes on television or online. Practicing yoga by taking a class once a week is a great way to manage stress, get in touch with your body, and increase flexibility. You may want to choose one or two yoga poses to use as short stress relievers during the day or when you wake up in the morning. Try the Sun Salutation when you get up each morning to start your day energized and relaxed (**Figure 15.4**).

Meditation Meditation is a mental exercise done for the purpose of achieving a heightened sense of spiritual awareness through quieting the mind. Meditation allows you to focus your thoughts and concentrate on your breathing or a mantra. A *mantra* is a sound, word, or group of words that has meaning to you. You may choose a mantra of "calm and peaceful today" to remind you that you want to stay in control of your stress. Meditation can help make your mind calmer and more focused and can help you turn negative thoughts into more positive ones.

To begin meditating, find a place that is quiet and free of distractions. This can be a chair, the floor, the library—

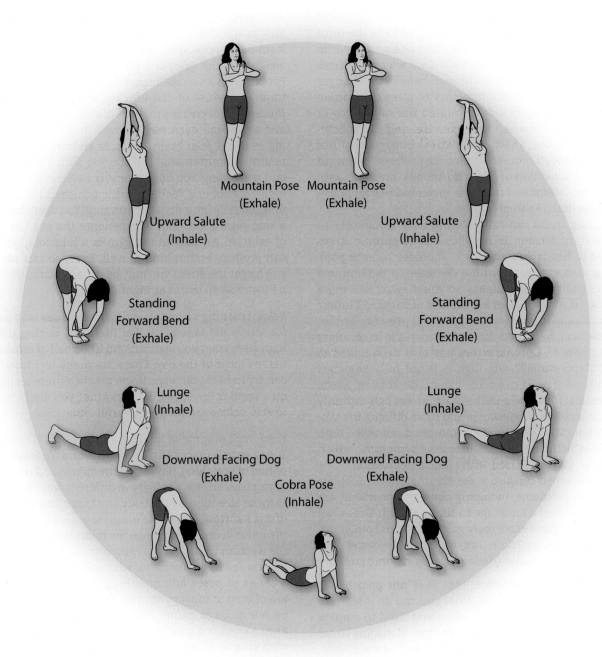

■ **Figure 15.4**

Sun Salutation

The sun salutation, or "salute to the sun," is traditionally done at sunrise facing the sun. It is a great way to start your day or to energize and relieve stress anytime.

Try Something New

Take a Deep Breath

Taking a breath is not something new. It is something you do every day—14,000 to 25,000 times a day, in fact. Although breathing is something you do naturally without giving it much thought, there are ways you can breathe that can help you relax or give you energy. Most people do not breathe as well as they could. As a result, you don't achieve all the benefits that proper breathing can bring. Most people tend to be shallow upper-chest breathers, using about half of the possible lung capacity. There is a proverb that states, "Life is in the breath. He who half-breathes, half-lives." Shallow breathing may provide you with enough oxygen, but it does not produce the benefits of deeper, slower breathing. Shallow breathing may even cause nervousness and keep you from thinking clearly.

The best way to breathe is abdominal breathing. Abdominal breathing uses the diaphragm, the muscle between your lungs and stomach. Breathing using your diaphragm draws air down into the bottom of your lungs. During abdominal breathing, your diaphragm should contract downward. Your lungs fill with air, but it should be your abdomen, not your chest, that moves. This may seem hard at first, especially if you have been a shallow breather for your entire life. Start with several deep breathing breaks a day; over time deep breathing will become more frequent and more natural.

Breathing for Relaxation
If you are having a stressful day or can't fall asleep, try this breathing technique. Sit on the floor, an armless chair, or the edge of the bed with your feet on the floor. Put your hands in your lap. Close your mouth. Close the right nostril using the middle finger of your right hand. Breathe in to the count of four using your diaphragm. Breathe out to the count of seven, pushing your diaphragm down. Do this three to four times and switch to the left nostril. You will feel your body relax and heart rate drop. You can add a mantra for even greater relaxation. When you breathe in say to yourself, "As I breathe in I am calm." When you breathe out say to yourself, "As I breathe out I am relaxed."

Breathing for Increased Energy
If you have been sitting in class or studying for hours and need a pick up, try this breathing technique before you head to the coffee shop. You can do this standing or sitting. Tilt your head slightly up and take a deep breath through your nose. Exhale forcefully through your mouth as you pull in your stomach and move your chin forward. You should be able to hear the air rush from your body. If you are not in public, try making a "ha" sound as you exhale. This breathing exercise releases all the excess carbon dioxide, which can make you feel sluggish.

wherever you can find quiet for even 5 minutes will do. Sit with your back straight and your eyes closed. The traditional posture for meditation is cross-legged on a cushion. However, as long as your back is straight (to prevent you from becoming groggy or sleepy) sit however is most comfortable for you. Relax the muscles in your face, arms, and legs. Turn your attention to your breathing and focus on nothing else. Your mind may want to go over your to-do list, the last conversation you had, or the test you have in a few hours; push those thoughts away and concentrate only on your breathing. You will become aware of just how busy your mind is when you try to calm it down. Gradually, with concentration, you will be able to settle your mind and think only of your breathing. Think about how your breathing feels coming in through your nostrils, filling your lungs, expanding your chest, then exhaling back through your nostrils. As your mind quiets, you may want to add a mantra that has meaning to you. So much of the stress you experience comes from your mind; just a few minutes of meditation per day can help reduce stress. You may find it helpful to make meditation a part of your daily routine.

Deep Breathing If you only have a few minutes and you find yourself in a stressful situation, don't forget to breathe. Taking deep breaths can clear your head and help you calm down in minutes.

Manage Your Time You most likely have multiple demands on you from school, work, family, volunteering, and personal interests. All of these demands can be overwhelming if you don't manage your time well. Managing your time does not mean scheduling every minute of every day with tasks just so you can get everything done. It means balancing your time so that you have time for all of the important things, including yourself. Start by taking a time audit. For two to three days write down everything you do in 15-minute blocks. This may help you identify where you could better use your time to get more done or have more time for the things you enjoy.

How you specifically manage your time is something that you will have to devise—what works for some may not work for you. However, you might want to try a number of time management strategies that work for many people.

Keep a detailed calendar so that you can keep track of all important deadlines. Whether you are using a smartphone, a laptop, an iPad, or a paper calendar, record your appointments, due dates for assignments, test dates, work schedule, birthdays, and so on. It is best to keep one calendar for everything as opposed to different calendars, one for work and school and another for your personal life. You can code things on your calendar accordingly, but having two calendars is just added stress. If other people need to see your calendar, you may want to use an online calendar system.

Make daily or weekly to-do lists, whatever works for you. Write down (or keep electronically) all of the tasks that you need to accomplish and put them in three different categories or color-code them. Category A is things that must be done immediately, or at least that day or week; category B is things that have a specific due date but are a little farther off; and category C is things that you would like to get done or even need to get done but don't have a due date. For large tasks, such as studying for an exam or writing a paper, break the task down into smaller pieces. For example, instead of just adding "study for chemistry exam" on your to-do list, break it down to:

1. Reread chapters 3 and 4 of the text.
2. Get notes from lecture that I missed.
3. Email the professor questions I have about oxidation.
4. Read class notes from the past month.

Keeping a detailed to-do list that is prioritized will help you keep everything on track. It will also help you see if you have too much to get done in a given day or week. You can then arrange your schedule accordingly or move tasks to a later date, if possible. You may need to get the oil changed in your car, but if this is an unusually packed week it may have to wait a few days. Similarly, if you have a week without a lot of pressing deadlines, this would be a good time to look at items in category C and get some of those done.

Using your to-do list, schedule your day using quarter-hour or half-hour segments. Block out the times that are set, like your class or work schedule. Then use your to-do list to add other tasks. Make sure to schedule personal time each day. Meditation, exercise, and shopping for groceries so you have healthy foods are not items that should get pushed aside, no matter how busy you are. Put them on the schedule first and schedule other tasks around them.

There are some common stumbling blocks to time management. Multitasking may appear on the surface to be a time-saver, but in reality it can actually take more time. Concentrate on one task at a time and then move on to the next task. Limit interruptions. When you are working on school or other important projects, ignore or silence your email and cell phone. Don't be a perfectionist. Do your best work, but don't let your tendency toward perfectionism slow you down to the point that you can't get all of your work done. Don't procrastinate. This is easier said than done sometimes, but if you can realize that procrastination often is the fear of putting your work out there to be judged it may be easier to get started. Do just one thing that will move the project ahead.

Know Your Limits

You may be a master at time management, but you still only have 24 hours in a day. You have to know your limits and learn when to back off, say no, or delegate tasks to someone else. Only you can say how much is too much to have on your to-do list. Taking on more than you can handle can cause overload or the feeling that there are too many demands on your time. If you feel you have taken on too much, evaluate what you can let go of to get your stress under control, or at least look at the short term of when your overload will be over. Sometimes just knowing and admitting, "It is going to be a busy and stressful time for the next two weeks until exams are over" will help you get past a tough time.

Get Adequate Sleep

You have a paper due tomorrow, but you have to work until 6 PM. You stay up late to finish your assignment and wake up exhausted. Too often sleep is treated as negotiable. If time is needed to complete a task, watch a favorite TV show, take care of a family obligation, or finally grab that one-hour of time for yourself, sleep is often sacrificed to get it all done.

For whatever reason, by choice or because of sleep difficulty, 30–40% of Americans do not get enough sleep.[18] Since the invention of the light bulb, sleep has decreased on average of two hours per night.[19] Getting enough sleep is often overlooked by healthcare providers and is not discussed as frequently as other aspects of health, such as diet and exercise.[20] However, sleep is a critical component to good health.

Abundant evidence indicates that inadequate sleep greatly impacts several aspects of health, including overall quality of life.[21–24] Not getting enough sleep has been identified as one risk factor for overweight and obesity in both adults and children.[25–33] The exact mechanism for this is unclear, but it may be related to the body's sense of needing energy to keep going; food replaces what is really needed, which is adequate sleep. Inadequate sleep may cause an imbalance in the hormones ghrelin and leptin.[34] Because these hormones are responsible for hunger and satiety, lack of sleep may cause cravings and increased appetite.

Inadequate sleep negatively affects the immune system.[32] Mood and cognitive performance are also altered by inadequate sleep.[35–38] Staying up late to study for an exam may be counterproductive if you are not rested enough to perform as you should during the test. Finally, inadequate sleep is a threat to public safety, increasing the risk of automobile accidents.[10,39]

How much sleep do you need for optimal health? How much sleep a person needs is largely dictated by age (**Figure 15.5**). Infants and children need more sleep than adults. Adults need anywhere from seven to nine hours a sleep per night.[11] Where you fall on the scale is largely dictated by genetics.[40] Short-sleeping runs in families, as

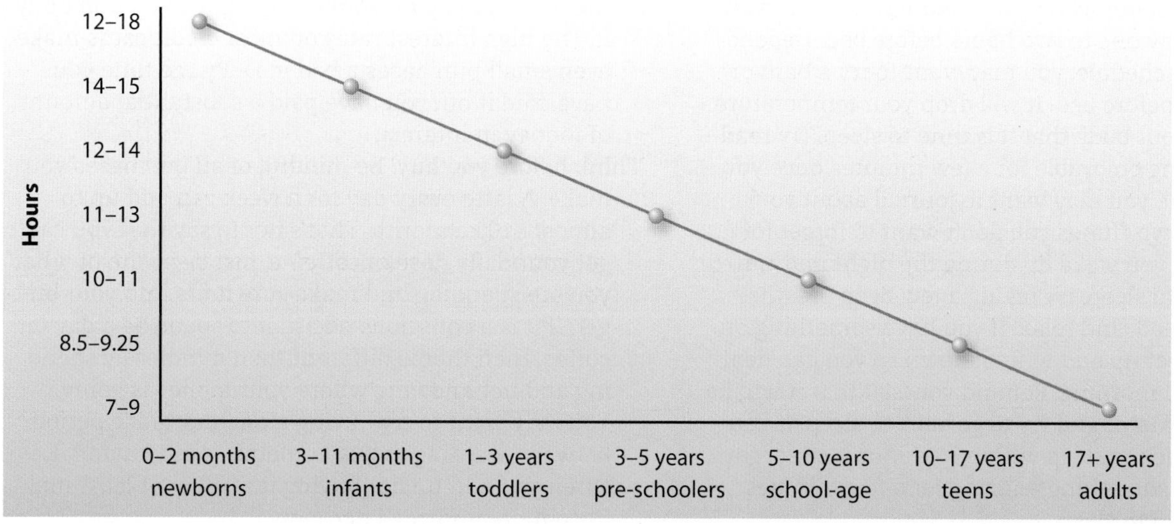

Figure 15.5
How Much Sleep Do We Need?
Source: Data from National Sleep Foundation. How much sleep do we really need? http://www.sleepfoundation.org/article/how-sleep-works/how-much-sleep-do-we-really-need. Accessed October 5, 2010.

does long-sleeping. To best estimate how much sleep you need, track the amount of sleep that you get when you are well rested. How many hours of sleep do you get before you wake up on your own without the alarm? How many hours of sleep do you need to feel well rested throughout the day?

You can take a number of steps to make sure that you get the sleep you need. Try these tips to get you into the routine of getting a good night's sleep.

Set a schedule. Set a time that you should go to sleep to get the number of hours you need. Try to go to bed and get up at approximately the same time every day, even on weekends. Don't take naps, this includes falling asleep in front of the TV. Getting your body into a sleep routine is a great first step to good overall sleep hygiene.

Avoid caffeine and alcohol. Don't consume caffeinated beverages after 1 or 2 PM. Stop consuming them earlier or avoid them altogether if you are especially sensitive to caffeine. Alcohol may make you drowsy and help you fall asleep, but when it wears off several hours later it can cause you to wake up. Alcohol also does not allow you to enter the deep sleep needed for a night of quality sleep. Keep alcohol consumption to a minimum and avoid it just before going to bed.

Don't eat too close to bedtime. Try to eat your evening meal at least three hours before bedtime. If you want an evening snack, choose something light and something that you know will not cause any gastrointestinal problems. Good choices for evening snacks include a small bowl of cereal with milk, yogurt, a banana, or graham crackers.

Exercise. One of the many benefits of an exercise routine is that it can help you sleep. If you are an evening exerciser, do so at least two hours prior to bed. Exercising closer to bedtime can make it more difficult to fall asleep.

Turn your bedroom into a sleep sanctuary. Your bedroom should be for sleep, meditation, intimacy, and reading for pleasure—that's it. If quality sleep is your goal, there should be no TV or computer in your bedroom. Watching TV just prior to bed is not a relaxing way to go to sleep. It is not recommended to fall asleep with the TV on. If you listen to music, choose music that is instrumental only. Lyrics can stimulate your mind and make it difficult to fall or stay asleep. Make sure your bedroom is cool, dark, and quiet. The best temperature for good sleep is 60–68 degrees. Try to get your bedroom as dark as possible. If your partner has a different sleep pattern than you or you cannot achieve total darkness in your bedroom, try a sleep mask to keep out the light. If a quiet bedroom is not possible due to city noise, family, or roommates, try a white noise machine or earplugs. The walls, furniture, and linens in your bedroom should be neutral colors. Your bedroom is not a good place for bold, bright colors.

Establish a bedtime routine. You cannot go from email, studying, or even a television drama directly to bed and expect to fall right to sleep. Get into a routine an hour of so prior to bed to prepare to sleep. Try not to use the computer just prior to bed. The light emitted from the computer can signal your brain to be awake. Put work away one to two hours before bed. Depending on your schedule, you may want to try a bath or shower just before bed. It will drop your temperature and signal your body that it is time to sleep. Try reading something enjoyable for a few minutes once you get in bed. Or, you may want to journal about your day or jot down things you don't want to forget for tomorrow. If you wake up during the night and cannot go back to sleep, try taking a few deep breaths, clear your head, and relax. If you have something on your mind, get up and write it down so you can deal with it in the morning. Remind yourself that it will be taken care of later and try to go back to sleep. If you cannot go back to sleep within 30 minutes or so, get up and read something relaxing for a few minutes then try again to sleep.

If you try all of the tips above and still have trouble falling asleep, staying asleep, or staying awake during the day, consult your physician. You may have a sleep disorder that requires medical attention.

Get Your Finances in Order

You have no doubt heard that money cannot buy happiness. True, but worrying about money may keep you from being happy. In fact, money worries and concerns about the economy have been identified as the top source of stress in America.[41] Although the economic well-being of the country is beyond your control, getting control of your financial matters can mean less stress. Whatever your income or money situation, living within your means will not only decrease your stress but help your financial health as well.

The following strategies can help you get your finances in order and potentially decrease your stress about money:

Create a budget. It does not have to be elaborate, just a small notebook or spreadsheet will do. Calculate all your expenses, living expenses, food, and so on. Make sure to include expenses that you may not pay monthly, such as car insurance. Calculate all of your income, including odd jobs that you pick up from time to time, funds given to you by family members, and so on. Subtract your expenses from your income. Whatever is left is what you have for discretionary spending. If you spend more than that each month, you are living beyond your means and are falling further into debt each month. Analyze your finances and take action to modify your spending habits before they are out of control.

Don't use credit cards. If you use credit cards for convenience and pay off the balance each month, fine. Otherwise, keeping a balance on your credit card and buying things that you don't have the cash for means you are living beyond your means. If you don't have the funds to pay for something right away, don't buy it. The high interest rates on most credit cards make even small purchases a bad idea. By the time you have paid it off, you have paid a substantial amount of money in interest.

Think before you buy. Be mindful of all purchases you make. A latte every day for a week can add up to almost $100 a month. That's not to say that you can't get your daily dose of caffeine, just be aware of what you are spending and make sure it fits into your budget. If it is a conscious decision to spend $4 a day on coffee, then that is different than mindlessly spending and not knowing where your money is going. You may want to try having a one-day grace period between wanting to buy something and buying it. Often you end up not buying it at all or at least making a more informed decision.

A detailed financial management plan is beyond the scope of this text. However, there are plenty of places to turn to for help. If you are in debt, talk with your financial institution to see what your options are. Ask if it offers any type of program or service to help you get out of debt quickly. If you are not in debt, stay that way. Learn to live within your means and begin to build your savings. Educate yourself about money matters. Check with your bank to see if it offers educational seminars about how to manage your money.

Find the Support You Need

Having support to help you handle stress, both good and bad, is essential. That support may come from your partner, family, friends, or faith community. If you are going through a really stressful time or just feel that you can't get your stress under control, you may find it helpful to talk with a mental health professional. A trained counselor or therapist can help you identify the source of stress and help find ways you can learn to cope. Check the resources you have through school or your community to see what is available.

Avoid Unhealthy Behaviors

Adopting healthy habits, including eating right, exercise, and managing stress, are the cornerstones of good health; however, there are also behaviors that you should avoid to achieve optimal health.

Don't Use Tobacco Tobacco use is the number one preventable risk factor for several major chronic diseases. Tobacco increases the risk for heart disease and several forms of cancer.[42–45] Regardless of the source—cigarettes, cigars, pipe, or smokeless—tobacco increases your risk of cancer and other health problems.[46] If you don't use tobacco, don't start. If you do use tobacco, stop. Quitting may not be easy but it is certainly worth the effort. Call 1.800.QUIT NOW or go to www.smokefree.gov for assistance to move towards becoming tobacco free.

How Policy and Environment Affect My Choices

Secondhand Smoke

You don't use tobacco, so you must be at a pretty low risk of lung cancer from exposure to smoke, right? Well, that depends. Exposure to secondhand smoke has been shown to increase the risk of lung and other forms of cancer.[47] How much risk depends on the level of exposure; however, research indicates that even brief exposure to secondhand smoke (30 minutes) can cause cell damage.[48] Secondhand, or passive, smoke is the smoke you experience by being in an environment with smokers. You yourself may not be holding a cigarette, but your body is being exposed to toxic carcinogens.

The dangers of secondhand smoke have triggered policies to protect you from smoke exposure. Most of these policies have been passed at the local or state level. Policies such as no smoking in public places, no smoking in public buildings, and no smoking in restaurants and bars are common across North America. These policies have been put in place to protect workers and consumers from being exposed to harmful smoke. Although these policies were once fodder for controversy, because some thought their rights were being taken away, they are now commonplace, and most consider them helpful for decreasing exposure to secondhand smoke. Smoke-free policies allow you to choose to work or shop or eat in a safer environment.

Alcohol Only in Moderation or Not at All Consume alcohol in moderation or not at all. The amount of alcohol that is recommended for consumption by adults by the *Dietary Guidelines for Americans* is one to two drinks per day for men and one drink per day for women.[49] The risks and benefits of alcohol are discussed in detail in Chapter 7. Although consuming moderate amounts of alcohol can be consistent with good health, overconsumption or abuse of alcohol is dangerous. If you are concerned that you, a friend, or a family member might have a drinking problem, consult your healthcare provider or campus health services or call the National Drug and Alcohol Treatment Referral Routing Service at 1-800-662-HELP.

Don't Abuse Drugs It goes without saying that abuse of drugs is not consistent with good health. Abuse of drugs includes taking prescribed or over-the-counter drugs in a manner not prescribed by a physician or as indicated on the label. Some prescription drugs, such as OxyContin or Vicodin, if taken in excess can have disastrous effects on a person's health. Drug abuse can also include using illegal substances, such as LSD or heroin. If you or someone you know is abusing drugs, taking drugs not prescribed to them by a physician, or taking drugs prescribed to them in excess, get help from a local substance abuse program or your healthcare provider.

Practice Safer Sex

Practice safer sex to protect yourself against sexually transmitted diseases (STDs). Use of condoms, even if you are using some other form of birth control, is standard practice to reduce the risk of STDs, including HIV. Condoms should be used for intercourse and for oral sex. Choose latex condoms and water-based lubricants, because petroleum-based lubricants can damage the condom. Use a new condom for every act of vaginal, anal, or oral sex. Put the condom on before there is any genital contact. Use of condoms shows you care about your health and the health of your partner. Of course, the one sure way to not acquire an STD is to abstain from sexual intercourse.

Avoid Overexposure to the Sun

Protect yourself from overexposure to the sun. Skin cancer is the most common form of cancer in the United States. The second most common forms of skin cancer, basal cell and squamous cell, are highly curable. The third form of skin cancer, melanoma, is much more dangerous and can result in death. Approximately 65–90% of melanomas are caused by exposure to the sun. Tanning beds have also been associated with an increased risk of skin cancer.[50] The younger you are when you start using tanning beds, the more likely you are to have sun damage, including melanoma.[51] To protect yourself from the sun, stay out of tanning beds and use sunscreen year round. Choose a sunscreen that has at least a sun protection factor (SPF) of 15 and that has both UVA and UVB protection. Throw away sunscreen that is past the expiration date displayed on the container. Wear clothing to protect against exposure, including a wide-brim hat and sunglasses. If you want a tan, try some of the sunless tanning products on the market.

Drive and Ride Safely

Motor vehicle–related injuries are the leading cause of death in the United States for people under age 35.[52] Many of these deaths could have been prevented. Seatbelts save thousands of lives each year. As a rider or driver, protect yourself by always wearing your seatbelt. Don't drive or ride with anyone under the influence of drugs or alcohol. Every 45 minutes someone in the United States dies in a motor vehicle crash that involves a driver who is under the influence of alcohol.[53] When you are behind the wheel, make sure that driving is your only task. Distracted driv-

Table 15.1

Screening Tests and Immunization Guidelines for Women

These charts are guidelines only. Your healthcare provider will personalize the timing of each test and immunization to meet your healthcare needs.

Screening Tests	Ages 18–39	Ages 40–49	Ages 50–64	Ages 65 and Older
General health: Full checkup, including weight and height	Discuss with your doctor or nurse.	Discuss with your doctor or nurse.	Discuss with your doctor or nurse.	Discuss with your doctor or nurse.
Thyroid (TSH) test	Discuss with your doctor or nurse.	Discuss with your doctor or nurse.	Discuss with your doctor or nurse.	Discuss with your doctor or nurse.
HIV test	Get the test at least once to find out your HIV status. Ask your doctor or nurse if and when you need the test again.	Get the test at least once to find out your HIV status. Ask your doctor or nurse if and when you need the test again.	Get the test at least once to find out your HIV status. Ask your doctor or nurse if and when you need the test again.	Discuss with your doctor or nurse.
Heart health: Blood pressure test	At least every 2 years	At least every 2 years	At least every 2 years	At least every 2 years
Cholesterol test	Start at age 20, discuss with your doctor or nurse.	Discuss with your doctor or nurse.	Discuss with your doctor or nurse.	Discuss with your doctor or nurse.
Bone health: Bone density screen		Discuss with your doctor or nurse.	Discuss with your doctor or nurse.	Get a bone mineral density test at least once. Talk to your doctor or nurse about repeat testing.
Diabetes: Blood glucose or A1c test	Discuss with your doctor or nurse.	Start at age 45, then every 3 years.	Every 3 years	Every 3 years
Breast health: Mammogram (x-ray of breast)		Every 1–2 years Discuss with your doctor or nurse.	Every 1–2 years Discuss with your doctor or nurse.	Every 1–2 years Discuss with your doctor or nurse.
Clinical breast exam	At least every 3 years starting in your 20s	Yearly	Yearly	Yearly
Reproductive health: Pap test	Every 2 years starting at age 21. Women 30 and older, every 3 years.	Every 3 years	Every 3 years	Discuss with your doctor or nurse.
Pelvic exam	Yearly beginning at age 21. Younger than 21 and sexually active, discuss with your doctor or nurse.	Yearly	Yearly	Yearly
Chlamydia test	Yearly until age 25 if sexually active. Age 26 and older, get this test if you have new or multiple partners.	Get this test if you have new or multiple partners.	Get this test if you have new or multiple partners.	Get this test if you have new or multiple partners.
Sexually transmitted infection (STI) tests	Both partners should get tested for STIs, including HIV, before initiating sexual intercourse.	Both partners should get tested for STIs, including HIV, before initiating sexual intercourse.	Both partners should get tested for STIs, including HIV, before initiating sexual intercourse.	Both partners should get tested for STIs, including HIV, before initiating sexual intercourse.
Mental health screening	Discuss with your doctor or nurse.	Discuss with your doctor or nurse.	Discuss with your doctor or nurse.	Discuss with your doctor or nurse.
Colorectal health: (use 1 of these 3 methods): Fecal occult blood test			Yearly	Yearly. Older than age 75, discuss with your doctor or nurse.
Flexible sigmoidoscopy (with fecal occult blood test)			Every 5 years	Every 5 years. Older than age 75, discuss with your doctor or nurse.
Colonoscopy			Every 10 years	Every 10 years. Older than age 75, discuss with your doctor or nurse.
Eye and ear health: Comprehensive eye exam	Discuss with your doctor.	Get a baseline exam at age 40, then every 2–4 years or as your doctor advises.	Every 2–4 years until age 55, then every 1–3 years until age 65, or as your doctor advises.	Every 1–2 years

Table 15.1

Screening Tests and Immunization Guidelines for Women *(Continued)*

Screening Tests	Ages 18–39	Ages 40–49	Ages 50–64	Ages 65 and Older
Hearing test	Starting at age 18, then every 10 years	Every 10 years	Every 3 years	Every 3 years
Skin health: Mole exam	Monthly mole self-exam; by a doctor or nurse as part of a routine full checkup starting at age 20.	Monthly mole self-exam; by a doctor or nurse as part of a routine full checkup.	Monthly mole self-exam; by a doctor or nurse as part of a routine full checkup.	Monthly mole self-exam; by a doctor or nurse as part of a routine full checkup.
Oral health: Dental exam	Routinely; discuss with your dentist.	Routinely; discuss with your dentist.	Routinely; discuss with your dentist.	Routinely; discuss with your dentist.
Immunizations: Seasonal influenza vaccine	Yearly	Yearly	Yearly	Yearly
Pneumococcal vaccine				One time only
Tetanus-diphtheria-pertussis booster vaccine	Every 10 years	Every 10 years	Every 10 years	Every 10 years
Human papillomavirus (HPV) vaccine	Up to age 26, if not already completed vaccine series; discuss with your doctor or nurse.			
Meningococcal vaccine	Discuss with your doctor or nurse if you are a college student or military recruit.			
Herpes zoster vaccine (to prevent shingles)			Starting at age 60, one time only. Ask your doctor or nurse if it is okay for you to get it.	Starting at age 60, one time only. Ask your doctor or nurse if it is okay for you to get it.

Source: US Department of Health and Human Services, Office on Women's Health. General screenings and immunizations for women. 2009. http://www.womenshealth.gov/prevention/general/general.pdf. Accessed October 6, 2010.

Table 15.2

Screening Tests and Immunization Guidelines for Men

These charts are guidelines only. Your healthcare provider will personalize the timing of each test and immunization to meet your healthcare needs.

Screening Tests	Ages 18–39	Ages 40–49	Ages 50–64	Ages 65 and Older
General health: Full checkup, including weight and height	Discuss with your doctor or nurse.	Discuss with your doctor or nurse.	Discuss with your doctor or nurse.	Discuss with your doctor or nurse.
HIV test	Get the test at least once to find out your HIV status. Ask your doctor or nurse if and when you need the test again.	Get the test at least once to find out your HIV status. Ask your doctor or nurse if and when you need the test again.	Get the test at least once to find out your HIV status. Ask your doctor or nurse if and when you need the test again.	Discuss with your doctor.
Heart health: Blood pressure test	At least every 2 years	At least every 2 years	At least every 2 years	At least every 2 years
Cholesterol test	Start at age 20, discuss with your doctor or nurse.	Discuss with your doctor or nurse.	Discuss with your doctor or nurse.	Discuss with your doctor or nurse.
Diabetes: Blood glucose or A1c test	Discuss with your doctor or nurse.	Start at age 45, then every 3 years.	Every 3 years	Every 3 years
Prostate health: Digital rectal exam (DRE)		Discuss with your doctor or nurse.	Discuss with your doctor or nurse.	Discuss with your doctor or nurse.
Prostate-specific antigen (PSA) test		Discuss with your doctor or nurse.	Discuss with your doctor or nurse.	Discuss with your doctor or nurse.

(continues)

Table 15.2

Screening Tests and Immunization Guidelines for Men *(Continued)*

Screening Tests	Ages 18–39	Ages 40–49	Ages 50–64	Ages 65 and Older
Reproductive health: Testicular exam	Discuss with your doctor or nurse.	Discuss with your doctor or nurse.	Discuss with your doctor or nurse.	Discuss with your doctor or nurse.
Sexually transmitted infection (STI) tests	Both partners should get tested for STIs, including HIV, before initiating sexual intercourse.	Both partners should get tested for STIs, including HIV, before initiating sexual intercourse.	Both partners should get tested for STIs, including HIV, before initiating sexual intercourse.	Both partners should get tested for STIs, including HIV, before initiating sexual intercourse.
Colorectal health: (use 1 of these 3 methods): Fecal occult blood test			Yearly	Yearly. Older than age 75, discuss with your doctor.
Flexible sigmoidoscopy (with fecal occult blood test)			Every 5 years	Every 5 years. Older than age 75, discuss with your doctor.
Colonoscopy			Every 10 years	Every 10 years. Older than age 75, discuss with your doctor.
Eye and ear health: Comprehensive eye exam	Discuss with your doctor.	Get a baseline exam at age 40, then every 2–4 years or as your doctor advises.	Every 2–4 years until age 55, then every 1–3 years until age 65, or as your doctor advises.	Every 1–2 years
Hearing test	Starting at age 18, then every 10 years	Every 10 years	Every 3 years	Every 3 years
Skin health: Mole exam	Monthly mole self-exam; by a doctor or nurse as part of a routine full checkup starting at age 20.	Monthly mole self-exam; by a doctor or nurse as part of a routine full checkup.	Monthly mole self-exam; by a doctor or nurse as part of a routine full checkup.	Monthly mole self-exam; by a doctor or nurse as part of a routine full checkup.
Oral health: Dental exam	Routinely; discuss with your dentist.	Routinely; discuss with your dentist.	Routinely; discuss with your dentist.	Routinely; discuss with your dentist.
Mental health screening	Discuss with your doctor or nurse.	Discuss with your doctor or nurse.	Discuss with your doctor or nurse.	Discuss with your doctor or nurse.
Immunizations: Seasonal influenza vaccine	Yearly	Yearly	Yearly	Yearly
Pneumococcal vaccine				One time only
Tetanus-diphtheria-pertussis booster vaccine	Every 10 years	Every 10 years	Every 10 years	Every 10 years
Meningococcal vaccine	Discuss with your doctor or nurse if you are a college student or military recruit.			
Herpes zoster vaccine (to prevent shingles)			Starting at age 60, one time only. Ask your doctor or nurse if it is okay for you to get it.	Starting at age 60, one time only. Ask your doctor or nurse if it is okay for you to get it.
Human papillomavirus (HPV) vaccine	Up to age 26, if not already completed vaccine series; discuss with your doctor or nurse.			

Source: US Department of Health and Human Services, Office on Women's Health. General screenings and immunizations for men. 2010. http://www.womenshealth.gov/prevention/men/men.pdf. Accessed October 6, 2010.

ing includes anything that takes your attention from the road, including eating, drinking, using a cell phone, using a GPS navigation system, adjusting the radio, or texting. Many states have laws that prohibit cell phone use in the car unless it is a hands-free device. Whatever your state law, be safe and don't text or use your cell phone while driving.

Practice Bicycle Safety

Bicycling for transportation or for recreation is a great way to stay physically active; however, you need to stay safe as well. Wherever you ride, on the road, trail, or greenway, always wear a well-fitting helmet with chinstrap. If you are riding on the road, you must obey all traffic laws and signal turns using your left hand. Ride on the right side with traffic, never ride away from traffic. Be careful when passing parked cars; an open door can lead to a crash. Avoid busy streets if at all possible. Know your ability. If you are a beginner rider, ride on trails and in neighborhoods until you build up your bicycling skills. Check with a local bike shop or your state's Department of Transportation to see if there are bicycle safety workshops in your area.

Get Proper Medical Care

Getting proper medical care throughout your life is critical. That means seeing a physician or other healthcare provider on a regular basis, not just when you are sick or have a medical problem. You should also see a healthcare provider to schedule appropriate screenings that can identify diseases before you have symptoms. Your healthcare provider can perform some critical tests to help you track your overall health over time.[54,55] It is your responsibility as a patient to take control of your own health care. Actively participate in decisions you and your healthcare provider make about your health care. Get and stay informed about what screenings are recommended. The U.S. Department of Health and Human Services Agency for Health Care Research and Quality offers the latest in healthcare information for consumers (www.healthfinder.gov).

Personal Health Check

Know Your Numbers

You should know some critical numbers about your health. Take note of where you are now and follow your numbers over time. If any of your numbers are not in line, take steps to get them there. First, you should know your height and weight, which can be used to calculate your BMI, as well as your waist circumference. You should also know your blood pressure; this can be taken at your doctor's office, a local health department, or a pharmacy. You should also know your total cholesterol, LDL cholesterol, HDL cholesterol, triglycerides, and fasting blood glucose. For these measures, you will have to have a small amount of blood drawn that can be analyzed in a lab. You can get these tests at your doctor's office or health department.

Know Your Numbers

Measure	Goal
BMI: weight in pounds × 703/(height in inches)^2	< 25
Waist circumference	< 35 inches
Blood pressure	< 120/80 mm Hg
Fasting glucose	< 100 mg/dL
Total cholesterol	< 200mg/dL
LDL (lousy) cholesterol	< 100 mg/dL
HDL (healthy) cholesterol	≥ 50 mg/dL

Ready to Make a Change

Are you ready to make a change, small or large, in your overall health and well-being? If you are not eating healthy and are not active on a regular basis, you should start there. If you use tobacco, the biggest step you can take to positively impact your health is to stop. What other steps can you take for wellness? Make the commitment to take the first step. Whether it is a small, medium, or large change, it is a step in the right direction toward overall health and wellness.

I commit to a small first step. Know your numbers.

I am ready to take the next step and make a medium change. Practice good sleep hygiene. Think about the amount and quality of sleep you currently get and work towards getting the proper amount of sleep.

I have been making changes for some time and am ready to make a large change in my overall health. Practice stress management. Stress can have a profound impact on your overall health. Use some of the strategies in this chapter to create a stress management plan that works for you.

Myth Versus Fact

Myth: Catching up on sleep on the weekend is a good way to get the amount of sleep you need.

Fact: Staying on a routine of getting enough sleep each night is important for good health.

Myth: Not getting enough sleep is just a fact of life when you are in college.

Fact: Although it may be common for college students to not get the sleep they need, it should not be the norm. To perform your best in school and have good overall health, getting enough sleep is critical.

Myth: My boyfriend smokes, but it is only his health he is hurting.

Fact: If your boyfriend chooses to smoke around you or you allow him to smoke around you, you are being exposed to harmful secondhand smoke.

Myth: Stress is just a part of life. There is nothing you can do about it.

Fact: While it is true that stress cannot be avoided, you can look for ways to manage stress so you can mitigate its negative effects over time.

Myth: I am healthy, so there is no need for me to see a doctor.

Fact: Several health screenings need to be performed throughout life to detect diseases, even before you begin to have symptoms.

Myth: Tanning is fine as long as I don't burn.

Fact: There is no such thing as a safe tan. Exposure to sun, outside or in a tanning bed, increases your risk of skin cancer.

Myth: Using a condom is not necessary if my girlfriend is using birth control pills.

Fact: Birth control pills do a great job at preventing pregnancy but they do not protect against STDs. Use a condom for vaginal and anal intercourse as well as oral sex to help prevent HIV and other sexually transmitted diseases.

Back to the Story

Britney has managed even with a hectic school and work schedule to find time to stay active and eat healthy. Thanks to these two positive health behaviors, she is a healthy weight. There are other aspects of health in Britney's life, however, that need attention. Even though she is healthy, she should see a physician for a routine checkup and make sure that she has the proper screenings and immunizations for her age. Because she has health insurance, part or all of the cost of this may be covered. She also could do a better job of balancing work, school, and a social life. Her heavy workload is more than likely causing her to be overly stressed. If this is temporary, such as during final exams, that may not be a major concern. However, if her life is constantly out of balance, stress will begin to take its toll on her overall health. She may want to consider scheduling her work and school so that at least one or two nights a week she has time for friends and family or just to do something she enjoys. She should examine the amount of sleep she is getting on a regular basis. Getting proper sleep will help her to perform better at work and school. She should look at scheduling proper sleep just as she does scheduling time for all her other responsibilities. What other suggestions could you make for Britney to help her address her overall health?

References

1. Cohen S, Kessler RC, Gordon UL. Strategies for measuring stress in studies of psychiatric and physical disorder. In: Cohen S, Kessler RC, Gordon UL, eds. *Measuring Stress: A Guide for Health and Social Scientists*. New York, NY: Oxford University Press, 1995:3–26.
2. McEwen BS. Protective and damaging effects of stress mediators. *N Engl J Med*. 1998;338(3):171–179.
3. Graham JE, Christian LM, Kiecolt-Glaser JK. Stress, age, and immune function: toward a lifespan approach. *J Behav Med*. 2006;29(4):389–400.
4. O'Leary A. Stress, emotion, and human immune function. *Psychological Bulletin*. 1990;108(3):363–382.
5. Krantz DS, McCeney MK. Effects of psychological and social factors on organic disease: a critical assessment of research on coronary heart disease. *Annu Rev Psychol*. 2002;53:341–369.
6. Kivimaki M, Virtanen M, Elovainio M, Kouvonen A, Vaananen A, Vahtera J. Work stress in the etiology of coronary heart disease—a meta-analysis. *Scand J Work Environ Health*. 2006;32(6):431–442.
7. Li J, Hansen D, Mortensen PB, Olsen J. Myocardial infarction in parents who lost a child: a nationwide prospective cohort study in Denmark. *Circulation*. 2002;106(13):1634–1639.
8. Hammen C. Stress and depression. *Annu Rev Clin Psychol*. 2005;1:293–319.
9. van Praag HM, de Koet ER, van Os J. *Stress, the Brain and Depression*. Cambridge, England: Cambridge University Press, 2004.
10. Connor J, Norton R, Ameratunga S, Robinson E, Civil I, Dunn R, Bailey J, Jackson R. Driver sleepiness and risk of serious injury to car occupants: population based case control study. *BMJ*. 2002;324:1125.
11. National Sleep Foundation. How much sleep do we really need? http://www.sleepfoundation.org/article/how-sleep-works/how-much-sleep-do-we-really-need. Accessed October 5, 2010.
12. Mayer EA, Naliboff BD, Chang L, Coutinho SV. Stress and the gastrointestinal tract v. stress and irritable bowel syndrome. *Am J Physiol Gastrointest Liver Physiol*. 2001;280:519–524.
13. Chen E, Miller GE. Stress and inflammation in exacerbations of asthma. *Brain, Behav Immun*. 2007;21(8):993–999.
14. Berger BG. Stress reduction through exercise: the mind–body connection. *Motor Skills: Theory into Practice*. 1983;7(2):31–46.
15. Berger BG. Facts and fancy: mood alteration though exercise. *J Phys Ed Rec Dance*. 1982;53(9):47–48.
16. Dishman RK. Biological influences on exercise adherence. *Res Quarterly Exercise Sport*. 1981;52(2):143–159.
17. Folkins, CH, Sime WE. Physical fitness training and mental health. *Am Psychologist*. 1981;36:372–389.
18. Hossain JL, Shapiro CM. The prevalence, cost implications, and management of sleep disorders: an overview. *Sleep Breath*. 2002;6:85–102.
19. Maas JB, Wherry ML. *Power sleep: the revolutionary program that prepares your mind for peak performance*. New York: Quill/HarperCollins, 2001.
20. Sorcher AJ. How is your sleep? a neglected topic for health care screening. *J Am Board Fam Med*. 2008;21:141–148.
21. Strine TW, Chapman DP. Associations of frequent sleep insufficiency with health-related quality of life and health behaviors. *Sleep Med*. 2005;6:23–7.
22. Haack M, Mullington JM. Sustained sleep restriction reduces emotional and physical well-being. *Pain*. 2005;119:56–64.
23. Hasler G, Buysse DJ, Gamma A, et al. Excessive daytime sleepiness in young adults: a 20-year prospective community study. *J Clin Psychiatry*. 2005; 66:521–9.
24. Baldwin CM, Griffith KA, Nieto FJ, O'Connor GT, Walsleben JA, Redline S. The association of sleep disordered breathing and sleep symptoms with quality of life in the sleep heart health study. *Sleep*. 2001;24:96–105.
25. von Kries R, Toschke AM, Wurmser H, Sauerwald T, Koletzko B. Reduced risk for overweight and obesity in 5- and 6-year-old children by duration of sleep—a cross-sectional study. *Int J Obes Relat Metab Disord*. 2002; 26:710–716.
26. Gangwisch JE, Malaspina D, Boden-Albala B, Heymsfield SB. Inadequate sleep as a risk factor for obesity: analysis of the NHANES I. *Sleep*. 2005;28:1289–1296.
27. Coughlin SR, Mawdsley L, Mugarza JA, Calverley PM, Wilding JP. Obstructive sleep apnoea is independently associated with an increased prevalence of metabolic syndrome. *Eur Heart J*. 2004;25(9):735–741.
28. Bass J, Turek FW. Sleepless in America: a pathway to obesity and the metabolic syndrome? *Arch Intern Med*. 2005;165(1):15–16.
29. Gami AS, Somers VK. Obstructive sleep apnoea, metabolic syndrome, and cardiovascular outcomes. *Eur Heart J*. 2004;25(9):709–711.
30. Gottlieb DJ, Punjabi NM, Newman AB, et al. Association of sleep time with diabetes mellitus and impaired glucose tolerance. *Arch Intern Med*. 2005;165:863–867.
31. Taheri S, Lin L, Austin D, Young T, Mignot E. Short sleep duration is associated with reduced leptin, elevated ghrelin, and increased body mass index. PLoS Med 2004;1(3):e62.
32. Vgontzas AN, Papanicolaou DA, Bixler EO, Kales A, Tyson K, Chrousos GP. Elevation of plasma cytokines in disorders of excessive daytime sleepiness: role of sleep disturbance and obesity. *J Clin Endocrinol Metab*. 1997;82:1313–1316.

33. Patel SR, Hu FB. Short sleep duration and weigh gain: a systematic review. *Obesity*. 2008;16:643–653.
34. Spiegel K, Tasali E, Penev P, VanCauter E. Brief communication: sleep curtailment in healthy young men is associated with decreased leptin levels, elevated ghrelin levels, and increased hunger and appetite. *Ann Intern Med*. 2004;141:846–850.
35. Ford DE, Kamerow DB. Epidemiologic study of sleep disturbances and psychiatric disorders. An opportunity for prevention? *JAMA*. 1989;262(11):1479–1484.
36. Baldwin DC Jr, Daugherty SR. Sleep deprivation and fatigue in residency training: results of a national survey of first- and second-year residents. *Sleep*. 2004;27:217–23.
37. Roth T, Roehrs T. Insomnia: epidemiology, characteristics, and consequences. *Clin Cornerstone*. 2003; 5:5–15.
38. Durmer JS, Dinges DF. Neurocognitive consequences of sleep deprivation. *Seminars in Neurology*. 2005;25(1):117–129.
39. Leger D. The cost of sleep-related accidents: a report for the national commission on sleep disorders research. *Sleep*. 1994;17:84–93.
40. Hor H, Tafti M. How much sleep do we need? *Science*. 2009;325:825–826.
41. American Psychological Association. Economy and money top causes of stress for Americans. http://www.apa.org/news/press/releases/2008/06/economy-stress.aspx. Accessed October 22, 2010.
42. Ockene IS, Miller NH. Cigarette smoking, cardiovascular disease, and stroke: a statement for healthcare professionals from the American Heart Association, American Heart Association Task Force on Risk Reduction. *Circulation*. 1997;96:3243–3247.
43. Barnoya J, Glantz SA. Cardiovascular effects of secondhand smoke: nearly as large as smoking. *Circulation*. 2005;111:2684–2698.
44. Khuder SA, Milz S, Jordan T, Price J, Silvestri K, Butler P. The impact of a smoking ban on hospital admissions for coronary heart disease. *Prev Med*. 2007;45(1):3–8.
45. Gandini S, Botteri E, Iodice S, et al. Tobacco smoking and cancer: a meta-analysis. *Int J Cancer*. 2008;122(1):155–164.
46. Boffetta P, Hecht S, Gray N, Gupta P, Straif K. Smokeless tobacco and cancer. *The Lancet Oncology*. 2008;9(7):667–675.
47. Oberg M, Jaakkola MS, Woodward A, Peruga A, Pruss-Ustun A. Worldwide burden of disease from exposure to second-hand smoke: a retrospective analysis of data from 192 countries. *Lancet*. 2011;377:139–146.
48. Heiss C, Amabile N, Lee AC, et al. Brief secondhand smoke exposure depress endothelial progenitor cells activity and endothelial function. *J Am Cardiol*. 2008;51:1760–1771.
49. US Department of Agriculture and US Department of Health and Human Services. *Dietary Guidelines for Americans, 2010*. 7th ed. Washington DC. US Government Printing Office, December 2010.
50. The International Agency for Research on Cancer Working Group on artificial ultraviolet (UV) light and skin cancer. The association of use of sunbeds with cutaneous malignant melanoma and other skin cancers: A systematic review. *Int J Cancer*. 2007;120:1116–1122.
51. Westerdahl J, Ingvar C, MasbackA. Jonsson N, Olsson H. Risk of cutaneous malignant melanoma in relation to use of sunbeds: further evidence for UV-A carcinogenicity. *Br J Cancer*. 2000;82:1593–1599.
52. Xu J, Kochanek KD, Murphy SL, Tejada-Vera B. Death: final data for 2007. *National Vital Statistics Reports*. 2010:58(19). http://www.cdc.gov/nchs/data/nvsr/nvsr58/nvsr58_19.pdf. Accessed December 10, 2010.
53. Dept of Transportation (US), National Highway Traffic Safety Administration (NHTSA). Traffic Safety Facts 2008: Alcohol-Impaired Driving. Washington, DC: NHTSA; 2009. http://www-nrd.nhtsa.dot.gov/Pubs/811155.PDF. Accessed December 9, 2010.
54. US Department of Health and Human Services, Office on Women's Health. General screenings and immunizations for women. 2009. http://www.womenshealth.gov/prevention/general/general.pdf. Accessed October 6, 2010.
55. US Department of Health and Human Services, Office on Women's Health. General screenings and immunizations for men. 2010. http://www.womenshealth.gov/prevention/men/men.pdf. Accessed October 6, 2010.

Appendix A

Vitamins and Minerals

Vitamin or Mineral	Best Sources	Function(s)	Deficiency Symptoms	Toxicity Symptoms	Notes
Fat-Soluble Vitamins					
Vitamin A RDA: Women: 700 micrograms Men: 900 micrograms UL: 3,000 micrograms	Carrots Sweet potatoes Winter squash Cantaloupe Spinach Broccoli Leafy greens Milk (fortified with vitamin A) Beef liver Chicken liver	Essential for healthy vision. Supports a healthy immune system. Needed for the formation and maintenance of mucous membranes, skin, and bones.	Rare in developed countries. Increased susceptibility of infection. Impaired vision, especially in dim light. Xerophthalmia, or night blindness, is caused by a vitamin A deficiency.	Vitamin A toxicity from foods is generally not a problem. Vitamin A in excess of the UL can cause fatigue, vomiting, bone and joint pain, skin disorders, and birth defects.	There are three active forms of vitamin A—retinol, retinal, and retinoic acid—referred to as the retinoids. Carotenoids are precursors for vitamin A and are powerful antioxidants. The body can use preformed vitamin A and beta-carotene to make the active form of vitamin A in the body. The amount of vitamin A in foods is expressed in retinol activity equivalents (RAE), which is a measure of the amount of active vitamin A that your body will get from that food.
Vitamin D AI: 200 IU UL: 2,000 IU	Exposure to sunlight Fortified foods, including milk and breakfast cereals	Essential for healthy bones. Increases absorption of calcium and phosphorus.	Rickets in children is a result of low vitamin D and is characterized by weak, deformed bones. Reduced calcium absorption in adults can result in osteoporosis.	Vitamin D in excess of the UL can cause nausea, vomiting, loss of appetite, or pain. Vitamin D in excess of the UL may be prescribed for some conditions or to address low vitamin D levels.	Poor vitamin D status is common, especially with advancing age.
Vitamin E RDA: 15 milligrams UL: 1,000 milligrams	Nuts Seeds Vegetable oils	Serves as an antioxidant. Helps in the formation of red blood cells.	Rare except in individuals with severe malnutrition or inability to absorb fat.	No adverse effects from consuming vitamin E in food. High doses of supplements can cause hemorrhage and interrupt blood coagulation.	Inconsistent and limited evidence to support vitamin E's role in cancer prevention. Conflicting results as to vitamin E's role in reducing risk of heart disease.
Vitamin K AI: Women: 90 micrograms Men: 120 micrograms	Green leafy vegetables Soybean oil Olive oil Canola oil	Necessary for normal blood clotting.	Impaired blood clotting. Deficiency is uncommon in healthy adults.	No known toxicity.	Can be made by the bacteria in the digestive tract.
Water-Soluble Vitamins					
Vitamin C RDA: Women: 75 milligrams Men: 90 milligrams UL: 2,000 milligrams	Citrus fruit Tomatoes Strawberries Cantaloupe Vegetables in the cabbage family (Brussels sprouts, cauliflower, broccoli)	Serves as an antioxidant. Needed for the synthesis of collagen, which helps in wound healing, bone formation, and strengthening blood vessel walls. Strengthens resistance to infection. Aids in iron absorption	Scurvy is the deficiency disease for vitamin C. It is characterized by anemia, depression, bleeding gums, loose teeth, and poor wound healing.	Nausea, diarrhea, headache, fatigue, increased risk for kidney stones.	Many believe that vitamin C can cure the common cold. Many well-controlled studies have proven otherwise, but despite this evidence people continue to take vitamin C when a cold strikes.

Vitamin or Mineral	Best Sources	Function(s)	Deficiency Symptoms	Toxicity Symptoms	Notes
Thiamin (B_1) RDA: Women: 1.1 milligrams Men: 1.2 milligrams	Meat Fish Poultry Whole grains Enriched breads, cereals, and grains Nuts Legumes	Aids in the release of energy from carbohydrates. Supports nervous system function.	Beriberi is the deficiency disease for thiamine. It is characterized by edema, heart irregularity, mental confusion, muscle weakness, and impaired growth.	No known toxicity.	
Riboflavin (B_2) RDA: Women: 1.1 milligrams Men: 1.3 milligrams	Milk and milk products Green leafy vegetables Whole grains Enriched breads, cereals, and grains	Aids in the release of energy from energy-providing nutrients. Promotes healthy skin. Promotes normal vision.	Skin problems, especially around the nose and mouth. Eye problems. Magenta tongue. Hypersensitivity to light.	No known toxicity.	Can be destroyed by sunlight or fluorescent lighting, which is why milk is usually sold in cardboard or opaque plastic containers as opposed to clear glass or plastic.
Niacin (B_3) RDA: Women: 14 milligrams Men: 16 milligrams UL: 35 milligrams	Meat Eggs Poultry Fish Whole grains Enriched breads, cereals, and grains Nuts Legumes	Aids in the release of energy from energy-providing nutrients. Promotes healthy skin.	Pellagra is the deficiency disease for niacin. It is characterized by flaky skin on skin exposed to the sun, loss of appetite, weakness, dizziness, fatigue, and indigestion.	Nausea, flushing, headaches, cramps, heartburn, liver damage.	Very high doses (10 times the RDA) have been shown to lower blood cholesterol. However, this produces side effects and can cause liver damage. High doses of niacin should only be taken under the care of a physician.
Vitamin B_6 RDA: Women: 1.3 milligrams Woman 51 and older: 1.7 milligrams Men: 1.3 milligrams Men 51 and older: 1.7 milligrams	Meat Poultry Fish Shellfish Legumes Whole grains Green leafy vegetables Fruit	Aids in the metabolism of protein and fat. Involved in the formation of antibodies. Involved in the formation of red blood cells.	Nervous disorders, skin rash, anemia, kidney stones.	Depression, fatigue, irritability, headaches, nerve damage.	High doses of B_6 have been used to treat carpal tunnel syndrome. However, there is no evidence that this is effective.
Vitamin B_{12} RDA: 2.4 micrograms	Meat Cheese Milk Poultry Eggs Products fortified with vitamin B_{12}	Helps maintain nerve cells. Involved in red blood cell formation.	Anemia, smooth red tongue, fatigue, nerve degeneration that can progress to paralysis.	No known toxicity.	Unlike other B vitamins in that it is not found in plants. The body stores large amounts of vitamin B_{12}.
Folate RDA: 400 micrograms	Legumes Green leafy vegetables Citrus fruits Melons Cereals fortified with folate	Essential for DNA synthesis and cell division. Needed for protein metabolism.	Anemia, diarrhea, smooth red tongue, depression, poor growth, increased risk of heart disease and certain forms of cancer.	People sensitive to folate may experience hives or respiratory distress when taking folate supplements.	Good folate status early in pregnancy greatly reduces the risk of neural tube defects. Because folate is needed so early in pregnancy, when women may be unaware that they are pregnant, several common foods are fortified with folic acid.
Pantothenic acid AI: 5 micrograms	Widespread in foods	Involved in energy metabolism.	Uncommon.	No known toxicity.	

Vitamin or Mineral	Best Sources	Function(s)	Deficiency Symptoms	Toxicity Symptoms	Notes
Biotin AI: 30 micrograms	Widespread in foods	Involved in energy metabolism.	Loss of appetite, nausea, depression, muscle pain.	No known toxicity.	
Macrominerals					
Sodium AI: Younger than age 51: 1,500 milligrams Ages 51–70: 1,300 milligrams Over age 70: 1,200 milligrams UL: Younger than age 51: 2,300mg; Ages 51 and older, African American, or those who have hypertension, diabetes, or chronic kidney disease: 1,500mg	Salt Soy sauce Condiments Processed foods	Helps maintain normal fluid and acid-base balance.	Muscle cramps and loss of appetite.	High blood pressure.	Getting enough sodium is not an issue for most people. Most people consume far too much sodium, which puts them at risk for high blood pressure.
Chloride AI: Younger than age 51: 2,300 milligrams Ages 51–70: 2,000 milligrams Over age 70: 1,800 milligrams UL: 3,600 milligrams	Salt Soy sauce Processed foods	Essential component of hydrochloric acid found in the stomach. Necessary for proper digestion. Essential for fluid balance.	Muscle cramps, growth failure in children, loss of appetite.	No known toxicity.	
Potassium AI: 4,700 milligrams	Meat Milk Fruits and vegetables Grains Legumes	Essential for fluid balance. Involved in muscle contraction.	Muscle weakness, paralysis, confusion; can cause death in severe cases.	Toxicity from potassium from food is rare. Potassium supplements should only be prescribed by a healthcare provider due to the potential of large amounts of potassium slowing or even stopping the heart.	Moderate potassium deficiency may increase risk of high blood pressure.
Calcium AI: Younger than age 51: 1,000 milligrams Age 51 and older: 1,200 milligrams UL: 2,500 mg	Milk and milk products Green leafy vegetables Soybeans Tofu processed with calcium carbonate	Essential for bone mineralization. Involved in muscle contraction. Needed for proper blood clotting.	Bone loss in adults (osteoporosis). Improper growth in children.	Toxicity is rare; however, calcium supplements may interfere with the absorption of other minerals, specifically iron, zinc, and magnesium.	The body keeps the calcium level in the blood constant. Even if calcium intake is very low, calcium will be pulled from the bones.

Vitamin or Mineral	Best Sources	Function(s)	Deficiency Symptoms	Toxicity Symptoms	Notes
Phosphorus RDA: 700 milligrams UL: 4,000 milligrams	Meat Poultry Milk and milk products Soft drinks Processed foods	Involved in the mineralization of bones and teeth. Essential for acid-base balance.	Uncommon.	Kidney stones.	
Magnesium RDA: Women: 320 milligrams Men: 420 milligrams UL: 350 milligrams from nonfood sources	Nuts Legumes Green leafy vegetables Seafood	Involved in bone mineralization. Essential for protein synthesis. Needed for muscle contraction.	Weakness, confusion, growth failure.	Uncommon.	Calcium can interfere with the absorption of magnesium. If you take a calcium supplement, be sure to regularly include foods high in magnesium in your diet.
Microminerals					
Iron RDA: Women younger than age 51: 18 milligrams Women 51 and over: 8 milligrams Men: 8 milligrams UL: 45 milligrams	Meat Seafood Spinach Lentils Cereals fortified with iron	Transports oxygen in the blood. Serves as a component of many enzymes.	Anemia.	Digestive problems. Accidental iron overdose is a leading cause of poising deaths in young children.	Cooking in an iron pan, especially acid foods, such as spaghetti sauce, can increase the iron content of food dramatically.
Zinc RDA: Women: 8 milligrams Men: 11 milligrams UL: 40 milligrams	Meat Fish Shellfish Poultry Cereals fortified with zinc	Helps stabilize cell membranes. Supports fertility and reproduction. Involved in cell growth and replication.	Uncommon.	Uncommon from food sources. High doses of zinc through supplements can cause a decrease in immune function.	Zinc lozenges are commonly used to decrease the duration of the common cold. There is conflicting evidence as to the effectiveness.
Copper RDA: 900 micrograms UL: 10,000 micrograms	Shellfish Sunflower seeds Hazelnuts Mushrooms Beans Peanuts	Helps make hemoglobin. Serves as a component of several enzymes.	Uncommon.	Uncommon.	
Manganese AI: Women: 1.8 milligrams Men: 2.3 milligrams UL: 11 milligrams	Green leafy vegetables Whole grains Sweet potatoes	Involved in energy metabolism. Serves as a component of several enzymes.	Uncommon.	Uncommon.	
Molybdenum RDA: 45 micrograms UL: 2,000 micrograms	Grains Nuts Legumes	Serves as a component of several enzymes.	Uncommon.	Uncommon.	

Vitamin or Mineral	Best Sources	Function(s)	Deficiency Symptoms	Toxicity Symptoms	Notes
Selenium RDA: 55 micrograms UL: 400 micrograms	Meat Seafood Whole grains Vegetables	Serves as a component of enzymes.	Impaired immune function; may increase the risk of some forms of cancer.	Brittle nails and hair, nausea, abdominal pain, liver and nerve damage.	The content of selenium in vegetables depends greatly on the amount of selenium in the soil where they are grown.
Iodine RDA: 150 micrograms UL: 1,100 micrograms	Iodized salt Seafood Bread Eggs	Essential component of thyroid hormones.	Low levels of thyroid hormones. Severe deficiency causes a goiter or enlargement of the thyroid gland—this is rare in North America.	Decreased thyroid activity.	
Fluoride AI: Women: 3 milligrams Men: 4 milligrams UL: 10 milligrams	Water, if fluoridated or naturally containing fluorine Tea Seafood	Needed for proper bone and teeth formation. Helps make teeth resistant to decay.	Susceptibility to tooth decay.	Discoloration of teeth (fluorosis), nausea, vomiting.	
Chromium AI: Women under age 51: 25 milligrams Women 51 and over: 20 milligrams Men: 35 milligrams Men 51 and over: 30 milligrams	Whole grains Meats Vegetable oil	Helps glucose move into the cell. Aids in lipid metabolism.	Abnormal glucose metabolism.	Only known toxicity is exposure to airborne chromium in industrial settings.	Chromium supplements are popular among athletes and body builders even though there is limited evidence of their effectiveness.

Appendix B

Nutrition and Health for Canadians

Contents

Canadian Guidelines for Nutrition

For more than 60 years, the Canadian government has worked to promote healthy and nutritious eating habits. In 1987, Health and Welfare Canada began a major review of the system for guiding Canadians on their food choices. To perform the review, the government appointed two advisory committees—the Scientific Review Committee and the Communications and Implementation Committee.

After examining research evidence available on nutrition and public health, the Scientific Review Committee issued a report in 1990 called *Nutrition Recommendations.* The report included both updated Recommended Nutrient Intakes (RNI) and a scientific description of a healthy dietary pattern that would deliver adequate nutrients for health and reduce the risk of nutrition-related chronic diseases.

Meanwhile, the Communications and Implementation Committee translated these scientific findings into understandable guidelines and outlined implementation strategies in a report called *Action Towards Healthy Eating: Technical Report* (1990). This report suggested that Canada develop a "total diet approach" towards healthy eating. A total diet approach would give consumers a better idea of eating patterns associated with reducing the risk of developing chronic diseases.

In 1990, the government issued *Nutrition Recommendations: A Call for Action*, a summary report produced jointly by the Scientific Review Committee and the Communications and Implementation Committee.

A Revised Food Guide

In accordance with the recommendations of its two advisory groups, the Health Department undertook to revise *Canada's Food Guide*. In 1992, the agency launched *Canada's Food Guide to Healthy Eating* and an explanatory document called *Using the Food Guide.* It promoted dietary diversity, a reduction in total fat intake, and an active lifestyle and offered consumers a pattern for establishing healthy eating habits in their daily selection of foods.

Moreover, the guide introduced a number of new concepts. A range of servings from the four food groups accommodated the wide range of energy needs for different ages, body sizes, activity levels, genders, and conditions such as pregnancy and nursing. The wide range of servings in grain products, vegetables, and fruits was designed to give consumers a better idea of the type of diet that would help reduce the risk of developing nutrition-related chronic diseases.

The guide also introduced a category of "other" foods such as sweets, fats such as butter, and drinks like coffee, that, though part of the diets of many Canadians, would traditionally not have been mentioned in a food guide. The guide recommended moderation in the consumption of these foods and acknowledged their role, along with the wide range of servings in grains, vegetables, and fruits, as a "total diet approach" to healthy eating.

A Work in Progress

Some groups and organizations challenged specific aspects of the government's *Nutrition Recommendations.* In a typically Canadian twist, the government responded to challengers by including them in the development process. When the Canadian Pediatric Society, for example, queried the dietary recommendations on fat consumption in children, the Society was invited to join Health Canada in researching the issue. The result was *Nutrition Recommendations Update: Dietary Fat and Children* (1993), which adjusted the recommendation of appropriate levels of dietary fat for growing children. In 1995, Health Canada issued *Canada's Food Guide to Healthy Eating: Focus on Preschoolers* as a background paper for educators and communicators.

A thorough review of the 1992 *Food Guide* began in 2002. Many strengths as well as some challenges in understanding and using the information from the 1992 *Food Guide* were identified. An assessment of the nutritional adequacy of the 1992 *Food Guide* using Dietary Reference Intakes was undertaken. The assessment also sought to address changes in the food supply and patterns of food use. Extensive stakeholder consultation was also carried out. Health Canada worked with three advisory groups, an external *Food Guide* Advisory Committee, an Interdepartmental Working Group, and the Expert Advisory Committee on Dietary Reference Intakes throughout the revision process. In 2007, Health Canada released *Eating Well with Canada's Food Guide*, which is available in 10 languages. In addition, *A Food Guide for First Nations, Inuit, and Métis,* which recognizes the cultural, spiritual, and physical importance of traditional aboriginal foods, was also released in 2007.

Health Canada has positioned nutrition in a broader health context, which includes physical activity and a positive outlook on life. One result of this comprehensive approach was the Vitality Leaders Kit (1994), intended to help community leaders promote healthy eating, active living, and positive self-image and body image in an integrated way. *Canada's Physical Activity Guidelines* were released in 2011.

Looking Ahead

The job of keeping Canada's nutrition policy and consumer guidelines up-to-date is an ongoing task. New scientific research on nutrition and health continually uncovers new relationships and connections between them. Consumer tastes in foods vary in response to prevailing fashions and shifting demographics. Global trade also influences the food choices that appear on the Canadian dinner table.

The science underlying nutrition recommendations knows no borders. An increasingly complex knowledge base on nutrients, food and health, global trade, and international agreements requires international efforts. Scientists from Canada and the United States worked with the National Academy of Sciences to develop the Dietary

Reference Intakes (DRIs), recommended nutrient intake levels for healthy people in the U.S. and Canada.

To keep abreast of the latest developments in Canada's nutrition policies, visit the Food and Nutrition area of the Health Canada website at: http://www.hc-sc.gc.ca.

Nutrient Intake Recommendations for Canadians

Health Canada has reviewed and made recommendations on nutrient requirements on a periodic basis since 1938. Known as the Recommended Nutrient Intakes, or RNI, these values were last published in 1990 as part of *Nutrition Recommendations: The Report of the Scientific Review Committee*. Since that time, there have been advances in science and by 1994, it was clear that it was time to initiate another review of the scientific data.

At the same time, the Food and Nutrition Board of the National Academy of Sciences was beginning a consultation process on the review of the Recommended Dietary Allowances, the nutrient recommendations used in the United States. Health Canada considered that participating in the U.S. review would offer several advantages to Canada. These were as follows:

- The science underlying nutrient requirements knows no borders and scientists everywhere are utilizing the same knowledge produced from studies conducted all over the world.
- The knowledge base on nutrients, foods, and health is increasing rapidly in scope and complexity. This increases the need for specialized expertise. Participating in the U.S. review permits Canada to expand the base of scientific expertise that could be utilized.
- International trade considerations, including NAFTA, suggest that the harmonization of the science base underlying nutrition policy will facilitate harmonization of such trade-related matters as nutrition labeling and food composition.

Canadian and American scientists establish Dietary Reference Intakes (DRIs) through a review process overseen by the Food and Nutrition Board of the Institute of Medicine, National Academy of Sciences. DRIs have replaced the RNIs and are found printed inside the covers of this text.

The National Academy of Sciences is an American private nonprofit society of distinguished scholars engaged in scientific and engineering research, dedicated to the advancement of science and technology and to their use for the general welfare. The Academy has a mandate that requires it to advise the U.S. federal government on scientific and technical matters.

The Food and Nutrition Board (FNB) is a unit of the Institute of Medicine, part of the National Academy of Sciences. The Board is a multidisciplinary group of biomedical scientists with expertise in various aspects of nutrition, food sciences, biochemistry, medicine, public health, epidemiology, food toxicology, and food safety. The major focus of the FNB is to evaluate emerging knowledge of nutrient requirements and relationships between diet and the reduction of risk of common chronic diseases and to relate this knowledge to strategies for promoting health and preventing disease.

Canada's Food Guide

Scientists have known for some time that adequate nutrition is essential for proper growth and development. More recently, healthy eating has been accepted as a significant factor in reducing the risk of developing nutrition-related problems, including heart disease, cancer, obesity, hypertension (high blood pressure), osteoporosis, anemia, dental decay, and some bowel disorders.

What "Reducing Risk" Means

Reducing risk means lowering the chances of developing a disease. It does not guarantee the prevention of a disease. Since the development of disease involves several factors, risk reduction usually involves several different strategies or approaches. Healthy eating is just one positive action that may help to avoid a potential problem.

Healthy Eating with Canada's Food Guide

The revised *Food Guide* was designed to meet the body's needs for vitamins, minerals, and other nutrients; to reduce the risk of obesity, type 2 diabetes, heart disease, and certain types of cancer and osteoporosis; and to enhance the overall health and vitality of Canadians over the age of 2. The *Food Guide* outlines the recommended number of servings from the different food groups based on age and gender. **Figure B.1** shows the current *Food Guide*.

Canada's Physical Activity Guidelines

High levels of physical inactivity are a serious threat to public health in Canada. Nearly two-thirds of Canadians are not active enough to achieve optimal health benefits. These Canadians are at risk for heart disease, obesity, high blood pressure, adult-onset diabetes, osteoporosis, stroke, depression, and colon cancer. Although physical activity levels increased during the 1980s and early 1990s, the progress has stalled. Health Canada estimates that physical inactivity results in at least 21,000 premature deaths annually.

Canada's Physical Activity Guidelines, produced by a joint effort of Health Canada and the Canadian Society for Exercise Physiology, provide guidelines for physical activity. It provides information to help Canadians understand how to achieve health benefits by being physically active. The guidelines complement the popular *Canada's Food Guide*

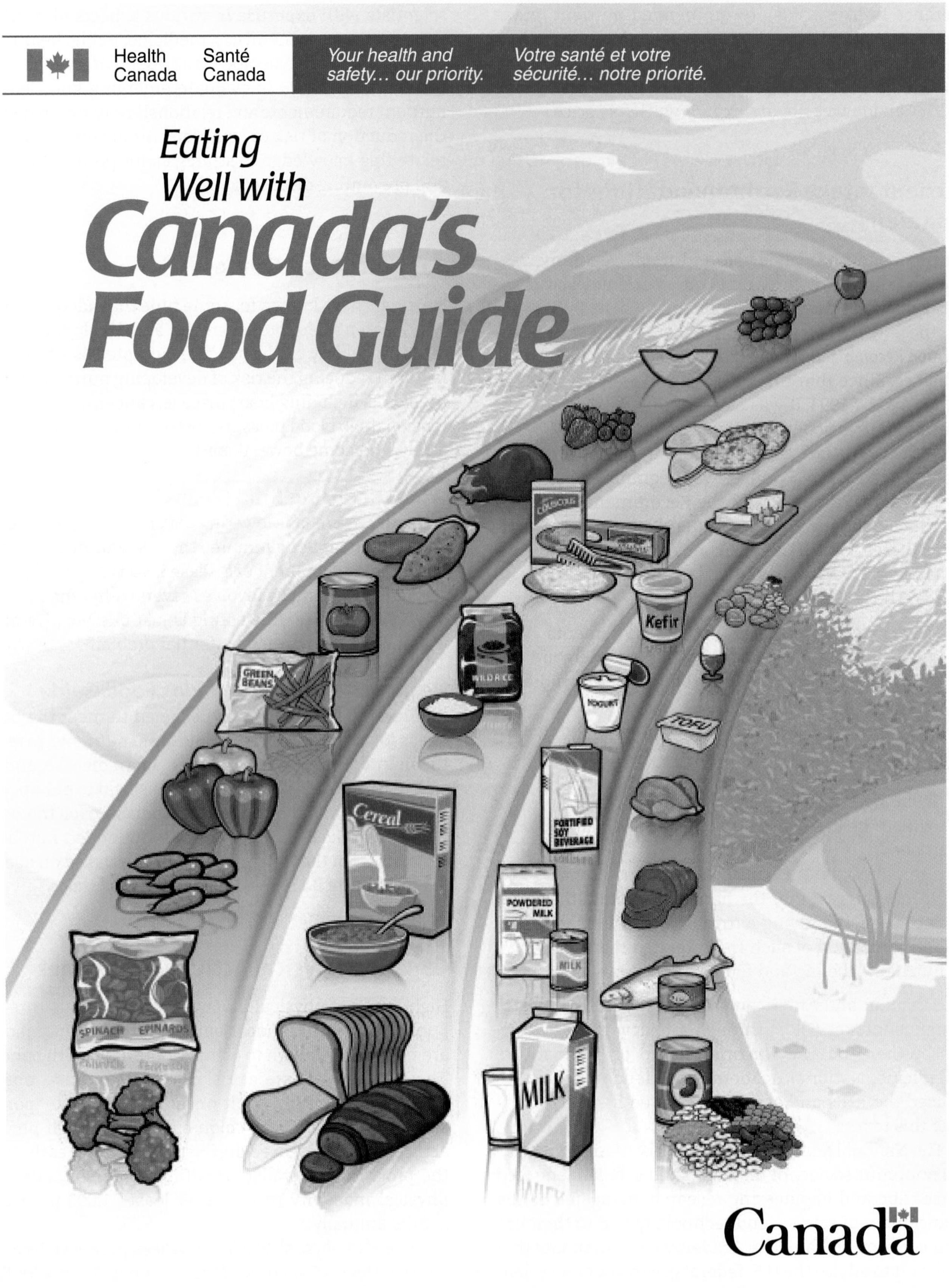

■ **Figure B.1**

Eating Well with Canada's Food Guide.

Source: © Canada's Food Guide. Health Canada, 2007. Reproduced with the permission of the Minister of Health, 2011.

Recommended Number of Food Guide Servings per Day

	Children			Teens		Adults			
Age in Years	2-3	4-8	9-13	14-18		19-50		51+	
Sex	Girls and Boys			Females	Males	Females	Males	Females	Males
Vegetables and Fruit	4	5	6	7	8	7-8	8-10	7	7
Grain Products	3	4	6	6	7	6-7	8	6	7
Milk and Alternatives	2	2	3-4	3-4	3-4	2	2	3	3
Meat and Alternatives	1	1	1-2	2	3	2	3	2	3

The chart above shows how many Food Guide Servings you need from each of the four food groups every day.

Having the amount and type of food recommended and following the tips in *Canada's Food Guide* will help:

- Meet your needs for vitamins, minerals and other nutrients.
- Reduce your risk of obesity, type 2 diabetes, heart disease, certain types of cancer and osteoporosis.
- Contribute to your overall health and vitality.

■ **Figure B.1**

Eating Well with Canada's Food Guide. (Continued)

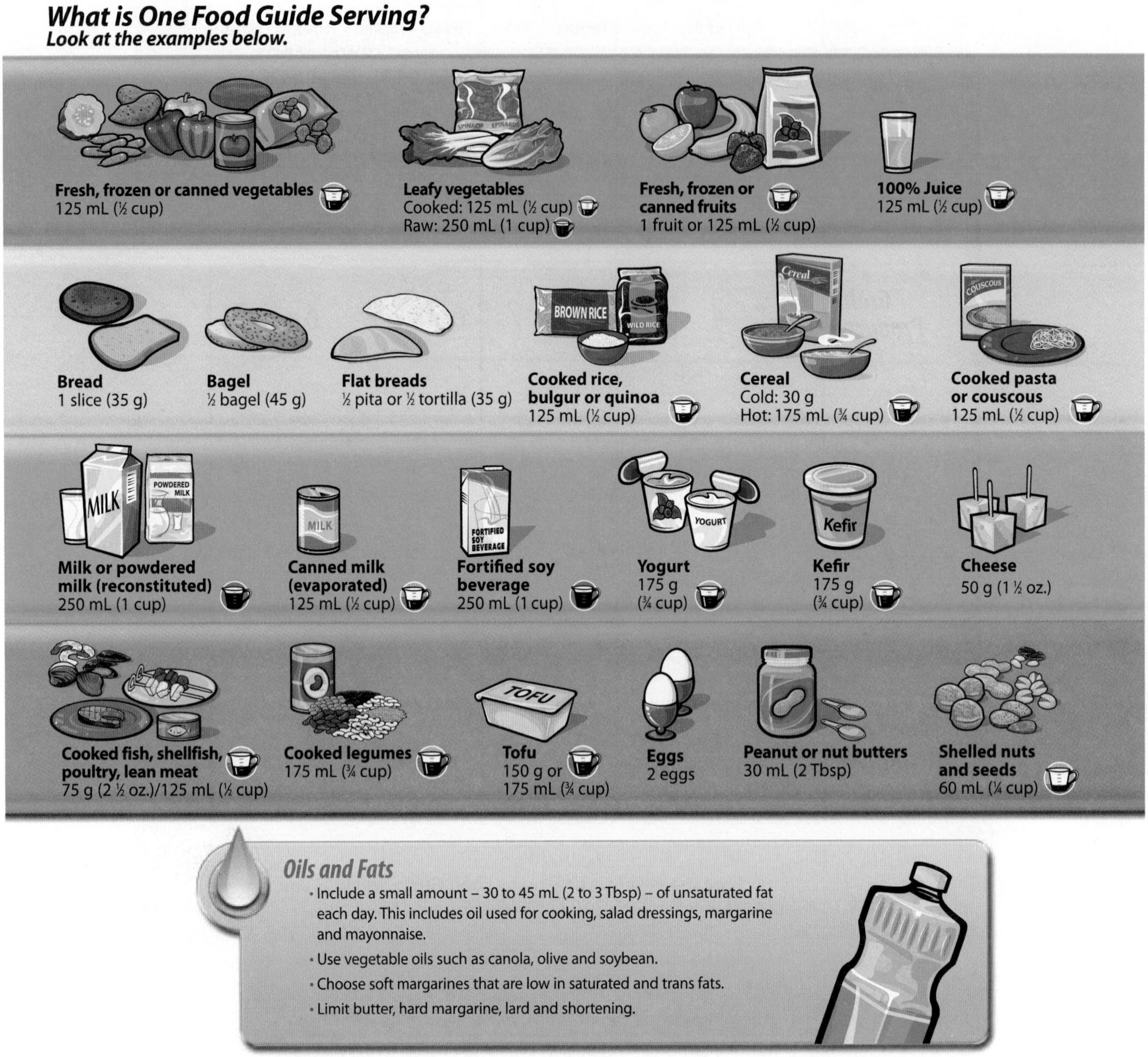
What is One Food Guide Serving?
Look at the examples below.
Fresh, frozen or canned vegetables
125 mL (½ cup)
Leafy vegetables
Cooked: 125 mL (½ cup)
Raw: 250 mL (1 cup)
Fresh, frozen or canned fruits
1 fruit or 125 mL (½ cup)
100% Juice
125 mL (½ cup)
Bread
1 slice (35 g)
Bagel
½ bagel (45 g)
Flat breads
½ pita or ½ tortilla (35 g)
Cooked rice, bulgur or quinoa
125 mL (½ cup)
Cereal
Cold: 30 g
Hot: 175 mL (¾ cup)
Cooked pasta or couscous
125 mL (½ cup)
Milk or powdered milk (reconstituted)
250 mL (1 cup)
Canned milk (evaporated)
125 mL (½ cup)
Fortified soy beverage
250 mL (1 cup)
Yogurt
175 g
(¾ cup)
Kefir
175 g
(¾ cup)
Cheese
50 g (1 ½ oz.)
Cooked fish, shellfish, poultry, lean meat
75 g (2 ½ oz.)/125 mL (½ cup)
Cooked legumes
175 mL (¾ cup)
Tofu
150 g or
175 mL (¾ cup)
Eggs
2 eggs
Peanut or nut butters
30 mL (2 Tbsp)
Shelled nuts and seeds
60 mL (¼ cup)
Oils and Fats
• Include a small amount – 30 to 45 mL (2 to 3 Tbsp) – of unsaturated fat each day. This includes oil used for cooking, salad dressings, margarine and mayonnaise.
• Use vegetable oils such as canola, olive and soybean.
• Choose soft margarines that are low in saturated and trans fats.
• Limit butter, hard margarine, lard and shortening.

■ **Figure B.1**

Eating Well with Canada's Food Guide. (Continued)

Make each Food Guide Serving count...
wherever you are – at home, at school, at work or when eating out!

- **Eat at least one dark green and one orange vegetable each day.**
  - Go for dark green vegetables such as broccoli, romaine lettuce and spinach.
  - Go for orange vegetables such as carrots, sweet potatoes and winter squash.
- **Choose vegetables and fruit prepared with little or no added fat, sugar or salt.**
  - Enjoy vegetables steamed, baked or stir-fried instead of deep-fried.
- **Have vegetables and fruit more often than juice.**

- **Make at least half of your grain products whole grain each day.**
  - Eat a variety of whole grains such as barley, brown rice, oats, quinoa and wild rice.
  - Enjoy whole grain breads, oatmeal or whole wheat pasta.
- **Choose grain products that are lower in fat, sugar or salt.**
  - Compare the Nutrition Facts table on labels to make wise choices.
  - Enjoy the true taste of grain products. When adding sauces or spreads, use small amounts.

- **Drink skim, 1%, or 2% milk each day.**
  - Have 500 mL (2 cups) of milk every day for adequate vitamin D.
  - Drink fortified soy beverages if you do not drink milk.
- **Select lower fat milk alternatives.**
  - Compare the Nutrition Facts table on yogurts or cheeses to make wise choices.

- **Have meat alternatives such as beans, lentils and tofu often.**
- **Eat at least two Food Guide Servings of fish each week.***
  - Choose fish such as char, herring, mackerel, salmon, sardines and trout.
- **Select lean meat and alternatives prepared with little or no added fat or salt.**
  - Trim the visible fat from meats. Remove the skin on poultry.
  - Use cooking methods such as roasting, baking or poaching that require little or no added fat.
  - If you eat luncheon meats, sausages or prepackaged meats, choose those lower in salt (sodium) and fat.

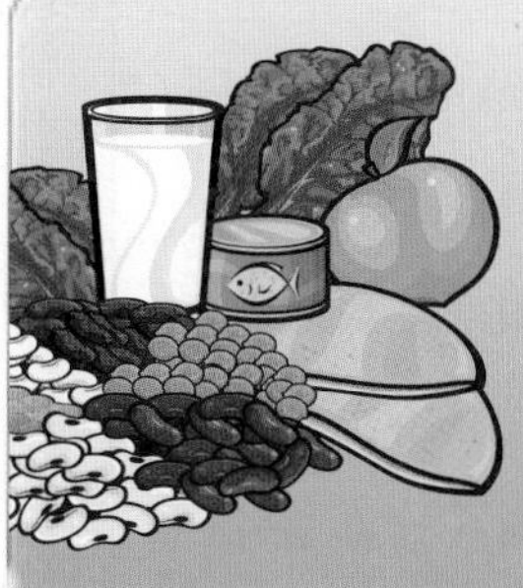

Enjoy a variety of foods from the four food groups.

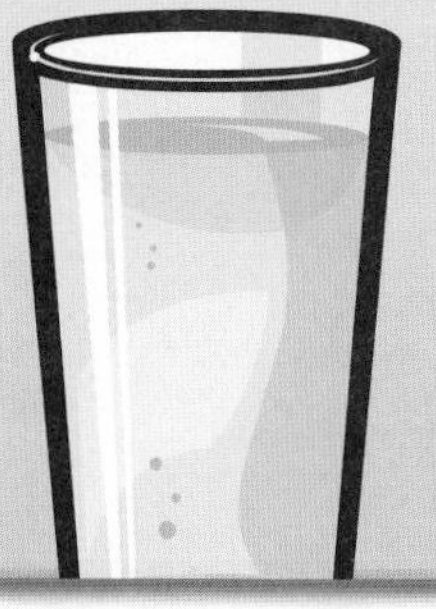

Satisfy your thirst with water!

Drink water regularly. It's a calorie-free way to quench your thirst. Drink more water in hot weather or when you are very active.

* Health Canada provides advice for limiting exposure to mercury from certain types of fish. Refer to www.healthcanada.gc.ca for the latest information.

Figure B.1

Eating Well with Canada's Food Guide. (Continued)

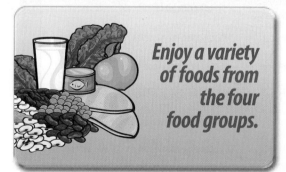

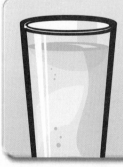

Advice for different ages and stages...

Children

Following *Canada's Food Guide* helps children grow and thrive.

Young children have small appetites and need calories for growth and development.

- Serve small nutritious meals and snacks each day.
- Do not restrict nutritious foods because of their fat content. Offer a variety of foods from the four food groups.
- Most of all... be a good role model.

Women of childbearing age

All women who could become pregnant and those who are pregnant or breastfeeding need a multivitamin containing **folic acid** every day. Pregnant women need to ensure that their multivitamin also contains **iron**. A health care professional can help you find the multivitamin that's right for you.

Pregnant and breastfeeding women need more calories. Include an extra 2 to 3 Food Guide Servings each day.

Here are two examples:

- Have fruit and yogurt for a snack, or
- Have an extra slice of toast at breakfast and an extra glass of milk at supper.

Men and women over 50

The need for **vitamin D** increases after the age of 50.

In addition to following *Canada's Food Guide*, everyone over the age of 50 should take a daily vitamin D supplement of 10 µg (400 IU).

How do I count Food Guide Servings in a meal?

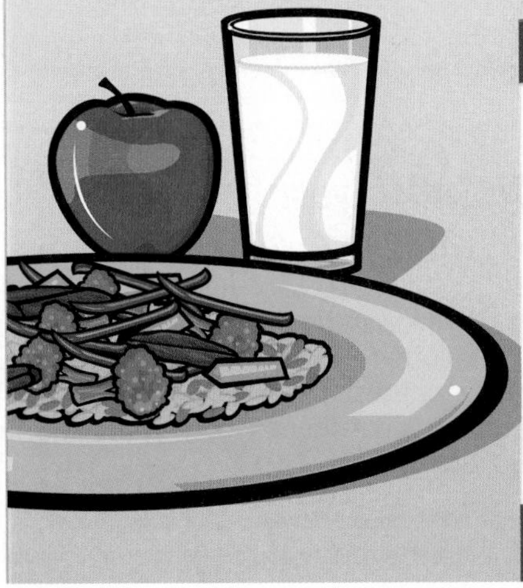

Here is an example:

Vegetable and beef stir-fry with rice, a glass of milk and an apple for dessert		
250 mL (1 cup) mixed broccoli, carrot and sweet red pepper	=	2 **Vegetables and Fruit** Food Guide Servings
75 g (2 ½ oz.) lean beef	=	1 **Meat and Alternatives** Food Guide Serving
250 mL (1 cup) brown rice	=	2 **Grain Products** Food Guide Servings
5 mL (1 tsp) canola oil	=	part of your **Oils and Fats** intake for the day
250 mL (1 cup) 1% milk	=	1 **Milk and Alternatives** Food Guide Serving
1 apple	=	1 **Vegetables and Fruit** Food Guide Serving

Figure B.1

Eating Well with Canada's Food Guide. (Continued)

Eat well and be active today and every day!

The benefits of eating well and being active include:

- Better overall health.
- Lower risk of disease.
- A healthy body weight.
- Feeling and looking better.
- More energy.
- Stronger muscles and bones.

Be active

To be active every day is a step towards better health and a healthy body weight.

Canada's Physical Activity Guide recommends building 30 to 60 minutes of moderate physical activity into daily life for adults and at least 90 minutes a day for children and youth. You don't have to do it all at once. Add it up in periods of at least 10 minutes at a time for adults and five minutes at a time for children and youth.

Start slowly and build up.

Eat well

Another important step towards better health and a healthy body weight is to follow *Canada's Food Guide* by:

- Eating the recommended amount and type of food each day.
- Limiting foods and beverages high in calories, fat, sugar or salt (sodium) such as cakes and pastries, chocolate and candies, cookies and granola bars, doughnuts and muffins, ice cream and frozen desserts, french fries, potato chips, nachos and other salty snacks, alcohol, fruit flavoured drinks, soft drinks, sports and energy drinks, and sweetened hot or cold drinks.

Read the label

- Compare the Nutrition Facts table on food labels to choose products that contain less fat, saturated fat, trans fat, sugar and sodium.
- Keep in mind that the calories and nutrients listed are for the amount of food found at the top of the Nutrition Facts table.

Nutrition Facts
Per 0 mL (0 g)

Amount	% Daily Value
Calories 0	
Fat 0 g	0 %
Saturates 0 g	0 %
+ Trans 0 g	
Cholesterol 0 mg	
Sodium 0 mg	0 %
Carbohydrate 0 g	0 %
Fibre 0 g	0 %
Sugars 0 g	
Protein 0 g	
Vitamin A 0 %	Vitamin C 0 %
Calcium 0 %	Iron 0 %

Limit trans fat

When a Nutrition Facts table is not available, ask for nutrition information to choose foods lower in trans and saturated fats.

Take a step today...

✓ Have breakfast every day. It may help control your hunger later in the day.

✓ Walk wherever you can – get off the bus early, use the stairs.

✓ Benefit from eating vegetables and fruit at all meals and as snacks.

✓ Spend less time being inactive such as watching TV or playing computer games.

✓ Request nutrition information about menu items when eating out to help you make healthier choices.

✓ Enjoy eating with family and friends!

✓ Take time to eat and savour every bite!

For more information, interactive tools, or additional copies visit Canada's Food Guide on-line at: www.healthcanada.gc.ca/foodguide

or contact:

Publications
Health Canada
Ottawa, Ontario K1A 0K9
E-Mail: publications@hc-sc.gc.ca
Tel.: 1-866-225-0709
Fax: (613) 941-5366
TTY: 1-800-267-1245

Également disponible en français sous le titre : Bien manger avec le Guide alimentaire canadien

This publication can be made available on request on diskette, large print, audio-cassette and braille.

HC Pub.: 4651 Cat.: H164-38/1-2007E ISBN: 0-662-44467-1

Figure B.1
Eating Well with Canada's Food Guide. (Continued)

to Healthy Eating and provide concrete examples of how to incorporate physical activity into daily life.

Designed for adults, the guide recommends 60 minutes of physical activity every day to stay healthy or improve your health. As a person progresses to more intense activity, he or she can cut down to 30 minutes, four days a week. The guide also suggests Canadians can add up their activities in periods of at least 10 minutes each, starting slowly and building up. **Figure B.2** shows the *Physical Activity Guidelines*.

Federal, provincial, and territorial governments are working to reduce the number of inactive Canadians. *Canada's Physical Activity Guidelines* are a major step toward building the knowledge and awareness necessary for all Canadians to become more active.

Canadian Physical Activity Guidelines

2011 SCIENTIFIC STATEMENTS

FOR CHILDREN - 5 – 11 YEARS

Preamble

These guidelines are relevant to all apparently healthy children (5-11 years), irrespective of gender, race, ethnicity or socio-economic status of the family. Children are encouraged to participate in a variety of physical activities that support their natural development and are enjoyable and safe.

Children should be physically active daily as part of play, games, sports, transportation, recreation, physical education, or planned exercise, in the context of family, school and community (e.g. volunteer, employment) activities. This should be achieved above and beyond the incidental physical activities accumulated in the course of daily living.

Following these physical activity guidelines can improve cholesterol levels, blood pressure, body composition, bone density, cardiorespiratory and musculoskeletal fitness, and aspects of mental health. The potential benefits far exceed the potential risks associated with physical activity.

These guidelines may be appropriate for children with a disability or medical condition; however, their parents or caregiver should consult a health professional to understand the types and amounts of physical activity appropriate for them.

For those who are physically inactive, doing amounts below the recommended levels can provide some health benefits. For these children, it is appropriate to start with smaller amounts of physical activity and gradually increase duration, frequency and intensity as a stepping stone to meeting the guidelines.

For guidance on decreasing sedentary behaviour please refer to Canada's Sedentary Behaviour Guidelines for Children and Youth.

Guidelines

- For health benefits, children aged 5-11 years should accumulate at least 60 minutes of moderate- to vigorous-intensity physical activity daily. This should include:
    - Vigorous-intensity activities at least 3 days per week.
    - Activities that strengthen muscle and bone at least 3 days per week.
- More daily physical activity provides greater health benefits.

CSEP | SCPE
THE GOLD STANDARD IN EXERCISE SCIENCE AND PERSONAL TRAINING
www.csep.ca/guidelines

■ **Figure B.2**

Canada's Physical Activity Guidelines.

Source: © Canadian Physical Activity Guidelines, © 2011. Used with permission from the Canadian Society for Exercise Physiology, www.csep.ca/guidelines.

Canadian Physical Activity Guidelines

2011 SCIENTIFIC STATEMENTS

FOR YOUTH - 12 – 17 YEARS

Preamble

These guidelines are relevant to all apparently healthy youth (12-17 years), irrespective of gender, race, ethnicity or socio-economic status of the family. Youth are encouraged to participate in a variety of physical activities that support their natural development and are enjoyable and safe.

Youth should be physically active daily as part of play, games, sports, transportation, recreation, physical education, or planned exercise, in the context of family, school and community (e.g. volunteer, employment) activities. This should be achieved above and beyond the incidental physical activities accumulated in the course of daily living.

Following these physical activity guidelines can improve cholesterol levels, blood pressure, body composition, bone density, cardiorespiratory and musculoskeletal fitness, and aspects of mental health. The potential benefits far exceed the potential risks associated with physical activity.

These guidelines may be appropriate for youth with a disability or medical condition; however, their parents or caregiver should consult a health professional to understand the types and amounts of physical activity appropriate for them.

For those who are physically inactive, doing amounts below the recommended levels can provide some health benefits. For these youth, it is appropriate to start with smaller amounts of physical activity and gradually increase duration, frequency and intensity as a stepping stone to meeting the guidelines.

For guidance on decreasing sedentary behaviour please refer to Canada's Sedentary Behaviour Guidelines for Children and Youth.

Guidelines

- For health benefits, youth aged 12-17 years should accumulate at least 60 minutes of moderate- to vigorous-intensity physical activity daily. This should include:
  - Vigorous-intensity activities at least 3 days per week.
  - Activities that strengthen muscle and bone at least 3 days per week.
- More daily physical activity provides greater health benefits.

CSEP | SCPE
THE GOLD STANDARD IN EXERCISE SCIENCE AND PERSONAL TRAINING
www.csep.ca/guidelines

Figure B.2
Canada's Physical Activity Guidelines. (Continued)

Canadian Physical Activity Guidelines

2011 SCIENTIFIC STATEMENTS

FOR ADULTS - 18 – 64 YEARS

Preamble

These guidelines are relevant to all apparently healthy adults aged 18-64 years, irrespective of gender, race, ethnicity or socio-economic status. Adults are encouraged to participate in a variety of physical activities that are enjoyable and safe.

Adults can meet these guidelines through planned exercise sessions, transportation, recreation, sports or occupational demands, in the context of family, work, volunteer and community activities. This should be achieved above and beyond the incidental physical activities accumulated in the course of daily living.

Following these guidelines can reduce the risk of premature death, coronary heart disease, stroke, hypertension, colon cancer, breast cancer, type 2 diabetes and osteoporosis and improve fitness, body composition and indicators of mental health. The potential benefits far exceed the potential risks associated with physical activity.

These guidelines may be appropriate for those who are pregnant, have a disability or have a medical condition; however, they should consult a health professional to understand the types and amounts of physical activity appropriate for them.

For those who are physically inactive, doing amounts below the recommended levels can provide some health benefits. For these adults, it is appropriate to start with smaller amounts of physical activity and gradually increase duration, frequency and intensity as a stepping stone to meeting the guidelines.

Guidelines

- To achieve health benefits, adults aged 18-64 years should accumulate at least 150 minutes of moderate- to vigorous-intensity aerobic physical activity per week, in bouts of 10 minutes or more.
- It is also beneficial to add muscle and bone strengthening activities using major muscle groups, at least 2 days per week.
- More physical activity provides greater health benefits.

CSEP | SCPE
THE GOLD STANDARD IN EXERCISE SCIENCE AND PERSONAL TRAINING
www.csep.ca/guidelines

Figure B.2
Canada's Physical Activity Guidelines. (Continued)

Canadian Physical Activity Guidelines

2011 SCIENTIFIC STATEMENTS

FOR OLDER ADULTS - 65 YEARS & OLDER

Preamble

These guidelines are relevant to all apparently healthy adults aged 65 years and older, irrespective of gender, race, ethnicity or socio-economic status. Older adults are encouraged to participate in a variety of physical activities that are enjoyable and safe.

Older adults can meet these guidelines through planned exercise sessions, transportation, recreation, sports or occupational demands in the context of family, work, volunteer and community activities. This should be achieved above and beyond the incidental physical activities accumulated in the course of daily living.

Following these guidelines can reduce the risk of chronic disease and premature death, maintain functional independence and mobility, as well as improve fitness, body composition, bone health, cognitive function and indicators of mental health. The potential benefits far exceed the potential risks associated with physical activity.

These guidelines may be appropriate for older adults with frailty, a disability or medical condition; however, they should consult a health professional to understand the types and amounts of physical activity appropriate for them based on their exercise capacity and specific health risks or limitations.

For those who are physically inactive, doing amounts below the recommended levels can provide some health benefits. For these adults, it is appropriate to start with smaller amounts of physical activity and gradually increase duration, frequency and intensity as a stepping stone to meeting the guidelines.

Guidelines

- To achieve health benefits and improve functional abilities, adults aged 65 years and older should accumulate at least 150 minutes of moderate- to vigorous-intensity aerobic physical activity per week, in bouts of 10 minutes or more.
- It is also beneficial to add muscle and bone strengthening activities using major muscle groups, at least 2 days per week.
- Those with poor mobility should perform physical activities to enhance balance and prevent falls.
- More physical activity provides greater health benefits.

CSEP | SCPE
THE GOLD STANDARD IN EXERCISE SCIENCE AND PERSONAL TRAINING
www.csep.ca/guidelines

■ **Figure B.2**
Canada's Physical Activity Guidelines. (Continued)

Canadian Physical Activity Guidelines

FOR CHILDREN - 5 – 11 YEARS

Guidelines

For health benefits, children aged 5-11 years should accumulate at least 60 minutes of moderate- to vigorous-intensity physical activity daily. This should include:

Vigorous-intensity activities at least 3 days per week.

Activities that strengthen muscle and bone at least 3 days per week.

More daily physical activity provides greater health benefits.

Let's Talk Intensity!

Moderate-intensity physical activities will cause children to sweat a little and to breathe harder. Activities like:

- Bike riding
- Playground activities

Vigorous-intensity physical activities will cause children to sweat and be 'out of breath'. Activities like:

- Running
- Swimming

Being active for at least **60 minutes** daily can help children:

- Improve their health
- Do better in school
- Improve their fitness
- Grow stronger
- Have fun playing with friends
- Feel happier
- Maintain a healthy body weight
- Improve their self-confidence
- Learn new skills

Parents and caregivers can help to plan their child's daily activity. Kids can:

☑ Play tag – or freeze-tag!
☑ Go to the playground after school.
☑ Walk, bike, rollerblade or skateboard to school.
☑ Play an active game at recess.
☑ Go sledding in the park on the weekend.
☑ Go "puddle hopping" on a rainy day.

60 minutes a day. You can help your child get there!

PARTICIPACTION

CSEP | SCPE
THE GOLD STANDARD IN EXERCISE SCIENCE AND PERSONAL TRAINING
www.csep.ca/guidelines

■ **Figure B.2**
Canada's Physical Activity Guidelines. (Continued)

Canadian Physical Activity Guidelines

FOR YOUTH - 12 – 17 YEARS

Guidelines

For health benefits, youth aged 12-17 years should accumulate at least 60 minutes of moderate- to vigorous-intensity physical activity daily. This should include:

Vigorous-intensity activities at least 3 days per week.

Activities that strengthen muscle and bone at least 3 days per week.

More daily physical activity provides greater health benefits.

Let's Talk Intensity!

Moderate-intensity physical activities will cause teens to sweat a little and to breathe harder. Activities like:

- Skating
- Bike riding

Vigorous-intensity physical activities will cause teens to sweat and be 'out of breath'. Activities like:

- Running
- Rollerblading

Being active for at least **60 minutes** daily can help teens:

- Improve their health
- Do better in school
- Improve their fitness
- Grow stronger
- Have fun playing with friends
- Feel happier
- Maintain a healthy body weight
- Improve their self-confidence
- Learn new skills

Parents and caregivers can help to plan their teen's daily activity. Teens can:

☑ Walk, bike, rollerblade or skateboard to school.
☑ Go to a gym on the weekend.
☑ Do a fitness class after school.
☑ Get the neighbours together for a game of pick-up basketball, or hockey after dinner.
☑ Play a sport such as basketball, hockey, soccer, martial arts, swimming, tennis, golf, skiing, snowboarding…

Now is the time. 60 minutes a day can make a difference.

PARTICIPACTION

CSEP | SCPE THE GOLD STANDARD IN EXERCISE SCIENCE AND PERSONAL TRAINING

www.csep.ca/guidelines

Figure B.2

Canada's Physical Activity Guidelines. (Continued)

Canadian Physical Activity Guidelines

FOR ADULTS - 18 – 64 YEARS

Guidelines

To achieve health benefits, adults aged 18-64 years should accumulate at least 150 minutes of moderate- to vigorous-intensity aerobic physical activity per week, in bouts of 10 minutes or more.

It is also beneficial to add muscle and bone strengthening activities using major muscle groups, at least 2 days per week.

More physical activity provides greater health benefits.

Let's Talk Intensity!

Moderate-intensity physical activities will cause adults to sweat a little and to breathe harder. Activities like:

- Brisk walking
- Bike riding

Vigorous-intensity physical activities will cause adults to sweat and be 'out of breath'. Activities like:

- Jogging
- Cross-country skiing

Being active for at least **150 minutes** per week can help reduce the risk of:

- Premature death
- Heart disease
- Stroke
- High blood pressure
- Certain types of cancer
- Type 2 diabetes
- Osteoporosis
- Overweight and obesity

And can lead to improved:

- Fitness
- Strength
- Mental health (morale and self–esteem)

Pick a time. Pick a place. Make a plan and move more!

☑ Join a weekday community running or walking group.
☑ Go for a brisk walk around the block after dinner.
☑ Take a dance class after work.
☑ Bike or walk to work every day.
☑ Rake the lawn, and then offer to do the same for a neighbour.
☑ Train for and participate in a run or walk for charity!
☑ Take up a favourite sport again or try a new sport.
☑ Be active with the family on the weekend!

Now is the time. Walk, run, or wheel, and embrace life.

PARTICIPACTION

CSEP | SCPE THE GOLD STANDARD IN EXERCISE SCIENCE AND PERSONAL TRAINING

www.csep.ca/guidelines

■ Figure B.2

Canada's Physical Activity Guidelines. (Continued)

Canadian Physical Activity Guidelines

FOR OLDER ADULTS - 65 YEARS & OLDER

Guidelines

To achieve health benefits, and improve functional abilities, adults aged 65 years and older should accumulate at least 150 minutes of moderate- to vigorous-intensity aerobic physical activity per week, in bouts of 10 minutes or more.

It is also beneficial to add muscle and bone strengthening activities using major muscle groups, at least 2 days per week.

Those with poor mobility should perform physical activities to enhance balance and prevent falls.

More physical activity provides greater health benefits.

Let's Talk Intensity!

Moderate-intensity physical activities will cause older adults to sweat a little and to breathe harder. Activities like:

- Brisk walking
- Bicycling

Vigorous-intensity physical activities will cause older adults to sweat and be 'out of breath'. Activities like:

- Cross-country skiing
- Swimming

Being active for at least **150 minutes** per week can help reduce the risk of:

- Chronic disease (such as high blood pressure and heart disease) and,
- Premature death

And also help to:

- Maintain functional independence
- Maintain mobility
- Improve fitness
- Improve or maintain body weight
- Maintain bone health and,
- Maintain mental health and feel better

Pick a time. Pick a place. Make a plan and move more!

☑ Join a community urban poling or mall walking group.
☑ Go for a brisk walk around the block after lunch.
☑ Take a dance class in the afternoon.
☑ Train for and participate in a run or walk for charity!
☑ Take up a favourite sport again.
☑ Be active with the family! Plan to have "active reunions".
☑ Go for a nature hike on the weekend.
☑ Take the dog for a walk after dinner.

Now is the time. Walk, run, or wheel, and embrace life.

PARTICIPACTION

CSEP | SCPE
THE GOLD STANDARD IN EXERCISE SCIENCE AND PERSONAL TRAINING
www.csep.ca/guidelines

Figure B.2

Canada's Physical Activity Guidelines. (Continued)

The Nutrition Facts Box

The Nutrition Facts box allows consumers to make informed choices.

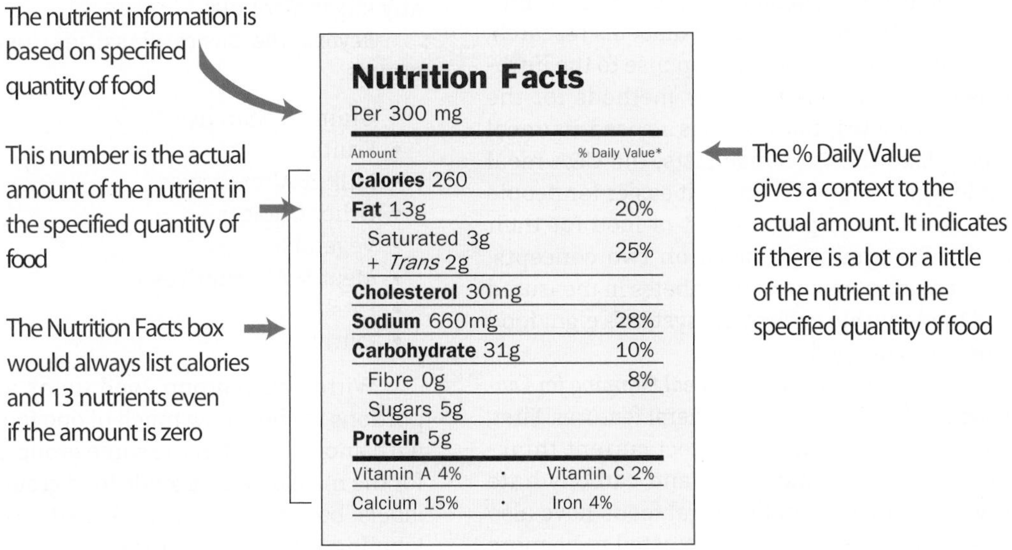
The nutrient information is based on specified quantity of food
This number is the actual amount of the nutrient in the specified quantity of food
The Nutrition Facts box would always list calories and 13 nutrients even if the amount is zero
Nutrition Facts
Per 300 mg
Amount
% Daily Value*
Calories 260
Fat 13g 20%
Saturated 3g
+ Trans 2g
25%
Cholesterol 30mg
Sodium 660mg 28%
Carbohydrate 31g 10%
Fibre 0g 8%
Sugars 5g
Protein 5g
Vitamin A 4% · Vitamin C 2%
Calcium 15% · Iron 4%
The % Daily Value gives a context to the actual amount. It indicates if there is a lot or a little of the nutrient in the specified quantity of food

■ **Figure B.3**
How to read a food label.

Nutrition Labeling for Canadians

The nutrition label is one of the most useful tools in selecting foods for healthy eating (**Figure B.3**). The *Food Guide* outlines a pattern of healthy eating; the nutrition label supports the *Food Guide* by helping consumers to choose foods according to healthy eating messages.

Consumers can use labels to compare products and make choices on the basis of nutrient content. For example, consumers can choose a lower-fat product based on the fat content given on the labels.

Consumers also can use label information to evaluate products in relation to healthy eating. For instance, the *Nutrition Recommendations* advise Canadians to get 30 percent or less of their day's energy (kilocalories/kilojoules) from fat. This translates into a range of fat, in grams, that can be used as a benchmark against which individual foods and meals can be evaluated. The *Food Guide* covers a range of energy needs from 1,800 to 3,200 kilocalories (7,500 to 13,400 kilojoules) per day. A fat intake of 30 percent or less of a day's calories means a fat intake between 60 and 105 grams of fat.

Label Claims

A claim on a food label highlights a nutritional feature of a product. It is known to influence consumers' buying habits. Manufacturers often position label claims in a bold, banner format on the front panel of a package or on the side panel along with the nutrition label. Because a label claim must be backed up by detailed facts relating to the claim, the consumer should look for the nutrition label for more information.

Nutrient Content Claims

A nutrient content claim describes the amount of a nutrient in a food. A food whose label carries the claim *high fibre* must contain 4 grams or more of fiber per reference amount and serving of stated size. A "sodium-free" food must contain less than 5 mg of sodium per reference amount and serving of stated size.

Diet-Related Health Claims

Optional health claims highlight the characteristics of a diet that reduces the chance of developing a disease such as cancer or heart disease. They also tell how the food fits into the diet.

Characteristic of the Diet:	Reduced Risk of:
Low in sodium and high in potassium	High blood pressure
Adequate in calcium and vitamin D	Osteoporosis
Low in saturates and trans fats	Heart disease
Rich in fruits and vegetables	Some types of cancer

For the latest information, visit the Nutrition Labeling area of the Health Canada website at: http://www.hc-sc.gc.ca/fn-an/label-etiquet/nutrition/index-eng.php.

Canadian Diabetes Association's Meal Planning Guide

The Canadian Diabetes Association (CDA) works to promote the health of Canadians through diabetes research, education, service, and advocacy. In response to the introduction of new medications and new methods for the management of diabetes, the CDA has revised its meal planning guide. Like the Exchange Lists, the CDA meal planning guide was designed to make it easier for people with diabetes to eat the right amount of food for their insulin supply. The system is based on two concepts: Most foods are eaten by people with diabetes in measured amounts, and foods within each of the system's eight food groups can be interchanged.

The new guide, *Beyond the Basics: Meal Planning for Diabetes Prevention and Management,* has several features. First, food items have been modified to reflect current thinking on heart health, glycemic index, and carbohydrate counting. A wider range of multicultural foods have also been added. Portion sizes have been adjusted to be more similar to *Canada's Food Guide,* and to the Quebec and U.S. meal planning systems. The guide also used color coding to help consumers: green for "choose more often" or "everyday" foods and amber for "choose less often" or "special occasion foods." The listed portions of all carbohydrate-rich foods now contain 15 grams of available carbohydrate (total carbohydrate minus fiber and half of any sugar alcohols).

Beyond the Basics classifies foods into eight food groups:

- Grains & Starches
- Fruits
- Milk & Alternatives
- Other Choices
- Vegetables
- Meat & Alternatives
- Fats
- Extras

Within each group, food items are listed along with portions to show how much of one food is interchangeable with another food in the same group. In the past, symbols for the meal planning guide food groups were used on food labels, but this has been phased out with the new food labeling regulations. However, the CDA partnered with Dietitians of Canada to develop *Healthy Eating Is in Store for You,* a nutrition labeling education program. For more information visit the CDA website: http://www.diabetes.ca/diabetes-and-you/nutrition/healthy-eating/.

Glossary

Acceptable Daily Intake (ADI) The amount of a substance in food (food additives) or drinking water that can be ingested on a daily basis over a lifetime without an appreciable health risk.

Acceptable Macronutrient Distribution Ranges (AMDRs) A set of values for carbohydrates, fat, and protein expressed as a percentage of total daily calorie intake. Ranges of intake are set to be consistent with the reduction of risk of chronic disease.

Adequate Intake (AI) Used when there is no Recommended Daily Allowance (RDA) established, but some data support an amount of a nutrient that is believed to be adequate for most people.

aerobic activity Physical activity that requires the heart and lungs to work harder to meet the body's oxygen demands; includes brisk walking, jogging, running, swimming, or other activity that uses the large muscle groups.

aflatoxin Toxin produced by food molds.

American Medical Association (AMA) Promotes the science and art of medicine. Disseminates information to its members and to the public on critical health issues.

amino acids Building blocks of proteins; have an acid on one end and a nitrogen-containing amine group on the other.

amniotic fluid The fluid that surrounds the fetus.

anorexia nervosa An eating disorder that involves an inability to stay at the minimum body weight considered to be healthy. Persons with this disorder may have an intense fear of weight gain, even when they are underweight. They may use extreme dieting, excessive exercise, or other methods to lose weight.

antibodies Proteins in the blood that fight infection.

antioxidants Substances that neutralize free radicals, thus protecting cells and tissues against damage from oxidation.

appetite The physiological desire to eat; not always accompanied by hunger.

basal metabolic rate (BMR) The amount of energy the body expends at rest to maintain bodily functions, such as breathing.

baseline activity Light-intensity activities performed in everyday life, such as standing, walking slowly, or lifting lightweight objects.

best if used by (or before) date A date usually found on nonperishable foods that indicates the date after which quality may be compromised; the date is not related to the safety of the food.

bile A mixture of compounds, including bile salts, bile acids, and lecithin, made by the liver and stored and concentrated in the gallbladder. Bile is secreted into the small intestine to help emulsify fats and transport them to the intestinal wall so they can be absorbed.

binge-eating disorder An eating disorder characterized by a loss of control over eating and recurring binge-eating episodes

biodynamic An organic farming method that treats the farm as an individual organism, emphasizing the interrelationships among soil, plants, and animals.

blood glucose level The amount of glucose present in the blood. Glucose is carried in the bloodstream to provide energy to all the cells.

body image A person's perception of his or her physical appearance.

body mass index (BMI) A measure of body fat based on height and weight.

bran The outer layer of a grain; it is high in fiber.

bulimia nervosa An eating disorder in which a person binges on food or has regular episodes of significant overeating and feels a loss of control. The affected person then uses various methods, such as vomiting or laxative abuse, to prevent weight gain.

caffeine A compound found naturally in coffee, tea, and chocolate and added to other foods and beverages; it acts as a central nervous system stimulant.

calorie balance The balance between calories consumed in foods and beverages and calories expended through physical activity and metabolic processes.

calories A unit used to measure energy in foods and beverages.

carbohydrates Organic compounds that contain carbon, hydrogen, and oxygen. Carbohydrates include sugars, starches, and fiber. They are a major source of energy for your body.

carotenoids Yellow, orange, and red pigments, many of which are precursors of vitamin A; they are found widely in fruits and vegetables.

Centers for Disease Control and Prevention (CDC) The federal agency that tracks and investigates public health trends. Promotes health and quality of life by preventing and controlling disease, injury, and disability.

cholecystokinin (CCK) A hormone produced by the intestine that stimulates the secretion of bile from the gallbladder and pancreatic lipase from the pancreas.

chylomicrons Large lipoprotein particles that allow fat to travel in the bloodstream. They contain triglycerides and small amounts of cholesterol and phospholipids and have an outer coating of protein.

circulatory system An organ system that connects all the cells in the body. Through the blood, it transports water, oxygen, and nutrients to all the cells of the body and carries away waste.

collagen The most abundant protein in the body; the primary protein in connective tissue.

community-supported agriculture (CSA) A community of individuals who pledge support to a farm operation; members of a CSA provide monetary support to a farmer and in return receive shares in the farm's production.

complete protein A protein that contains all of the essential amino acids; proteins from animal sources and soy are complete proteins.

complete streets Streets designed and operated to accommodate all users, including bicyclists, public transportation vehicles and riders, and pedestrians of all ages and abilities.

complex carbohydrates Long chains of sugars (oligosaccharides or polysaccharides) arranged as starch or fiber.

congregate nutrition sites Provide hot lunches to seniors aged 60 and older.

cruciferous vegetables Members of the mustard family; they are rich sources of sulfur-containing compounds known as glucosinolates that may help protect against cancer.

dehydration Situation that arises when your body does not have as much water as it needs; can be caused by losing too much fluid, not drinking enough water or fluids, or both.

denaturation Change in the three-dimensional structure of a protein caused by agitation, heat, or acidity.

Department of Health and Human Services (DHHS) The primary federal agency for protecting the health of all Americans and for providing essential human services.

diabetes mellitus A chronic condition where the uptake of glucose into the cells is impaired, resulting in too much glucose in the blood.

Dietary Guidelines for Americans Provides evidence-based nutrition information and advice for people age 2 and older. It serves as the basis for federal food and nutrition education programs.

Dietary Reference Intakes (DRIs) Nutrition recommendations used in the United States and Canada.

distress A level of stress that is too high and can cause emotional and physical problems.

diuretic Drug or other substance that promotes the formation of urine by the kidneys.

electrolytes Substances that separate into charged particles (ions) when dissolved in water; they can conduct an electrical current.

endosperm Starchy portion of a grain.

energy density The number of calories a food contains in a given weight. Foods high in water, such as fruits and vegetables, have lower energy density than foods high in fat and sugar. High-energy-density foods have a lot of calories in a small package.

Environmental Protection Agency (EPA) Federal agency founded to protect human health and to safeguard the natural environment, including air, water, and land.

enzymes Proteins that speed up chemical reactions. Enzymes are found throughout the body and are especially important in digestion.

essential fatty acids Fatty acids that are needed but cannot be made by the body and must be obtained in the diet.

Estimated Average Requirement (EAR) Average daily nutrient intake level estimated to meet the needs of 50% of the people in a particular age/gender group.

Estimated Energy Expenditure (EEE) The amount of energy you use to carry out bodily functions and activity.

eustress A level of stress that is healthy and gives you a feeling of fulfillment.

exercise A type of physical activity that is planned, structured, repetitive, and done for the purpose of improving physical fitness, physical performance, or health.

Expanded Food and Nutrition Education Program (EFNEP) A federally funded educational program conducted through the Cooperative Extension Service in every state and U.S. territory. Families receive education about nutrition, food safety, and how to make the most of their food dollar.

fats (lipids) Organic compounds that contain carbon, hydrogen, and oxygen. Fats provide structure for your cells, carry fat-soluble vitamins into your body, and are a component of many hormones.

fiber Carbohydrate found in plants that is not digestible by humans.

flavonoids Polyphenol compounds that act as powerful antioxidants; found in fruits and vegetables and in high concentration in tea.

flexibility activities Physical activity done to increase the ability of a joint to move through a range of motion, such as bending, reaching, or stretching.

food allergy An abnormal immune response that occurs when the immune system produces antibodies and histamines in response to a specific food.

Food and Drug Administration (FDA) The federal agency that has oversight for the approval of new drugs, medical devices, cosmetics, and food additives. Provides regulation and oversight for food labeling. The FDA is also responsible for advancing the public health by helping to speed innovations that make medicines and foods safer, more effective, and more affordable and aiding the public in getting the accurate, scientific information they need to use medicines and foods to improve their health.

food aversion Dislike of a particular food.

food bank An agency or center that collects food and distributes it to the needy.

foodborne illness Any illness that is caused by consuming food that is contaminated by a pathogen; commonly called *food poisoning*.

Food Code Guidelines released by the FDA every four years as a model for food safety for the retail and food service industry; used by local and state regulators to develop or update their own food safety rules to be consistent with national food regulatory policy.

food desert Area that lacks access to affordable fruits, vegetables, whole grains, low-fat milk, and other foods that make up the full range of a healthy diet.

food insecurity Uncertainty of having or inability to acquire enough food to meet the needs of all members of the household due to insufficient money or other resources for food.

food intolerance A nonallergic, negative reaction to a food.

food irradiation A food safety technology that eliminates pathogens from foods by treating food with ionizing radiation.

Food Quality Protection Act Federal law that mandates health-based standards for pesticides used in foods.

free radicals Highly reactive, unstable compounds created by the body as a result of chemical reactions involving oxygen; can damage cells and tissues.

fructose A monosaccharide found in fruits and honey.

galactose A monosaccharide similar to glucose, usually found joined with other monosaccharides.

gallbladder A nonessential organ that stores and concentrates bile from the liver.

gastric lipase An enzyme secreted by the stomach that breaks down triglycerides into diglycerides and fatty acids.

gastrointestinal (GI) tract A long hollow tube that starts at your mouth and ends at your anus. The organs that comprise the GI tract are the mouth, esophagus, stomach, small intestine, large intestine (also called the colon), rectum, and anus.

Generally Regarded as Safe (GRAS) Designation that a substance that is added to food is considered safe by experts. Any substance added to food must meet this standard.

genetically engineered food A food that has been produced using plant or animal ingredients that have been modified using biotechnology.

germ The inner part of a whole grain; contains nutrients and fat.

gestational diabetes A diabetic condition that results in high blood glucose levels during pregnancy.

gleaning The act of collecting useful leftover crops from the fields or orchards that have been commercially harvested.

glucagon A hormone that promotes the breakdown of glycogen to glucose to maintain blood glucose levels.

glucose A monosaccharide and source of energy in the body.

glycogen Storage form of carbohydrate in the body composed of chains of glucose; stored in the liver and muscle.

Health Canada A federal department responsible for helping Canadians maintain and improve their health, while respecting individual choices and circumstances.

health-enhancing physical activity Physical activity beyond baseline physical activity that produces health benefits.

heme iron Iron from animal sources.

high-density lipoprotein (HDL) Often referred to as "good cholesterol," it is high in protein and picks up cholesterol from inside the arteries. Remember *H* for *healthy* cholesterol.

high fructose corn sweetener (HFCS) A sweetener made by processing corn syrup to increase the level of fructose; used extensively as a sweetener in processed foods and soft drinks.

hunger The physiological drive to eat. A term used to describe the problem of lack of food and nutrients.

hydrogenation A process by which hydrogen is added to liquid fat to produce a more saturated fat; the result is a trans fat.

hyperglycemia A condition that occurs when blood glucose levels are higher than normal.

hypoglycemia A condition that occurs when blood glucose levels are lower than normal.

immunocompromised A person who is less capable of fighting infection due to an immune system that is impaired because of illness, life stage, or treatment for illness.

insoluble fiber Fiber that does not dissolve in water; includes cellulose and hemicelluloses found in bran, vegetables, seeds, and whole grains.

Institute of Medicine (IOM) Reviews research and conducts policy studies on health issues.

insulin Hormone secreted by the pancreas that is involved in regulating carbohydrate and fat metabolism. Insulin allows for glucose to enter the cells and signals the liver and muscles to store glycogen.

iron-deficiency anemia A decrease in the number of red cells in the blood caused by too little iron.

isoflavones A phytoestrogen found in soy.

keratin The primary protein in hair, nails, and the outer layer of the skin.

ketone bodies Molecules formed from breakdown of fats; occurs when there is not enough carbohydrate available.

ketosis Presence of high levels of ketones in the urine; caused when fats are broken down for energy in absence of carbohydrates; can cause dehydration and acidify the blood.

kwashiorkor A type of protein-energy malnutrition (PEM) where adequate calories are present in the diet but protein intake is inadequate.

lacto-ovo vegetarian Person who consumes no meat, poultry, or fish but does consume dairy products and eggs.

lactose intolerant An inability to digest lactose, or milk sugar, caused by inadequate lactase production.

legumes A category of plants with edible seed pods that split into two halves, such as beans, peas, lentils, and soybeans.

limited evidence Reflects either a small number of studies, studies of weak design, and/or inconsistent results.

lingual lipase An enzyme secreted by the salivary glands that begins the breakdown of fat in the mouth.

live active cultures The bacteria *Lactobacillus bulgaricus* and *Streptococcus thermophilus* that convert milk to yogurt during fermentation. These can be killed if the yogurt is heat-treated during processing.

low-density lipoprotein (LDL) Often referred to as "bad cholesterol," it transports cholesterol and triglycerides from the liver to other tissues. Remember *L* for *lousy* cholesterol.

lutein A yellow pigment found in yellow, orange, and green fruits and vegetables; has antioxidant properties and may protect against macular degeneration.

lycopene Red pigment found predominantly in tomatoes; has antioxidant properties and may help promote health and protect against heart disease and some forms of cancer.

lymph system Part of the immune systems, it is composed of a network of lymphatic vessels that carry lymph (a clear fluid) toward the heart.

malnutrition Under- or overconsumption of energy or nutrients, resulting in compromised health.

marasmus A type of protein-energy malnutrition (PEM) where protein and calories are inadequate in the diet.

Meals on Wheels A nonprofit organization that delivers hot meals to the elderly and homebound.

micelle Monoglycerides and free fatty acids surrounded by bile. Micelles allow for the transport of fat to the intestinal wall.

mindfulness A state of active attention to the present, having greater awareness of moment-to-moment thoughts, feelings, and actions. Mindfulness means living in the moment and being aware of everything that makes up your day.

minerals Inorganic substances that help regulate body processes and provide structure to the body.

moderate evidence Reflects somewhat less evidence or less consistent evidence. The body of evidence may include studies of weaker design and/or some inconsistency in results. The studies may be susceptible to some bias, but not enough to invalidate the results, or the body of evidence may not be as generalizable to the population of interest.

monounsaturated fatty acid A fatty acid with one double bond between two carbon atoms. Monounsaturated fats are found in peanuts, peanut oil, safflower oil, olives, olive oil, canola oil, and avocados and are liquid at room temperature.

muscle-strengthening activity Sometimes called *resistance training*; a type of physical activity that engages the muscles to do more work than they are used to doing, such as when lifting weights or using stretch bands.

musculoskeletal All of the muscles, bones, joints, and related structures that function in the movement of the body.

MyPlate A graphic that illustrates the five food groups using a familiar mealtime visual—a place setting. The graphic is part of a larger communications initiative to help consumers make better food choices. MyPlate is designed to remind you to eat healthfully.

National Center for Complementary and Alternative Medicine (NCCAM) The federal government's lead agency for scientific research on the diverse medical and healthcare systems, practices, and products that are not generally considered part of conventional medicine.

National School Breakfast Program A federally funded program that provides cash assistance to states to operate nonprofit breakfast programs in schools and residential childcare institutions.

National School Lunch Program (NSLP) A federally funded program that provides free or reduced-price school lunches to eligible students based on family income levels.

neophobia Dislike of anything new or unfamiliar.

nonheme iron Iron from plant sources.

nutrient dense Foods and beverages that provide vitamins, minerals, and other substances and that may have positive health effects with relatively few calories.

nutrients Substances in food that the body uses for energy, growth, tissue repair, or regulation of body processes.

nutrition The science of food and its components, including food's relationship to health and disease.

obese For adults, a BMI of 30 or higher. For children under the age of 20, a BMI for age at or greater than the 95th percentile.

omega-3 fatty acid A polyunsaturated fatty acid that has the first double bond three carbons from the endmost (omega) carbon in the chain. Omega-3 fatty acids are found in fatty fish and flaxseed.

omega-6 fatty acid A polyunsaturated fatty acid that has the first double bond six carbons from the endmost (omega) carbon in the chain. Omega-6 fatty acids are found in most vegetable oils.

organically grown foods Food grown by farmers who emphasize the use of renewable resources and the conservation of soil and water to enhance environmental quality for future generations.

organically produced meat Meat produced without the use of antibiotics or growth hormones and fed only organic feed.

osteopenia A bone mineral density that is lower than normal but not low enough to be classified as osteoporosis.

osteoporosis Thinning of the bones with reduction in bone mass caused by loss of calcium and protein from bone, which leads to the bone becoming fragile and, in turn, increasing the risk in fractures.

overweight For adults, a BMI between 25.0 and 29.9. For children under the age of 20, a BMI for age that is greater than the 85th percentile but less than the 95th percentile.

oxalates Substances in vegetables, especially spinach, that are capable of forming an insoluble salt with calcium, thus interfering with its absorption.

pancreas An organ that produces digestive enzymes and hormones, including insulin.

pancreatic lipase An enzyme secreted by the pancreas into the small intestine that breaks down triglycerides and diglycerides into monoglycerides and free fatty acids.

pasteurization A method of treating food by heating it to a certain point to kill disease-causing organisms, but not change the flavor or quality of the food. Milk is pasteurized by heating it to about 145° F for 30 minutes or to 160° F for 15 minutes. This technique also used with beer, wine, fruit juices, cheese, and egg products.

pathogen An agent, such as a bacteria or virus, that causes disease or illness.

pescatarian Person who does not consume meat or poultry but does consume fish; may or may not consume dairy products and eggs.

pH A measure of the degree of the acidity or alkalinity of a solution.

physical activity Any movement that works the muscles and uses more energy than when the body is at rest.

physical fitness A state of well-being with low risk of premature health problems and energy to participate in a variety of physical activities; includes cardiorespiratory endurance, muscular endurance, muscular strength, and flexibility.

phytates Substances in vegetables and grains that are capable of forming an insoluble salt with calcium, zinc, iron, and other nutrients, thus interfering with their absorption.

phytoestrogens A group of chemicals found in plants that can have estrogen-like effects in the body.

phytonutrients (phytochemicals) Compounds found in plants that may help promote health and reduce risk of some chronic diseases.

placenta The organ that develops during pregnancy that connects the fetus to the mother. It allows for nutrients and gases to pass to the fetus and for waste to be removed from the fetus.

polychlorinated biphenyls (PCBs) A chemical once used as a coolant or lubricant. Although no longer produced in the United States, it still exists as an environmental pollutant. It is a known carcinogen.

polyunsaturated fatty acid A fatty acid with two or more double bonds between two carbon atoms. Polyunsaturated fats are found in fatty fish, nuts, most vegetable oils, and soybeans and are liquid at room temperature. There are different types of polyunsaturated fats depending on where the double bonds between the carbon atoms are located.

portion distortion The perception that large portions are appropriate amounts to eat at one sitting; caused by the increase in portion sizes served primarily in restaurants and fast-food outlets.

preeclampsia A condition in pregnancy that is characterized by high blood pressure, edema, and protein in the urine.

probiotics Microorganisms thought to be beneficial to health; commonly consumed as part of fermented foods such as yogurt.

protein-energy malnutrition (PEM) A long-term deficiency of protein, energy, or both. PEM results in wasting of body tissue, impaired body function, and increased susceptibility to infection.

proteins Organic compounds that contain carbon, hydrogen, nitrogen, and oxygen. Proteins differ from other energy-providing nutrients in that they contain nitrogen. Proteins are made of smaller building blocks called amino acids. Proteins can provide energy but are unique in their function of maintaining body structure and regulating many processes in the body.

Recommended Dietary Allowance (RDA) Daily dietary intake level of a nutrient sufficient to meet 97–98% of healthy individuals in a particular age/gender group.

resveratrol An antioxidant found in many plants, it is found in especially high concentrations in the skin of grapes; its ability to protect against heart disease and cancer is still under investigation.

retinol activity equivalents (RAE) A unit of measure of

the amount of vitamin A in a food; 1 RAE = 1 microgram of retinol.

rickets Softening of bones in children or adolescents usually caused by extreme and prolonged vitamin D deficiency.

saturated fatty acid A fatty acid with the maximum possible number of hydrogen atoms. Saturated fats are usually solid at room temperature and are found in meat, poultry, dairy products, and tropical oils (coconut and palm).

sell-by date The date printed on a package of perishable food that indicates the date after which it should not be offered for sale.

semi-vegetarian Person who limits meat or does not consume red meat; sometimes called a *part-time vegetarian* or a *flexitarian*.

simple carbohydrates Sugars composed of one sugar molecule (monosaccharides) or two sugar molecules (disaccharides).

soluble Fiber that dissolves or swells in water; includes pectins, gums, mucilages, and beta-glucans found in fruits, vegetables, legumes, and oats.

starch The major form of carbohydrate stored in plants; it is composed of long chains of glucose molecules.

stress Your body's reaction to a change that requires a physical, mental, or emotional adjustment or response. Stress can come from any situation or thought that makes you feel frustrated, angry, nervous, or anxious.

stressor An external stimulus that causes stress.

strong evidence Reflects consistent, convincing findings derived from studies that use a robust methodology and that are relevant to the population of interest.

subcutaneous fat Body fat that acts as insulation, protecting the body from extreme heat and cold.

Supplemental Nutrition Assistance Program (SNAP) Formerly called Food Stamps, this federal assistance program provides low-income people with funds to purchase food.

Tolerable Upper Intake Level (UL) Set to caution against excessive intake of nutrients that can be harmful in large amounts.

trans fat A type of fat that is formed when hydrogen is added to a liquid fat to form a solid or semisolid fat. Trans fats are also found naturally in small amounts in dairy and meat. Consumption of trans fats is linked to an increased risk of heart disease.

type 1 diabetes A type of diabetes that occurs when the cells in the pancreas that produce insulin are damaged or destroyed; usually diagnosed in childhood or early adulthood.

type 2 diabetes Form of diabetes usually diagnosed later in life whereby the body does not make enough insulin or the cells do not respond as they should to insulin.

undernourished Underconsumption of calories or nutrients that leads to disease or susceptibility to disease.

United States Department of Agriculture (USDA) The federal agency that is responsible for the development and execution of policy on farming, agriculture, and food. The agency ensures that the United States has a safe food supply and that natural resources are protected.

United States Pharmacopeia (USP) A nongovernmental, official public standards–setting authority for prescription and over-the-counter medicines and other healthcare products manufactured or sold in the United States.

vegan Person who consumes no meat, poultry, fish, eggs, milk, or anything made with animal products.

very-low-density lipoprotein (VLDL) A type of lipoprotein very high in triglycerides that releases triglycerides to cells.

vitamins Organic substances that help regulate hundreds of processes in the body. Although they provide no energy, they help your body use the energy in the foods you eat.

Women, Infants, and Children Program (WIC) A federally funded program that provides nutritious foods, nutrition education, and referrals and access to health care to low-income pregnant women, new mothers, and infants and children at nutritional risk. WIC participants now receive a new healthier WIC food package that includes, fruits, vegetables, low-fat milk, and whole-grain bread.

World Health Organization The public health arm of the United Nations; monitors disease outbreaks and assesses the performance of health systems around the world.

Chapter 1

Food: Why You Eat What You Eat

Personal Health Check

What Influences Your Food Choices?

Examine what influences your food choices. Have you become a creature of habit, eating the same things day in and day out just because that is what you have always eaten? Have you allowed a tight food budget to send you to the fast-food restaurant more than you should, rather than taking the time to prepare simple foods at home? What are the major influences on your food choices?

Once you have determined what influences your food choices, break out of your mold and expand your choices to include foods you may have never tried or take a trip to a nearby farm stand where you have never shopped. If you often rely on prepackaged foods, try making food from scratch some of the time. Expanding your food choices will help you have a more varied, interesting diet. How can you expand your food choices?

Try Something New

External Cues to Eat

You have just had lunch, and you feel full. On your walk back to class, you pass a bakery and are struck by the smell of warm chocolate chip cookies. The familiar smell causes your mouth to water. Before you know it, you are diving into a bag of just-baked goodness. Were you driven by hunger to eat, or did the smell of something you knew would taste good stimulate your appetite? How susceptible are you to external cues to eat?

Often, external stimuli to eat, such as smelling, seeing, or even talking about food, override your need for calories. In other words, you may eat because the food tastes good, not because you are hungry. Even though you may salivate at the sight of a favorite food, it does not mean you should eat it. External cues may be signaling you to eat, but are you really hungry?

Use the chart below to keep track of how hungry you are each time you eat for the next few days. Use the hunger scale below as a guide. This will help you be more mindful of eating when you are hungry, not just when you are prompted to by external cues.

1. **Weak and light-headed** — your stomach is churning
2. **Ravenous** — you are irritable and cannot concentrate
3. **Hungry** — your stomach is rumbling
4. **Slightly hungry** — beginning to feel the signs of hunger
5. **Neutral** — you could eat more but are not hungry
6. **Satisfied** — perfectly comfortable
7. **Full** — a little uncomfortable
8. **Stuffed** — uncomfortably full
9. **Bloated** — need to loosen clothing
10. **Nauseous** — so full you may be sick

Hunger Scale

You should only eat when you are at a 1, 2, 3, or 4 on the scale. Put down your fork when you get to a 5 or 6.

Day 1		Day 2		Day 3	
	Breakfast		Breakfast		Breakfast
	Lunch		Lunch		Lunch
	Dinner		Dinner		Dinner
	Snacks		Snacks		Snacks

Critical Analysis

1. What are some solutions to domestic and global hunger?

2. Should companies be allowed to advertise and market unhealthy foods? Should they be able to advertise such foods directly to children?

3. Assess your environment. Is it supportive of healthy eating? What access do you have to a grocery store, cooking facilities, and restaurants that serve healthy foods?

Chapter 2

Eating Healthy: Tools to Help You Choose

Personal Health Check

Food Tracker

Tracking what you eat and how you move even for a few days will give you an estimate of how you are doing with respect to eating healthy and being active. It will give you a starting point from which you can begin to make any needed changes to improve the healthfulness of the foods you select and your physical activity level. Use the Food Tracker at www.ChooseMyPlate.gov for a few days and see how you do. Because the tracker is based on your age, gender, weight, height, and activity level, you will have a personalized account of how close your diet and activity levels are to what is recommended for good health.

Try Something New

Compare Your Choices

Next time you are at the grocery store choose one food that you buy on a regular basis and examine the Nutrition Facts panel. A good place to start would be breakfast cereal or yogurt. Check out the serving size, calories per serving, and % Daily Value for fat and sodium. Compare that product to similar products. Does the product you usually consume have more or less of any nutrient than you thought? Were there products that were similar that may be a better choice for your overall diet? If so, give the new product a try; you may be willing to make a trade-off to make your usual choice the healthier choice.

Compare Breakfast Cereals

	My Usual Cereal	Cereal #2	Cereal #3
Serving size			
Calories per serving			
Fat grams			
Sodium milligrams			

Compare Yogurts

	My Usual Yogurt	Yogurt #2	Yogurt #3
Serving size			
Calories per serving			
Fat grams			
Sodium milligrams			

Based on what you found in this activity, will you change the cereal or yogurt you usually buy? If so, why?

Critical Analysis

1. Do health claims on a label, such as "may reduce the risk of certain cancers," help consumers choose healthy foods, or do they create more confusion?

2. MyPlate has replaced MyPyramid. Compare these two food guidance systems. Which one do you think is more helpful in aiding the general public choose a healthier diet? Why?

Test Your Skills

Use the Daily Food Plan interactive tool at www.ChooseMyPlate.gov to estimate your daily nutrition needs. Record your recommended nutrition information below.

Food Group	Amount Needed Each Day
Grains	
Vegetables	
Fruits	
Dairy	
Protein Foods	
Other Notes	

Chapter 3

Eating Out or Eating In: Where You Eat Affects What You Eat

Personal Health Check

What's in Your Favorite Restaurant Meals?

You don't have to stop eating out altogether to eat healthy. Prepare and eat more meals at home, and when you do go out choose healthy options. A good way to start is to find out how your favorite meals eaten away from home stack up nutritionally. Write down the three restaurants you go to most and list what you usually order. Use the Internet to find out the calories and fat in your favorite meals. If you choose a local restaurant without nutritional information, you may have to choose a similar meal from a chain restaurant that offers nutritional information. If the meals that you normally order are higher in calories than they should be, look for other menu items that you could order instead. Check the restaurant's website to see if it offers any healthy alternatives; many do. Now you are ready to dine out without breaking the calorie bank.

My Usual Meal from Restaurant #1

Food	Calories	Fat	Sodium

My Usual Meal from Restaurant #2

Food	Calories	Fat	Sodium

My Usual Meal from Restaurant #3

Food	Calories	Fat	Sodium

Did what you discover change any of your ordering habits? If so, how?

____

____

____

____

____

Try Something New

Make a Weekly Plan

How do you decide what you are going to eat for dinner? Often a plan can make the difference between having a healthy meal or reaching for fast food. Making a weekly plan for at least your evening meal will help you steer clear of unhealthy options like the number one value meal from a fast-food restaurant. Once you get the hang of it, it does not take too much time or effort. The time you do invest pays big dividends in meals that promote health and help you maintain a healthy weight.

Start by making a list of the simple, healthy entrees and side dishes that you know how to make and that you and your family and friends enjoy. Sometime during the week, set aside 30 minutes to plan for the next week. Make a list of the main dish and the side dishes that you will make each day of the week. You may make roast chicken on Sunday and then plan to eat the leftovers ("planned-overs") on Wednesday. If you know your week will be especially hectic, you may want to cook more than one meal ahead of time so that it is ready to reheat and eat.

For inspiration, look at cookbooks, websites, or grocery store flyers. Keep it simple; choose recipes with five or fewer ingredients. Choose one-pot entrees, such as stir-fry or stew. Use time savers such as bagged salad or precut or frozen vegetables. Be sure to include quick dinner ideas as part of your plan. Each week, you could have one night that is soup and sandwich and/or one night that is a cheese omelet and toast. Now that you have your plan for the week, make your shopping list so you will have the foods you need on hand to follow your plan.

Meals to Remember

Sometimes the hardest part about fixing dinner is figuring what to make. List the meals you and your family enjoy to help you plan your week. Post the list in a handy spot like the inside door of a cabinet. Keep adding new favorites.

MAIN DISH (chicken, beef, pork, fish, pasta, beans, etc.)	SIDE DISH (salad, vegetables, fruit, potatoes, rice, etc.)

Plan your dinners for the week. It will help with shopping and save time.

What's for Dinner?

Monday ______

Tuesday ______

Wednesday ______

Thursday ______

Friday ______

Saturday ______

Sunday ______

Critical Analysis

1. Use the 10 keys to cooking smart to analyze your cooking style and cooking facilities. How are you doing? Do you have the basics to eat and prepare more meals at home?

   1: Keep it simple ______

   2: Make room to cook ______

   3: Clean as you go ______

   4: *Mise en place* ______

   5: Develop your own style ______

   6: Go slow ______

   7: Trust your instincts ______

   8: Organize your recipes ______

   9: Find the joy ______

   10: Plan ______

2. Restaurants with 20 or more locations are now required to post the calories contained in each menu item. Based on what you have learned, do you think this will help consumers choose foods from restaurants more wisely?

Test Your Skills

1. Try packing your lunch for one week instead of grabbing fast food or eating out. How did this impact what you ate?

2. Use the sample policy on page 43 to help a group or club of which you are a member serve healthier items.

Chapter 4

Digestion and Absorption: How Your Body Uses the Food You Eat

Personal Health Check

Screening for Colorectal Cancer

Although the exact cause of colorectal cancer is not known, we do know that the earlier it is caught the better a person's chance for a full recovery. It is recommended that screenings for colon cancer begin at age 50 and continue through age 75.[21] A number of different screening methods are available. Testing your stool for blood is the most noninvasive method of testing. Another test for colon cancer is the flexible sigmoidoscopy. With this test, a thin, flexible, lighted tube is inserted into the rectum so that a physician can check for polyps or cancer in the lower third of the colon. A colonoscopy is similar to a flexible sigmoidoscopy, but it enables the physician to view the entire colon.

If you are older than age 50, you should check with your physician about the right time to begin screening. Not quite to 50 yet? Then mark your calendar to start screenings when you hit the half-century mark. In the meantime, eat a healthy diet, maintain an ideal weight, engage in regular physical activity, and don't smoke to decrease your risk of colorectal cancer.

Critical Analysis

1. Research popular detox diets on the Internet and examine the tactics they use to promote the practice of detox. Is there truth to their claims? Is detoxing necessary for optimal gastrointestinal health? Why or why not?

2. Now that you know about digestion and absorption, what changes can you make in your diet or exercise routine to improve the overall health of your gastrointestinal system?

Chapter 5

Carbohydrates: Skip the Simple, Add More Complex

American Diabetes Association.

ALERT!DAY

ARE YOU AT RISK?

DIABETES RISK TEST

Calculate Your Chances for Type 2 or Pre-Diabetes

The American Diabetes Association has revised its Diabetes Risk Test according to a new, more accurate statistical model. The updated test includes some new risk factors, and projects risk for pre-diabetes as well as diabetes.

This simple tool can help you determine your risk for having pre-diabetes or diabetes. Using the flow chart, answer the questions until you reach a colored shape. Match that with a risk message shown below.

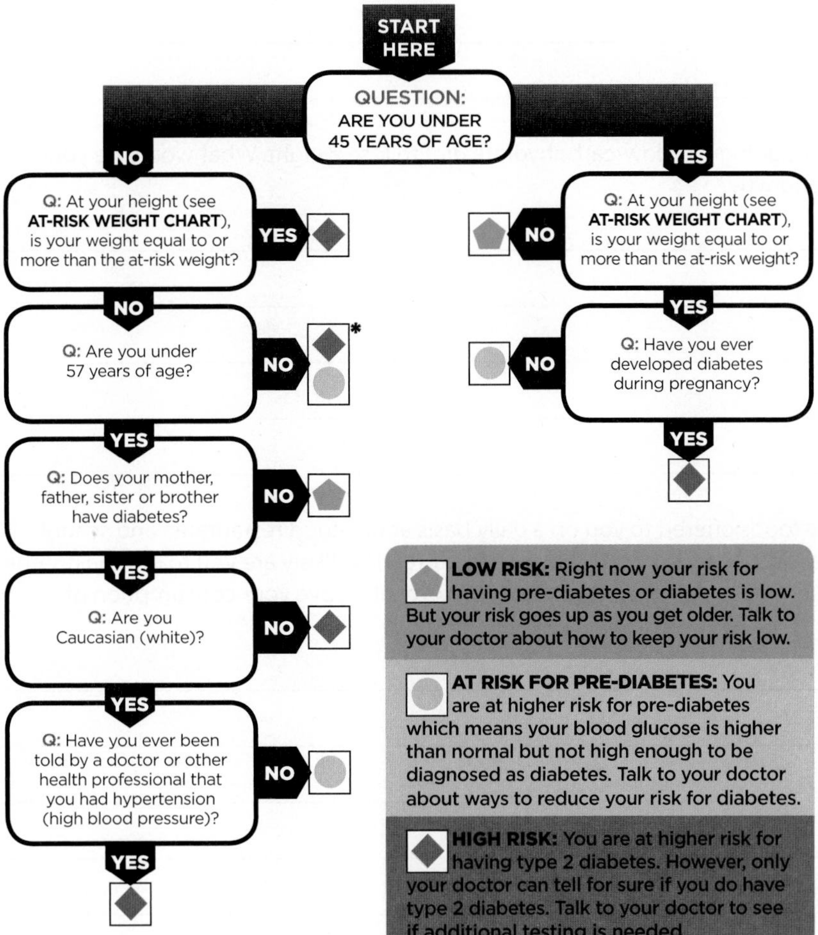
START HERE
QUESTION: ARE YOU UNDER 45 YEARS OF AGE?
NO
YES
Q: At your height (see AT-RISK WEIGHT CHART), is your weight equal to or more than the at-risk weight?
YES
NO
Q: Are you under 57 years of age?
NO
*
YES
Q: Does your mother, father, sister or brother have diabetes?
NO
YES
Q: Are you Caucasian (white)?
NO
YES
Q: Have you ever been told by a doctor or other health professional that you had hypertension (high blood pressure)?
NO
YES
Q: At your height (see AT-RISK WEIGHT CHART), is your weight equal to or more than the at-risk weight?
NO
YES
Q: Have you ever developed diabetes during pregnancy?
NO
YES

LOW RISK: Right now your risk for having pre-diabetes or diabetes is low. But your risk goes up as you get older. Talk to your doctor about how to keep your risk low.

AT RISK FOR PRE-DIABETES: You are at higher risk for pre-diabetes which means your blood glucose is higher than normal but not high enough to be diagnosed as diabetes. Talk to your doctor about ways to reduce your risk for diabetes.

HIGH RISK: You are at higher risk for having type 2 diabetes. However, only your doctor can tell for sure if you do have type 2 diabetes. Talk to your doctor to see if additional testing is needed.

AT-RISK WEIGHT CHART

HEIGHT	WEIGHT
4'10"	148 LBS
4'11"	153 LBS
5'0"	158 LBS
5'1"	164 LBS
5'2"	169 LBS
5'3"	175 LBS
5'4"	180 LBS
5'5"	186 LBS
5'6"	192 LBS
5'7"	198 LBS
5'8"	203 LBS
5'9"	209 LBS
5'10"	216 LBS
5'11"	222 LBS
6'0"	228 LBS
6'1"	235 LBS
6'2"	241 LBS
6'3"	248 LBS
6'4"	254 LBS
6'5"	261 LBS

STOP DIABETES.
1-800-DIABETES
diabetes.org/risktest

*Your risk for diabetes or pre-diabetes depends on additional risk factors including weight, physical activity and blood pressure.

Source: American Diabetes Association, diabetes.org/risktest.

Try Something New

Try a New Grain

Some of the whole grains in Table 5.5 may not be familiar to you. In the United States, we do not usually consume grains such as millet, bulgur, or quinoa. However, they can add variety, interest, and a healthy dose of whole grain to your diet. One in particular that you may want to try is quinoa, pronounced "keen-wah." Quinoa is a great alternative to rice and has a mild nutty flavor. Quinoa is available in some grocery stores and in many health food stores. It is easy to cook: just use 2 cups of water to 1 cup of quinoa, bring to a boil, cover, and lower the heat. Quinoa cooks fast; only 15 minutes and it will be done. You can use it as-is for a side dish as you would rice or potatoes or you can add it to a recipe. To make a quick salad, cook 1 cup of quinoa and then chill it. Add 2 cups of chopped vegetables, your choice. Good vegetables to choose include mild onions, tomatoes, bell peppers, and carrots. Mix in 1/4 cup of chopped parsley or other herb. Toss with your favorite Italian dressing or oil and vinegar. This salad will keep for several days in the refrigerator and makes a great light lunch.

Critical Analysis

1. How does the Farm Bill affect what you pay for food? Does it affect all food prices?

____

____

____

____

____

2. A friend is thinking about going on a low-carbohydrate diet to lose weight. What would be your advice for your friend, and why?

____

____

____

____

____

3. Take a closer look at the foods offered to you on a daily basis at fast-food restaurants and school dining facilities and the foods you choose at the grocery store. How likely are you to get the number of servings of whole grains you need each day? How could you improve your consumption of whole-grain foods?

____

____

____

____

____

Test Your Skills

1. Go to the grocery store and choose a healthier breakfast cereal and a healthier breakfast bar based on the following criteria:

   Choose a breakfast cereal that has:

   - Less than 200 calories per serving
   - Less than 6 grams sugar per serving
   - At least 3 grams dietary fiber per serving

   Cereals that fit the criteria:

   ____

   ____

   ____

   ____

   Choose a breakfast bar that has:

   - Less than 200 calories per bar
   - Less than 6 grams sugar per 100 calories
   - At least 3 grams dietary fiber per bar

   Breakfast bars that fit the criteria:

   ____

   ____

   ____

   ____

2. Go to the grocery store and use the ingredient label to choose a bread that is a good source of whole grain. How do you know this bread is a good whole-grain choice? Can you find a whole-grain bread that is moderate in calories (50–70 per slice)?

   ____

   ____

   ____

   ____

   ____

Chapter 6

Fruits and Vegetables: Eat All the Colors

Personal Health Check

How Is Your Fruit and Vegetable Intake?

We know from national surveys that most of us do not get enough fruits and vegetables on a daily basis. Assess your own fruit and vegetable intake. Keep a fruit and vegetable food diary for three days. Make sure that one of those days is a weekend day. Keep track of all of the fresh, frozen, canned, raw, cooked—any kind—of fruits and vegetables you eat. Keep track of the amount, the preparation method, and any condiments or sauces added. Once you have your diary, add the number of cups of fruit and vegetables you consumed each day and find the average for the three days. How did you do? What are some ways you can increase your consumption if you are below the recommended amounts?

Day	Food Log	Cups of Fruits and Vegetables
Day 1		
Day 2		

Day	Food Log	Cups of Fruits and Vegetables
Day 3		
	Total Cups of Fruits and Vegetables:	
	Average Cups of Fruits and Vegetables per Day	

Analysis:

____

____

____

____

____

Try Something New

Create Your Own Stir-Fry Mix

Stir-frying is an easy, quick, and healthy way to cook vegetables. To make stir-fry convenient, try making your own stir-fry mix. Select four or five vegetables; pick your favorites and/or what is on sale that week. Wash and cut the vegetables into bite size pieces and place them in a plastic bag or plastic sealable container. Choose vegetables that all cook in about the same time or keep those that need shorter cooking time, such as mushrooms, separate. Having your stir-fry mix ready to go makes it easy to grab the vegetables you need and have stir-fried vegetables in a matter of minutes. Choose a sauce or just salt and pepper to taste. You don't need a specialty pan to stir-fry vegetables. A skillet works just as well as a wok or stir-fry pan.

Critical Analysis

1. Do you buy organic fruits and vegetables? Justify your answer using scientific evidence.

2. What strategies can you use to make sure that you get adequate fruits and vegetables, even if you are on a tight budget?

3. How does consuming fruits and vegetables contribute to weight loss and/or weight maintenance?

Test Your Skills

1. Survey the environment near your school or where you live. How many farm stands or farmers' markets are available? Visit one or more and investigate if the produce it sells is produced locally.

2. Compare the price and nutritional content of frozen, canned, and fresh fruits and vegetables. Include one that is in-season and one that is out-of-season.

In-season fruit or vegetable: ____________________

	Fresh	Canned	Frozen
Price per cup or unit			
Calories			
Fat			
Sodium			

Out-of-season fruit or vegetable: ____________________

	Fresh	Canned	Frozen
Price per cup or unit			
Calories			
Fat			
Sodium			

For both examples, which would you buy and why?

____

____

____

____

____

____

____

____

____

____

Chapter 7

Beverages: Rethink Your Drink

Personal Health Check

Create a Personal Beverage Clock

For the next 24 hours, keep a beverage clock. Write down all the beverages you consume, the amount, the kind, and the time of day. Use the tracker at www.choosemyplate.gov to estimate the number of calories you consume in a day of beverages. Make a list of changes you would be willing to try in the next week to make your beverage clock healthier. Repeat the above exercise and see how you were able to make some positive changes. Remember, you don't have to make all the changes at once. Taking it one beverage at a time is a step in the right direction.

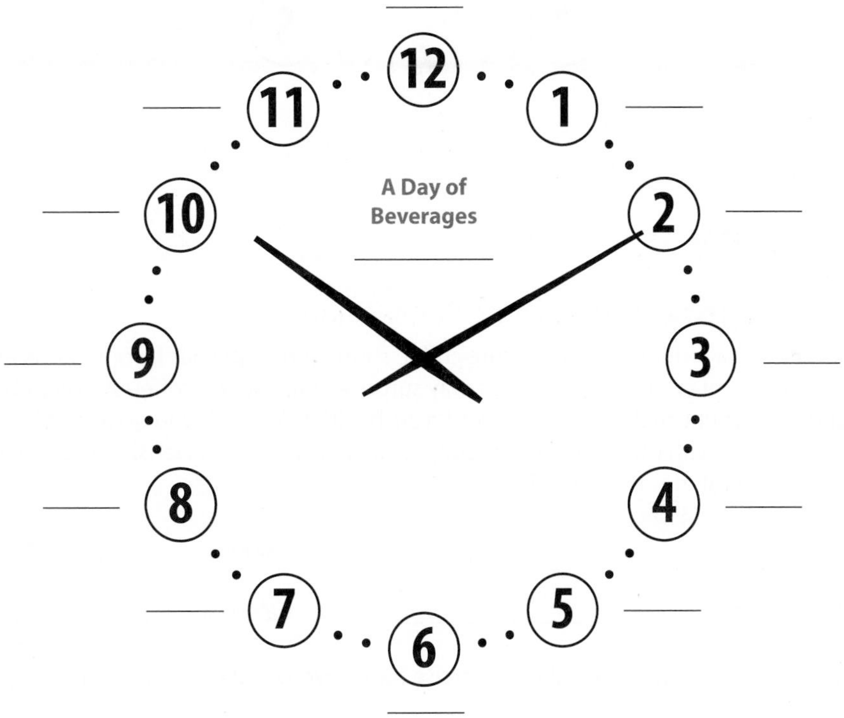

Make a list of changes you would be willing to try in the next week to make your beverage clock healthier.

____

____

____

____

____

Repeat the activity to see if you were able to make some positive changes. Remember, you don't have to make all the changes at once. Taking it one beverage at a time is a step in the right direction.

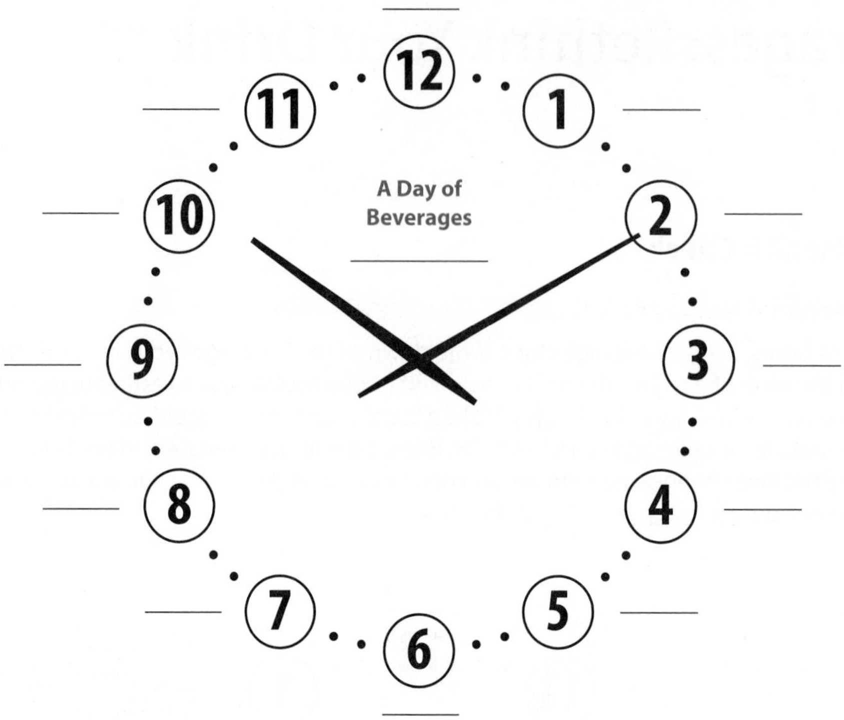

Try Something New

Order Something New at Your Favorite Coffee Shop

Break out of your mocha routine at your favorite coffee shop. Although your favorite drink at the coffee shop may sound innocent enough, the calories may surprise you. Use the coffee shop's website to get the calories and fat in your usual order and in your new, healthier order. If you go to a coffee shop that does not have a website with nutrition information, use a national chain's website to get at least an estimate of the fat and calories in your order.

My usual order: ________________________ Calories: __________ Fat: __________

My new, healthier order: ____________________ Calories: __________ Fat: __________

If you don't drink coffee, complete the above exercise for a beverage that you consume on most days of the week.

Critical Analysis

1. Are sugar-sweetened beverages contributing to the obesity crisis? If so, how? If not, why not?

2. Assess the beverage options on campus. Are there calorie-free options available at the same or lower cost as high-calorie, high-sugar beverages? What size beverages are offered? Are sugar-sweetened beverages marketed heavily on campus (i.e., drink machines with beverage logos, events sponsored by beverage companies, etc.)? How might all of these factors affect your own or other students' beverage consumption?

Test Your Skills

Assess your environment for healthy beverage choices. What is available in your home and at school, work, friends' homes, and so on? Are most of the beverage choices sugar-sweetened, or are calorie-free beverages available as well? Are there vending machines on campus that promote sugar-sweetened beverage consumption?

Chapter 8

Protein: More Is Not Always Better

Personal Health Check

How Much Protein Do You Need Each Day?

Use the following formula to calculate the amount of protein you need each day:

_____ body weight in pounds ÷ 2.2 = _____ body weight in kilograms

_____ body weight in kilograms × 0.8 = _____ RDA for protein

Example:

22-year-old man who weighs 165 pounds.

165 pounds ÷ 2.2 = 75 kilograms

75 kilograms × 0.8 = 60 grams of protein per day

Note: Use ideal body weight.

Protein Food Diary

Record what you eat on a typical day or for several days. Use the Food Tracker at www.ChooseMyPlate.gov to enter your food intake and analyze the amount of protein you are eating.

Food	Amount	Protein

Decision-Making Workbook

How did you do? Where did most of your protein come from (i.e., animal or vegetable sources)? If you were too low in protein (which is doubtful), how can you make sure you get enough in the future? If you ate too much protein, how can you bring your protein intake in line with recommendations? If most of the protein you consume is from animal sources, can you try consuming more protein from vegetable sources, such as beans?

Try Something New

Beans

Beans are certainly not new. However, they don't make their way into the diet of many Americans on a regular basis. Beans are an inexpensive high-protein, low-fat, high-fiber food that can easily be added to your diet. Beans and rice make a great substitute for meat, bean soup will warm you up on a cold winter day, and bean tacos are great to serve friends while watching the game. Beans are easy to prepare as well. Canned beans are quick and convenient. For a real money saver, try dried beans. For a couple of dollars you get a pound of dried beans that makes about 8 cups of beans. Just soak the beans overnight in the refrigerator. Pour off the water the next morning. Add the beans to a large pot, add water and seasonings, and cook. The cooking time will depend on the type of bean; just check the package for details. If you have a slow cooker (crock pot) it is even easier. Just put the soaked beans in the slow cooker in the morning; add water to cover, plus about 2 inches; incorporate seasonings, such as onion or chili powder; and cook on low for eight hours. When you get home that evening, you'll have beans that are ready to eat. Add a little more water, and you'll have bean soup.

Black Bean Soup

Ingredients

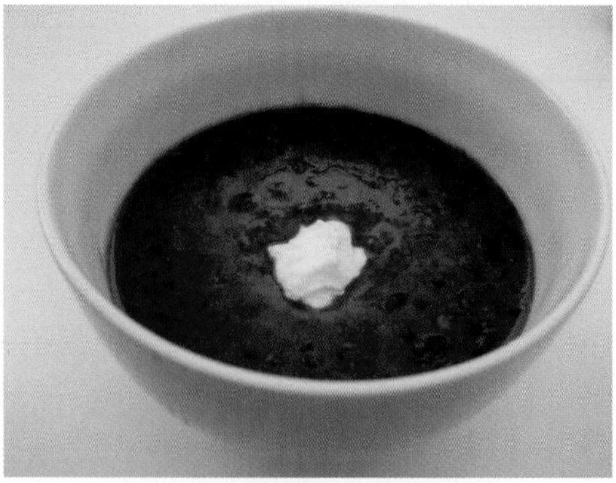

1 tablespoon olive oil
1 medium onion, chopped
1 tablespoon ground cumin or chili powder
2, 14.5-ounce cans black beans, drained
2 cups chicken broth or water
Salt and pepper to taste
Sour cream or cheese for topping (optional)

Instructions

1. Sauté the onion in olive oil in a large pot.
2. After two minutes, add the cumin or chili powder.
3. Add one can of beans and broth or water.
4. Cook for four to five minutes on medium heat, stir occasionally.
5. Remove from heat and use a hand blender to puree ingredients or transfer to a blender and puree.
6. Add the second can of beans to the pot and cook over medium heat three to four minutes or until bubbly.
7. Taste and add salt and pepper as needed.
8. Serve topped with sour cream and/or cheese (optional).

Critical Analysis

1. How can your choice of dietary protein affect the environment? Is there a difference in the environmental impact of the production of animal versus vegetable protein?

2. What are the advantages and disadvantages of a vegetarian diet?

3. What advantage, if any, would there be to go meatless for one or more days a week (part-time vegetarian)?

Test Your Skills

Choose one day a week to go meatless. Meatless Monday (or whatever day you choose) will help you break out of an animal protein rut and experiment with the wide variety of plant proteins. Record what you eat that day and check your protein intake. Were you still within what is recommended for you?

Chapter 9

Milk and Dairy: Not Just for Kids

Personal Health Check

Do You Need a Calcium Supplement?

The first step to answering the question of whether you need a calcium supplement is to examine your diet and assess how much calcium you currently consume. Use the calcium wheel below for a rough estimate of how much calcium you get on a regular basis. If you do not consume dairy products on a regular basis, or consume them in small amounts, you may need a supplement. Keep in mind that although there are other foods that contain calcium, in addition to dairy products, the amount you would need to consume to get close to the recommended amounts is very high. This makes it very difficult to get enough calcium without consuming dairy products.

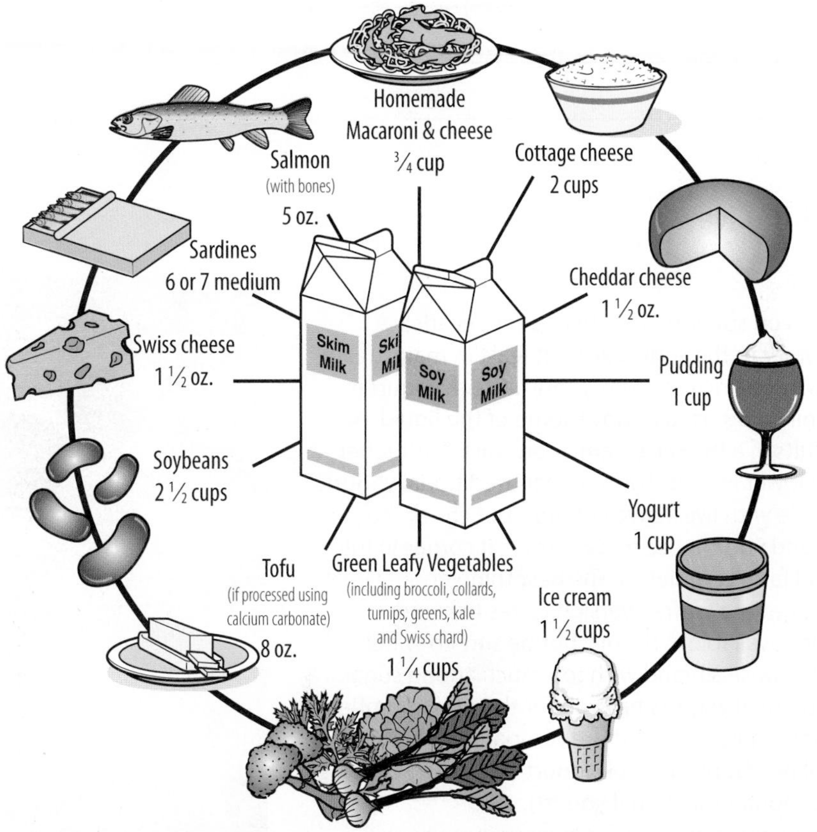

If you decide that you would like to try a calcium supplement, several are on the market from which to choose. The most common forms of calcium supplements are calcium carbonate and calcium citrate. Both are absorbed at similar rates. Some people have fewer digestive issues with calcium citrate. The body absorbs calcium carbonate best when consumed with food. Consumption of food has no effect on the absorption of calcium from calcium citrate. Calcium phosphate is also a supplemental form of calcium, but it is less available and more expensive than either calcium carbonate or calcium citrate. The following are some factors to consider when choosing a calcium supplement:

- **Dose:** The maximum dose of calcium that should be taken at one time is 500 milligrams. If you want to take more, break it up over the course of the day.
- **Vitamin D:** Vitamin D will help with calcium absorption. Choose a calcium supplement that also contains vitamin D.
- **Tolerance:** Calcium carbonate can cause side effects such as gas, bloating, or constipation in some people. If these side effects occur, try a different type of calcium supplement or a different brand. Calcium citrate is an alternative that does not cause constipation.
- **Purity:** Many calcium supplements are on the market. You should choose a familiar brand name that has the United States Pharmacopeia (USP) symbol on the box or bottle. Don't choose supplements made from unrefined oyster shells, bone meal, or dolomite. These supplements do not have the USP symbol, and they may contain high levels of lead or other toxic metals.
- **Price:** Calcium supplements vary in price. Chelated calcium supplements have higher absorption rates but are much more expensive. Calcium carbonate tends to be less expensive than calcium citrate. Choose a calcium supplement that can be tolerated by both your budget and your stomach.

Notes:

Try Something New

Greek Yogurt

Yogurt has been on supermarket shelves for decades. A relative newcomer to the yogurt aisle, at least in mainstream grocery stores in America, is Greek yogurt. Greek yogurt is made by straining yogurt to remove some of the liquid, or whey. This results in a thicker, creamier product. It is higher in protein and lower in carbohydrate than traditional yogurt. It usually is made with live active cultures, but check the label of the brand you choose to be certain. It comes in full-fat, low-fat, and fat-free varieties. The best thing about Greek yogurt is that even the fat-free version tastes rich and creamy. It is also available in flavors, but be sure to watch that you don't choose a brand with too much added sugar. Greek and traditional yogurts have about the same number of calories when similar products are compared (120 calories for 8 ounces of nonfat plain Greek yogurt versus 100 calories for 8 ounces of nonfat traditional yogurt).

Even if you are not a big fan of regular yogurt you will want to give Greek yogurt a try. Its rich, thick, creamy taste may make you a yogurt convert. If you are already a yogurt fan, try Greek yogurt for a change of pace. The extra protein helps to keep hunger away. You may also want to try Greek yogurt if you are lactose intolerant, because it typically has less lactose than traditional yogurt.

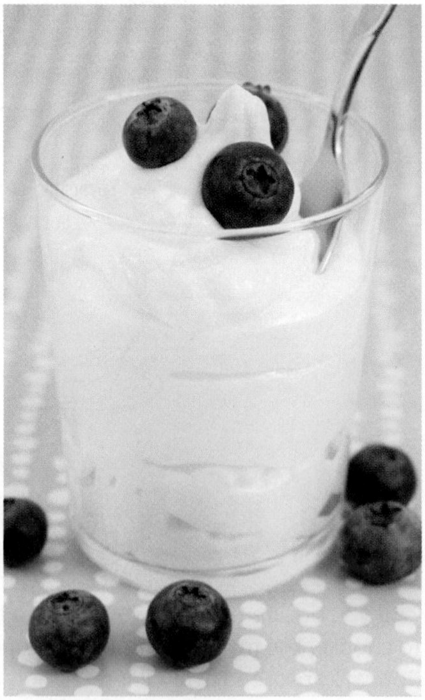

Greek Yogurt Is Thicker and Creamier Than Traditional Yogurt

Critical Analysis

1. Some experts argue that the only creature that should consume cow's milk is a baby cow. Do you agree? Why or why not? If dairy products are off the menu, how could someone get adequate calcium?

2. Organic milk is now available in most grocery stores. Is it worth the extra money? Why or why not?

Chapter 10

Fats and Oils: A Little Goes a Long Way

Personal Health Check

Does Low Fat Mean Low Calorie?

In some cases, choosing the low-fat option results in a significant difference in fat and calories. Other times, however, the low-fat or fat-free versions of a food are very similar in calories to the regular version. You still need to read the whole label carefully. The bottom line is that you may want to ignore what is on the front of the package and go straight to the Nutrition Facts label and the ingredient list. *Fat free*, *reduced fat*, and *low fat* may sound healthy, but these foods may still be loaded with sugar and calories. Examine two foods and their low-fat or fat-free counterparts to see just how much fat and calories you are saving. Make sure you compare similar serving sizes.

Low-Fat (or Fat-Free) Versus Regular Cookies

	Name	Serving Size	Calories	Fat
Low-fat or fat-free:				
Regular:				

Low-Fat (or Fat-Free) Versus Regular Salad Dressing

	Name	Serving Size	Calories	Fat
Low-fat or fat-free:				
Regular:				

Try Something New

Choose Low-Fat Dressings

Salads are a great way to add lots of vegetables to your diet. They also can be a low-fat addition; that is, unless you drown them in high-fat dressing. Many low-fat and fat-free dressings are available in restaurants and grocery stores. When you eat out, ask for low-fat or fat-free dressing. At home, try making your own fat-free dressing. Experiment with your own favorites. It will keep for several days in the refrigerator.

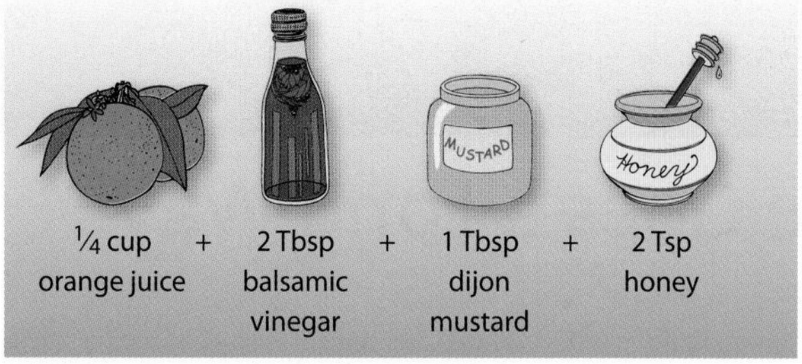
MUSTARD
Honey
¼ cup orange juice
+
2 Tbsp balsamic vinegar
+
1 Tbsp dijon mustard
+
2 Tsp honey

Make Your Own Oil-Free Dressing

Blend the ingredients together in a small container. It will keep for several days in the refrigerator.

Critical Analysis

1. Are foods labeled 0 grams of trans fat on the front of the label free of trans fats? If not, why not?

2. Eggs are high in cholesterol but are considered by some to be a healthy food. Why?

3. Discuss how both the quality and quantity of fat you consume is important in reducing your risk of chronic disease.

Chapter 11

Physical Activity and Exercise: Move More Every Day

Personal Health Check

How Many Steps Do You Get Each Day?

If you are on the go all day running from home to school to work, you may feel that you get plenty of activity. Using a pedometer can help you assess just how many steps you take during the day. A pedometer is a small device that is worn on your waistband or belt that counts the number of steps you take. A good goal is to get 10,000 steps per day, the equivalent of 5 miles. Pedometers are inexpensive and available at sporting goods or discount stores. Purchase a pedometer, wear it for a week, and record how many steps you take each day. If you are under 10,000 steps for most days, think about adding some additional activity to your schedule.

Day	Steps
Monday	
Tuesday	
Wednesday	
Thursday	
Friday	
Saturday	
Sunday	

Take the President's Challenge Adult Fitness Test

Knowing where you are with your level of fitness will help you set your physical activity goals. The President's Challenge Adult Fitness Test will help you estimate your level of aerobic fitness, muscular strength and endurance, flexibility, and body composition. To assess your aerobic fitness, you will participate in either a 1-mile walk or a 1.5-mile run. Push-ups and sits-ups done in a one-minute time span will help you estimate your muscular strength and endurance. Flexibility is tested by measuring your reach in a sit-and-reach position. Finally, your BMI and waist circumference are used to estimate your body composition. Specifics on how to do the tests properly for an accurate measure can be found at www.adultfitnesstest.org. You should only complete this test if you are in good health. Once you have completed the tests, record your results in the following form. Enter your data online for an instant estimate of your fitness level. How did you do? Use the information to set fitness goals for the next month, year, or longer.

THE PRESIDENT'S CHALLENGE

ADULT FITNESS TEST

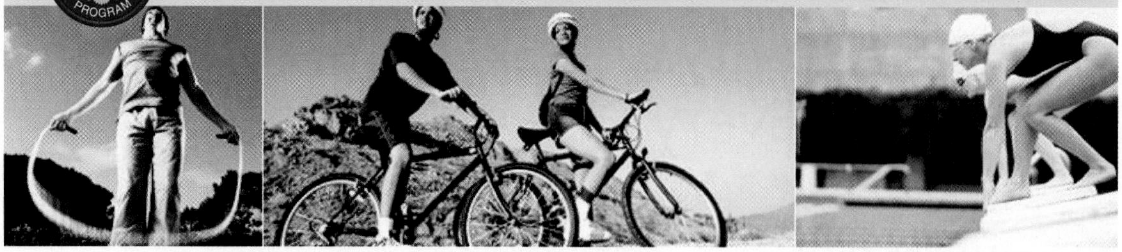

Get Your Adult Fitness Test Score!

As you complete each of the testing events, enter your data into the fields below. When all testing events are completed, transfer the data to the online data entry form and submit your data.

Please complete the form below. Mandatory fields are marked *

PERSONAL INFORMATION

State*

Gender * ❑ Male ❑ Female

Age * ____ yrs

AEROBIC FITNESS

Must enter either a 1-mile walk time and heart rate or enter a 1.5-mile run time.

Mile Walk Time ____ minutes ____ seconds

Heart Rate (after walk) ____ beats per minute

Weight ____ lbs required for result calculation

OR

1.5-Mile Run Time ____ minutes ____ seconds

MUSCULAR STRENGTH

Half Sit-Ups ____ (in one minute)

Push-Ups ____

FLEXIBILITY

Sit and Reach ____ inches

BODY COMPOSITION

BMI/BODY MASS INDEX

Enter height in feet AND inches.

Height ____ feet ____ inches

Weight ____ lbs

Waist Measurement ____ inches

Source: © The President's Council on Fitness, Sports & Nutrition. The President's Challenge Adult Fitness Test. www.adultfitnesstest.org Accessed April 10, 2011.

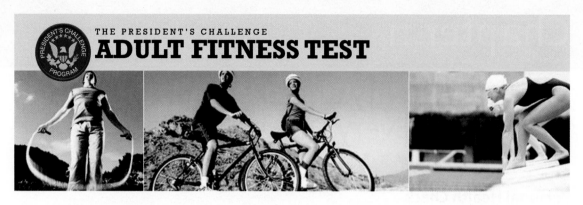

Try Something New

Try a New Physical Activity

If you think running on a treadmill is boring or that your same old gym workout has you in a rut, try something new. There are many different types of physical activity that are fun and provide a great workout. Find what appeals to you and is available in your area. Keep your physical activity routine interesting by varying it regularly. Here are a few ideas:

Boxing. You don't have to be a fighter to train like one. Find a boxing class in your area. There are two basic types of boxing classes; those that use air-boxing techniques without the use of boxing gloves or a bag and those that use gloves and a heavy bag. A one-hour boxing class not only burns lots of calories but is also a fun way to get both muscle-building and aerobic physical activity.

Pilates. A physical fitness system developed by Josef Pilates that promotes the use of core muscles to keep the body balanced. Pilates teaches awareness of breath and alignment of the back to develop strong muscles in the abdomen. Classes can be taught using only your body and a mat or through the use of specialized apparatus.

Martial arts. You can learn self-defense and get a good workout at the same time. There are many different forms of martial arts from which to choose. Check with your college physical education department or local parks and recreation to see if they offer classes.

Group fitness classes. Most gyms and many colleges offer group fitness classes. Group fitness can be aerobic, as with step aerobics or spin, or a combination of muscle-building and aerobic classes that use weights in addition to a cardio workout.

What is your plan to add something new to your workout routine?

Critical Analysis

1. Does the way neighborhoods and communities are designed affect physical activity?

2. Should schools be responsible for providing all the physical activity a child needs each day? Should the physical activity opportunities in elementary, middle, or high school differ?

Test Your Skills

1. Assess your neighborhood for walkability, a measure of how friendly it is for walking. Are there sidewalks, crosswalks, and ways to safely move from where you live to stores and services in the area? Can you walk, run, or bike for exercise? Use www.walkscore.com to assess the walkability of where you live.

2. What opportunities for physical activity are there on your campus? Are there intramural sports, group fitness classes, and access to physical activity facilities?

Chapter 12

Overweight and Obesity: The Public Health Crisis of Our Time

Personal Health Check

Your BMI and Daily Calorie Needs

What Is Your BMI?

Height \ Weight	100	110	120	130	140	150	160	170	180	190	200	210	220	230	240	250	260	270	280	290	300	310	320	330
5'0	20	21	23	25	27	29	31	33	35	37	39	41	43	45	47	49	51	53	55	57	59	61	63	65
5'1"	19	21	23	25	27	28	30	32	34	36	38	40	42	44	45	47	49	51	53	55	57	59	61	62
5'2"	18	20	22	24	26	27	29	31	33	35	37	38	40	42	44	46	48	49	51	53	55	57	59	60
5'3"	18	19	21	23	25	27	28	30	32	34	36	37	39	41	43	44	46	48	50	51	53	55	57	59
5'4"	17	19	21	22	24	26	28	29	31	33	34	36	38	40	41	43	45	46	48	50	52	53	55	57
5'5"	17	18	20	22	23	25	27	28	30	32	33	35	37	38	40	42	43	45	47	48	50	52	53	55
5'6"	16	18	19	21	23	24	26	27	29	31	32	34	36	37	39	40	42	44	45	47	49	50	52	53
5'7"	16	17	19	20	22	24	25	27	28	30	31	33	35	36	38	39	41	42	44	46	47	49	50	52
5'8"	15	17	18	20	21	23	24	26	27	29	30	32	34	35	37	38	40	41	43	44	46	47	49	50
5'9"	15	16	18	19	21	22	24	25	27	28	30	31	33	34	36	37	38	40	41	43	44	46	47	49
5'10"	14	16	17	19	20	22	23	24	26	27	29	30	32	33	35	36	37	39	40	42	43	45	46	47
5'11"	14	15	17	18	20	21	22	24	25	27	28	29	31	32	34	35	36	38	39	41	42	43	45	46
6'0"	14	15	16	18	19	20	22	23	24	26	27	29	30	31	33	34	35	37	38	39	41	42	43	45
6'1"	13	15	16	17	19	20	21	22	24	25	26	28	29	30	32	33	34	36	37	38	40	41	42	44
6'2"	13	14	15	17	18	19	21	22	23	24	26	27	28	30	31	32	33	35	36	37	39	40	41	42
6'3"	13	14	15	16	18	19	20	21	23	24	25	26	28	29	30	31	33	34	35	36	38	39	40	41
6'4"	12	13	15	16	17	18	20	21	22	23	24	26	27	28	29	30	32	33	34	35	37	38	39	40

Height / Weight

Underweight · Healthy Weight · Overweight · Obese · Severely Obese

What Is Your BMI?

Source: Data from Eat Smart, Move More North Carolina. http://www.eatsmartmovemorenc.com. Accessed April 10, 2011.

Record your BMI: ______________________

Circle your weight category:

Underweight   Healthy Weight   Overweight   Obese   Severely Obese

If you are not in the healthy weight category, how many pounds would you need to gain or lose to move into the green zone? ______________________

Set a SMART (Specific, Measurable, Attainable, Realistic, and Timely) goal to move toward a healthy weight if you are not in the healthy weight zone. If you are already in the healthy weight zone, set a healthy eating SMART goal.

SMART goal: ____

____

List at least three strategies you will use to help you reach your SMART goal.

1. ____

____

____

2. ____

____

____

3. ____

____

____

How Many Calories Do You Need Each Day?

Use the following equations to determine how many calories you need each day.

total daily energy expenditure = BMR × physical activity multiplier

1. Calculate your BMR.

Female BMR:

BMR = −161 + 10(weight in pounds ÷ 2.2) + 6.25(height in inches × 2.54) − 5(age)

BMR = −161 + 10(_____ ÷ 2.2) + 6.25 (_____ × 2.54) − 5(_____)

Male BMR:

BMR = 5 + 10(weight in pounds ÷ 2.2) + 6.25(height in inches × 2.54) − 5(age)

BMR = 5 + 10(_____ ÷ 2.2) + 6.25(_____ × 2.54) − 5(_____) = BMR

My BMR is _____.

2. Assess your physical activity level and calculate your physical activity multiplier.

Physical Activity Multiplier

Sedentary = BMR × 1.2 (little or no exercise, desk job)

Light activity = BMR × 1.375 (light exercise/sports 1–3 days/week)

Moderate activity = BMR × 1.55 (moderate exercise/sports 3–5 days/week)

Very active = BMR × 1.75 (hard exercise/sports 6–7 days/week)

Extremely active = BMR × 1.9 (hard daily exercise/sports and physical job OR twice daily athletic training)

My physical activity multiplier is ______________________

3. Calculate total daily energy expenditure by multiplying BMR by the appropriate physical activity multiplier:

BMR _____ × Physical Activity Multiplier _____ = _____ Total Daily Energy Expenditure

My total daily energy expenditure is _____ calories.

Source: Mifflin MD, St Jeor ST, Hill LA, Scott BJ, Daugherty SA, Koh YO. A new predictive equation for resting energy expenditure in healthy individuals. *Am J Clin Nutr.* 1990;51:241–247.

Try Something New

Mindful Eating

Too often meals are eaten in such a hurry that we don't even realize what we are eating or how it tastes. Eating mindfully means eating with awareness of what is on your plate and of the entire eating experience. Mindful eating is being present in the moment and enjoying every aspect of the meal you are eating.

Simple Steps for Mindful Eating

- Eat without distractions—no cell phone, TV, work, computer, newspaper, etc.
- Don't eat while driving or working at your desk.
- Eat sitting down.
- Eat slowly and enjoy every bite.
- Try to make each meal last at least 20 minutes.

Suggested Activity

Use a raisin to learn about mindful eating.

1. Put a raisin in your mouth and close your eyes. Do not begin chewing yet.
2. Try not to pay attention to the ideas running through your mind, just focus on the raisin. Notice its texture, temperature, and taste.
3. Begin chewing slowly. Notice what it feels like. If you find your mind wandering away from the raisin and on to other things, gently bring your thoughts back to the raisin.
4. Notice how your jaw moves each time you chew.
5. Swallow slowly and sense the movement of muscles in your throat and tongue.
6. Take a deep breath and open your eyes.

Try using this technique for the first few bites of each meal to bring your awareness to what you are eating.

Critical Analysis

1. Is fast food to blame for the overweight and obesity crisis? Why or why not?

2. If someone lives more than a mile from a grocery store and does not have transportation every day, what effects could this have on the person's eating habits?

3. Analyze what foods are available to you on campus in dining facilities, convenience stores, and vending machines. Do you have access to fruits, vegetables, whole grains, fat-free dairy, and lean protein?

Test Your Skills

You now have an estimate of your calorie needs each day. Keep a food record for a few days and analyze the calories you are consuming, on average. How close are you to eating what you need to maintain your current weight? If you are trying to lose weight, you should be eating fewer calories than you need without going below 1,200 to 1,400 calories. If you are trying to gain weight, you should be eating more calories than you need.

Use the following table to record what you eat. You can also use the Tracker at www.ChooseMyPlate.gov.

Day 1

Food	Calories
Total Daily Calories:	

Day 2

Food	Calories
Total Daily Calories:	

Day 3

Food	Calories
Total Daily Calories:	

Day 4

Food	Calories
Total Daily Calories:	

Day 5

Food	Calories
Total Daily Calories:	

Chapter 13

Lifecycle Nutrition: Eating Smart Across the Life Span

Personal Health Check

Are You Eating Right for Your Stage in Life?

Be mindful of your stage in life and how that may affect what you should be eating. Healthy eating is not something with which you are ever finished. It is something you do each day and can change from year to year. As you transition from one stage of life to another, changes that occur may require you to adjust your eating habits. Think about the stage of life you are in now, what are your specific nutrition needs? How will your needs change as you think about starting a family or get older? If you have children or plan to, how can you help them develop healthy eating habits?

Create several SMART (Specific, Measurable, Attainable, Realistic, and Timely) goals for your current lifecycle stage related to healthy eating and/or physical activity.

Goal 1: ____________________

How will this goal change as you age? ____________________

____

Goal 2: ____________________

How will this goal change as you age? ____________________

____

Goal 3: ____________________

How will this goal change as you age? ____________________

____

Goal 4: ____________________

How will this goal change as you age? ____________________

____

Critical Analysis

1. The number of children who are overweight or obese continues to rise. What can parents do to help their children create healthy eating habits?

____

____

____

2. What are some barriers to serving healthy foods in school cafeterias? How can those barriers be overcome?

3. The media often perpetuates the idea that ultra thin is beautiful. What effect can this have on the body image of young women? What can be done to counteract this? Does the media perpetuate unattainable bodies for young men as well?

Test Your Skills

Find out about community gardens in your area. How can you become involved? How would you go about starting a community garden?

Chapter 14

Safety of the Food Supply: Keep Your Food Safe

Personal Health Check

Analyze Your Food Safety Practices

You can take many steps at home to keep food safe for you, your family, and your friends. Take the Home Food Safety Inspection Quiz and see how you do. Do you need to adjust some of your food safety practices?

Home Food Safety Inspection Quiz

Answer the questions below based on your usual practices in the kitchen. If you answer any of the questions NO, change your kitchen habits to keep food safe.		
Yes	**No**	
		I wash my hands before I begin to prepare food.
		I wash my hands during food preparation if I handle raw meat or poultry.
		I don't prepare food when I am sick.
		I have hand soap in my kitchen.
		I have soap for washing dishes in my kitchen.
		Pets do not walk on countertops.
		I wash dishes, pots, and pans as I use them and don't pile them in the sink.
		My sink is clean and does not have bits of food.
		I change the dishtowel and dishcloth often.
		I wash the cutting board with soapy water in-between uses and after cutting raw meat or poultry.
		I don't put cooked food onto a plate that held raw foods without washing it first.
		The shelves and drawers in the refrigerator are clean and don't have spills, mold or bits of food.
		I refrigerate food quickly after a meal.
		I thaw meat in the refrigerator or microwave and not on the counter.

Use a Food Thermometer

Using a thermometer may seem overwhelming and not something you need to do as a novice cook. You may think it is just easier to estimate when meats are done. However, it is very difficult, if not impossible, to tell if meat and poultry are cooked as well as they should be. Using the color of meat as a guide to doneness is not effective. Using a thermometer takes the guessing out of cooking and provides you with instant information as to the internal temperature of the food you are cooking. Although it will make sure you cook foods long enough to achieve a safe temperature, using a thermometer will also help you not overcook foods, which can make them dry.

Your first step is to get a good thermometer. Tip-sensitive, instant-read, digital thermometers are the most accurate and are recommended by food safety experts. These are available at most discount stores or grocery stores.

How to Use a Food Thermometer

1. Use a digital, instant-read thermometer to check the internal temperature near the end of the cooking time, but before the food is expected to be done.
2. The food thermometer should be placed in multiple places in the thickest parts of the food and should not be touching bone, fat, or gristle. The thermometer should be inserted slowly to reveal if there are any cold spots.
3. Compare your thermometer reading to the temperatures in Table 14.3 to determine if your food has reached a safe temperature.
4. Make sure to clean you food thermometer with soapy water before and after each use.

There are many types of food thermometers. Follow the instructions for your specific food thermometer.

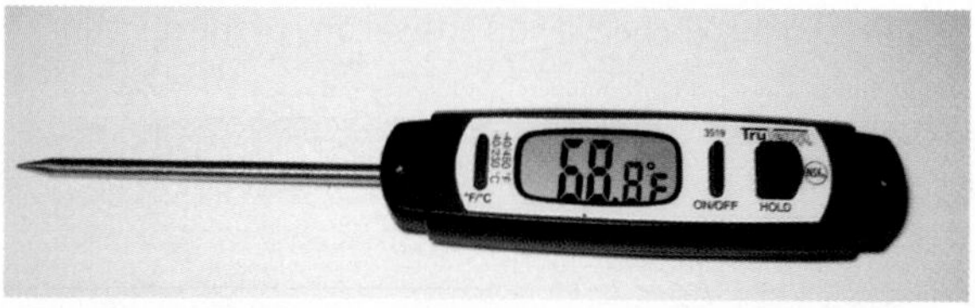

Food Thermometer

Use a tip-sensitive, digital thermometer to accurately gauge the internal temperature of meat, poultry, seafood, and leftovers.

Record your experience with using a food thermometer. Did the thermometer help you better gauge when your food was done but not overdone?

____

____

____

____

____

Critical Analysis

1. If you want to pack your lunch to take with you to school or work, how can you make sure that it is safe to eat? Your answer should begin with the purchase of food and end with consumption.

   ____

   ____

   ____

   ____

   ____

2. You purchase raw chicken at the grocery store, bring it home, cook it on the grill, eat it for dinner, store the leftovers, and take the leftovers for lunch the next day. Outline how you will complete these tasks to decrease your risk of foodborne illness.

Test Your Skills

Next time you go to a restaurant, observe the food safety practices that you can see as a patron, such as how the server handles the food or notations on the menu with respect to undercooked foods. Did you observe anything that could increase your risk of foodborne illness? Do the same next time you observe a friend or family member prepare food. Were there practices that could be improved to decrease the risk of foodborne illness?

Chapter 15

Beyond Eating Smart and Moving More: Other Components of a Healthy Life

Know Your Numbers

There are some critical numbers that you should know about your health. Take note of where you are now and follow your numbers over time. If any of your numbers are not in line, take steps to get them there. First, you should know your height and weight, which can be used to calculate your BMI, as well as your waist circumference. You should also know your blood pressure; this can be taken at your doctor's office, a local health department, or a pharmacy. You should also know your total cholesterol, LDL cholesterol, HDL cholesterol, triglycerides, and fasting blood glucose. For these measures, you will have to have a small amount of blood drawn that can be analyzed in a lab. You can get these tests at your doctor's office or health department.

Measure	Goal	Actual #1	Actual #2	Actual #3
BMI	< 25			
Waist circumference	< 35 inches			
Blood pressure	< 120/80 mm Hg			
Fasting glucose	< 100 mg/dL			
Total cholesterol	< 200mg/dL			
LDL (lousy) cholesterol	< 100 mg/dL			
HDL (healthy) cholesterol	≥ 50 mg/dL			

For any number above the acceptable range, work with a health care professional to create a SMART (Specific, Measurable, Attainable, Realistic, and Timely) goal to help you get that number in line.

Try Something New

Take a Deep Breath

Taking a breath is not something new. It is something you do every day—14,000 to 25,000 times a day, in fact. Although breathing is something you do naturally without giving it much thought, there are ways you can breathe that can help you relax or give you energy. Most people do not breathe as well as they could. As a result, you don't achieve all the benefits that proper breathing can bring. Most people tend to be shallow upper-chest breathers, using about half of the possible lung capacity. There is a proverb that states, "Life is in the breath. He who half-breathes, half-lives." Shallow breathing may provide you with enough oxygen, but it does not produce the benefits of deeper, slower breathing. Shallow breathing may even cause nervousness and keep you from thinking clearly.

The best way to breathe is abdominal breathing. Abdominal breathing uses the diaphragm, the muscle between your lungs and stomach. Breathing using your diaphragm draws air down into the bottom of your lungs. During abdominal breathing, your diaphragm should contract downward. Your lungs fill with air, but it should be your abdomen, not your chest, that moves. This may seem hard at first, especially if you have been a shallow breather for your entire life. Start with several deep breathing breaks a day; over time deep breathing will become more frequent and more natural.

Breathing for Relaxation

If you are having a stressful day or can't fall asleep, try this breathing technique. Sit on the floor, an armless chair, or the edge of the bed with your feet on the floor. Put your hands in your lap. Close your mouth. Close the right nostril using the middle finger of your right hand. Breathe in to the count of four using your diaphragm. Breathe out to the count of seven, pushing your diaphragm down. Do this three to four times and switch to the left nostril. You will feel your body relax and heart rate drop. You can add a mantra for even greater relaxation. When you breathe in say to yourself, "As I breathe in I am calm." When you breathe out say to yourself, "As I breathe out I am relaxed."

Breathing for Increased Energy

If you have been sitting in class or studying for hours and need a pick up, try this breathing technique before you head to the coffee shop. You can do this standing or sitting. Tilt your head slightly up and take a deep breath through your nose. Exhale forcefully through your mouth as you pull in your stomach and move your chin forward. You should be able to hear the air rush from your body. If you are not in public, try making a "ha" sound as you exhale. This breathing exercise releases all the excess carbon dioxide, which can make you feel sluggish.

Critical Analysis

1. Describe what *wellness* means to you.

____

____

____

____

____

2. Why is it important to see a healthcare provider on a regular basis even if you are not sick?

____

____

____

____

____

Test Your Skills

Select the statement after each health behavior that best describes you.

Emotional support:

a. I have friends and family that provide support in good times and bad.

b. I have some friends and family, but they are not always there for me.

c. I don't really have a support system.

Stress:

a. I manage my stress well and keep my life relatively balanced.
b. I feel my stress levels are sometimes out of control.
c. I feel my stress levels are often out of control.

Sleep:

a. I get seven to eight hours of sleep most nights.
b. I sometimes get seven to eight hours of sleep.
c. I rarely get seven to eight hours of sleep.

Sexual health:

a. I do not engage in sexual activity. OR, I always use safer sex practices.
b. I use safer sex practices most of the time.
c. I rarely use safer sex practices.

Sun exposure:

a. When I am out in the sun, I use sunscreen with an SPF of 30 or higher.
b. When I am out in the sun, I use sunscreen with an SPF of 30 or higher some of the time, but not always.
c. When I am out in the sun, I rarely use sunscreen.

Bicycle safety:

a. I do not ride a bicycle. OR, when I ride a bicycle I always wear a helmet.
b. When I ride a bicycle I sometimes wear a helmet.
c. When I ride a bicycle I rarely wear a helmet.

Automobile safety:

a. I always wear a seatbelt.
b. I sometimes wear a seatbelt.
c. I rarely wear a seatbelt.

Tobacco use:

a. I do not use tobacco.
b. I sometimes use tobacco.
c. I use tobacco.

Secondhand smoke exposure:

a. I avoid secondhand smoke exposure.
b. I am sometimes exposed to secondhand smoke.
c. I am often exposed to secondhand smoke.

Alcohol use:

a. I do not consume alcohol or only do so in moderation (one drink per day for women; two drinks per day for men).
b. I sometimes consume more alcohol than would be considered moderate.
c. I often consume more alcohol than would be considered moderate.

Medical care:

a. I see a medical professional at least every two years for a checkup.
b. I see a medical professional only when I am sick.
c. I rarely seek medical attention even when I am sick.

Financial health:

a. I have enough money to pay my bills without going into debt.
b. I sometimes don't have enough money to pay my bills and have to use credit cards or loans.
c. I rarely have enough money to pay my bills and have to use credit cards or loans.

What Your Answers Mean

An answer of A means you are on track with that particular health behavior. If you answered B, you have some room for improvement. An answer of C indicates that this is an area of health that is relatively far away from what is recommended. For the areas of health that you have a B or C answer, create a SMART goal for how you will begin to move towards what is recommended for that health behavior.

Example: An answer of C for secondhand smoke indicates that I am often exposed. A SMART goal might be: I will decrease my exposure to second hand smoke starting today by not going to restaurants/bars that allow smoking and by asking friends that smoke not to smoke in my apartment.

SMART goal: ____

____

How I will achieve my goal: ____

____

____

____

____

____

____

____

____

____

____

____

____

____

Index

D

G

P

R

S

Photo Credits

Chapter 1

Opener © Stockdisc/age fotostock; 1.1 (photo) © LiquidLibrary; 1.2 (left) © straga/ShutterStock, Inc.; (middle left) © Maksymilian Skolik /ShutterStock, Inc.; (middle) © Photodisc; (middle right) © photokup/ShutterStock, Inc.; (right) © Shebeko/ShutterStock, Inc.; 1.3 (left) © Artistic Endeavor/ShutterStock, Inc.; (middle left) © AGfoto /ShutterStock, Inc.; (middle) © Thomas M Perkins /ShutterStock, Inc.; (middle right) © Lorraine Kourafas/ShutterStock, Inc.; (right) © Mark Stout Photography/ShutterStock, Inc.

Chapter 2

Opener © Noel Hendrickson/Digital Vision /Thinkstock; page 28 © dbvirago/Fotolia.com

Chapter 3

Opener © Lev Olkha/ShutterStock, Inc.; 3.5 (cereal bowl) Courtesy of Communication Services, NC State University; 3.6 (cereal bowl) Courtesy of Communication Servics, NC State University; 3.7 Courtesy of Shree Vodicka

Chapter 4

Opener © Brand X Pictures/Jupiterimages /Thinkstock

Chapter 5

Opener © Mircea BEZERGHEANU/ShutterStock, Inc.; 5.2 (top) © Lepas/ShutterStock, Inc.; (middle) © Skyline/ShutterStock, Inc.; (bottom) © Imageman /ShutterStock, Inc.; 5.11 Courtesy of Communication Services, NC State University

Chapter 6

Opener © Serg64/ShutterStock, Inc.; 6.1 (top) © optimarc/ShutterStock, Inc.; (middle top) © photosync/ShutterStock, Inc.; (middle) © XuRa /ShutterStock, Inc.; (middle bottom) © Aleksandr Bryliaev/ShutterStock, Inc.; (bottom) © spinetta /ShutterStock, Inc.; 6.2 (top) © Elena Schweitzer /ShutterStock, Inc.; (middle) © Elena Schweitzer /ShutterStock, Inc.; (bottom) © Lepas/ShutterStock, Inc.; 6.3 (beans) © Lepas/ShutterStock, Inc.; (corn) © Danny Smythe/ShutterStock, Inc.; (apple) © Photodisc; (grapefruit) © Zloneg/ShutterStock, Inc.; (orange) © atoss/ShutterStock, Inc.; (berries) © AGfoto/ShutterStock, Inc.; (canned fruit) © Fotaw/ShutterStock, Inc.; 6.4, 6.5 Courtesy of Communication Services, NC State University; 6.6 (nacho chips) © James E. Knopf/ShutterStock, Inc.; (apple) © Andresr/ShutterStock, Inc.; (cookies) © cristi180884/ShutterStock, Inc.; (banana) © Tatiana Popova/ShutterStock, Inc.; (candy) © charles taylor /ShutterStock, Inc.; (grapes) © Evgeniya Uvarova /ShutterStock, Inc.; (rice) © piyato/ShutterStock, Inc.; (broccoli, rolls) © Hemera/Thinkstock; (tomato) © Galina Mikhalishina/ShutterStock, Inc.; (chips) © Bragin Alexey/ShutterStock, Inc.; (celery and carrot) © Charlotte Lake/ShutterStock, Inc.; 6.7 (left) © SunnyS/ShutterStock, Inc.; (middle) © adsheyn /ShutterStock, Inc.; (right) © Barbro Bergfeldt /ShutterStock, Inc.

Chapter 7

Opener © mikeledray/ShutterStock, Inc.; 7.2 (photo) © johnfoto18/ShutterStock, Inc.; 7.6 (left) © Loskutnikov/ShutterStock, Inc.; (middle) © Evgeny Karandaev/ShutterStock, Inc.; (right) © atoss/ ShutterStock, Inc.; 7.9 (photos) © Photodisc

Chapter 8

Opener © iStockphoto/Thinkstock; page 146 (left) © U.S. Fish & Wildlife Service; (middle) © maya13/ShutterStock, Inc.; (right) © Evlakhov Valeriy/ShutterStock, Inc.; page 147 (black beans) © Galayko Sergey/ShutterStock, Inc.; (black-eyed peas) © Lusoimages/ShutterStock, Inc.; (chickpeas) © Elena Elisseeva/ShutterStock, Inc.; (kidney beans) © jeehyun/ShutterStock, Inc.; (lentils) © Imageman/ShutterStock, Inc.; (pinto beans) © Ivaylo Ivanov/ShutterStock, Inc.; (split peas) © iStockphoto/Thinkstock; (navy beans) © Oliver Hoffmann/ShutterStock, Inc.; page 151 (soy beans) © Photodisc; (tofu) © Ruben Paz/ShutterStock, Inc.; (soy milk) © Patty Orly/ShutterStock, Inc.; (miso) © deepblue-photographer/ShutterStock, Inc.; (tempeh) © Christy Liem/ShutterStock, Inc.; (burger) © aguilarphoto/ShutterStock, Inc.; 8.6 © Lasse Kristensen/ShutterStock, Inc.; 8.7 © Comstock/Thinkstock

Chapter 9

Opener © CandyBox Images/ShutterStock, Inc.; 9.1 © TGPRN Milk Processor Education Program/AP Photos; 9.3 (top) © Comstock/Thinkstock; (bottom left) © Reika/ShutterStock, Inc.; (bottom right) © Anna Hoychuk/ShutterStock, Inc.; page 169 © Jupiterimages/Creatas/Thinkstock; page 171 (left) © Anna Hoychuk/ShutterStock, Inc.; (right) © Preserve, Gimme 5; page 173 (photo) © Dr. Michael Klein/Peter Arnold, Inc.

Chapter 10

Opener © Laurent Renault/ShutterStock, Inc.

Chapter 11

Opener © Frances L Fruit/ShutterStock, Inc.; 11.1 (left) © Photos.com; (middle left) © Geanina Bechea/ShutterStock, Inc.; (middle) © Comstock Images/Thinkstock; (middle right) © stefanolunardi/ShutterStock, Inc.; (right) © Andres Rodriguez/Dreamstime.com; 11.3 (photo) © Creatas Image/Jupiterimages; 11.4 (photo) © Photodisc; 11.5 © Shariff Che' Lah/Dreamstime.com; 11.6 © Stockbyte/Thinkstock; 11.8 © Frances L Fruit/ShutterStock, Inc.; 11.10 © markjb/ShutterStock, Inc.; 11.11 © ARENA Creative/ShutterStock, Inc.; page 219 (top) © Dan Burden/Walkable and Livable Communities Institute; (bottom) © Walkable and Livable Communities Institute

Chapter 12

Opener © Ã?mit Erdem/Thinkstock; 12.6 (rice) © Bassittart/ShutterStock, Inc.; (salad) © Olga Lyubkina/ShutterStock, Inc.; (berries) © matin/ShutterStock, Inc.; (milk) © Horiyan/ShutterStock, Inc.; (stir fry) © keko64/ShutterStock, Inc.; 12.7 (left) © Nattika/ShutterStock, Inc.; (middle) © Courtesy of Renee Comet/National Cancer Institute; (right) © Albo003/ShutterStock, Inc.

Chapter 13

Opener © Subbotina Anna/ShutterStock, Inc.; 13.2 (newborn) © Photodisc; (head up) © Barbara Penoyar/Photodisc/Getty Images; (supported sitter) © Stuart Pearce/age fotostock; (independent sitter) © Maureen Lawrence/StockImage/age fotostock; (crawler) © Picture Partners/age fotostock; (begin to walk) © Tom Grill/age fotostock; (toddler) © Picture Partners/age fotostock

Chapter 14

Opener © Payless Images/ShutterStock, Inc.; 14.1 (groceries) © SFC/ShutterStock, Inc.; (meat and eggs) © Sergej Razvodovskij/ShutterStock, Inc.; (water) © ILYA AKINSHIN/ShutterStock, Inc.; (clipboard) © Fotoline/ShutterStock, Inc.; (restaurant grade) © Bebeto Matthews/AP Photos; (microscope) © Johanna Goodyear/ShutterStock, Inc.

Chapter 15

Opener © Comstock/Thinkstock; 15.2 (photo) © iStockphoto/Thinkstock

Workbook

Page 374 © Anna Hoychuk/ShutterStock, Inc.

Tolerable Upper Intake Levels (UL[1])

Life stage group	Vitamin A[2] (µg/d)	Vitamin D (µg/d)	Vitamin E[3,4] (mg/d)	Niacin[4] (mg/d)	Vitamin B_6 (mg/d)	Folate[4] (µg/d)	Vitamin C (mg/d)	Choline (g/d)	Calcium (g/d)	Phosphorus (g/d)	Magnesium[5] (mg/d)	Sodium (g/d)
Infants												
0-6 mo	600	25	ND[7]	ND	ND	ND	ND	ND	ND	ND	ND	ND
7-12 mo	600	25	ND	ND	ND	ND	ND	ND	ND	ND	ND	ND
Children												
1-3 y	600	50	200	10	30	300	400	1.0	2.5	3	65	1.5
4-8 y	900	50	300	15	40	400	650	1.0	2.5	3	110	1.9
Males, females												
9-13 y	1,700	50	600	20	60	600	1,200	2.0	2.5	4	350	2.2
14-18 y	2,800	50	800	30	80	800	1,800	3.0	2.5	4	350	2.3
19-70 y	3,000	50	1,000	35	100	1,000	2,000	3.5	2.5	4	350	2.3
>70 y	3,000	50	1,000	35	100	1,000	2,000	3.5	2.5	3	350	2.3
Pregnancy												
≤18 y	2,800	50	800	30	80	800	1,800	3.0	2.5	3.5	350	2.3
19-50 y	3,000	50	1,000	35	100	1,000	2,000	3.5	2.5	3.5	350	2.3
Lactation												
≤18 y	2,800	50	800	30	80	800	1,800	3.0	2.5	4	350	2.3
19-50 y	3,000	50	1,000	35	100	1,000	2,000	3.5	2.5	4	350	2.3

Life stage group	Iron (mg/d)	Zinc (mg/d)	Selenium (µg/d)	Iodine (µg/d)	Copper (µg/d)	Manganese (mg/d)	Fluoride (mg/d)	Molybdenum (µg/d)	Boron (mg/d)	Nickel (mg/d)	Vanadium[6] (mg/d)	Chloride (g/d)
Infants												
0-6 mo	40	4	45	ND	ND	ND	0.7	ND	ND	ND	ND	ND
7-12 mo	40	5	60	ND	ND	ND	0.9	ND	ND	ND	ND	ND
Children												
1-3 y	40	7	90	200	1,000	2	1.3	300	3	0.2	ND	2.3
4-8 y	40	12	150	300	3,000	3	2.2	600	6	0.3	ND	2.9
Males, females												
9-13 y	40	23	280	600	5,000	6	10	1,100	11	0.6	ND	3.4
14-18 y	45	34	400	900	8,000	9	10	1,700	17	1.0	ND	3.6
19-70 y	45	40	400	1,100	10,000	11	10	2,000	20	1.0	1.8	3.6
>70 y	45	40	400	1,100	10,000	11	10	2,000	20	1.0	1.8	3.6
Pregnancy												
≤18 y	45	34	400	900	8,000	9	10	1,700	17	1.0	ND	3.6
19-50 y	45	40	400	1,100	10,000	11	10	2,000	20	1.0	ND	3.6
Lactation												
≤18 y	45	34	400	900	8,000	9	10	1,700	17	1.0	ND	3.6
19-50 y	45	40	400	1,100	10,000	11	10	2,000	20	1.0	ND	3.6

[1] UL = The maximum level of daily nutrient intake that is likely to pose no risk of adverse effects. Unless otherwise specified, the UL represents total intake from food, water, and supplements. Due to lack of suitable data, ULs could not be established for vitamin K, thiamin, riboflavin, vitamin B_{12}, pantothenic acid, biotin, or carotenoids. In the absence of ULs, extra caution may be warranted in consuming levels above recommended intakes.

[2] As preformed vitamin A (retinol) only.

[3] As α-tocopherol; applies to any form of supplemental α-tocopherol.

[4] The ULs for vitamin E, niacin, and folate apply to synthetic forms obtained from supplements, fortified foods, or a combination of the two.

[5] The ULs for magnesium represent intake from a pharmacological agent only and do not include intake from food and water.

[6] Although vanadium in food has not been shown to cause adverse effects in humans, there is no justification for adding vanadium to food and vanadium supplements should be used with caution. The UL is based on adverse effects in laboratory animals and these data could be used to set a UL for adults but not children or adolescents.

[7] ND = Not determinable due to lack of data on adverse effects in this age group and concern with regard to lack of ability to handle excess amounts. Source of intake should be from food only to prevent high levels of intake.

Sources: Data compiled from *Dietary Reference Intakes for Calcium, Phosphorus, Magnesium, Vitamin D, and Fluoride*. Washington, DC: National Academies Press; 1997. *Dietary Reference Intakes for Thiamin, Riboflavin, Niacin, Vitamin B_6, Folate, Vitamin B_{12}, Pantothenic Acid, Biotin, and Choline*. Washington, DC: National Academies Press; 1998. *Dietary Reference Intakes for Vitamin C, Vitamin E, Selenium, and Carotenoids*. Washington, DC: National Academies Press; 2000. Institute of Medicine, Food and Nutrition Board. *Dietary Reference Intakes for Vitamin A, Vitamin K, Arsenic, Boron, Chromium, Copper, Iron, Manganese, Molybdenum, Nickel, Silicon, Vanadium, and Zinc.* Washington, DC: National Academies Press, 2000. *Dietary Reference Intakes for Water, Potassium, Sodium, Chloride, and Sulfate.* Washington, DC: National Academies Press; 2005. These reports may be accessed via http://nap.edu.